Neurovascular Neuropsychology

Joanne R. Festa · Ronald M. Lazar
Editors

Neurovascular Neuropsychology

Foreword by J.P. Mohr

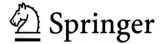 Springer

Editors

Joanne R. Festa
Columbia University
College of Physicians
 and Surgeons
New York, NY, USA
jf2128@columbia.edu

Ronald M. Lazar
Columbia University
College of Physicians
 and Surgeons
New York, NY, USA
ral22@columbia.edu

ISBN 978-0-387-70713-6   e-ISBN 978-0-387-70715-0
DOI 10.1007/978-0-387-70715-0

Library of Congress Control Number: 2008942051

Printed on acid-free paper

springer.com

To Gloria, Jason and Ethan, whose unending support has given me the opportunity to learn and to grow from my patients and their families.

–RML

To Ron for sharing his visionary concept of a neurovascular neuropsychology.

To Lyle, for his love and support, and to all the Festas and Baroncellis who are my foundation.

–JRF

Foreword

This book provides a major step in the direction of a new subspecialty, neurovascular neuropsychology. For too long the emphasis has been on seemingly compartmentalized cerebral functions which, caused by disease, have carried names like the aphasias, apraxias, agnosias, even motor-system disorders, deafness, and blindness. The purpose of this book is to present methodology and data that support the use of neuropsychological techniques as a means of shedding light on cerebral localization, plasticity and vascular pathophysiology. The authors have demonstrated how unique insights into brain mechanisms are derived from observing the neuropsychological outcomes of systematic investigation of hemodynamics, neurotransmitter systems, blood oxygenation levels and cardiac failure. The implications of these findings bear directly on our understanding of the nature and extent of disease, disease progression, treatment efficacy, and prognosis for recovery or disease recurrence.

If anything is emerging from modern studies it is how tightly integrated is much of the brain's function in health, and even after focal lesions. Watching and measuring the changes from the acute stage into the weeks, months, even years make it difficult to apply former notions of 'pure word deafness', semantic aphasia, ideomotor dyspraxia. We are increasingly concerned with more complex integrative cognition, like executive function or multi-tasking, affected both by direct structural injury and by physiological abnormalities of more remote origin. The emerging activation of perilesional and contrahemispheral systems on imaging and the subsidence of some activations, with the strengthening of others, is awe-inspiring to witness. There is a long path ahead before these observations gain the structure needed for a comprehensive understanding of the rules at work behind such changes. Whatever else is happening, simplistic notions of 'recovery' are now outmoded.

Doris & Stanley Tananbaum   JP Mohr
Stroke Center, Neurological
Institute, Columbia
University College of
Physicians & Surgeons
New York, NY 10032

Preface

Working in stroke and critical care at a large academic medical center, I examine and study patients with large and small-vessel stroke, intracranial hemorrhage, hemodynamic compromise from carotid disease, and major cardiac conditions. Because of the nature of this setting, my colleagues ask questions less about the characterization of cognitive deficits and more about what causes them. After all, medical and surgical treatment is an institutional mission. And so I began to realize several things: First, behavior could be an index of disease severity and progression, pathophysiology, and treatment efficacy often more sensitive than physical signs and symptoms; and second, that factors involving the blood supply to the brain represent a common thread among many of the cognitive syndromes that are brought to my attention. The notion of *neurovascular neuropsychology* was borne out of this experience.

The goal of this book is to provide a model for neuropsychology, as a discipline, in which the investigational focus is as much on causal mechanisms as it is on the exquisite measurement of cognitive and behavioral outcomes. It seems to me that the intimate relationship between the brain and its blood supply provides a unique opportunity to expand the role of neuropsychological inquiry. The concentration here is on adult neurovascular conditions, leaving to others similar afflictions that concern children.

To this end, we first present an historical perspective, followed by a primer of neurovascular anatomy and the diagnostic modalities most frequently used to measure structural integrity. We then begin the journey along the continuum of neurovascular injury, starting first with the focal disease that encompasses ischemic and hemorrhagic stroke, and local vascular anomalies such as cerebral aneurysms and brain arteriovenous malformations. But focal disease spread across critical brain regions can also have a cognitive effect greater than the sum of affected tissue, disturbing more integrative functions such as mental speed and decision-making. In this regard, vascular dementia and its precursor vascular cognitive impairment are discussed, as well as the consequences of the genetic mutations associated with CADA-SIL and MELAS. At a more macroscopic level, we progress to vascular hemispheral conditions in which there is obstruction of the carotid arterial system. We consider here both the direct effects of stenosis and occlusion, as well as the consequences of treatment, such as surgical bypass, and angioplasty and stenting. At the global level, we consider abnormalities of cardiopulmonary origin, examining cardiac arrest, congestive heart failure, cardiac surgery and pulmonary disease as pathophysiologies that have a significant cognitive impact on millions of individuals world-wide. There are also chronic systemic diseases and conditions, such as diabetes and hypertension, which affect cognition either by directly altering the structural nature of blood vessels or by providing the route of pathogenic dissemination in the blood supply. Sometimes entities, like collagen vascular diseases (e.g., systemic lupus), can do both. We also consider the high frequency and impact of mood disorders, particularly depression, on cognition and recovery in neurovascular disease.

But so as not to leave the reader without hope, it is also important to present the increasing recognition that the adult human brain is far more plastic than previously thought, and that an understanding of neurotransmitter systems and principles of brain reorganization is leading to new treatments and to greater expectations of recovery.

In the end, neurovascular neuropsychology is less a sub-specialty than an approach to our field. It broadens our purview into patient care by allowing us to ask questions about the physiologic reasons for behavioral change which are potentially treatable. For many of us, that is the reason why we entered this field in the first place.

Levine Cerebral Localization Laboratory   Ronald M. Lazar, PhD
Neurological Institute
Columbia University College
  of Physicians and Surgeons
New York, NY

Contents

Contributors

Michael Alexander Behavioral Neurology Unit, Departments of Neurology, Beth Israel Deaconess Medical Center and Harvard Medical School, Boston, MA, USA

Craig S. Anderson Neurological and Mental Health, The George Institute for International Health, Royal Prince Alfred Hospital, Sydney, Australia

Anna M. Barrett Kessler Medical Rehabilitation Research and Education Center, Departments of Physical Medicine and Rehabilitation, Neurology and Neurosciences, The University of Medicine and Dentistry, The New Jersey Medical School, West Orange, NJ, USA

Sarah Benisty Department of Geriatric Medicine and Neurology, Hopital Lariboisiere-Fernand-Widal, Paris, France

Robin L. Brey University of Texas Health Science Center at San Antonio, Department of Medicine/Neurology, San Antonio, TX, USA

Donna K. Broshek Neurocognitive Assessment Laboratory, Brain Injury and Sports Concussion Institute, University of Virginia School of Medicine, Charlottesville, VA, USA

Hughes Chabriat Service de Neurologie, Hopital Lariboisière, Paris, France

Mohamad Chmayssani Stroke and Critical Care Division, Department of Neurology, Neurological Institute, New York Presbyterian Hospital, Columbia University, College of Physicians and Surgeons, New York, NY, USA

Giuseppe Colloca Centro Medicina dell'Invecchiamento, Università Cattolica del Sacro Cuore, Policlinico A. Gemelli, Roma, Italy

John DeLuca Neuropsychology and Neuroscience Laboratory Kessler Medical Rehabilitation Research and Education Center, West Orange, NJ, USA; New Jersey Medical School University of Medicine and Dentistry of New Jersey, Newark, NJ, USA

Gail A. Eskes Departments of Psychiatry, Psychology and Medicine (Neurology), Brain Repair Centre, Dalhousie University, Halifax, Nova Scotia, Canada

Joanne R. Festa Stroke and Critical Care Division, Department of Neurology, Neurological Institute, New York Presbyterian Hospital, Columbia University, College of Physicians and Surgeons, New York, NY, USA

Steven R. Flanagan New York University School of Medicine, Rusk Institute of Rehabilitation Medicine, NYU-Langone Medical Center, New York, NY, USA

Wayne A. Gordon Department of Rehabilitation Medicine, Mount Sinai School of Medicine, New York, NY, USA

Rebecca F. Gottesman Cerebrovascular Division, Department of Neurology, Johns Hopkins University School of Medicine, Baltimore, MD, USA

Bret Haake London Health Sciences Centre, University Hospital, London, ON, Canada

Vladimir Hachinski London Health Sciences Centre, University Hospital, London, ON, Canada

Maree L. Hackett The George Institute for International Health, Sydney, Australia

Stephen L. Holliday University of Texas Health Science Center, San Antonio, TX, USA

Howard S. Kirshner Department of Neurology, Vanderbilt University Medical Center, Nashville, TN USA

Joel H. Kramer Department of Neurology, University of California, **San Francisco,** Memory and Aging Center, San Francisco, CA, USA

Ronald M. Lazar Stroke and Critical Care Division, Departments of Neurology and Neurological Surgery, Neurological Institute, New York Presbyterian Hospital, Columbia University, College of Physicians & Surgeons, New York, NY, USA

Emily R. Lantz Stroke and Critical Care Division, Department of Neurology, Neurological Institute, New York Presbyterian Hospital, Columbia University, College of Physicians and Surgeons, New York, NY, USA

Lenore J. Launer Neuroepidemiology Section, Laboratory of Epidemiology, Demography and Biometry, National Institute on Aging, Bethesda, MD, USA

David J. Libon Department of Neurology, Drexel University College, Philadelphia, PA, USA

Chun Lim Behavioral Neurology Unit, Beth Israel Deaconess Medical Center, Boston, MA, USA

Victor W. Mark Department of Physical Medicine and Rehabilitation, University of Alabama at Birmingham, Birmingham, AL, USA

Randolph S. Marshall Stroke Division, Department of Neurology, Neurological Institute, New York Presbyterian Hospital, Columbia University, College of Physicians & Surgeons, New York, NY, USA

José G. Merino Suburban Hospital Stroke Program Bethesda, MD, USA

Dana Penney Department of Neurology, Lahey Clinic Medical Center, Burlington, MA, USA; Tufts University School of Medicine, Boston, MA, USA

Alfio Pennisi New Jersey Institute for Successful Aging, University of Medicine and Dentistry of New Jersey – School of Osteopathic Medicine, Newark, NJ, USA

Charles J. Prestigiacomo Department of Neurological Surgery and Radiology, New Jersey Medical School, University of Medicine and Dentistry of New Jersey, Newark, NJ, USA

Catherine C. Price Department of Health Psychology, University of Florida, Gainesville, FL, USA

Mark D. Robbins Neurocognitive Assessment Laboratory, University of Virginia Health System, Charlottesville, VA, USA

Ola A. Selnes Division of Cognitive Neuroscience, Department of Neurology, Johns Hopkins University School of Medicine, Baltimore, MD, USA

George W. Shaver Neurocognitive Assessment Laboratory, University of Virginia Health System, Charlottesville, VA, USA

Rodney A. Swenson Department of Neuroscience, University of North Dakota School of Medicine and Health Sciences, Grand Forks, ND, USA

Matteo Tosato Department of Gerontology, Catholic University of the Sacred Heart, Rome, Italy

Margaret E. Wetzel Department of Neurology, University of California, San Francisco, CA, USA

Clinton Wright Evelyn F. McKnight Center for Age Related Memory Loss, Division of Cognitive Disorders, Department of Neurology, Miller School of Medicine, University of Miami, Miami, FL, USA

Giuseppe Zuccalà Department of Gerontology, Catholic University of the Sacred Heart, Rome,Italy

Chapter 1
Historical Perspective

José G. Merino and Vladimir Hachinski

The idea that brain softening leads to cognitive decline dates at least from the 19th century (Ball & Chambard, 1881; Browne, 1874; Durand-Fardel, 1843; Rostan, 1823). The study of patients with stroke has provided important insights on how the brain functions, but over the past 150 years many issues about the relationship between cerebrovascular disease and cognitive decline have been, and still are, hotly debated.

A key question has been the mechanism through which cerebrovascular disease leads to cognitive decline: some writers postulated that dementia due to cerebrovascular disease is a question of strokes while others supported the idea that chronic ischemia is the main pathogenic mechanism. Current views hold that strokes, chronic ischemia, and other mechanisms play a role.

Another important topic of debate has been whether cerebrovascular disease is the major cause of cognitive decline in the elderly or whether it is only the culprit in a small proportion of cases. In the first half of the 20th century, most causes of dementia were considered to be arteriosclerotic; from 1920 to 1947, for example, several editions of "[Osler's] Principles and Practice of Medicine" included

Alzheimer's disease in the section on "Senile Arteriosclerosis" (Denning, 1995). However, by 1973, Fields (1973) could write that cerebral arteriosclerosis was a "non-cause" of dementia. Recently, the pendulum has swung again with the recognition of the high prevalence of cerebrovascular disease in patients with clinical and pathologic features of neurodegenerative dementia, the synergistic role of different pathologies, and the effects of ischemia on neurodegeneration (de la Torre, 2002). Furthermore, in a historical paper it is difficult to precisely define dementia because the term has been used differently at various times. Around the turn of the last century, for example, it had a much broader meaning than the DSM conceptualization of a disorder leading to decline in social and occupational functioning.

Stroke and Clinical-Anatomic Cognitive Syndromes

C. Miller Fisher reputedly said that students learn neurology "stroke by stroke" (Adams, Victor, & Ropper, 1997). This is particularly true for the study of brain-behavior relationships; the detailed study of patients with stroke has been critical in the development of neuropsychology and behavioral neurology (Graff-Radford & Biller, 1992). Monsieur Leborgne, immortalized by Broca's description of his language deficits, had a left frontal

J.G. Merino (✉)
Section on Stroke Diagnostics and Therapeutics, National Institute of Neurological Disorders and Stroke, National Institutes of Health, Bethesda, MD, USA
e-mail: merinoj@ninds.nih.gov

J.R. Festa, R.M. Lazar (eds.), *Neurovascular Neuropsychology*, DOI 10.1007/978-0-387-70715-0_1,
© Springer Science+Business Media, LLC 2009

stroke (Broca, 1861; Castaigne, Lhermitte, Signoret, & Abelanet, 1980) and Herr Ochs, Lieppmann's famous patient with apraxia and agraphia, had a stroke of the corpus callosum (Liepmann & Maas, 1907). Babinski first described anosognosia in a patient with a stroke in the right hemisphere (Heilman, 2002) and the first callosal syndrome—alexia without agraphia—was described by Dejerine (1892) after he saw a patient with a stroke in the distribution of the left posterior cerebral artery. Many other classical syndromes were initially described in patients with stroke, and to this day, the study of patients with focal ischemic and hemorrhagic strokes continues to generate important insights into the function of the brain (Heilman, 2002).

Strokes have been implicated in more than the genesis of circumscribed cognitive syndromes. Since early in the 19th century, several physicians recognized the effect of apoplexy on cognition. Durand-Fardel (1843), for example, wrote that changes of the intellect were among the most interesting features of apoplexy, and could progress to "une véritable démence." While Ball and Chambard (1881), who coined the term "apoplectic dementia," considered that persistent cognitive impairment was frequent after an ischemic stroke, Charcot emphasized red softening or hemorrhage (Berrios, 1995). In the next few years, the view that cerebral atherosclerosis and chronic brain ischemia rather than strokes were the culprit of the dementia became dominant, and while there were critics of this view, it was not until the 1950s that strokes took center stage again, and with growth of the concept of multi-infarct dementia (Hachinski, Lassen, & Marshall, 1974) became a central part of the semiology.

From Arteriosclerotic Dementia to Vascular Cognitive Impairment

In the second half of the 19th century, syphilis of the central nervous system was a major cause of dementia and insanity, and pathological analysis of brains infected with *T. pallidum* often had evidence of vessel narrowing or occlusion and focal areas of ischemia. Cerebrovascular disease was considered a contributor to the cognitive and behavioral changes (Berchtold & Cotman, 1998). In 1894, in an attempt to distinguish between purely cerebrovascular pathology from general paresis, Binswanger (1894) described the clinical and pathological features of two subtypes of dementia due to atherosclerosis of the cerebral vessels: encephalitis subcorticalis chronica progressiva and arteriosclerotic cerebral degeneration (Blass, Hoyer, & Nitsch, 1991). The following year, Alzheimer (1895) wrote about "arteriosclerotic atrophy of the brain," and later (Alzheimer, 1898, 1902) characterized two additional pathologic forms of focal cerebral disease leading to arteriosclerotic dementia: perivascular gliosis in the territory of the great vessels and senile sclerosis of the cerebral cortex due to degeneration of small cortical vessels. For Binswanger and Alzheimer, however, chronic ischemia and not discrete ischemic or hemorrhagic strokes was the cause of the dementia (Alzheimer, 1902; Mast, Tatemichi, & Mohr, 1995).

The idea that dementia was due to chronic hemodynamic failure secondary to arteriosclerosis of the cerebral vessels became dominant in the first half of the 20th century. In textbooks, dementias were classified as "mental disorders of cerebral arteriosclerosis" (Barrett, 1913; Osler & McCrae, 1921). The unitary view that considered post-apoplectic and arteriosclerotic dementias as the same entity prevailed for decades (Denning, 1995). Ferraro (1959), for example, wrote that arteriosclerotic dementia was due to "the gradual strangulation of the cerebral circulation... The mental symptoms in cerebral arteriosclerosis may develop in an insidious and gradual manner, or may be acute after an apoplectic attack..." The semiology of arteriosclerotic dementia focused on vague mental symptoms—mental lassitude, loss of memory for recent events, anxiety, emotional instability, confusion—and "strokes were [considered] but the culmination of a process started years before" (Barrett, 1913; Berrios, 1995; Denning & Berrios, 1991). Don Santiago Ramón y Cajal (1941), in his book "The World Seen at Eighty, Memoirs of an Arteriosclerotic," describes how the process of arteriosclerotic dementia was conceived in the first half of the century:

> I must abstain even of thoughtful and prolonged conversation. Woe to me if, giving in to temptation, I get caught up in pedantic philosophical or scientific conversation! The face and brain blush, memory fails, as if blocked by an insurmountable obstacle, words become hesitant, the imagination becomes labored and unruly; saintly equanimity, the treasure of the prudent and discrete, is lost. And, with all this, verbal flow continues unstoppable. Alienated, the spirit ignores that internal voice, anguished protest of the over-excited brain, which reminds us, with clemency, of the danger of the hemorrhage and sudden paralysis. And, threatened by Damocles' sword, we, the old arteriosclerotic, are reduced, finally warned, to inertia and indolence... Allow me here to recall briefly how this process began in me or, at least, the clear conscience of it, since it is a slowly incubated lesion... It was about thirteen years ago. From day to day I noticed, on leaving the gatherings at the cafe... that my head was ablaze, and walking or absolute silence could not suppress it. One day, after a photographic session [in the heat], the cerebral congestion was such that I was forced to consult the wise and pleasant Doctor Achúcaro, my laboratory companion. He examined me, and after some oratorical precautions, hurled the terrible verdict: My friend, the cerebral arteriosclerosis of senility has set in...[1]

By the early 1950s, the clinical and pathologic criteria for the diagnosis of the senile dementias "remained nebulous and confusing" (Fisher, 1951). Mental deterioration after ischemic or hemorrhagic stroke was termed arteriosclerotic. Clinically, cases of slowly progressive cognitive deterioration that began around age 50 were classified as Alzheimer's or Pick's disease "although neither has specific clinical or pathological features." When the deterioration occurred at a later age, the patient was diagnosed with arteriosclerotic or senile dementia.

---
[1] Our translation

In 1951, Fisher described several cases of dementia associated with occlusion of one or both carotid arteries, even in the absence of atherosclerosis of the cerebral vasculature. Based on observations by Kety (1950), who had found a 25% decrease in the cerebral blood flow in patients with senile dementia, he postulated that carotid occlusion may be a cause for the diminution in blood flow, and that unilateral occlusion of the internal carotid, particularly the left, may be causally related to dementia. He proposed that some cases of senile dementia may be due to chronic ischemia caused by occlusion of the carotid tree. In a subsequent report (Fisher, 1954) he acknowledged, however, that "the association of dementia and carotid occlusion...may be entirely fortuitous, and care must be exercised in drawing conclusions." Other investigators (Kapp, Cook, & Paulson, 1966; Sours, 1964) described cognitive and behavioral symptoms and syndromes associated with carotid occlusion, including "chronic brain syndrome associated with cerebral arteriosclerosis."

There was, however, gradual acknowledgement that discrete infarcts could be the main cause of the mental deterioration. In 1954, Mayer-Gross, Slater, and Roth considered that half the patients with arteriosclerotic psychosis had hypertension and that gradual "personality change" and "anxious self-scrutiny" could precede the cognitive changes. In a subsequent edition of their textbook, Slater and Roth (1969) expanded the prodromal symptoms to include memory decline, anxiety, blackouts, giddiness, headache, sexual disinhibition, and "a caricature of one or more conspicuous personality traits." They considered that lasting intellectual deficits rarely developed until clinical evidence of focal infarction appeared; often more than one stroke was required. In addition to cognitive impairment, the syndrome was characterized by a fluctuating course, somatic symptoms, and neurological abnormalities such as hemiparesis, aphasia, or field defects. They gradually shifted the focus from general ischemia to focal strokes. This semiology was important for the development of the Ischemic Score and the concept of multi-infarct dementia (Hachinski, Lassen et al., 1974).

This idea that dementia was due to stroke and not to global ischemia gained popularity in the next decade. In 1968, Fisher affirmed that "cerebrovascular disease is therefore a very common cause of dementia...for all major middle cerebral strokes...bring some measurable loss of cortical function and the same is only slightly less true for anterior cerebral and posterior cerebral strokes" and that "cerebrovascular dementia is a matter of strokes large and small." Fisher had changed his point of view since 1959, and in 1968 he wrote that it was a mistake to think that hardening of the arteries was a cause of dementia. He thought atherosclerosis led to dementia in so far as it led to infarcts. The gradual loss of memory and capabilities was not due to atherosclerosis of the cerebral arteries but to a neurodegenerative process—Alzheimer's disease—which was not related to cerebral ischemia.

Tomlinson, Blessed, and Roth (1968, 1970) studied the differences between neurodegenerative and vascular processes. They compared the pathological findings in 28 non-demented and 50 demented elderly patients and found that the degree of pathological changes (cerebral atrophy, ventricular dilatation, senile plaques, neurofibrillary tangles, granulovacuolar degeneration, and cerebral softening) was much greater in patients with dementia. In most cases they found purely neurodegenerative pathology: they diagnosed arteriosclerotic dementia in only nine brains and mixed dementia in another nine. They concluded that from a clinical perspective, vascular dementia was over-diagnosed. Their results lent support to the idea that both pathologies were distinct and that arteriosclerotic dementia was less common than previously believed. In the 1970s, elderly patients with dementia were increasingly diagnosed with Alzheimer's disease, even though clinical criteria to differentiate both types of dementia were not well defined, and relied mostly on the exclusion of a history of stroke. Hachinski, Lassen, and Marshal, in 1974, coined the term "multi-infarct

dementia" to refer to dementia due to the accumulation of cerebral infarcts. They considered that arteriosclerosis did not play an important role in the development of the progressive dementia of the elderly that was associated with Alzheimer type changes in the brain. A year later they described differences in blood flow between patients with "multi-infarct" and "primary degenerative" dementia, and described an Ischemic Scale that could be used to classify patients in each group based on historical and clinical criteria (Hachinski, Iliff, et al., 1975); the scale incorporates the criteria delineated by Mayer-Gross, Slater, and Roth (1954).

The concept of multiple-infarct dementia rapidly became popular, but the use of brain imaging showed that infarcts due to cardiac embolism of carotid plaques were only one of several possible etiologies of dementia due to cerebrovascular disease (Loeb & Meyer, 1996; Rivera, 1975). The term "vascular dementia" was coined to capture the complexity of this heterogeneous syndrome (Loeb, 1985). In contrast to the dominant unitary view that was popular a few decades earlier, several etiologic subtypes were described: multi-infarct dementia (Hachinski, Lassen et al., 1974), strategic infarct dementia (Tatemichi, Desmond, & Prohovnik, 1995), small vessel dementia (Mohr, 1982), hypoperfusion dementia (Brun, 1994), and hemorrhagic dementia (Cummings, 1994). In the 1980s, several diagnostic criteria for vascular dementia were proposed: these were commonly used despite being based on expert opinion and not on data.(American Psychiatric Association, 1987, 1994; Chui et al., 1992; Roman et al., 1993; World Health Organization, 1993). All of these criteria rely on memory impairment as the cardinal feature for the diagnosis of vascular dementia despite the fact that the cognitive impairment seen in patients with cerebrovascular disease preferentially affects other cognitive domains (Del Ser et al., 1990).

The pendulum has swung again, and many experts believe that vascular factors play an important role in the development of cognitive impairment in many, if not most, patients with dementia because Alzheimer-type and vascular pathology often coexist and have synergistic effects on cognitive decline. Furthermore, in recent years there has been a shift of focus toward early identification of people who are at risk of developing dementia. The concept of vascular cognitive impairment (VCI) broadens the idea of vascular dementia and "brain at risk" and includes the whole spectrum of cognitive impairment, from mild to frank dementia, that is associated with vascular risk factors and cerebrovascular disease (Hachinski, 1992). The alterations in cognitive function may be milder than those produced by a focal syndrome. While the classical syndromes may be part of VCI, VCI may be diagnosed in the absence of these deficits.

To avoid many of the pitfalls of earlier diagnostic schemes, prospective population-based data collection of the specific clinical, psychological, radiological, and pathological features of cognitive impairment and dementia in patients with cerebrovascular disease is required before any diagnostic criteria can be established. As an initial step, a panel convened recently by the National Institute of Neurological Disorders and Stroke and the Canadian Stroke Network (Hachinski, Iadecola et al., 2006) identified a minimal set of clinical, neuropsychological, radiological, and pathological data that should be prospectively collected in all studies of VCI to enable data sharing and comparison between studies, with the hope that further advances in the field will be driven by solid research data.

References

Adams, R., Victor, M., & Ropper, A. (1997). *Principles of neurology* (6th ed.). New York: McGraw-Hill.

Alzheimer, A. (1895). Die arteriosklerotische Atrophie des Gehirns. *Allgemeine Zeitschrift für Psychiatrie, 51*, 809–811.

Alzheimer, A. (1898). Baitrag zur pathologischen Anatomie der Saeelenstorungen des Greisenalters. *Allgemeine Zeitschrift für Psychiatrie, 56*, 272–273.

Alzheimer, A. (1902). Die Seellenstoerungen auf arteriosclerotischer Grundlage. *Allgemeine Zeitschrift für Psychiatrie, 59*, 695–711.

American Psychiatric Association (1987). *Diagnostic and statistical manual of mental disorders* (3rd revised ed.). Washington, D.C.:Author.

American Psychiatric Association (1994). *Diagnostic and statistical manual of mental disorders* (4th ed.). Washington, D.C.:Author.

Ball, B., & Chambard, E. (1881). Démence. In A. Dechambre & L. Lereboullet (Eds.), *Dictionnaire encyclopédique des sciences médicales* (pp. 559–605). Paris: Masson.

Barrett, A. (1913). Presenile, atherosclerotic and senile disorders of the brain and cord. In W. White & S. Jelliffe (Eds.), *The modern treatment of nervous and mental diseases* (pp. 675–709). London: Kimpton.

Berchtold, N. C., & Cotman, C. W. (1998). Evolution in the conceptualization of dementia and Alzheimer's disease: Greco-Roman period to the 1960s. *Neurobiol Aging, 19*(3), 173–189.

Berrios, G. (1995). Dementia. In G. Berrios & R. Porter (Eds.), *A history of clinical psychiatry* (pp. 34–62). London: The Athlone Press.

Binswanger, O. (1894). Die Abgrenzung der allgemeinen Paralyse. *Allgemeine Zeitschrift für Psychiatrie, 51*, 804–805.

Blass, J. P., Hoyer, S., & Nitsch, R. (1991). A translation of Otto Binswanger's article: 'The delineation of the generalized progressive paralyses' (1894). *Archives of Neurology, 48*(9), 961–972.

Broca, P. (1861). Perte de la parole, ramollissement chronique et destruction partielle du lobe antérieur du cerveau. *Bulletin de la Société d'Anthropologie de Paris, 2*, 235–238.

Browne, J. (1874). Clinical lectures on mental and cerebral disease: V. Senile dementia. *British Medical Journal, 1*, 601–603.

Brun, A. (1994). Pathology and pathophysiology of cerebrovascular dementia: pure subgroups of obstructive and hypoperfusive etiology. *Dementia, 5*(3–4), 145–147.

Castaigne, P., Lhermitte, F., Signoret, J. L., & Abelanet, R. (1980). Description et étude scannographique du cerveau de Leborgne. *Revista de Neurologia (Paris), 136*(10), 563–583.

Chui, H. C., Victoroff, J. I., Margolin, D., Jagust, W., Shankle, R., & Katzman, R. (1992). Criteria for the diagnosis of ischemic vascular dementia proposed by the State of California Alzheimer's Disease Diagnostic and Treatment Centers. *Neurology, 42*(3 Pt 1), 473–480.

Cummings, J. L. (1994). Vascular subcortical dementias: Clinical aspects. *Dementia, 5*(3–4), 177–180.

de la Torre, J. C. (2002). Alzheimer disease as a vascular disorder: nosological evidence. *Stroke, 33*(4), 1152–1162.

Dejerine, J. (1892). Des différentes variétés de cécité verbale. *Mémoires de la Société de Biologie, 3*, 1–30.

del Ser, T., Bermejo, F., Portera, A., Arredondo, J. M., Bouras, C., & Constantinidis, J. (1990). Vascular dementia: A clinicopathological study. *Journal of the Neurological Sciences, 96*(1), 1–17.

Denning, T. (1995). Stroke and other vascular disorders. In G. Berrios & R. Porter (Eds.), *A history of clinical psychiatry*. (pp. 72–85). London: Athlone.

Denning, T., & Berrios, G. (1991). The vascular dementias. In G. Berrios & H. Freeman (Eds.), *Alzheimer and the dementias* (pp. 66–76). London: Royal Society of Medicine.

Durand-Fardel, M. (1843). *Traité du ramollissement du cerveau*. Paris: Baillière.

Ferraro, A. (1959). Psychoses with cerebral arteriosclerosis. In S. Arieti (Ed.), *American handbook of psychiatry* (Vol. 2, pp. 1078–1108). New York: Basic Books.

Fields, W. (1973). Presenile dementia – a vascular (arteriosclerotic) disease? Cerebral arterioslerosis. A "non-cause" of dementia. In J. Meyer, H. Lechner, M. Reivich, & O. Eichorn (Eds.), *Cerebrovascular diseases. Sixth International Conference, Salzburg 1972* (pp. 197–199). Stuttgart: Georg Thieme Publishers.

Fisher, CM. (1951). Senile dementia- a new explanation of its causation. *Canadian Medical Association Journal*, 65(1), 1–7.

Fisher, CM. (1954). Occlusion of the carotid arteries: Further experiences. *AMA Archives of Neurology and Psychiatry*, 72(2), 187–204.

Fisher, CM. (1968). Dementia in cerebrovascular disease. In J. Toole, R. Siekert, & J. Whisnant (Eds.), *Cerebrovascular disease. The 6th Princeton Conference* (pp. 232–241). New York: Grune & Stratton.

Graff-Radford, N. R., & Biller, J. (1992). Behavioral neurology and stroke. *The Psychiatric Clinics of North America*, 15(2), 415–425.

Hachinski, V. (1992). Preventable senility: a call for action against the vascular dementias. *Lancet, 340* (8820), 645–648.

Hachinski, V., Iadecola, C., Petersen, R.C., Breteler, M.M., Nyenhuis, D.L., Black, S.E., et al. (2006). National Institute of Neurological Disorders and Stroke—Canadian stroke network vascular cognitive impairment harmonization standards. *Stroke, 37*, 2220–2241.

Hachinski, V., Iliff, L. D., Zilhka, E., Du Boulay, G. H., McAllister, V. L., Marshall, J. et al. (1975). Cerebral blood flow in dementia. *Archives of Neurology, 32*(9), 632–637.

Hachinski, V., Lassen, N. A., & Marshall, J. (1974). Multi-infarct dementia. A cause of mental deterioration in the elderly. *Lancet, 2* (7874), 207–210.

Heilman, K. (2002). *Matter of mind. A neurologist's view of brain-behavior relationships.* New York: Oxford University Press.

Kapp, J., Cook, W., & Paulson, G. (1966). Chronic brain syndrome. Arteriographic study in elderly patients. *Geriatrics, 21*(9), 174–181.

Kety, S. S. (1950). Circulation and metabolism of the human brain in health and disease. *The American Journal of Medicine, 8*(2), 205–217.

Liepmann, H., & Maas, O. (1907). Fall von linkseitiger Agraphie und Apraxie bei rechtseitiger Lahmung. *Z Psychiatrie, Neurologie, 10*, 214–227.

Loeb, C. (1985). Vascular dementia. In J. Fredericks (Ed.), *Handbook of clinical neurology* (Vol. 2: Neurobehavioral Disorders, pp. 353–369). Amsterdam: Elsevier.

Loeb, C., & Meyer, J. S. (1996). Vascular dementia: still a debatable entity? *Journal of Neurological Sciences, 143*(1–2), 31–40.

Mast, H., Tatemichi, T. K., & Mohr, J. P. (1995). Chronic brain ischemia: the contributions of Otto Binswanger and Alois Alzheimer to the mechanisms of vascular dementia. *Journal of Neurological Sciences, 132*(1), 4–10.

Mayer-Gross, W., Slater, E., & Roth, M. (1954). *Clinical psychiatry*. London: Cassell & Co.

Mohr, J. P. (1982). Lacunes. *Stroke, 13*(1), 3–11.

Osler, W., & McCrae, T. (1921). *The principles and practice of medicine* (9th ed.). New York: Appleton.

Ramon y Cajal, S. (1941). *El mundo visto a los ochenta años. Impresiones de un arterioesclerótico.* Madrid: Espasa-Calpe.

Rivera, V. (1975). Dementia and cerebrovascular disease. In J. Meyer (Ed.), *Modern concepts of cerebrovascular disease* (pp. 135–158). New York: Spectrum Publishers.

Roman, G. C., Tatemichi, T. K., Erkinjuntti, T., Cummings, J. L., Masdeu, J., Garcia, J. H., et al. (1993). Vascular dementia: diagnostic criteria for research studies. Report of the NINDS-AIREN International Workshop. *Neurology, 43*(2), 250–260.

Rostan, L. (1823). *Recherches sur le ramollissement du cerveau* (2. édition). Paris: Béchet, Gabon, Crévot.

Slater, E., & Roth, M. (1969). *Mayer-Gross, Slater and Roth clinical psychiatry* (3rd ed.). London: Bailliere, Tindal & Carssell.

Sours, J. A. (1964). Neuropsychiatric findings in internal carotid artery occlusive disease with cerebrovascular damage. Report of nine cases and review of the literature. *Psychiatr Q, 38*, 405–423.

Tatemichi, T. K., Desmond, D. W., & Prohovnik, I. (1995). Strategic infarcts in vascular dementia. A clinical and brain imaging experience. *Arzneimittelforschung, 45*(3A), 371–385.

Tomlinson, B. E., Blessed, G., & Roth, M. (1968). Observations on the brains of non-demented old people. *Journal of Neurological Sciences, 7*(2), 331–356.

Tomlinson, B. E., Blessed, G., & Roth, M. (1970). Observations on the brains of demented old people. *Journal of Neurological Sciences, 11*(3), 205–242.

World Health Organization. (1993). *The ICD-10 classification of mental and behavioral disorders. Diagnostic criteria for research.* Geneva: Author.

Chapter 2
Neurovascular Geography and Mapping the Consequences of Its Injury

Ronald M. Lazar and Joanne R. Festa

As with any organ in the body, the brain depends upon the integrity of its blood supply to maintain normal function. Despite the fact that it only constitutes about 2% of body weight, however, it needs about 20% of the cardiac output and a comparable proportion of the total amount of oxygen used by the body. To understand the cognitive and behavioral consequences of an interruption of normal blood flow, it is important to provide first a general description of the geography of the cerebral circulatory system. The purpose of this chapter is to provide this overview and then to describe the diagnostic tools that reveal the effects of diseases and conditions that disrupt supply. For a more detailed anatomical description of this system and investigative modalities, the reader is referred to *Stroke: Pathophysiology, Diagnosis and Management* (Mohr, Choi, Grotta, Weir, & Wolf, 2004).

Neurovascular Anatomy

The brain is fed by two main arterial sources: the internal carotid arteries and the vertebral arteries. The ascending aorta arises out of the

left ventricle of the heart and from the aortic arch come the brachiocephalic trunk and then the subclavian artery. From the brachiocephalic comes the carotid system with a left and right common carotid artery, and the subclavian artery, which gives rise to the left and right vertebral. Each common carotid artery splits, with the left and right internal carotid supplying the anterior cerebral circulation, about 80% of the brain's blood supply. The vertebral arteries unite at the border of the pons to form the basilar artery that supplies 20% of the brain's blood volume via the posterior cerebral circulation.

At the medial base of the cerebral hemispheres is a unique arterial ring, the circle of Willis, formed by early segments of the anterior, middle, and posterior cerebral arteries (PCAs) and the anterior and posterior communicating arteries. Figure 1 shows the distribution territories of the three major cerebral arteries.

The left and right anterior cerebral arteries (ACAs) arise from the anterior portion of the circle of Willis and are connected by the anterior communicating artery (ACoA). The ACoA, as well as small branches from the ACA, penetrate the brain to supply blood to the fornix, septal regions, anterior perforated substance, optic chiasm, optic tract, optic nerve, and suprachiasmatic area (Dunker & Harris, 1976). The ACA starts at the bifurcation of the internal carotid, entering the interhemispheric fissure, and then proceeding

R.M. Lazar (✉)
Stroke and Critical Care Division, Departments of Neurology and Neurological Surgery, Neurological Institute, New York Presbyterian Hospital, Columbia University, College of Physicians & Surgeons, New York, NY, USA
e-mail: ral22@columbia.edu

J.R. Festa, R.M. Lazar (eds.), *Neurovascular Neuropsychology*, DOI 10.1007/978-0-387-70715-0_2,
© Springer Science+Business Media, LLC 2009

Lateral View

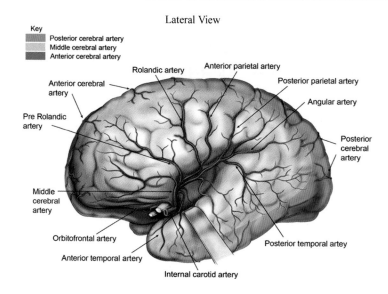

Medial View

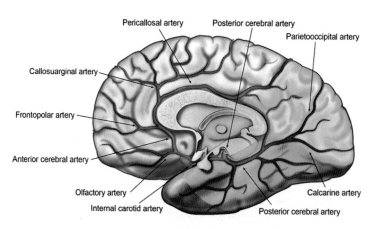

Fig. 1 Lateral (above) and medial (below) views of the major arterial territories in the cerebral hemispheres. (From Festa, J. F., Lazar, R. M., Marshall, R. S., Ischemic Stroke and Aphasic Disorders, in Ischemic stroke and aphasic disorders. In Textbook of Clinical Neuropsychology, J. E. Morgan, J. H. Rickers (eds). London: Taylor & Francis, 2008, with permission)

anteriorly and upward, and then posteriorly as it continues over the superior surface of the corpus callosum. Branches off the early segments of the ACA (e.g., Heubner's artery) supply the head of the caudate, the anterior part of the internal capsule, anterior globus pallidus, olfactory regions, and hypothalamus. The ACA gives rise to the medial striate artery, orbital branches, frontopolar branches, the pericallosal artery, and the callosomarginal

artery. Important brain regions supplied by these branches include the superior frontal gyrus, cingulate gyrus, and the premotor, motor, and sensory areas of the paracentral lobule.

The left and right middle cerebral arteries (MCAs) represent the largest of the major branches of the internal carotid arteries and supply most of the convex surface of the brain. Off the stem of the MCA are the lenticulostriate branches, named for the structures comprising the lentiform nucleus and striatum (caudate and putamen), and the internal capsule. As the MCA begins its course over the cortical surface, it then subdivides into several different branch configurations, but the most common pattern is a birfurcation into an upper and lower division. The initial segments in these two divisions supply the insula region, before proceeding over a large expanse of the lateral surfaces of frontal, parietal, and temporal lobes, much in the fashion of a candelabra. In the upper, or superior, division there is supply to the frontal lobe, including the orbital region, the inferior and middle frontal gyri, the pre- and post-central gyri, as well as the superior and inferior parietal lobules. The lower or inferior division of the MCA provides circulation to the parietal and temporal opercula, the posterior temporal, posterior parietal, and temporo-occipital regions. The MCA can also exist in a trifurcation pattern so that the orbitofrontal, prefrontal, and precentral branches comprise an upper division, the rolandic, anterior parietal, and angular branches make up a middle division, and the inferior division mainly consists of supply to the temporal lobe, and to the temporo-occipital region (Mohr, Lazar, Marshall, & Hier, 2004).

The vertebral arteries, as they course up the spine into the skull, provide arterial supply to the brain stem and cerebellum, before merging into the basilar artery at the level of the pons. The posterior cerebral arteries (PCA's) are typically formed by the bifurcation of the basilar artery at the circle of Willis where they are connected by the posterior communicating artery (PCoA). The PCAs continue to course superiorly along the lateral part of the brainstem, with penetrators supplying segments of the thalamus, before turning posterior as they pass over the tentorium and onto the medial and inferior surfaces of the temporal and occipital lobes. The nomenclature for the cortical branches of the PCA seems to vary, but in general there are vessels that subdivide into those that feed the ventral temporal surface, the occipito-temporal region, and those that supply the calcarine cortex. There is a variant of the PCA, called a "fetal" PCA, in which it arises directly from the internal carotid artery, and occurs in 5–10% of cases.

In addition to the three major cerebral arterial territory distributions, there are so-called "central arteries" that provide penetrating branches into deep brain. Among these are the anterior and posterior choroidal arteries. The anterior choroidal artery, usually arising from the internal carotid artery, courses from the lateral and then to the medial optic tract until the lateral geniculate body where is splits into many small branches before entering the temporal horn and the choroid plexus of the lateral ventricle. It supplies the optic tract, lateral geniculate body, medial temporal lobe, and the anterior one third of the hippocampus, the uncus, and part of the amygdala. Some of the perforating branches also feed the posterior limb of the internal capsule, optic radiations, the basal ganglia, and the ventrolateral region of the thalamus. Arising from the PCA, the posterior choroidal artery has one medial and two lateral branches and collectively feed superior and medial parts of the thalamus, the choroid plexus of the lateral ventricle, and the posterior two thirds of the hippocampus.

Autoregulation

In order to survive, the neurons and supportive tissue in the brain rely on a steady supply of oxygen and glucose via the circulatory system. Autoregulation occurs so that neither too little (hypoperfusion) nor too much (hyperperfusion) supply occurs. Depending on the degree and duration of disruption of the cerebral blood supply, the neuron undergoes a well-described series of pathophysiological steps in metabolic function before permanent cell death, or infarction, takes place. To maintain adequate function as long as possible, there are compensatory mechanisms that take place in response to disrupted blood flow.

Under normal circumstances, about one third of the oxygen and one tenth of the glucose circulating through the brain's circulation is metabolized (Zazulia, Markham, & Power, 2004) so that there is a uniform fraction of the available oxygen and glucose utilized, based on the amount needed for the resting metabolic rate of tissue. Autoregulation is the brain's ability to maintain cerebral perfusion pressure (CPP) when oxygen and glucose are not sufficient to meet its metabolic needs. Protection against abnormal blood flow begins to occur when the partial pressure of oxygen in the blood falls to about 50–60 mmHg (Buck et al., 1998). When the CPP falls, CBF can be maintained by dilation of the cerebral arterioles and recruitment of collateral vascular channels (Marshall et al., 2001). Adequate blood flow across the circle of Willis, for example, can serve this purpose, either from the ACoA or the PCoA bringing flow from the vertebro-basilar system. The state of maximal vasodilation has been referred to as Stage 1 hemodynamic failure. If the CPP continues to fall and there is maximal dilatation of the arteries, autoregulation induces an increase in the oxygen extraction fraction (OEF). When the arterioles are maximally dilated and OEF is increasing, then Stage II hemodynamic failure, or "misery perfusion," is said to occur. If there is a restoration of normal CBF before OEF reaches its maximum level, then there can be good recovery of neuronal function. But once maximal OEF occurs, ischemia begins and has a direct impact on neuronal function. Even after 30 s of ischemia, glucose metabolism is reduced to 15% of normal levels (Pulsinelli, Levy, & Duffy, 1982). If ischemia occurs for a critical period of time, a breakdown of cell function will occur and neurons will sustain permanent injury or death. In human stroke, the CBF is very low in the ischemic core, but can be high enough in the surrounding region, known as the ischemic penumbra, so that hemodynamic rescue via thrombolysis (e.g., rTPA) or mechanical removal of clot may be achieved. In general, the brain can function for only 6–8 min if oxygen or glucose is reduced below critical levels.

Diagnostic Studies

Brain Imaging

Since there are multiple causes for similar clinical manifestations of neurological dysfunction, differentiating vascular from non-vascular causes (e.g., tumor, infection, demyelination), hemorrhage from ischemia, and ischemic subtypes is critical for diagnosis and treatment. Among diagnostic modalities, modern brain imaging represents a key investigative modality that can identify the presence of neurovascular diseases and conditions.

Computerized Tomography

Computerized tomography (CT) of the brain is the most common imaging modality in cerebrovascular disease. Separating anatomy at different depths, a CT of the head uses moving sources of X-rays and detectors that measure the ability of tissue to block X-ray beams, with data that are reconstructed by computer into 5–7 mm slices oriented to the orbitomeatal plane, or about 15° from the horizontal plane. An example of a CT showing an ischemic stroke is shown in Fig. 2.

A CT scan of the head still represents the best way of distinguishing ischemic from hemorrhagic stroke: Low density signal attenuation suggests ischemia while high density indicates blood. Smaller hemorrhages may gradually lose signal intensity over 1 week but larger hemorrhages will produce high density signal changes that can persist for much longer durations. But within the acute period, the ability of CT to detect blood associated with parenchymal hemorrhage or subarachnoid hemorrhage makes it the radiographic modality of choice over MRI (Williams & Snow, 1995). The disadvantage of CT is that bone within the posterior fossa makes detection of signal changes in the brainstem more difficult.

With regard to ischemic brain injury, acute infarction can be detected as early as 3 h, with half of the cases positive at 12 h, and in some

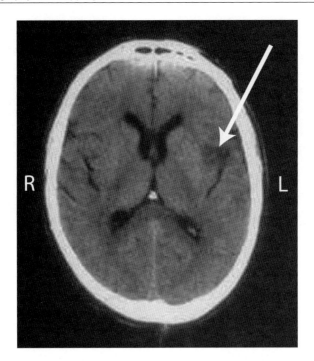

Fig. 2 A computerized tomographic (CT) image of the head without injection of contrast material. The top of the figure represents anterior and the bottom posterior locations in the brain. The arrow points to an ischemic infarct in the left hemisphere. L = Left, R = Right

instances, taking up to 3 days. But within 1 h after the onset of stroke symptoms, there is often loss of delineation between gray and white matter (Tomura et al., 1988). Ischemia resulting from embolic infarction seems more apparent on CT than ischemia associated with perfusion failure (Schuknecht, Ratzka, & Hofmann, 1990). With regard to the identification of ischemic changes in brain tissue supplied by small-vessel vessels, CT is capable of localizing injury as small as 1–2 mm.

Magnetic Resonance Imaging

Magnetic resonance imaging (MRI) has become an important technique in the visualization of cerebrovascular disease because of its ability to depict the brain in any plane, including top to bottom (axial), side to side (saggital), and front to back (coronal), and its superiority of resolution when compared to CT. Another advantage of MRI is that it does not use ionizing radiation or radioactive tracers.

The physics underlying MRI reveals that certain nuclei in tissue, mainly water and fat protons, when placed in a magnetic field align themselves with it. When radiofrequency (RF) pulses are then delivered, these nuclei absorb energy and then transfer energy back to a nearby detector coil at the same frequency. Over time, MR signal slowly fades away (relaxes) and the time constant for this decay varies in different tissues. The greater contrast resolution of MRI is based on its ability to detect the tissue-specific behavior of protons in different planes relative to the magnetic field. There are a number of different pulse sequences that have been used in MR imaging to assess cerebrovascular diseases and conditions; the most commonly used ones are described here. As of the moment, the magnetic strength of most clinical scanners ranges between 1.5 and 3.0 Tesla, although more powerful magnets, now used only for research, will likely be used in the future.

A T_1-weighted image (see Fig. 3, Left) is based on the relaxation time when protons

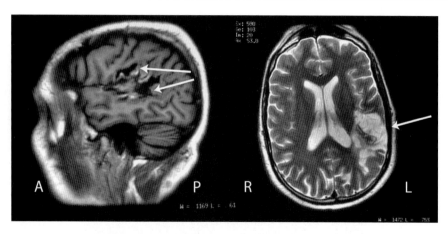

Fig. 3 Magnetic resonance images (MRI) of the brain. The left panel is a saggital (lateral view) T_1-weighted image of an ischemic infarct in the left hemisphere. A = Anterior, P = Posterior. The right panel is an axial T_2-weighted image of the same infarct

are aligned with the main (longitudinal) magnetic field. The T_1 image depicts white matter as brighter than gray matter. The cerebrospinal fluid (CSF) has low signal intensity so that it appears dark. Because of the water content in ischemic infarcts, it is therefore not surprising that they appear as hypointense on the T_1 image. In general, anatomy is more clearly defined with this pulse sequence.

A *T_2-weighted* image (see Fig. 3, Right) is derived when the RF pulses are delivered to hydrogen protons whose rotational spins are then flipped into the transverse plane relative to the main magnetic field. T_2 relaxation refers to the energy emitted back from the protons as they become re-aligned with the main magnetic field. The T_2 image shows CSF as a hyperintense (bright) signal. Ischemic brain lesions also appear hyperintense.

Fluid-attenuated inversion recovery (FLAIR) images (see Fig. 4, Left) involve the delivery of another RF pulse sequence that has the ability to suppress the CSF hyperintense signal so that it appears dark like in a T_1

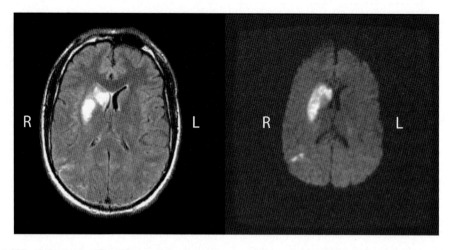

Fig. 4 MRI of the brain. The left panel is an axial fluid-attenuated inversion recovery (FLAIR) image of a subcortical stroke in the right hemisphere. The right panel is an axial, diffusion-weighted image (DWI) of the same clinical event

sequence but at the same time lesions appear bright like those in T_2 images. The result is an image that shows with greater contrast the presence of lesions. Another advantage of FLAIR imaging is excellent visualization of extra-axial blood, such as might be seen in subarachnoid hemorrhage or subdural hematoma (Noguchi et al., 1994).

The development of *diffusion-weighted imaging (DWI)*, and more recently *perfusion-weighted imaging (PWI)*, have improved identification of stroke in the acute phase, leading to a better understanding of acute pathophysiology and improving decision-making in acute stroke management (see Fig. 4, Right). The detection of the DWI signal is based on the presence of cytotoxic edema in the extracellular space arising from ischemic tissue. Areas of hyperintensity most often represent areas of infarction. Comparing sensitivity in detecting acute clinical stroke within 3 h after symptoms onset, Chalela et al. showed that DWI was superior to CT (Chalela et al., 2007). The sensitivity of DWI is such that nearly one-half of transient ischemic attack cases, defined by negative CT and a syndrome lasting less than 24 h, are DWI positive and therefore are reclassified as ischemic stroke (Kidwell et al., 1999).

Requiring the intravenous injection of the contrast agent gadolinium, PWI has the property of detecting the total brain volume of hemodynamically-compromised tissue, regardless of whether it is infarcted or compromised by ischemia but capable of recovery (Quast, Huang, Hillman, & Kent, 1993; Schlaug et al., 1999). The signs and symptoms of acute stroke have been shown to correspond with the total region of hemo-dynamically-compromised tissue, without distinguishing between the infarcted and the ischemic, still viable brain tissue. By assessing the volume of infarcted tissue as defined by the DWI image, and subtracting that from the PWI image, the DWI/PWI mismatch provides a visual representation of the tissue that is compromised but still capable of returning to normal function if blood flow could be restored. This border zone

between infarcted tissue and normally-appearing tissue is commonly referred to as the "ischemic penumbra," and is the target for acute reperfusion therapy. When reperfusion of the ischemic territory has taken place, either naturally or from intervention, the lingering clinical deficits correspond only to the residual region of infarction (Lee, Kannan, & Hillis, 2006).

One of the most recent developments in MRI sequencing is *diffusion tensor imaging (DTI)*. Although a thorough discussion of DTI is beyond the scope of this chapter, it takes advantage of edema detected in DWI by assessing the movement of water molecules in a region in which there are constraints in the direction of movement, such as in an intact white-matter tract in which the cell membrane constrains movement in the direction of that tract. The process of reconstructing the vector of the diffusion of these molecules is the basis of DTI tractography and holds promise for delineating the integrity of white matter in ischemic disease (Sotak, 2002).

Finally, another technique that holds promise in neurovascular disease but as yet largely remains investigative is *magnetic resonance spectroscopy (MRS)*, which measures the regional concentration of metabolites associated with, in this case, brain function. For example, Proton MRS has demonstrated that following middle cerebral artery stroke, there was a relative decrease in *N*-acetyl aspartate (associated with axonal myelin sheaths) and an increase in lactate in the regions of T_2 hyperintensity, compared to the contralesional side (Gillard, Barker, van Zijl, Bryan, & Oppenheimer, 1996). More recently MRS, used to assess the efficacy of hyperbaric oxygen treatment for neuroprotection in acute stroke, demonstrated improved aerobic metabolism and preserved neuronal integrity (Singhal et al., 2007).

Functional magnetic resonance imaging (fMRI), correlating some form of behavior during MRI with changes in oxygenated hemoglobin, is increasingly used in cerebrovascular disease and will be discussed in the chapter on stroke recovery (Chapter 17).

Other Imaging Studies of Blood Flow and Metabolism

Single photon emission computed tomography (SPECT) involves the measurement of cerebral blood flow (CBF) in tomographic reconstruction of brain images following the injection of a radionuclide, most frequently 99mTc-HMPAO. Alteration in CBF is thought to arise as a result its coupling to local brain metabolism and energy use, the pattern of which has been used to distinguish between dementia arising from Alzheimer's disease and that of vascular origin. More commonly, however, SPECT has been used to document CBF changes distal to stenosis or occlusion, or to visualize the effects of vascular anomalies, such as the brain arteriovenous malformation shown in Fig. 5(B). In this fashion, it becomes possible to dissociate the effects of focal ischemia arising from embolism from syndromes associated with perfusion failure from a more proximal location.

Positron emission tomography (PET), like SPECT, requires the injection of a radioactive tracer isotope. Whereas CBF is an indirect measurement of brain metabolism in SPECT, PET directly assesses neuronal integrity. Unfortunately, the agent most commonly used for this purpose is fluorodeoxyglucose (FDG), a glucose compound containing a radionuclide whose half-life is only a few hours and therefore requires a nearby cyclotron. PET can detect alterations in regional neuronal metabolism as well as determine the cerebral metabolic rate of oxygen. At this point, largely because of its limited availability, its application has largely been as a research tool with limited use in actual clinical practice in neurovascular disease.

Cerebral Angiography

In contrast to imaging brain tissue, the role of angiography is to visualize the inside of major vessels supplying to or returning blood from the brain as well as the cerebral vessels within the brain itself. The purpose is to ascertain whether there are any physical restrictions that could impede normal flow and to determine the presence of anomalies such as aneurysms and vascular malformations. The three principal methods are catheter-based digital subtraction angiography (DSA), magnetic resonance angiography (MRA), and CT angiography (CTA).

In DSA (see Fig. 6), a short catheter, or sheath, is placed into the common femoral artery, allowing the introduction of smaller catheters and guidewires that allow catheterization of the aortic arch and ultimately the

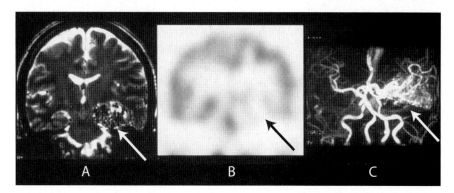

Fig. 5 Three images depicting a left medial temporal arteriovenous malformation (AVM). (A) A coronal (front view) T$_2$-weighted image. (B) A single photon emission computed tomographic (SPECT) image showing diminished cerebral blood flow in the left temporal region. (C) A magnetic resonance angiogram (MRA) of the brain AVM

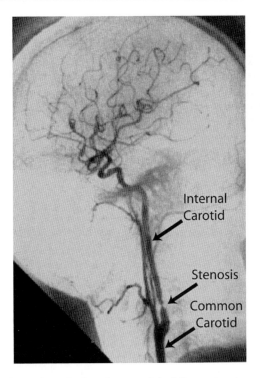

Internal
Carotid

Stenosis

Common
Carotid

Fig. 6 A cerebral angiogram of the left anterior circulation demonstrating a severe stenosis in the left internal carotid artery

carotid arteries and the anterior cerebral circulation, or the vertebrobasilar system and the posterior cerebral circulation. Contrast material which absorbs X-rays is injected at the target site, and the X-ray image maps the distribution of the contrast agent as it courses through the vascular territory. Superselective angiography entails the use of microcatheters, which can be placed further into the circulation and permit a more detail visualization of smaller defects. This technique represents the gold-standard of depicting vessels because of its high degree of resolution and its ability to show detail in vessels smaller than can be seen with any other angiographic method. There are, however, more risks associated with DSA. Among these include puncture of the blood-vessel wall, dislodgement of material adhered to the inner walls of vessels that can be carried downstream by the blood supply as emboli and cause ischemic stroke, and allergic reaction to the contrast agent. These risks have

been declining, mainly due to the development of new kinds of contrast materials and innovative catheter designs.

By changing the way RF pulses are delivered and the data are processed, it has become possible to use movement of blood to visualize large cerebral vessels during MRI, with the advantage that neither catheterization nor radiation is needed. MRA can render images in two dimensions, or as is more common, in three dimensions, which gives better spatial resolution (see Fig. 5c). In some settings, the comparability of conventional angiography and MRA is quite high.

Finally, new CT-based technology has enabled scanners to acquire blood flow data after the injection of a contrast agent. In addition to not requiring the use of a catheter, CTA has the significant advantage of being able to acquire images faster than other methods on scanners that are widely available.

Duplex and Transcranial Doppler Ultrasonography

First introduced in the 1970's, Doppler ultrasonography techniques are now commonly used to assess hemodynamics in the intracranial and extracranial arteries. A diagnostic imaging technology based on the analysis of high-frequency sound waves, Doppler ultrasonography is a rapid, non-invasive, portable, and low-cost means of assessing cerebral blood flow and is often employed as the initial screen for carotid disease and other suspected cerebrovascular disorders. Ultrasound can determine the patency of blood vessels, from stenosis to occlusion, the direction and velocities of blood flow through the vasculature, and the presence of vascular anomalies.

The Duplex test is a combination of ultrasound B-mode imaging, the black and white anatomic imaging, and color Doppler technology that can detect the movement of blood through the vessels by bouncing sound waves off blood cells. Using specified frequencies, the

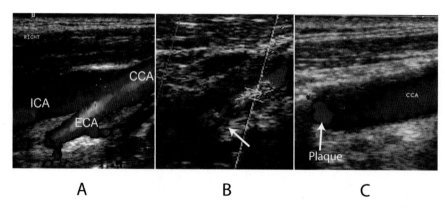

Fig. 7 Duplex Doppler ultrasonography of the carotid bifurcation in three different patients. (A) Normal blood flow through the common carotid artery (CCA), internal carotid artery (ICA), and external carotid artery (ECA) arteries; (B) blood flow through a stenotic segment of artery with arrow pointing to the area of stenosis; (C) total artery occlusion with arrow pointing to the occluding plaque

speed of blood flow in relation to the probe causes phase shifts with increases or decreases in sound frequency. The change in frequency directly correlates with the speed of blood flow. Typically used to assess the carotid and extracranial vertebral arteries, the Duplex test results in an image of the artery, any plaque causing stenosis, as well as a wave form that indicates blood velocity and other flow characteristics. Velocities determine the degree of artery stenosis and when no velocity is detected, the artery is considered occluded (see Fig. 7).

Transcranial Doppler (TCD) sonology uses the same technology to assess the intracranial vasculature through the transtemporal, transorbital, and transnuchal bone windows (see Fig. 8). The skull bones hamper ultrasound transmission so insonation of windows (areas with thinner walls) must be utilized, such as the temporal region in front of the ear. Certain patient demographics, such as age, gender, and race affect bone thickness and composition, and thus the ability to obtain data. The ability to accurately locate target vessels through these windows is highly dependent on individual training and experience. TCDs can be useful in identifying intracranial stenosis or occlusion, evaluation of collateral circulation, detection of intracranial aneurysms and AVMs, detection of vasospasm in SAH, and assessment of cerebral autoregulation (Mohr, Choi et al., 2004). TCD monitoring may also be used in detecting microemboli entering the cerebral circulation from a proximal source such as the heart, or during vascular procedures.

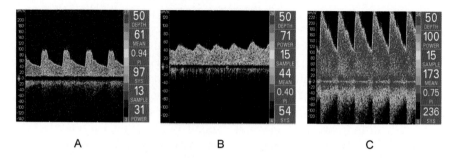

Fig. 8 Transcranial Doppler (TCD) ultrasonography of the middle cerebral artery. (A) Normal wave form; (B) blunted wave form representing flow distal to a stenosis; (C) accelerated wave form of flow through the stenotic segment of the vessel

References

Buck, A., Schirlo, C., Jasinksy, V., Weber, B., Burger, C., von Schulthess, G. K., et al. (1998). Changes of cerebral blood flow during short-term exposure to normobaric hypoxia. *Journal of Cerebral Blood Flow and Metabolism, 18* (8), 906–910.

Chalela, J. A., Kidwell, C. S., Nentwich, L. M., Luby, M., Butman, J. A., Demchuk, A. M., et al. (2007). Magnetic resonance imaging and computed tomography in emergency assessment of patients with suspected acute stroke: a prospective comparison. *Lancet, 369* (9558), 293–298.

Dunker, R. O., & Harris, A. B. (1976). Surgical anatomy of the proximal anterior cerebral artery. *Journal of Neurosurgery, 44* (3), 359–367.

Gillard, J. H., Barker, P. B., van Zijl, P. C., Bryan, R. N., & Oppenheimer, S. M. (1996). Proton MR spectroscopy in acute middle cerebral artery stroke. *AJNR American Journal of Neuroradiology, 17* (5), 873–886.

Kidwell, C. S., Alger, J. R., Di Salle, F., Starkman, S., Villablanca, P., Bentson, J., et al. (1999). Diffusion MRI in patients with transient ischemic attacks. *Stroke, 30* (6), 1174–1180.

Lee, A., Kannan, V., & Hillis, A. E. (2006). The contribution of neuroimaging to the study of language and aphasia. *Neuropsychology Review, 16* (4), 171–183.

Marshall, R. S., Lazar, R. M., Pile-Spellman, J., Young, W. L., Duong, D. H., Joshi, S., et al. (2001). Recovery of brain function during induced cerebral hypoperfusion. *Brain, 124* (Pt 6), 1208–1217.

Mohr, J. P., Choi, D. W., Grotta, J. C., Weir, B., & Wolf, P. A. (2004). *Stroke: Pathophysiology, diagnosis, and management* (4th ed.). New York: Churchill Livingston.

Mohr, J. P., Lazar, R. M., Marshall, R. S., & Hier, D. B. (2004). Middle cerebral artery disease. In J. P. Mohr, D. W. Choi, J. C. Grotta, B. Weir, & P. A. Wolf (Eds.), *Stroke: pathophysiology, diagnosis, and management* (4th ed.). New York: Churchill-Livingston.

Noguchi, K., Ogawa, T., Inugami, A., Toyoshima, H., Okudera, T., & Uemura, K. (1994). MR of acute subarachnoid hemorrhage: a preliminary report of fluid-attenuated inversion-recovery pulse sequences. *AJNR American Journal of Neuroradiology, 15* (10), 1940–1943.

Pulsinelli, W. A., Levy, D. E., & Duffy, T. E. (1982). Regional cerebral blood flow and glucose metabolism following transient forebrain ischemia. *Annals of Neurology, 11* (5), 499–502.

Quast, M. J., Huang, N. C., Hillman, G. R., & Kent, T. A. (1993). The evolution of acute stroke recorded by multimodal magnetic resonance imaging. *Magnetic Resonance Imaging, 11* (4), 465–471.

Schlaug, G., Benfield, A., Baird, A. E., Siewert, B., Lovblad, K. O., Parker, R. A., et al. (1999). The ischemic penumbra: operationally defined by diffusion and perfusion MRI. *Neurology, 53* (7), 1528–1537.

Schuknecht, B., Ratzka, M., & Hofmann, E. (1990). The "dense artery sign" – major cerebral artery thromboembolism demonstrated by computed tomography. *Neuroradiology, 32* (2), 98–103.

Singhal, A. B., Ratai, E., Benner, T., Vangel, M., Lee, V., Koroshetz, W. J., et al. (2007). Magnetic resonance spectroscopy study of oxygen therapy in ischemic stroke. *Stroke, 38* (10), 2851–2854.

Sotak, C. H. (2002). The role of diffusion tensor imaging in the evaluation of ischemic brain injury – a review. *NMR in Biomedicine, 15* (7–8), 561–569.

Tomura, N., Uemura, K., Inugami, A., Fujita, H., Higano, S., & Shishido, F. (1988). Early CT finding in cerebral infarction: obscuration of the lentiform nucleus. *Radiology, 168* (2), 463–467.

Williams, J. P., & Snow, R. D. (1995). Brain Imaging. In J. P. Mohr & J. C. Gautier (Eds.), *Guide to Clinical Neurology* (pp. 127–146.). New York: Churchill-Livingstone.

Zazulia, A. R., Markham, J., & Power, W. J. (2004). Cerebral blood flow and metabolism in human cerebrovascular disease. In J. P. Mohr, D. W. Choi, J. C. Grotta, B. Weir, & P. A. Wolf (Eds.), *Stroke: Pathophysiology, Diagnosis, and Management* (4th ed., pp. 799–819). New York: Churchill-Livingstone.

Chapter 3
Ischemic and Intracerebral Hemorragic Stroke

Howard Kirshner and Victor Mark

Introduction

Historically, stroke has been the source of much of our knowledge about the localization of higher cognitive functions in the brain. C. Miller Fisher, one of the founders of the field of vascular neurology, taught "We learn Neurology stroke by stroke." Stroke can be considered an "experiment of nature," in which one part of the nervous system is damaged, while the rest remains intact. Nineteenth century neurologists studied their patients in detail at the bedside, waited for them to die, and then correlated the syndrome described in life with the anatomy of the damage seen in the brain at autopsy.

In recent years, advances in brain imaging technologies have provided more immediate correlation of structure with function in the living patient. Computed tomographic (CT) and magnetic resonance imaging (MRI) scans reveal the anatomic areas damaged by stroke. Functional brain imaging with positron emission tomography (PET) single photon emission computed tomography (SPECT), and functional magnetic resonance imaging (fMRI) can delineate the areas of the brain that activate during a cognitive function, revealing not only single brain regions active in specific functions, but also networks of functionally-connected neurons. These techniques can be used in normal subjects to study where specific functions take place in the brain, but they are also being used increasingly in stroke patients. Such techniques can identify which components of a network are rendered dysfunctional after a stroke, including both areas directly damaged and those rendered metabolically less active because of damage to functionally connected structures. We can study how the brain recovers: do the same areas of the brain active in normal subjects recover function or do new areas of the brain become recruited to regain the function? Are the new areas on the same side of the brain or are they in the contralateral hemisphere? These questions underlie the study of brain imaging in patients with cerebrovascular disease.

Pathophysiology of Stroke Syndromes

A stroke, in general, is characterized by the abrupt onset of a focal neurological deficit in an awake patient. A stroke syndrome refers to the neurobehavioral and neurological symptoms and signs produced by the stroke. Syndromes tend to be relatively stereotyped, both because of consistencies between subjects in the organization of neurobehavioral functions in the brain and because of the

H. Kirshner (✉)
Department of Neurology, Vanderbilt University
Medical Center, Nashville, TN, USA
e-mail: howard.kirshner@vanderbilt.edu

stereotyped nature of vascular territories. It is important to recognize, however, that there are individual variations in both brain organization and in vascular territories. In addition, stroke syndromes are moving targets, evolving in the early minutes and hours of the stroke, with areas of ischemia becoming infarcted or recovering, and with the development of edema. During recovery, individuals vary in the plasticity of brain areas that might potentially take over lost functions.

This chapter is organized along the lines of the neurobehavioral features of the major stroke syndromes. Our approach will be to describe the major neurobehavioral deficits of each syndrome and correlate them with specific distributions and pathological mechanisms of ischemic and hemorrhagic strokes. This chapter will consider intracerebral hemorrhages, but syndromes related to subarachnoid hemorrhage, aneurysms, and arteriovenous malformations will be discussed in Chapters 4 and 5. We shall start with a brief review of the major arterial distributions of the brain and the major vascular pathologies underlying stroke syndromes.

Vascular Structures and Territories

The internal carotid artery is the site of atherosclerotic plaque formation, with the potential to occlude, leading to infarction in the distal territories of the vessel because of hemodynamic compromise, or to embolization and occlusion of intracranial branches. A stroke caused by occlusion of the internal carotid artery can vary from a large infarction of both the anterior cerebral artery (ACA) and middle cerebral artery (MCA) territory to a very small infarction in a branch of either the ACA or MCA territory, or in the "watershed" area between the two. Strokes related to carotid occlusive disease are frequently associated with transient ischemic attacks (TIAs) preceding the actual stroke, waxing and waning or stepwise progression of symptoms once the stroke begins, and onset

during sleep or in the early morning hours. Carotid artery strokes can evolve over a period of 1–2 days before stabilizing.

The intracranial branches of the internal carotid artery, especially the MCA, are less likely to be the site of atherothrombotic stroke, but more likely to be affected by emboli from more proximal sources such as the heart. In addition to the major branches, the ACA, MCA, and PCA, the deep structures of the brain are supplied by smaller arteries. A small branch of the ACA called the recurrent artery of Heubner, which arises from the ACA just after the ACoA, supplies parts of the caudate nucleus, anterior limb of internal capsule, and hypothalamus. Occlusion of the recurrent artery of Heubner may cause a stroke syndrome of faciobrachial weakness and dysarthria, occasionally accompanied by frontal lobe-like behavioral deficits (see below). Many small branches arise from the major intracranial arteries. The most commonly affected are the lenticulostriate branches of the MCA, which supply the basal ganglia and internal capsule. Similar branches called anterior striates arise from the ACA, and penetrating branches of the PCA supply the thalamus and midbrain. The anterior choroidal artery (AChA) is most often a branch of the internal carotid artery, just before its bifurcation into the ACA and MCA, though occasionally it arises from the proximal MCA or even the posterior communicating artery. This artery has a long territory extending posteriorly, supplying not only the choroid plexus, but also often the globus pallidus, internal capsule, anterior hippocampus, lateral thalamus and lateral geniculate body, optic radiation, and midbrain. The stroke syndrome resulting from occlusion of this artery is variable but can include contralateral hemiparesis, hemisensory loss, hemianopia, and if on the left side, aphasia. This is a major stroke syndrome occasioned by occlusion of a very small artery, and the infarction on CT or MRI can also be small. The posterior choroidal artery, a branch of the PCA, may anastomose with the AChA, but it rarely causes a stroke syndrome of its own.

The vertebrobasilar circulation consists of the two vertebral arteries, their junction to form the basilar artery, and the branches arising from the basilar artery. The vertebral arteries usually have only one branch, the posterior inferior cerebellar artery, supplying the lateral medulla and the inferolateral cerebellar hemisphere. The basilar artery gives rise to the anterior inferior cerebellar artery, supplying mostly the pons and cerebellum, and the superior cerebellar artery supplies the midbrain and upper portion of the cerebellum. There are also many small, penetrating branches, similar to the lenticulostriate arteries, arising from the basilar artery. Finally, the two PCAs typically arise from the top of the basilar, though the PCAs also receive collateral blood in most individuals from the carotid circulation via the posterior communicating artery.

Occasional strokes are associated with venous rather than arterial thrombosis and occlusion. Venous sinus and cortical vein thrombosis cause stroke syndromes, often in association with symptoms and signs of increased intracranial pressure. These strokes are also more likely to develop secondary hemorrhagic transformation than arterial strokes. Since these strokes are much less common than arterial strokes, we shall not discuss them further in this chapter.

Primary hemorrhage is a different vascular pathology from ischemic strokes. Most intracerebral hemorrhages occur deep in the brain, in the territory of small, penetrating arteries such as the lenticulostriates. Hemorrhages can also occur into cortical structures. These hemorrhages are less likely to be the direct result of hypertension and are more likely to be associated with amyloid angiopathy or cortical vascular pathologies such as arteriovenous malformations.

In addition to the dysfunction of the specific part of the brain affected by the stroke, which will be the major focus of this chapter, clinical features may suggest a specific type of vascular pathology. Large vessel atherothrombotic strokes, such as those in the internal carotid or vertebrobasilar circulation, are likely to be preceded by TIAs, and are likely to fluctuate or worsen in stepwise fashion in the 24–48 h after onset. Small vessel ischemic strokes may likewise be preceded by TIAs and may worsen in stepwise fashion. Thrombotic strokes of both types often occur during sleep or in the early AM hours. Small vessel strokes are especially likely to be associated with severe hypertension. Embolic strokes occur suddenly, without prior TIAs, and often with the deficit maximal at onset. They are likely to occur during waking activity. Hemorrhages often develop abruptly, but then worsen gradually over the next few hours. Hemorrhages are more likely to be associated with symptoms and signs of increased intracranial pressure such as headache, nausea, vomiting, and decreased level of consciousness. Hemorrhages are also often associated with severe elevations of blood pressure.

Specific Stroke Syndromes

Left Internal Carotid Stroke

The left internal carotid artery is particularly likely to cause aphasia as a part of the symptom complex. Aphasia is the loss of language function secondary to acquired brain disease. Aphasia has been described in historical writings as early as ancient Egypt, but in the nineteenth century through the work of Paul Broca, the language system was specifically related to dysfunction of the left cerebral hemisphere. Virtually 99% of right-handed persons have at least relative language dominance in the left cerebral hemisphere, and studies of left-handers have suggested that a majority also have relative left hemisphere dominance for language. Most aphasia syndromes result from damage in the distribution of the left MCA. While the subject of aphasia has always seemed complex, language disorders do have practical usefulness in localizing lesions and in defining stroke syndromes. A French study of 107 stroke patients, all documented with MR imaging, confirmed the general localizations of clinical studies over the past 140 years: frontal lesions were associated with nonfluent aphasia, whereas posterior temporal lesions affected comprehension (Kreisler et al., 2000).

Broca's Aphasia

Broca's aphasia is characterized by reduced fluency or difficulty getting words out. Many patients have associated dysarthria, or misarticulation of phonemes, and some have apraxia of speech, defined as an inconsistent pattern of articulatory errors, in addition to the aphasia or language disorder. The patient with Broca's aphasia has nonfluent speech productions, both spontaneously and during attempts to repeat. Naming is also impaired, with long pauses for word finding, but patients do respond to cues such as the initial sound or phoneme of the correct word. Auditory comprehension is usually functional for simple communication such as following simple commands or engaging in conversations, but with more detailed testing, deficits are apparent in the comprehension of complex syntax. Reading aloud is hesitant and reading for meaning is often more impaired than auditory comprehension. Writing is affected at least as severely as spontaneous speech.

The lesion localization in Broca's aphasia is usually in the left inferior frontal cortex, anterior to the motor strip. Patients with lesions restricted to this area usually recover well, whereas patients with lasting Broca's aphasia usually have larger frontoparietal lesions (Mohr et al., 1978). Alexander, Naeser, and Palumbo (1990) reported from their analysis of patients with left frontal infarctions that the full syndrome of Broca's aphasia required a lesion of the frontal operculum (Brodmann Areas 44 and 45), together with the lower motor cortex or motor face area. Patients with only the Area 44 and 45 lesions had a deficit in speech initiation of speech, but not a full-blown Broca's aphasia. Patients with involvement of only the lower motor cortex

had only hesitant speech and dysarthria. In terms of vascular anatomy, Broca's aphasia of the more severe, chronic type often results from occlusion of the internal carotid artery, with a large area of MCA territory infarction. The more isolated syndrome of Broca's aphasia, soon after onset, may reflect an embolus of cardiac origin to a frontal lobe branch of the MCA or an embolus arising from a plaque in the internal carotid artery. Naeser Palumbo, Helm-Estabrooks, Stiassny-Eder, and Albert (1989) reported that lesions associated with chronic nonfluent aphasia and poor recovery always include, in addition to the cortical frontal damage, subcortical damage in the "subcallosal fasciculus" deep to Broca's area and the periventricular white matter along the body of the left lateral ventricle.

Case 1: An 82-year-old lady presented with nonfluent speech and both dysarthria and inconsistent phoneme errors (speech apraxia), only mild comprehension disturbance, and a mild right hemiparesis, affecting the arm more than the leg. During a rehabilitation hospital admission, she regained independent ambulation with a cane and recovered partial use of the right arm and hand. Her speech fluency remained impaired at discharge. Figure 1 shows an MR image, indicating infarction of a small area of the left inferior frontal cortex, with involvement of the subjacent insula.

The apraxia of speech seen with Broca's aphasia has been the subject of conflicting anatomical analysis. In the series of Dronkers (1996), an overlapping lesion analysis pointed to the left insula as the structure correlating most consistently with apraxia of speech. In the more recent series of Hillis, Work et al. (2004), involving patients studied very acutely after stroke onset, the traditional Broca's area in the left frontal lobe correlated more closely with apraxia of speech.

Case 2: This 38-year-old male truck driver with a history of elevated blood pressures and smoking, presented with difficulty speaking, followed by the onset of right arm and leg weakness. He recalled two or three episodes of dim vision in his left eye over the preceding

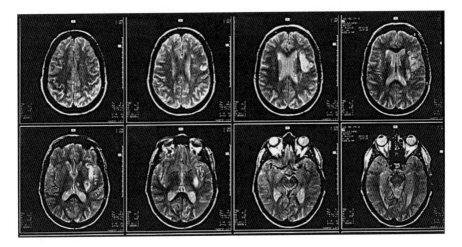

Fig. 1 Broca's aphasia with apraxia of speech

weeks, but he did not seek medical attention because of these. In the Emergency Department, he developed worsening inability to speak, combined with comprehension disturbance and increasing right hemiparesis. MRI (Fig. 2) showed an evolving infarction in the left frontoparietal region. MRA (Fig. 3) suggested severe stenosis of the left internal carotid artery. This was confirmed by arteriography (Fig. 4). The patient underwent carotid

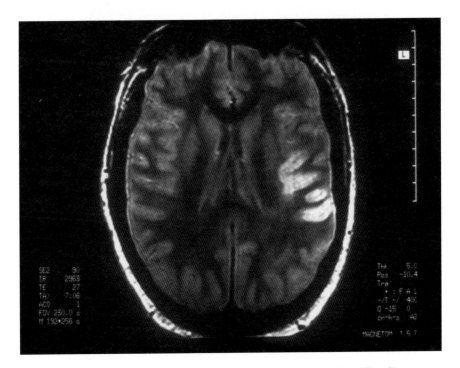

Fig. 2 Diffusion weighted MR image showing L posterior frontal acute infarction (Case 2).

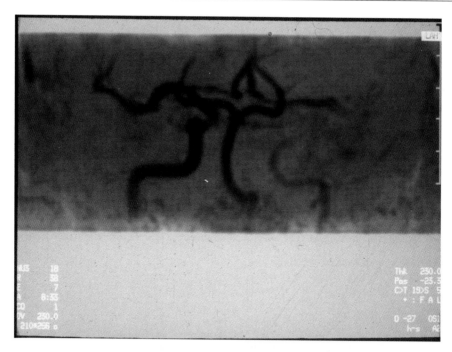

Fig. 3 MR angiogram, showing very little flow in the distal left internal carotid artery, reduced flow in the left MCA (Case 2).

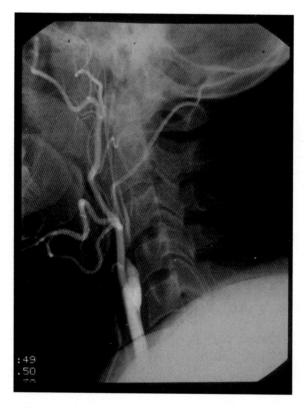

Fig. 4 Carotid arteriogram demonstrating severe stenosis of the left internal carotid artery just above the carotid bifurcation (Case 2).

endarterectomy but was left with residual aphasia and right hemiparesis.

A variant of Broca's aphasia is the more restricted syndrome now referred to as "aphemia" (Schiff, Alexander, Naeser, & Galaburda, 1983). Although Broca originally intended to use the term "aphemie" to describe the articulatory disorder later renamed "Broca's aphasia," "aphemia" is now used to designate a syndrome of nonfluent speech, with normal comprehension and writing. Patients with aphemia are often mute initially, with hesitant speech emerging over the next few days, often with prominent phonemic errors.

Patients with aphemia often have right facial weakness but no major motor deficits, and their comprehension, reading, and writing are largely normal. The lesions may involve the face area of the motor cortex (Alexander et al., 1990). Alexander, Benson, and Stuss (1989) equated aphemia with isolated apraxia of speech. In stroke terms, aphemia usually results from a cortical infarct, likely the result of an embolus to a frontal branch of the LMCA.

Wernicke's Aphasia

Wernicke's aphasia is a fluent aphasia syndrome, in which paraphasic errors make the utterances difficult for the listener to understand. Auditory comprehension is also affected, sometimes to a severe degree. Naming is usually impaired; whereas the Broca's aphasic struggles to get out phonemes, the patient with Wernicke's aphasia might effortlessly utter a completely incorrect name. Repetition is typically affected as well. Reading is typically affected much like auditory comprehension, but exceptional cases have been described in which either auditory comprehension or reading comprehension is relatively spared. It is important to look for such discrepancies in order to find a channel of communication for the patient. Writing is often produced with good penmanship, but the written productions have spelling errors, nonwords, and nonsensical constructions,

much like the speech. The errors in spelling may be a clue to a mild Wernicke's aphasia.

Wernicke's aphasia typically involves an infarction in the left superior temporal region, sometimes extending into the inferior parietal lobule. This is the territory of the inferior branches of the MCA, and Wernicke's aphasia classically results from an embolic stroke of cardiac origin. Rarely, a hemorrhage into the temporal lobe might produce Wernicke's aphasia. One personal case had a temporal lobe AVM that presented with hemorrhage and Wernicke's aphasia.

Studies have shown that destruction of Wernicke's area is most likely to result in lasting loss of auditory comprehension (Naeser, Helm-Estabrooks, Haas, Auerbach, & Srinivasan, 1987), though other authors have stressed the coexistence of lesions in the adjacent cortex of the temporal and inferior parietal lobes (Selnes, Niccum, Knopman, & Rubens, 1984; Kertesz, Lau, & Polk, 1993). Cases with disproportionately impaired auditory comprehension have lesions restricted to the temporal lobe, while those with more severe reading comprehension deficits may have lesions involving the parietal lobe (Kirshner, Casey, Henson, & Heinrich, 1989). Recently, Hillis, Wityk et al. (2001) have shown in a series of acute stroke patients that the degree of impairment of auditory word-picture matching correlated with the degree of hyperperfusion of Wernicke's area on perfusion weighted MR imaging (PWI). This study suggested that imaging in the acute phase of stroke may show less variability between subjects than imaging performed weeks or months into recovery.

Lazar, Marshall, Prell, and Pile-Spellman (2000) explored the subjective experience of a patient who had transient Wernicke's aphasia during a Wada test (amobarbital infusion into the inferior division of the LMCA) for planned resection of a left temporal arteriovenous malformation. The patient recalled the episodes afterwards, and he appeared to understand questions: "In general, my mind seemed to work except that words could not be found or had turned into other words. I also perceived throughout this procedure what a terrible disorder that would be if it were not reversible."

Case 3: A 51-year-old lady was admitted to the hospital for elective total knee replacement. She had no history of vascular risk factors except for obesity, smoking, and hormone replacement therapy. On the evening after the procedure she was reported by the nurse to be "confused" and not expressing herself clearly. The next morning, she had fluent, paraphasic speech and severely impaired auditory language comprehension, without any facial or extremity weakness. MRI (Fig. 5) showed a left superior temporal lesion by diffusion weighted imaging.

Global Aphasia

Global aphasia is the complete loss of language function, including nonfluent expressive speech, as in Broca's aphasia, and poor comprehension, as in Wernicke's aphasia, with severe impairment also of naming, repetition, reading, and writing. The lesion is typically large, involving most of the left MCA territory in the left frontal, parietal, and temporal lobes. Most patients have associated deficits such as right hemiparesis and right hemisensory deficits, though occasional patients may have lesions sparing the motor area, without hemiparesis (Legatt, Rubin, Kaplan, Healton, & Brust, 1987; Tranel, Biller, Damasio, Adams, & Cornell, 1987). Patients with mixed expressive and receptive deficits but not the severe impairment of global aphasia are sometimes referred to as "mixed aphasia."

With regard to stroke mechanism, global aphasia can be caused by a complete occlusion of the left internal carotid artery, or an embolus of cardiac origin that lodges in the left MCA stem. Finally, large subcortical lesions such as we see in large left basal ganglia intracerebral hemorrhages can also produce the syndrome of global aphasia. This syndrome is thus less helpful in identifying the stroke mechanism than some other syndromes.

Conduction Aphasia

Conduction aphasia is a syndrome of fluent speech, sometimes with frequent literal

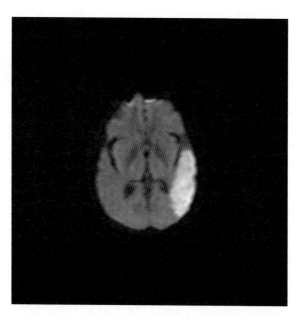

Fig. 5 Diffusion weighted MRI showing acute left superior temporal lobe infarction (Case 3).

paraphasic substitutions, preserved comprehension, but impaired repetition. Repetition is often the most severely impaired language modality in these patients, though naming, reading, and writing may also be impaired. By classical aphasia localization, this syndrome reflects a lesion that does not damage either Wernicke's or Broca's areas, but rather disconnects the two. Patient studies have not always supported this simple localization. Cases of conduction aphasia have been reported with either temporal or parietal lesions, and many of the parietal lesions involve the cortex of the inferior parietal lobule, especially the supramarginal gyrus (Benson et al., 1973; Damasio, Damasio, 1980). The inferior parietal lobule, particularly the supramarginal gyrus, appears to play a role in the perception of sounds and in the generation of phonemes (Hickok and Poeppel, 2000), perhaps explaining the frequent occurrence of phonemic paraphasic errors in the speech of patients with conduction aphasia. In terms of stroke syndromes, conduction aphasia can reflect a stage of recovery from a Wernicke's aphasia of embolic origin, or it may reflect an embolus to a left MCA branch supplying the parietal lobe.

Anomic Aphasia

Anomic aphasia is a syndrome in which naming is the language function most severely affected, with fluent expression, intact repetition and comprehension, intact ability to read and write, except for the naming difficulty. Anomic aphasia is not commonly seen as an acute stroke syndrome. It can be a stage in recovery of almost any of the aphasias, since naming is affected by lesions in the frontal, temporal, and parietal lobes. The patient mentioned above, under Wernicke's aphasia, with a temporal lobe AV malformation, had a nearly pure anomic aphasia after several months of recovery from Wernicke's aphasia. When last seen, she had recovered to a very mild naming deficit. In some studies, naming

of verbs is more affected by frontal lesions, naming of nouns more in temporal lesions. Anomic aphasia is also seen as a part of acute confusional states and dementing illnesses, again indicating that anomic aphasia is less localizing in terms of vascular diseases than the other aphasia syndromes.

Transcortical Aphasias

Transcortical aphasias make up the remaining syndromes of the eight classical aphasia syndromes described in the nineteenth century. They all share the sparing of repetition. In anatomic terms, this means that the "perisylvian language circuit," involving Wernicke's area and its connections to Broca's area, is not affected. The lesion lies outside this perisylvian circuit in an area referred to by Lichtheim (1885) as the "area of concepts," and which we now think of as the various association cortices that project into the language system.

Transcortical Motor Aphasia

Transcortical motor aphasia (TCMA) is a syndrome in which speech is nonfluent, as in Broca's aphasia, but repetition is preserved. The patient often pauses before responding to a question, may answer in one word utterances, but usually can communicate major concepts. Auditory comprehension is also preserved. The lesions typically involve the left frontal lobe, but the lesion may involve the prefrontal cortex anterior to Broca's area, the cortex of the medial frontal lobe (such as the supplementary motor area), or the deep frontal white matter. All of these lesion localizations are within the territory of the ACA (Masdeu, Schoene, & Funkenstein, 1978; Alexander and Schmitt, 1980; Freedman, Alexander, & Naeser, 1984). From a stroke standpoint, therefore, this syndrome is distinct from all of the syndromes of the left MCA. The vascular disorder underlying TCMA can be an embolus to the ACA, atherosclerotic disease in the LACA, or deep ischemia in the ACA territory from small vessel disease. Rarely, a frontal lobe hemorrhage could present with TCMA. Associated findings in the LACA territory ischemic stroke syndrome are quite different from those of LMCA territory stroke. The leg is typically weaker than the arm, and the shoulder is weaker than the hand. Many patients have an involuntary grasp response in the affected hand.

Transcortical Sensory Aphasia

Transcortical sensory aphasia (TCSA) is a syndrome of fluent but paraphasic speech output, impaired comprehension, but unlike Wernicke's aphasia, the patient is able to repeat. The lesions lie in the confluence of the temporal, parietal, and occipital lobes (Kertesz, Sheppard, & MacKenzie, 1982). TCSA is not a common stroke syndrome, though it can occur in watershed infarctions between the left middle and posterior cerebral artery territories.

Mixed Transcortical Aphasia

Mixed transcortical aphasia, or the "syndrome of the isolation of the speech area," is a rare syndrome in which the patient acts like a global aphasic yet can repeat. The patient has no propositional expressive speech, does not comprehend either spoken or written language, yet he or she can repeat flawlessly and even complete familiar utterances (such as "Roses are red, violets are..."). In a classical case (Geschwind, Quadfasel, & Segarra, 1968), the etiology of the syndrome was a very large watershed infarction in both hemispheres secondary to carbon monoxide poisoning. The patient had an intact perisylvian language circuit, but it was not connected to the association cortex in order for spontaneous speech or comprehension to take place in a meaningful way. This syndrome has also been reported in advanced dementing illnesses such as Alzheimer's disease.

Subcortical Aphasias

Aphasias do not always reflect disease of the left hemisphere perisylvian cortex. Lesions in the left hemisphere subcortical areas can also cause aphasia. The history of such lesions, however, is that lesions mapped by brain imaging studies led to the delineation of the subcortical aphasia syndromes, rather than analysis of symptoms and signs alone, as was the case with the cortical aphasia syndromes. In vascular terms, the subcortical lesions generally involve the distribution of proximal, lenticulostriate branches of the left MCA. Aphasia was first described with hemorrhages of the left basal ganglia, usually beginning in the putamen or internal capsule and involving a severe right hemiparesis and a prominent dysarthria, along with language disturbance (Alexander & Loverme, 1980). Patients with basal ganglia hemorrhages are often mute initially; later, varying degrees of aphasia remain, often with relatively preserved comprehension and repetition. The aphasia characteristics in lateral basal ganglia hemorrhage vary with the exact location and size of the bleed, varying from dysarthria and mild aphasia to severe global aphasia.

More recently, an aphasia syndrome has been described with infarctions of the anterior limb of the internal capsule, caudate head, and anterior putamen. This syndrome has been referred to as the "anterior subcortical aphasia syndrome." Features of this syndrome include dysarthria and decreased fluency, resembling Broca's aphasia, but typically with more dysarthria and greater fluency. Comprehension and repetition are usually less affected as compared to Broca's aphasia (Alexander, Naeser, & Palumbo, 1987). Most patients have an associated right hemiparesis. Recovery is typically quite good. Writing may also be affected more than expected in lesions of the internal capsule and putamen (Tanridag & Kirshner, 1985). The neuroanatomy of this syndrome likely involves disruption in the caudate nucleus or anterior limb of fibers projecting to the caudate from the auditory cortex, and from the caudate to the globus pallidus, ventrolateral thalamus, and premotor cortex.

Case 4: A 56-year-old lady walked into the outpatient clinic after noting difficulty with expressive speech, without any hemiparesis, on the day prior to the visit. She had a history of hypertension and hyperlipidemia. On examination, she was alert, but she had hesitant, nonfluent speech, with some dysarthria. Naming was also slow, with some deficits. She had similar difficulty with repetition, but her comprehension was excellent. Figure 6 shows an MRI scan from this patient. This is an example of the anterior subcortical aphasia syndrome, but a relatively mild version. She made a gradual recovery with outpatient speech therapy. She has had a permanent, mild dysfluency and anomia, present especially when she is fatigued, but she has been able to resume her normal life activities.

Subcortical aphasia syndromes are the subject of ongoing research. Published case studies differ, perhaps relating to the use of CT in earlier studies, which might have failed to detect cortical involvement. A good summary of correlations of strokes involving subcortical structures is that of Alexander and colleagues (1987). They reported that lesions restricted to the putamen or head of the caudate nucleus were not associated with language disturbance, or at worst mild anomia. Lesions of the anterior limb of the internal capsule were associated with language disturbance only if the adjacent structures of the caudate and putamen were also involved (anterior subcortical aphasia syndrome). Lesions involving the more posterior putamen were associated with hypophonia. Dysarthria was prominent if the damage extended to the white matter of the periventricular region or the genu of the internal capsule. Lesions located more posteriorly, converging on the temporal isthmus, produced fluent aphasia, neologisms, and impaired comprehension, resembling Wernicke's aphasia. Lesions involving both areas, including the anterior caudate and putamen, internal capsule, periventricular white matter, and temporal isthmus, produced global aphasia. Finally, lesions more laterally placed, involving the insular cortex, extreme capsule, claustrum, and internal capsule, produced a good mimic of conduction aphasia, with phonemic paraphasias and impaired repetition. A variety of syndromes can thus be associated with subcortical lesions, including imitators of most of the cortical aphasia syndromes. These relatively uncommon syndromes should not detract from the more

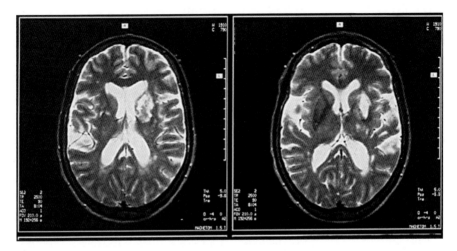

Fig. 6 T2-weighted MRI cuts demonstrating infarction of the left head of caudate, anterior limb of internal capsule, and anterior putamen (Case 4).

typical conclusion that a stroke causing aphasia is likely to involve the language cortex.

Another neurobehavioral syndrome associated with a subcortical lesion localization is a frontal-like syndrome associated with caudate lesions. Patients may show impaired attention, sequencing, and planning (Mendez, Adams, & Lewandowski, 1989). The caudate has extensive connections to the frontal lobe.

The basis of subcortical aphasia likely involves connections between the basal ganglia and the cortex. Motor speech is likely similar in its organization to the general motor control system, involving a feedback loop from the cerebral cortex to the striatum (putamen and caudate), then to the globus pallidus, then via projections to the lateral thalamus, via the anterior limb of internal capsule, back to the cerebral cortex. This loop is familiar to neurologists from discussion of movement disorders and Parkinson's disease. There are clear analogies between the motor and speech systems. The hesitancy and reduced fluency of speech parallel the abnormal limb control seen in basal ganglia disorders. Hesitancy, initiation difficulty, and disturbed motor control can be seen in the dysarthrias and aphasias, just as limb movements and gait are deranged in basal ganglia disorders.

A very separate type of subcortical aphasia is "thalamic aphasia." Like the anterior subcortical aphasia syndrome, thalamic aphasia was first described in patients with thalamic hemorrhage (Fisher, 1959; Reynolds, Turner, Harris, Ojemann, & Lavis, 1979, Mohr, Watters, & Duncan, 1975). The aphasia pattern usually associated with thalamic damage is fluent, with paraphasic errors, but with less impairment of comprehension and repetition as compared to Wernicke's aphasia. Mohr and colleagues described a "dichotomous" state in which patients fluctuate between relatively normal, intelligible speech when they are alert, but mumbling unintelligibly when they are somnolent. Luria (1977) called thalamic aphasia a "quasiaphasic disturbance of vigilance," meaning a failure of the alerting

mechanism of the thalamus in activating the temporal cortex; the posterior thalamus has extensive projections to Wernicke's area, and the anterior and paramedian thalamic nuclei connect to structures involved in memory and attention (Crosson, 1985). Thalamic aphasia also has implications for cerebral dominance. Hemorrhages in the right thalamus have produced aphasia in left-handed patients, indicating that language dominance in one hemisphere extends down to the level of the thalamus (Kirshner and Kistler, 1982).

More precise anatomic localization in thalamic aphasia has come from cases of ischemic infarction of the thalamus, since ischemic strokes are associated with less swelling and mass effect than hemorrhages. Bogousslavsky, Miklossy, et al. (1988) and Bogousslavsky, Regli, and Uske (1988) in a study of 40 cases of thalamic infarction, distinguished four separate vascular territories, later updated by Schmahmann (2003) and Carrera, Michel, and Bogousslavsky (2004). Aphasia correlated best with infarctions in the territory of the tuberothalamic artery, which supplies the anterior thalamus, including the ventral anterior and part of the ventral lateral nuclei. Strokes in this vicinity were associated with hypophonia, verbal paraphasias, impaired comprehension, and intact repetition. Strokes in this location on either side are also associated with apathy, personality changes, and impaired memory. Similar aphasic deficits occurred in patients with paramedian thalamic infarcts, within the territory of the thalamoperforating artery (now referred to as the "paramedian artery"), sometimes associated with depressed level of consciousness. The other two thalamic syndromes, posterior choroidal artery infarcts with infarction of the lateral geniculate body and ventroposterolateral infarcts in the territory of the inferolateral arteries, were associated with hemianopia and hemisensory loss, respectively, without language disturbance. Graff-Radford, Eslinger, Damasio, and Yamada (1984) also described fluent aphasia, anomia, perseveration, reduced comprehension, preserved reading, and intact repetition in cases of thalamic infarction. Deficits in short-term memory and attention have also been reported in cases of paramedian thalamic infarction (Stuss Guberman, Nelson, & Larochelle, 1988; Fensore, Lazzarino,Nappo, & Nicolai, 1988; Schmahmann, 2004). Carrera et al. (2004) stated that anteromedian thalamic infarcts were often cardioembolic in origin, central thalamic infarcts were often lacunar, and posterolateral infarctions were either cardioembolic or artery-to-artery emboli.

Pure Alexia with Agraphia

Traditionally, the alexias are divided into three categories: pure alexia with agraphia, pure alexia without agraphia, and alexia associated with aphasia ("aphasic alexia"). The syndrome of pure alexia with agraphia, described by the French physician Dejerine (1891), is an acquired illiteracy. Reading and writing are disrupted more than other language modalities, though many patients with alexia with agraphia have some degree of paraphasic speech and dysnomia. Repetition and auditory comprehension are preserved. Occasional cases of alexia with agraphia evolve from an initial deficit of Wernicke's aphasia, with some impairment of auditory comprehension as well as reading. Both reading words aloud and reading comprehension are abnormal. The patient cannot understand words spelled orally, though exceptional cases with sparing of oral spelling have been reported. Writing is also severely impaired, such that the patient cannot write or spell even single words. This difficulty with words and letters is also reflected in difficulties with numbers and calculations (acalculia), as well as musical notation. Other associated neurological deficits in alexia with agraphia include a right hemianopsia or inferior quadrantanopsia; sensory and motor signs are usually mild or completely absent. Other features of the Gerstmann syndrome (see below) may be associated.

The lesions in alexia with agraphia involve the left inferior parietal lobule, especially the left angular gyrus. Dejerine conceived of the angular gyrus as a "visual word center," important to the understanding of visual language symbols. Current models consider the inferior parietal lobule a "heteromodal cortex" involved in cross-associations between different sensory modalities, such as auditory and visual language symbols. The syndrome of alexia with agraphia is not a common stroke syndrome, but it may be seen in infarctions involving the inferior division of the left MCA or a "watershed" infarct between the left middle and posterior cerebral arteries. Hemorrhages in the left parietal lobe can also be associated with the syndrome of alexia with agraphia.

Gerstmann and Angular Gyrus Syndromes

Gerstmann (1930) associated four cognitive deficits with left parietal lesions: agraphia, right-left confusion, acalculia, and finger agnosia. Finger agnosia refers to a topographical difficulty with body parts, tested by having the patient point to specific fingers on his or her or the examiner's hand on either side. Gerstmann's syndrome has become controversial, but most recent studies have reconfirmed its validity, at least as a collection of symptoms that can occur in varying combination with lesions in the inferior parietal region. Other deficits, including deficits in reading and naming, often accompany the four cardinal elements of the Gerstmann syndrome.

Benson, Cummings, and Tsai (1982) described the "angular gyrus syndrome" as a variant of Gerstmann's syndrome and a mimicker of dementia. A patient with a single lesion in the left angular gyrus, documented by PET scan but not by CT, had combined deficits of anomia, fluent aphasia, alexia, agraphia, acalculia, right-left disorientation, finger agnosia, and constructional apraxia. These multiple cognitive impairments mimicked a generalized dementia, though the absence of a lesion on CT makes this questionable. This multiplicity of deficits also underlines the importance of the inferior parietal region as a "heteromodal" association cortex. The inferior parietal association cortex, along with the prefrontal cortex, has expanded the most of any brain region in comparing ape to human brains.

Pure Alexia Without Agraphia

Dejerine (1892) also described the syndrome of pure alexia without agraphia, also called pure alexia, pure word blindness, and letter-by-letter alexia. Patients with pure alexia have little abnormality of spoken language modalities. They can speak fluently, name objects (though sometimes not colors), repeat, and understand spoken language, even words spelled orally to them. Strikingly, they can write; the hallmark of this syndrome is the paradoxical inability of the patients to read words they have just written. Pure alexia is a true "word blindness," in which printed words have lost their meaning, though the patient is not blind. Initially, patients may be unable to read at all. Over time they may regain the ability to recognize letters and to spell words out, letter-by-letter (hence the name "letter-by-letter alexia"; Patterson & Kay, 1982). During recovery, patients with pure alexia learn to read silently, but still slowly. Reading remains effortful, and patients rarely read for pleasure again. Some patients make visual errors in reading; they perceive the beginning letters of the word and then guess the rest, incorrectly. For example, the patient may read the word "automatic" as "automobile." Patients with pure alexia are not illiterate, as in alexia with agraphia, but they act as if they have a linguistic blindfold.

Associated symptoms and signs in pure alexia include an almost invariable right visual field defect, either a hemianopsia or right upper quadrantanopsia. Occasional patients have intact visual fields; some of these lose color vision in the right visual field

("hemiachromatopsia"; Damasio & Damasio, 1983). Primary motor and sensory deficits are usually absent, though mild right hemiparesis or hemisensory loss may be present. Associated neurobehavioral deficits in pure alexia include color anomia and memory loss. The inability of these patients to name colors is not a perceptual problem; as described by Geschwind and Fusillo (1966), they can match and sort colors normally, indicating that the deficit is not a problem of visual perception. They can also name colors in the abstract, such as the color of a banana or a schoolbus, excluding an anomia. The deficit is an inability to associate a perceived color with its name, a deficit called "color agnosia." Occasionally, the deficit in naming colors may extend to pictures or objects, in which case the patient has visual agnosia; usually, visual agnosias develop only in patients with bihemispheral lesions. Deficits in memory may manifest initially as an acute confusional state; as the sensorium clears, a pure short-term memory impairment remains (Benson, Marsden, & Meadows, 1974; Von Cramon, Hebel, & Schuri, 1988). Immediate memory and memory for remote events are preserved in patients with PCA infarctions. Patients with pure alexia typically have no parietal lobe signs such as calculation difficulty or the other elements of the Gerstmann and angular gyrus syndromes.

Pure alexia without agraphia correlates with strokes in the distribution of the left posterior cerebral artery, involving the medial occipital and medial temporal lobes, and the splenium of the corpus callosum. The left occipital lobe lesion produces a right homonymous hemianopia, while the lesion in the corpus callosum prevents visual information from the right occipital lobe from reaching left hemisphere language centers. Alexia without agraphia is one of the syndromes referred to by Geschwind (1965) as "disconnection syndromes." The features of pure alexia without agraphia correlate with specific branches of the posterior cerebral artery; alexia correlates with the medial occipital and splenial lesion;

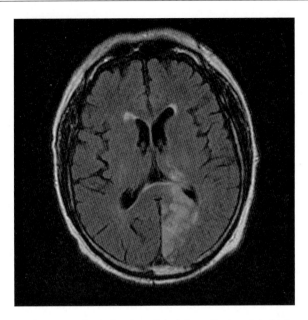

Fig. 7 MRI (FLAIR image) demonstrating infarction of the left medical occipital lobe, splenium, and thalamus, PCA territory (Case 5).

motor and sensory involvement, when present, correlates with involvement of proximal branches to the thalamus and cerebral peduncle. The short-term memory loss correlates with medial temporal involvement, especially the hippocampus. In the study of Von Cramon et al. (1988) of 30 PCA territory infarctions, verbal short-term memory impairment correlated with left sided strokes, and in particular, infarction of the posterior parahippocampal gyrus and collateral isthmus, disrupting afferent and efferent connections to the hippocampus. Patients with more lateral occipital infarctions, sparing the splenium and medial occipital and temporal regions, have a more partial or transient alexia, sparing letters, and often sparing memory, color-naming, and visual field deficits (Damasio and Damasio, 1983).

Case 5: This 81-year-old man with atrial fibrillation developed the abrupt onset of a mild confusional state, with memory difficulty and visual disturbance. On examination, he spoke fluently and named objects well, though he was totally unable to read, and he had difficulty naming colors. He could write sentences, but he could not read them later. His short-term memory was mildly impaired. He had a dense R homonymous hemianopsia. He had no motor or sensory disturbance. MRI scan (Fig. 7) showed a left occipital infarction, with infarction of the splenium of the corpus callosum.

Disorders of the Right Hemisphere

The right hemisphere is often dismissively referred to as the "minor" or "nondominant" hemisphere because it does not play a critical role in language function in most people. The right hemisphere, however, carries out very important neurobehavioral functions. Right hemisphere strokes are very disabling and can cause cognitive, behavioral, and personality changes. Right hemisphere neurobehavioral impairments include constructional and dressing difficulties, spatial and topographical disorientation, inattention to the left side of the body and of space, neglect and denial of neurological deficits, emotional disturbances, and alterations in the emotional aspect of communication.

With regard to stroke syndromes, the right MCA is the cause of most of the deficits to be discussed. Stroke syndromes involving the right ACA territory, posterior cerebral artery territory, and deep structures will be discussed in passing.

Neglect, Anosognosia

One of the most striking deficits exhibited by patients with cerebrovascular disease is the neglect of the left side of the body and of the deficit itself. An acute right hemisphere stroke patient may lie with the head and eyes turned to the right, turning toward stimuli or people on the right but completely ignoring stimuli on the left. The patient may neglect the left side of the body when dressing or shaving, may eat the food on the right side of the plate but leave the left side untouched. If the patient is ambulatory, he or she may bump into obstacles on the left side; when reading, she may omit words at the left side of a line; when driving, she may fail to notice oncoming vehicles on the left. Hemineglect is very disabling deficit.

The patient may or may not have a left hemianopsia; some patients can see stimuli in the left visual field but pay no attention to them ("visual neglect"). Neglect can involve the left side of the body or the left side of space (Calvanio, Petrone, & Levine, 1987; Heilman, Valenstein, & Watson, 2000). Neglect can affect all sensory modalities. One aspect of the neglect phenomenon is "extinction" of left-sided stimuli when bilateral stimuli are presented (Critchley, 1966). Some patients grimace when pinched on the left limbs but cannot localize the source of pain. Occasional patients with right hemisphere lesions experience peculiar sensations of the left limbs, e.g., amputation or phantom limb feeling or the presence of "extra" limbs or even an extra person in the bed. Functional MRI studies have indicated that the right occipital cortex is activated in response to left-sided visual stimuli, even when they are "extinguished" and not consciously seen by the subject; these stimuli are perceived in the visual cortex but not made available to conscious awareness (Rees et al., 2000).

Neglect of the deficit itself in a patient with a right hemisphere stroke was termed "anosognosia" by Babinski. Patients with acute right hemisphere strokes may be completely unaware of their paralysis. When asked to lift up both arms, the patient may lift only the right arm, yet the patient may deny being weak. He or she seems unconcerned about the paralysis ("anisodiaphoria"). In the most severe form of the neglect syndrome, the patient may even deny his own left arm or leg or claim that his left arm is the examiner's arm. As neglect improves, recovery occurs in stages. After a few days, the patient no longer denies the hemiparesis and may acknowledge both the stroke and the left-sided weakness. The patient may still not be fully aware of the deficit, however, attempting to get up and falling; right hemisphere stroke patients are major fall risks. Patients may also speak of the deficit in neutral terms, such as "They say my left side is paralyzed." Finally, in the mildest stage of neglect, the patient is aware of the deficit but seems inappropriately unconcerned, joking or asking when he or she can go home, despite deficits that render a patient unable to walk or to work. Such unawareness of functional disability is an interfering factor with rehabilitation (Denes, Semenza, Stoppa, & Lis, 1982).

In terms of stroke anatomy, a number of separate lesion sites can produce neglect behavior. An extensive classical literature links neglect to the right parietal lobe, and particularly the inferior parietal lobule (Critchley, 1966; Denny-Brown and Chambers, 1958). In the study of Hier, Mondlock, and Caplan (1983), those patients with strokes associated with neglect and denial of deficit had large infarcts, usually involving much of the parietal lobe, but the lesion diagrams in this study largely represented the distribution of large RMCA infarctions. Samuelsson, Jenson, Ekholm, Naver, and Blomstrand (1997) correlated visuospatial neglect with lesions of the middle temporal gyrus and temporoparietal paraventricular white matter; 12/18 right hemisphere stroke patients with neglect had lesions involving one or both of these areas, whereas 1/35 patients without neglect had a lesion of these areas. Another CT scan study (Egelko et al., 1988), however, found that visual neglect correlated only with right hemisphere lesions; the parietal lobe had no more association with visual neglect than did the temporal and occipital lobes. Isolated right frontal lesions have also been associated with neglect (Heilman and Valenstein, 1972; Damasio et al., 1980). The lesions in these cases involved either the medial or dorsolateral surfaces of the frontal lobe or the cingulate gyrus. Thus the right ACA territory is also a source of neglect syndromes. Deep, subcortical strokes in the right hemisphere, specifically in the striatum and deep white matter (Damasio et al.; Bogousslavsky, Miklossy et al., 1988; Bogousslavsky, Regli et al., 1988), posterior limb of the internal capsule (Ferro & Kertesz, 1984), and thalamus (Watson, Valenstein, & Heilman, 1981) have been associated with left-sided neglect. As with syndromes of aphasia associated with left hemisphere subcortical lesions, these right hemisphere subcortical lesions may produce their effect partly by disrupting the function of the cortex by mass effects or by interruption of ascending and descending connections. SPECT studies in patients with subcortical neglect (Bogousslavsky, Miklossy et al., 1988; Bogousslavsky, Regli et al., 1988) have shown hypoperfusion of the right parietal lobe as well as of the subcortical structures directly involved in CT scans.

Mechanism of Hemineglect

Many theories have been advanced to explain the cerebral mechanisms underlying neglect and hemi-inattention (Heilman and Valenstein, 1979). Early theories emphasized afferent sensory defects, including altered sensation or disordered body schema. Accounts of neglect based on sensory abnormalities, however, cannot explain impaired motor acts, such as denial of hemiparesis or omission of the left side of a drawing.

A second possible mechanism of neglect is a disorder of attention. Both Brain (1941) and Critchley (1966) early cited the importance of right hemisphere function in maintaining attention. Heilman and colleagues developed an "attention-arousal" hypothesis, involving right hemisphere dominance for attention. Anatomically, the attentional system in the brain involves the ascending reticular activating system and its connections to the frontal and inferior parietal cortices. Disruption of this ascending system may explain the neglect seen with thalamic and other subcortical strokes (Watson et al., 1981). Evidence for the dominance of the right hemisphere for attention has come from measures of reaction time, galvanic skin response, and EEG desynchronization in right hemisphere stroke patients.

A third cerebral mechanism related to neglect is unilateral hypokinesia, or decreased spontaneous motor use of either the left limbs or of all limbs in the left side of space. This mechanism can be thought of as the "motor" aspect of neglect, or "intentional" as opposed to "attentional" neglect. Some right hemisphere stroke patients spontaneously move the left limbs much less than the right, even in the absence of weakness or sensory extinction (Valenstein and Heilman, 1981). Hemiakinesia may also explain the omission of left-sided details in the spontaneous drawings of patients with right hemisphere lesions. In clinical usage, line bisection tasks are thought to show attentional neglect, whereas "cancellation tasks" (cross out all of the letter "S's" in a display of letters) reveal intentional deficits (Na et al., 1998). Coslett and Heilman (1989) suggested that the right hemisphere is dominant for motor intention of both sides, whereas the left hemisphere is dominant only for motor intention of the right side of the body. These authors matched nine patients with similar infarcts in the MCA territory of the right and left hemispheres; the right hemisphere group had much less elevation of the contralateral shoulder when subjects were asked to lift both shoulders than did the left.

Experimental evidence also favors motor akinesia as a factor in neglect behavior. Heilman and colleagues demonstrated unilateral or hemispatial hypokinesia in three separate experimental paradigms. First, patients were tested on a line bisection task after being asked to read a letter on the right or left end of the line. Looking to the left or right before bisecting the line had very little effect on performance, whereas moving the entire line into the subject's left hemispace produced much more neglect than placement of the line in the midline or to the right. The authors interpreted these findings as more consistent with hemispatial hypokinesia than with a sensory or attentional mechanism (Heilman and Valenstein, 1979). Second, patients were asked to point directly in front of their chests, with their eyes closed, to what they thought was the midline. In this task, patients with right hemisphere lesions erred more to the right of midline than those with left hemisphere lesions erred to the left. The authors again interpreted this result as a motor phenomenon, as the task, in their opinion, did not require any visual or somatosensory input from the left side (Heilman, Bowers, and Watson, 1983). The third experimental model involved monkeys with lesions in either the right frontal (Watson, Miller, and Heilman, 1978) or right temporoparietal (Valenstein et al., 1982) cortex, both of which produced neglect but no paralysis. The animals were required to move the right upper limb, ipsilateral to the lesion, when stimulated on the left, and the contralateral (left) upper limb when stimulated on the right. Only stimulation on the side ipsilateral to the lesion produced abnormal motor responses. Because the ipsilateral side would be expected to have normal sensation, this deficit too appeared more consistent with hypokinesia than with sensory loss as the mechanism of neglect. Husain and colleagues (2000) have also confirmed the role

of the parietal lobe in planning motor reaching to the contralateral space, from human stroke cases as well as animal models.

Mesulam (1981) synthesized the behavorial and neuroanatomical data on neglect into a "network" approach. In this model, the right inferior parietal region contains the sensory schema for the contralateral body, and hence right parietal lesions produce sensory inattention, extinction, and abnormalities of spatial and topographical function. The frontal lobe subserves movement and exploration in contralateral space, and hence right frontal lesions produce inattention and hypokinesia. The cingulate gyrus, a limbic structure also implicated in neglect (Heilman and Valenstein, 1972), relates to the motivation to explore or attend to contralateral space. The cingulate gyrus has extensive connections to other limbic structures thought related to motivation and rewards. Finally, the reticular activating system in the brain stem and thalamus is necessary for arousal, vigilance, and attention, especially as directed to the contralateral body and space. Support for a right hemisphere network subserving attention has also come from PET studies (Fiorelli, Blin, Bakchine, Laplane, & Baron, 1991), which showed hypometabolism throughout the frontal, temporal, and parietal cortex and subcortical structures in right hemisphere stroke patients with neglect, even if the anatomic lesion was much smaller. This "network" theory brings together the three mechanisms of sensory alteration, inattention, and hypokinesia, and takes into account much of the clinical and experimental evidence relating to neglect.

Recovery and Therapy of Hemineglect

Neglect is a disabling deficit in patients with strokes and other right hemisphere injuries. Frequently, progress in rehabilitation is minimal until the patient can recognize the deficits in the neglected side of the body and work actively to correct them. Neglect is often variable, coming and going in the same patient on the same tests (Small and Ellis, 1994), perhaps related to alertness, fatigue, motivation, and presence of other stimuli on the left side (Seki K et al., 1996). Neglect is temporarily reduced by vestibular stimulation via cold liquids infused into the ear canal (Cappa, Sterzi, Vallar, & Bisiach, 1987; Rode, Perenin, Honore, & Boisson, 1998). A study of recovery of visual neglect after stroke (Stone, Patel, Greenwood, & Hallligan, 1992) found that most patients had recovered from neglect at three months post-onset. The most rapid recovery occurred in the first 10 days. Amphetamine stimulation may facilitate motor recovery, possibly via alleviation of neglect (Crisostomo, Duncan, Propst, Dawson, & Davis, 1988; Walker-Batson, Smith, Curtis, Unwein, & Greenlee, 1995; Grade, Redford, Chrostowski, Toussaint, & Blackwell, 1998). These and other methods are used in rehabilitation programs to help patients overcome neglect.

Post Stroke Delirium

A syndrome occasionally seen in acute right hemisphere stroke patients is delirium, with agitation, disorientation, and hallucinations. Acute confusional states can occur shortly after a right MCA territory stroke (Mesulam et al., 1976) or after recovery (Levine and Finklestein, 1982). Factors associated with the occurrence of delirium in right hemisphere stroke patients include seizures (Levine and Finklestein) and preexisting cerebral atrophy, as seen on CT or MRI scans (Levine and Grek, 1984). Rabins, Starkstein, and Robinson (1991) found the following associations between delusions and hallucinations in stroke patients: older age; family history of psychiatric disorder; right hemisphere lesions, particularly involving the temporo-parieto-occipital junction; cortical atrophy; and seizures. Caplan and colleagues (1986) described agitated delirium in association with acute

infarction of the inferior division of the right MCA, a stroke syndrome often not associated with hemiparesis. The authors called this the "mirror image of Wernicke's aphasia" in the left hemisphere. Acute confusional states have also been described in patients with right posterior cerebral artery territory strokes.

Constructional Impairment

Patients with right parietal infarctions often have deficits on bedside tests of constructional function, such as drawing and copying figures such as a clock or a house, or even the intersecting pentagon figure from the Mini Mental State Examination. These functions are more elaborately tested by neuropsychologists in measures such as the block design subtest of the Wechsler Adult Intelligence Scale, the Bender Gestalt drawings, the Rey-Osterreith figure, and the Benton Visual Retention Test (Lezak, 1983).

Patients with RMCA territory strokes frequently fail on copying drawings both because they cannot perceive spatial relationships and because they do not pay attention to the left side of space or of a figure. Figure 8 shows drawings of a clock and a Greek cross by a patient with a right parietal stroke; the patient's CT scan is shown in Fig. 9. All 12 clock numbers are crowded into the right side of the clock face and the left side of the cross is missing. Drawings of patients with right hemisphere lesions also frequently contain misplaced lines or misaligned spatial relationships in two-dimensional geometric forms.

The deficits seen in these visuoconstructional tasks probably reflect a variety of behavioral impairments: altered visuospatial perception, poor conceptualization of spatial relationships, left-sided inattention, motor difficulties in the execution of drawings, and impersistence or inability to sustain attention to a task. The anatomic localization of constructional impairment is most typically in the right parietal lobe. Several studies have

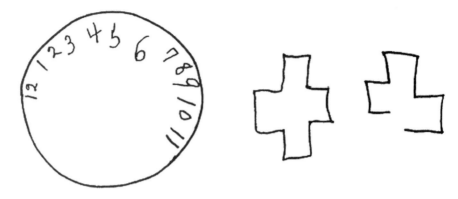

Fig. 8 Clock drawing and copying of a Greek cross

documented that constructional impairment occurs with lesions of either hemisphere, more with posterior than anterior lesions (Benton, 1967, 1973; Black & Strub, 1976). Constructional impairment from left hemisphere lesions correlates closely with receptive language deficits and is infrequent with purely expressive or no language dysfunction (Benton, 1973). More complex visuoconstructional tasks, such as the copying of drawings or three-dimensional block designs, are impaired more frequently by right than left hemisphere lesions, though deficits in simple block design may occur with equal incidence in the presence of lesions of the two hemispheres (Benton, 1975). In a CT scan study of neuropsychological

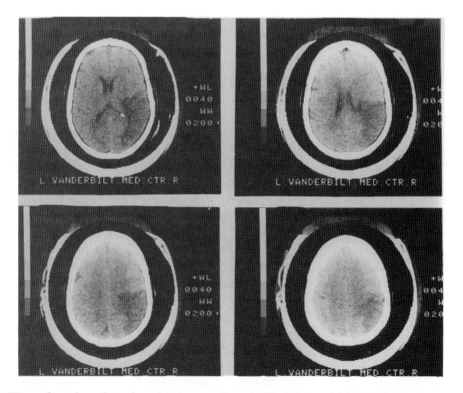

Fig. 9 CT scan from the patient whose drawings are shown in Fig. 8 (left parietal infarction)

deficits in 41 right hemisphere stroke patients, Hier et al. (1983) found a close correlation among impaired block design, poor performance on the Rey figure, and unilateral neglect in drawing; all three deficits were associated with right parietal lesions posterior to the rolandic fissure.

Constructional impairment is a common accompaniment of right hemisphere lesions, occurring in 36–93% of patients (Benton, 1967; Hier et al., 1983). Constructional impairment can be taken to indicate a disorder of the right parietal lobe, until proved otherwise.

Dressing Impairment

Patients with right hemisphere lesions frequently have difficulty with dressing or getting garments onto their bodies. This deficit has traditionally been referred to as "dressing apraxia," but the deficit seems to stem more from a perceptual difficulty than a true apraxia. Dressing impairment is largely related to an inability to conceive the spatial relationships of garments to parts of the body, though neglect of the left side may also play a role (Brain, 1941). Whereas constructional impairment must be detected by bedside testing, dressing impairment is apparent to the patient and family, and it is often mentioned in the history. Dressing apraxia correlates most closely with strokes involving the right parietal lobe. In the study of Hier et al. (1983), dressing impairment correlated with both left-sided neglect and visuospatial and visuoconstructional deficits and the localization by CT scan was nearly always right parietal.

Spatial and Topographical Impairment

Patients with right hemisphere lesions frequently manifest spatial disorientation for both the body image and external space. Stroke rehabilitation patients often become lost in trying to wheel themselves to the cafeteria or back to their rooms. Patients also manifest topographical impairment when drawing maps and locating cities on a map, or on bedside tests such as the Judgment of Line Orientation Test (Benton et al., 1975). Spatial and topographical deficits have a strong association with right parietal lesions, though they do occur occasionally in left hemisphere stroke patients (Benton, Levin, and Van Allen, 1974). As in constructional and dressing impairments, left neglect contributes to this deficit. In addition, the right parietal lobe appears to have direct involvement in the sense of topographical relationships between the body and space. Takahashi, Kawamura, Shiota, Kasahata, and Hirayama (1997) described three patients with focal intracerebral hemorrhages in the retrosplenial area of the right medial occipital lobe, extending into the medial parietal lobe. These patients lost the ability to recall the spatial relationships of streets and buildings, though they recalled the streets and buildings themselves. The retrosplenial region of the right occipital lobe, within the territory of the posterior cerebral artery, appears to be involved in topographical sense.

Another right parietal deficit is "reduplicative paramnesia," a syndrome in which patients are aware of their correct location but also say that they are at or near home. The patient may be oriented in other respects and not globally confused. This syndrome, named by Benson and colleagues in 1976, may reflect right parietal or bilateral posterior hemisphere lesions (Benson, Gardner, & Meadows, 1976). A patient in our hospital manifested prolonged and consistent reduplicative paramnesia, thinking he was both in our hospital in Nashville but also in his hometown of Knoxville, Tennessee. He repeatedly said that Vanderbilt Hospital was in Knox County. This patient had suffered a single, right MCA territory infarction.

Bisiach and Luzzatti (1978) studied the neglect of visual space in imaginary, as opposed to actual visual situations. These investigators asked patients to describe, from memory, the Piazza del Duomo in Milan, Italy. Patients described more details on the imagined right side of the Piazza than on the left. When they were asked what they imagined from a vantage point at the other end of the Piazza, however, they then described the buildings on the side of the square that they had previously neglected. Marshall and Halligan (1993) have shown that neglect of actual and imaginary spaces do not necessarily parallel each other; neglect can be selective for either actual or imagined space. Beschin, Cocchini, Della Sala, & Logie (1997) have also reported a patient with "representative" or imaginary neglect, without neglect for actually perceived scenes.

Motor Impersistence

Another neurobehavioral deficit described in association with right hemisphere strokes is "motor impersistence," a tendency for patients to stop performing a motor task even when asked to continue it. Such impersistence is seen even in simple tasks such as closing the eyes or protruding the tongue (Kertesz, Nicholson, Cancelliere, Kassa, & Black, 1985). Hier et al. (1983) tested motor impersistence in their study of right hemisphere stroke patients; like neglect, motor impersistence correlated with right parietal lesions. Motor impersistence is a functionally important deficit because it can interfere with activities of daily living and job responsibilities.

Right Hemisphere Language and Communication Impairments

Although the left hemisphere is dominant for language in most people, the right hemisphere plays important roles in communication. Aside from left-handed patients, a minority of whom have partial or complete right

hemisphere dominance for language, and the rare, right-handed patients with "crossed" aphasia after right hemisphere strokes, the right hemisphere plays important roles in communication even in right-handed people. The right hemisphere is especially involved in "extralinguistic," emotional aspects of communication. Patients with right hemisphere strokes may understand "what is said but not how it is said" (Tucker, Watson, and Heilman, 1977). Heilman and colleagues used the term "affective agnosia" to denote the inability of right hemisphere stroke patients to understand the emotional tone of dictated sentences, tested by having the patient match the intoned emotion to emotional drawings of faces. Left hemisphere stroke patients, even those with aphasia, performed the task well (Heilman, Scholes, and Watson, 1975). Subsequent studies demonstrated that right hemisphere stroke patients are impaired in both the expression and the comprehension of emotional tone (Tucker, Watson, and Heilman; Ross and Mesulam, 1979). Ross refers to deficits in the emotional aspect of communication as "aprosodias," and he has divided the aprosodias into expressive and receptive subtypes, similar to the classification of the aphasias. They are more selective syndromes, analogous to the categories of aphasia (Ross, 1981). We found that all 20 of a sample of right hemisphere stroke patients had affective prosody disturbance, but there were only weak correlations between expressive and receptive aprosodia and lesion localization (Wertz, Henschel, Auther, Ashford, & Kirshner, 1998). Prosody of speech involves not only emotional tone, but also such elements of speech as the placement of stress or emphasis within a sentence (Weintraub, Mesulam, & Kramer, 1981). Right hemisphere stroke patients also have problems in understanding humor or irony (Wapner, Hamby, & Gardner, 1981). These extralinguistic and "pragmatic" aspects of communication, such as intonation, emphasis, context, humor, turn-taking in conversation, and emotional tone place right hemisphere stroke patients at a disadvantage in interpersonal communication. Rehabilitative therapies should address these communication difficulties (Kirshner, Alexander, Lorch, & Wertz, 1999).

Short-Term Memory Impairments

Students of neurology are familiar with a bihemispheral system called "Papez's circuit," which is involved in memory. Classically, memory loss results when parts of this system are damaged on both sides, resulting in the "amnestic syndrome," classically described in patients with Wernicke-Korsakoff encephalopathy, Herpes simplex encephalitis, and bilateral surgical ablations of the hippocampus. In stroke, bilateral infarctions within the posterior cerebral artery territory cause a permanent amnestic syndrome. Many such patients are also cortically blind, from bilateral occipital damage. Unilateral PCA territory strokes can also be associated with less severe impairments of short-term memory. Left PCA strokes, as discussed earlier in this chapter, frequently result in a short-term memory loss as well as right hemianopsia, alexia without agraphia, and color naming deficits. Unilateral RPCA territory strokes produce left hemianopsia, and often a degree of nonverbal memory difficulty.

A final stroke syndrome associated with impairment of short-term memory is that of patients with ruptured aneurysms of the anterior communicating artery, with damage in the medial frontal or septal region. This syndrome will be discussed in Chapter 4.

Bilateral Syndromes

Bifrontal damage, from stroke or more frequently from traumatic brain injury, is associated with a state of reduced motor output and behavior, often with preserved alertness. This state is called "akinetic mutism" or "abulia." Less severe degrees of frontal damage result in apathetic states, or occasionally in disinhibited behavior.

Cortical Auditory Syndromes

Cortical Deafness

Cortical deafness is classically caused by bilateral lesions of the temporal lobe, as caused, for example, by bilateral infarctions in the MCA territory. In fact, very few such patients are completely deaf to pure tones. In most cases, patients have more selective deficits for understanding spoken words (pure word deafness), understanding nonverbal noises such as animal cries (auditory nonverbal agnosia), and recognizing familiar voices (phonagnosia) (Polster and Rose, 1998). Pure word deafness typically arises from bilateral temporal lesions; one such patient was reported to be able to learn over 100 signs of American sign language and communicate via visual language modalities (Kirshner and Webb, 1981). Cases with unilateral temporal lesions have been reported (Takahashi, Kawamura, Shinotou et al., 1992; Stefanatos, Gershkoff, and Madigan, 2005). Geschwind interpreted pure word deafness as a disconnection syndrome, in which both primary auditory cortices ("Heschl's gyrus," part of the superior temporal gyrus) were cut off from Wernicke's area, such that sounds could be heard but not processed as language. A unilateral left temporal stroke could conceivably create a similar disconnection from the auditory cortices. More likely, however, unilateral left temporal strokes, without parietal damage, can affect the auditory comprehension modality disproportionately, as in Wernicke's aphasia (Kirshner et al., 1989).

Case 6: This 51-year-old man, a television executive, had a Tetralogy of Fallot repaired at age 17. He had reportedly suffered ischemic events involving transitory symptoms of headache and memory disturbance, without any obvious neurological residua. CT and MRI scans showed an infarction in the right temporal lobe. A few months later, he developed an acute, left hemisphere stroke. His INR was subtherapeutic, and he received intravenous tPA. Initially, he had a severe, Wernicke-type aphasia, as well as right hemiparesis. Over time, his hemiparesis resolved, and his ability to read and write returned, but he was left with a nearly complete inability to speak or to understand spoken language. He describes his difficulty with hearing: "I hear all sounds at the same time with the same volume. I can't ignore subtle sounds, like computer fans, air conditioning."

On examination, the patient was alert and cooperative. He sent several e-mails of 2–3 paragraphs, with only minor spelling errors. By contrast, he could not speak intelligibly, producing sounds but no fully formed words. His auditory comprehension was severely impaired. He failed to match spoken words to pictures. He was not deaf; he could identify nonverbal sounds, such as snapping fingers or the bark of a dog, with his eyes closed. He followed printed commands, wrote answers to printed questions, and wrote the names of pictures. His cranial nerve, motor, and sensory examinations were essentially normal. CT and MRI scans showed bilateral temporal lobe infarctions. Pure tone hearing on audiography showed minimal impairment. This is a classic case of pure word deafness secondary to bilateral infarctions involving the temporal lobes.

Figure 10 is a CT scan from another case of bilateral temporal infarctions and pure word deafness.

Cortical Blindness, Visual Agnosia, Prosopagnosia, Optic Aphasia

As in the auditory system, several syndromes can result from bilateral lesions of the occipital lobe. Bilateral primary visual cortex lesions do produce complete cortical blindness. Some

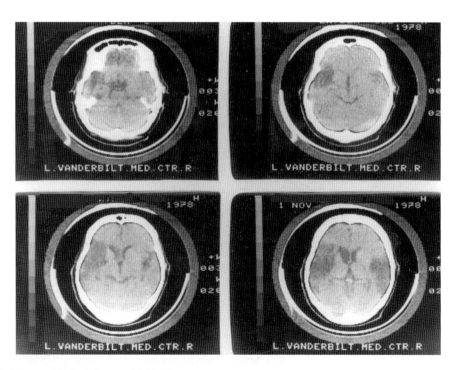

Fig. 10 CT scan, bilateral temporal infarctions

patients are unaware that they are blind, a syndrome called "Anton's syndrome." In other cases, patients report not seeing anything, yet they can avoid obstacles and occasionally react as if they have seen objects. Such unconscious visual processing is called "blindsight."

Balint's Syndrome

Another variation of cortical blindness is Balint's syndrome, in which a patient can see small visual details but fail to perceive the overall object, or literally, the patient "cannot see the forest for the trees." This deficit is related to descriptions of inability to perceive two visual stimuli simultaneously ("simultanagnosia"). Balint's syndrome is a triad of visual agnosia, optic ataxia, and ocular apraxia. In addition to the visual disorder, the patient cannot scan a scene or picture, gazing at only one part of the display, and the patient cannot visually guide the reaching for an object with either hand. The syndrome is usually seen with bilateral lesions, but usually not involving the visual cortex. The lesions are often bilateral parietal in location, but other combinations of lesions have been reported (can be occipital, parietal, or even frontal (Rizzo & Vecera, 2002). This syndrome is not always seen in strokes; any bihemispheral disease process can be associated.

Prosopagnosia

Prosopagnosia refers to the inability to recognize faces. Descriptions of this syndrome have involved either bilateral or unilateral, right hemisphere lesions, most often involving the fusiform ("fusiform face area") or inferior occipital gyri ("occipital face area"). Studies suggest a feed-forward processing of faces from the occipital cortex to the fusiform cortex, with involvement also of the anterior temporal lobe for memory of specific faces (Barton

and Cherkasova, 2003; Rossion et al., 2003; Steeves et al., 2006). The syndrome can occur in unilateral right hemisphere strokes, though congenital cases and progressive syndromes related to neurodegenerative disorders of the temporal or occipital lobes have been reported. A striking example, reported by Semenza, Sartori, and D'Andrea, (2003), was a patient who could look at a Venetian vase and name the artist, but he could not name a picture of the Pope.

Bithalamic Syndromes

Strokes involving the left thalamus are involved in subcortical aphasia, and those involving the right thalamus are implicated in neglect, as discussed earlier in this chapter. Less commonly seen are ischemic strokes involving both thalami. These occur in patients who have a single artery, sometimes termed the artery of Percheron, arising off the basilar artery or one posterior cerebral artery. The resultant infarction involves paramedian areas of the thalamus on both sides, and sometimes the upper midbrain as well. The resultant syndrome can involve coma, somnolence, akinetic mutism, extraocular and pupillary abnormalities if the midbrain is involved, and often profound apathy and deficits in short term memory (Meissner, Sapir, Kokmen, & Stein, 1987; Schmahmann, 2003). As patients with this bithalamic syndrome awaken, they sometimes become impulsive and aggressive, even physically violent. Rarely, bilateral thalamic infarctions can result from venous thrombosis in the deep cerebral venous system.

Case 7: A 42-year-old man was found slumped over the steering wheel in his car, which was pulled off the road onto a median. He had been expected to pick up his child after soccer practice, and he failed to appear. His family indicated that he had suffered a myocardial infarction in the past and that he was a smoker. He had been told of high blood pressure as well, but he was not on medications. On

arrival in the emergency room, he was comatose, without meaningful response to stimuli.
His pupils were midposition and only slug-
gishly reactive, but he moved all limbs to
pinch, reflexes were symmetric, and his plan-
tars were downgoing. A head CT was negative.
The initial impression of the Emergency
Department resident was that he might have
a drug overdose or metabolic encephalopathy.
Initial laboratory studies were unremarkable,
as was a drug screen. Over several hours, he
did not awaken, and a neurological consultant
found that he had horizontal eye movements
by oculocephalic maneuver, but no upward
gaze could be induced. An MRI was then
done (figure 11). This indicated a bilateral paramedian thalamic and upper midbrain infarction. His subsequent course was one of gradual
improvement in alertness, and in the Rehabilitation Unit he became fully ambulatory, but he
remained disoriented and completely amnestic
for the events leading up to hospitalizations, as
well as for ongoing events. He became agitated
at times, angry with his family for not taking
him home. He ultimately required placement in
a psychiatric facility. Figure 11 is an MRI showing bithalamic infarctions.

Cerebellar Syndromes

Most strokes involving the brainstem and cerebellum do not produce major cognitive or
behavioral changes. A growing literature,
however, has documented cognitive changes
with cerebellar infarctions. One study found
cognitive deficits in both isolated brainstem
and cerebellar infarctions, though no characteristic syndrome was reported (Hoffman
and Schmitt, 2004). A recent study found
greater cognitive and memory impairment
with infarctions in the territory of the posterior
inferior cerebellar artery than in the superior
cerebellar artery (Exner, Weniger, & Irle,
2004). Hokkanen, Kauranen, Roine, Salonen,
and Kotila (2006) reported verbal memory
impairment related to right cerebellar infarctions, and visuospatial deficits related to left
cerebellar lesions, reflecting the crossed input
between the cortex and cerebellum. Most
patients recovered well by 3 months after
stroke. Schmahmann (2004) and Schmahmann
and Caplan (2006) has described a "cerebellar
cognitive affective syndrome" including impairments in executive function, visuospatial tasks,
verbal memory and language ability, and

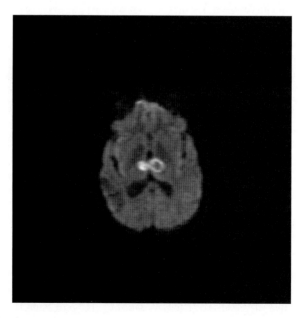

Fig. 11 Bithalamic infarctions

affective changes such as depression and emotional blunting. Schmahmann also refers to "dysmetria of thought." The lesions correlating with this syndrome are mainly in the posterior lateral cerebellar hemisphere and also the vermis. Disruption of cortical-cerebellar loops is presumably the basis of the syndrome. Lesions of the right cerebellum have also been linked to deficits in motor speech.

References

Alexander, M. P., Benson, D. F., & Stuss, D. (1989) Frontal lobes and language. *Brain and Language, 37*, 656–691.

Alexander, M. P., & LoVerme, S. R. (1980) Aphasia after left hemispheric intracerebral hemorrhage. *Neurology,* 1193–1202.

Alexander, M. P., Naeser, M. A., & Palumbo, C. L. (1987) Correlations of sub-cortical CT lesion sites and aphasia profiles. *Brain, 110*, 961–991.

Alexander, M. P., Naeser, M. A., & Palumbo, C. (1990) Broca's area aphasias: aphasia after lesions including the frontal operculum. *Neurology, 40*, 353–362.

Alexander, M. P., & Schmitt, M. A. (1980) The aphasia syndrome of stroke in the left anterior cerebral artery territory. *Archives of Neurology, 37*, 97–100.

Barton, J. J., & Cherkasova, M. (2003) Face imagery and its relation to perception and covert recognition in prosopagnosia. *Neurology, 61*, 220–225.

Benson, D. F., Cummings, J. C., & Tsai, S. I. (1982) Angular gyrus syndrome simulating Alzheimer's disease. *Archives of Neurology, 39*, 616–620.

Benson, D. F., Gardner, H., & Meadows, J. C. (1976). Reduplicative paramnesia. *Neurology (NY), 26*, 147–151.

Benson, D. F., Marsden, C. D., & Meadows, J. C. (1974) The amnestic syndrome of posterior cerebral artery occlusion. *Acta Neurologica Scandinavica, 50*, 133–145.

Benson, D. F., Sheremata, W. A., Bouchard, R., Segarra, J. M., Price, D., & Geschwind, N. (1973) Conduction aphasia: a clinicopathological study. *Archives of Neurology, 28*, 339–346.

Benton, A. L. (1967) Constructional apraxia and the minor hemisphere. *Confinia Neurologica, 29*, 1–16.

Benton, A. L. (1973) Visuoconstructive disability in patients with cerebral disease: its relationship to side of lesion and aphasic disorder. *Documenta Ophthalmologica, 34*, 67–76.

Benton, A. L., Levin, H.S., & Van Allen, M.W. (1974) Geographic orientation in patients with unilateral cerebral disease. *Neuropsychologia, 12*, 183–191.

Beschin, N., Cocchini, G., Della Sala, S., Logie, R. H. (1997) What the eyes perceive, the brain ignores: a case of pure unilateral representational neglect. *Cortex, 33*, 3–26.

Bisiach, E., & Luzzatti, C. (1978) Unilateral neglect of representational space. *Cortex, 14*, 129–133.

Black, F. W., & Strub, R.L. (1976) Constructional apraxia in patients with discrete missile wounds of the brain. *Cortex, 12*, 212–220.

Bogousslavsky, J., Miklossy, J., Regli, F., Deruaz, J.-P., Assal, G., & Delaloye. B. (1988) Subcortical neglect: Neuropsychological, SPECT, and neuropathological correlations with anterior choroidal artery territory infarction. *Annals of Neurology, 23*, 448–452.

Bogousslavsky, J., Regli, F., & Uske, A. (1988) Thalamic infarcts: clinical syndromes, etiology, and prognosis. *Neurology, 38*, 837–848.

Brain, W. R. (1941) Visual disorientation with special reference to lesions of the right cerebral hemisphere. *Brain, 64*, 244–272.

Calvanio, R., Petrone, P. N., & Levine, D. N. (1987) Left visual spatial neglect is both environment-centered and body-centered. *Neurology, 37*, 1179–1183.

Caplan, L. R., Kelly, M., & Kase, C. S., et al (1986) Infarcts of the inferior division of the right middle cerebral artery: Mirror image of Wernicke's aphasis. *Neurology, 36*, 1015–1020.

Cappa, S., Sterzi, R., Vallar, G., & Bisiach, E. (1987) Remission of hemineglect and anosognosia during vestibular stimulation. *Neuropsychologia, 25*, 775–782.

Carrera, E., Michel, P., & Bogousslavsky, J. (2004) Anteromedian, central, and posterolateral infarcts of the thalamus. Three variant types. *Stroke, 35*, 2826–2831.

Coslett, H. B., & Heilman, K. M. (1989) Hemihypokinesia afer right hemisphere strokes. *Brain Cogn, 9*, 267–278.

Crisostomo, E., Duncan, P., Propst, M., Dawson, D. V., & Davis, J. N. (1988) Evidence that amphetamine with physical therapy promotes recovery of motor function in stroke patients. *Annals of Neurology, 23*, 94–97.

Critchley, M. (1966) The parietal lobes. New York: Hafner.

Crosson, B. (1985) Subcortical functions in language: a working model. *Brain and Language, 25*, 257–292.

Damasio, A. R. (1992) Aphasia. *The New England Journal of Medicine, 326*, 531–539.

Damasio, H., & Damasio, A. R. (1980) The anatomical basis of conduction aphasia. *Brain, 103*, 337–350.

Damasio, A. R., & Damasio, H. (1983) The anatomic basis of pure alexia. *Neurology, 33*, 1573–1583.

Damasio, A. R., Damasio, H., & Chui, H. C. (1980) Neglect following damage to frontal lobe or basal ganglia. *Neuropsychologia, 18*, 123–132.

Denes, G., Semenza, C., Stoppa, E., & Lis, A. (1982) Unilateral spatial neglect and recovery from hemiplegia. *Brain, 105*, 543–552.

Denny-Brown, D., & Chambers, R. A. (1958) The parietal lobe and behavior. *Proceedings of the Association for Research in Nervous and Mental Disease*, *36*, 35–117.

Dejerine, J. (1891) Sur un cas de cecite verbale avec agraphie, suivi d'autopsie. *Mémoires de la Société de Biologie*, *3*, 197–201.

Dejerine, J. (1892) Contribution a l'etude anatomo-pathologique et clinique des differentes varietes de cecite verbale. *Mémoires de la Société de Biologie*, *4*, 61–90.

Dronkers, N. F. (1996) A new brain region for coordinating speech articulation. *Nature*, *384*, 159–161.

Egelko, S., Gordon, W. A., Hibbard, M. R., Diller, L., Lieberman, A., & Holliday, R., et al. (1988) Relationship among CT scans, neurological exam, and neuropsychological test performance in right brain-damaged stroke patients. *Journal of Clinical and Experimental Neuropsychology*, *10*, 539–564.

Exner, C., Weniger, G., & Irle, E. (2004) Cerebellar lesions in the PICA but not SCA territory impair cognition. *Neurology*, *63*, 2132–2135.

Fensore, C., Lazzarino, L. G., Nappo, A., & Nicolai, A. (1988) Language and memory disturbances from mesencephalothalamic infarcts. A clinical and computed tomographic study. *European Neurology*, *28*, 51–56.

Ferro, J. M., & Kertesz, A. (1984) Posterior internal capsule infarction associated with neglect. *Archives of Neurology*, *41*, 422–424.

Fiorelli, M., Blin, J., Bakchine, S., Laplane, D., & Baron, J. C. (1991) PET studies of diaschisis in patients with motor hemi-neglect. *Journal of the Neurological Sciences*, *104*, 135–142.

Fisher, C. M. (1959) The pathological and clinical aspects of thalamic hemorrhage. *Transactions of the American Neurological Association*, *84*, 56–59.

Freedman, M., Alexander, M. P., & Naeser, M. A. (1984) Anatomic basis of transcortical motor aphasia. *Neurology*, *34*, 409–417.

Gerstmann J. (1930) Zur symptomatologie der Hirnlasion en im Ubergangsgebier der unteren Parietal- und mittlerin Occipital windung (Das Syndrom Fingeragnosie, Rechts-Links-Storung, Agraphie, Akalkulie). Nervenartzt, 691–695.

Geschwind, N. (1965) Disconnection syndromes in animals and man. *Brain*, *88*, 237–294, 585–644.

Geschwind, N., & Fusillo, M. (1966) Color-naming defects in association with alexia. *Archives of Neurology*, *15*, 137–146.

Geschwind, N., Quadfasel, F., & Segarra, J. (1968) Isolation of the speech area. *Neuropsychologia*, *6*, 327–340.

Grade, C., Redford, B., Chrostowski, J., Toussaint, L., & Blackwell, B. (1998) Methylphenidate in early post-stroke recovery: a double blind, placebo-controlled study. *Archives of Physical Medicine and Rehabilitation*, *79*, 1047–1050.

Graff-Radford, N. R., Eslinger, P. J., Damasio, A. R., & Yamada, T. (1984) Nonhemorrhagic infarction of the thalamus: behavioral, anatomic, and physiologic correlates. *Neurology*, *34*, 14–23.

Heilman, K. M., & Valenstein, E. (1972) Frontal lobe neglect in man. *Neurology (NY)*, *22*, 660–664.

Heilman, K. M., & Valenstein, E. (1979) Mechanisms underlying hemispatial neglect. *Annals of Neurology*, *5*, 166–170.

Heilman, K. M., Bowers, D., & Watson, R. T. (1983) Performance on hemispatial pointing task by patients with neglect syndrome. *Neurology*. *33*, 661–664.

Heilman, K. M., Valenstein, E., & Watson, R. T. (2000) Neglect and related disorders. *Seminars in Neurology*, *20*, 463–470.

Heilman, K. M., Scholes, R., & Watson, R. T. (1975) Auditory affective agnosia: disturbed comprehension of affective speech. *Journal of Neurology, Neurosurgery, and Psychiatry*, *38*, 69–72.

Hickok, G., & Poeppel, D. (2000) Towards a functional neuroanatomy of speech perception. *Trends in Cognitive Sciences*, *4*, 131–138.

Hier, D. B., Mondlock, J., & Caplan, L. R. (1983) Behavioral abnormalities after right hemisphere stroke. *Neurology (NY)*, *33*, 337–344.

Hillis, A. E., Wityk, R. J., Tuffiash, E., Beauchamp, N. J., Jacobs, M. A., & Barker, P. B., et al. (2001) Hypoperfusion of Wernicke's area predicts severity of semantic deficit in acute stroke. *Annals of Neurology*, *50*, 561–566.

Hillis, A. E., Work, M., Barker, P. B., Jacobs, M. A., Breese, E. L., & Maurer, K. (2004) Re-examining the brain regions crucial for orchestrating speech articulation. *Brain*, *127*, 1479–1487.

Hoffman, M., & Schmitt, F. (2004) Cognitive impairment in isolated subtentorial stroke. *Acta Neurologica Scandinavica*, *109*, 14–24.

Hokkanen, L. S., Kauranen, V., Roine, R. O., Salonen, O., & Kotila, M. (2006) Subtle cognitive deficits after cerebellar infarcts. *European Journal of Neurology*, *13*, 161–170.

Husain, M., Mattingley, J. B., Rorden, C., Kennard, C., & Driver, J. (2000) Distinguishing sensory and motor biases in parietal and frontal neglect. *Brain*, *123*, 1643–1659.

Kertesz, A., Lau, W. K., & Polk, M. (1993) The structural determinants of recovery in Wernicke's aphasia. *Brain and Language*, *44*, 153–164.

Kertesz, A., Nicholson, I., Cancelliere, A., Kassa, K., & Black, S. E. (1985) Motor impersistence: a right-hemisphere syndrome. *Neurology*, *35*, 662–666.

Kertesz, A., Sheppard, A., & MacKenzie, R. (1982) Localization in transcortical sensory aphasia. *Archives of Neurology*, *39*, 475–478.

Kirshner, H. S., Alexander, M., Lorch, M. P., & Wertz, R. T. (1999) Disorders of speech and language. *Continuum*, *5*, 1–237.

Kirshner, H. S., Casey, P. F., Henson, J., & Heinrich, J. J. (1989) Behavioural features and lesion localization in Wernicke's aphasia. *Aphasiology, 3*, 169–176.

Kirshner, H. S., & Kistler, K. H. (1982) Aphasia after right thalamic hemorrhage. *Archives of Neurology, 39*, 667–669.

Kirshner, H., & Webb, W. (1981) Selective involvement of the auditory-verbal modality in an acquired communication disorder: benefit from sign language therapy. *Brain and Language, 13*, 161–170.

Kreisler, A., Godefroy, O., & Delmaire, C., Debachy, B., Leclercq, M., Pruvo, J.-P., et al. (2000) The anatomy of aphasia revisited. *Neurology, 54*, 1117–1123.

Lazar, R. M., Marshall, R. S., Prell, G. D., & Pile-Spellman, J. (2000) The experience of Wernicke's aphasia. *Neurology 55*, 1222–1224.

Legatt, A. D., Rubin, M. J., Kaplan, L. R., Healton, E. B., & Brust, J. C. (1987) Global aphasia without hemiparesis: multiple etiologies. *Neurology, 37*, 201–205.

Levine, D. N., & Finklestein, S. (1982) Delayed psychosis after right temporoparietal stroke or trauma: relation to epilepsy. *Neurology, 32*, 267–273.

Levine, D. N., & Grek, A. (1984) The anatomic basis of delusions after right cerebral infarction. *Neurology, 34*, 577–582.

Lezak, M. (1983) Neuropsychological Assessment. Second Edition. New York: Oxford University Press.

Lezak, M. D., Howieson, D. B., & Doring, D. W., et al. (2004) Neuropsychological assessment (4th ed., pp. 1–1016). Oxford: Oxford University Press.

Lichtheim, L. (1885) On aphasia. *Brain, 7*. 433–484.

Luria, A. R. (1977) On quasi-aphasic speech disturbances in lesions of the deep structures of the brain. *Brain and Language, 4*, 432–459.

Marshall, J. C., & Halligan, P. W. (1993) Imagine only the half of it. *Nature, 364*, 193–194.

Masdeu, J. C., Schoene, W. C., & Funkenstein, H. (1978) Aphasia following infarction of the left supplementary motor area. A clinicopathologic study. *Neurology, 28*, 1220–1223.

Meissner, I., Sapir, S., Kokmen, E., & Stein, S. D. (1987) The paramedian diencephalic syndrome: a dynamic phenomenon. *Stroke, 18*, 380–385.

Mendez, M. F., Adams, N. L., & Lewandowski, K. S. (1989) Neurobehavioral changes associated with caudate lesions. *Neurology, 39*, 349–354.

Mesulam, M.-M. (1981) A Cortical network for directed attention and unilateral neglect. *Annals of Neurology, 10*, 309–325.

Mesulam, M. M., Waxman, S. G., Geschwind, N., & Sabin, T. D. (1976) Acute confusional states with right middle cerebral artery infarctions. *J Neurol Neurosurg Psychiatry, 39*, 84–89.

Mohr, J. P., Pessin, M. S., Finklestein, S., Funkenstein, H. H., Duncan, G. W., & Davis, K. R. (1978) Broca aphasia: pathologic and clinical. *Neurology, 28*, 311–324.

Mohr, J. P., Watters, W. C., & Duncan, G. W. (1975) Thalamic hemorrhage and aphasia. *Brain and Language, 2*, 3–17.

Na, D. L., Adair, J. C., Williamson, D. J., Schwartz, R. L., Haws, B., & Heilman, K. M. (1998) Dissociation of sensory-attentional from motor-intentional neglect. *Journal of neurology, neurosurgery, and psychiatry, 64*, 331–338.

Naeser, M. A., Helm-Estabrooks, N., Haas, G., Auerbach, S., & Srinivasan, M. (1987) Relationship between lesion extent in "Wernicke's area" on CT scan and predicting recovery of comprehension in Wernicke's aphasia. *Archives of Neurology, 44*, 73–82.

Naeser, M. A., Palumbo, C. L., Helm-Estabrooks, N., Stiassny-Eder, D., & Albert, M. L. (1989) Role of the medial subcallosal fasciculus and other white matter pathways in recovery of spontaneous speech. *Brain, 112*, 1–38.

Patterson, K., & Kay, J. (1982) Letter-by letter reading: psychological descriptions of a neurological syndrome. *The Quarterly Journal of Experimental Psychology, 34A*, 411–441.

Polster, M. R., & Rose, S. B. (1998) Disorders of auditory processing: evidence for modularity in audition. *Cortex, 34*, 47–65.

Rabins, P. V., Starkstein, S. E., & Robinson, R. G. (1991) Risk factors for developing atypical (schizophreniform) psychosis following stroke. *J Neuropsychiatry Clin Neurosci, 3*, 36–39.

Rees, G., Wojciulik, E., Clarke, K., Husain, M., Frith, C., & Driver, J. (2000) Unconscious activation of visual cortex in the damaged right hemisphere of a parietal patient with extinction. *Brain, 123*, 1624–1633.

Reynolds, A. F., Turner, P. T., Harris, A. B., Ojemann, G. A., & Lavis, L. E. (1979) Left thalamic hemorrhage with dysphasia: a report of five cases. *Brain and Language, 7*, 62–73.

Rizzo, M., & Vecera, S. P. (2002) Psychoanatomical substrates of Balint's syndrome. *Journal of Neurology, Neurosurgery, and Psychiatry, 72*, 162–178.

Rode, G., Perenin, M. T., Honore, J., & Boisson, D. (1998) Improvement of the motor deficit of neglect patients through vestibular stimulation: evidence for a motor neglect component. *Cortex, 34*, 253–261.

Ross, E. D. (1981) The aprosodias: functional-anatomic organization of the affective components of language in the right hemisphere. *Archives of Neurology, 38*, 561–569.

Ross, E. D., & Mesulam, M.-M. (1979) Dominant language functions of the right hemisphere?

Prosody and emotional gesturing. *Archives of Neurology, 36*, 144–148.

Rossion, B., Caldara, R., Seghier, M., Schuller, A. M., Lazeyras, F., & Mayer, E. (2003) A network of occipito-temporal face-sensitive areas besides the right middle fusiform gyrus is necessary for normal face processing. *Brain, 126*, 2381–2395.

Samuelsson, H., Jenson, C., Ekholm, S., Naver, H., & Blomstrand, C. (1997) Anatomical and neurological correlates of acute and chronic visuospatial neglect following right hemisphere stroke. *Cortex, 33*, 271–285.

Small, M., & Ellis, S. (1994) Brief remission periods in visuospatial neglect: evidence from long-term follow-up. *Eur Neurol, 34*, 147–154.

Schiff, H. B., Alexander, M. R., Naeser, M. A., & Galaburda, A. M. (1983) Aphemia: clinical-anatomic correlations. *Archives of Neurology, 40*, 720–727.

Schmahmann, J. D. (2004) Disorders of the cerebellum: ataxia, dysmetria of thought, and the cerebellar cognitive affective syndrome. *The Journal of Neuropsychiatry and Clinical Neurosciences, 16*, 367–378.

Schmahmann, J. D. (2003) Vascular syndromes of the thalamus. *Stroke, 34*, 2264–2278.

Schmahmann, J. D., & Caplan, D. (2006) Cognition, emotion and the cerebellum. *Brain, 129*, 290–292.

Seki, K., Ishiai, S., Koyama, Y., & Fujimoto, Y. (1996) Appearance and disappearance of unilateral spatial neglect for an object: influence of attention-attracting peripheral stimuli. *Neuropsychologia, 34*, 819–826.

Selnes, O. A., Niccum, N., Knopman, D. S., & Rubens, A. B. (1984) Recovery of single word comprehension:, C. T.-scan correlates. *Brain and Language, 21*, 72–84.

Semenza, C., Sartori, G., & D'Andrea, J. (2003) He can tell which master craftsman blew a Venetian vase, but he can not name the Pope: a patient with a selective difficulty in naming faces. *Neuroscience Letters, 352*, 73–75.

Steeves, J. K., Culham, J. C., Duchaine, B. C., Pratesi, C. C., Valyear, K. F., & Schindler, I., et al. (2006) The fusiform face area is not sufficient for face recognition: evidence from a patient with dense prosopagnosia and no occipital face area. *Neuropsychologia, 44*, 594–609.

Stefanatos, G. A., Gershkoff, A., & Madigan, S. (2005) On pure word deafness, temporal processing and the left hemisphere. *Journal of the International Neuropsychological Society, 11*, 456–470.

Stone, S. P., Patel, P., Greenwood, R. J., & Halligan, P. W. (1992) Measuring visual neglect in acute stroke and predicting its recovery: the visual neglect recovery index. *Journal of Neurology, Neurosurgery, and Psychiatry, 55*, 431–436.

Stuss, D. T., Guberman, A., Nelson, R., & Larochelle, S. (1988) The neuropsychology of paramedian thalamic infarction. *Brain and Language, 8*, 348–378.

Takahashi, N., Kawamura, M., Shinotou, H., Hirayama, K., Kaga,. K., & Shindo, M. (1992) Pure word deafness due to left hemisphere damage. *Cortex, 28*, 295–303.

Takahashi, N., Kawamura, M., Shiota, J., Kasahata, N., & Hirayama, K. (1997) Pure topographic disorientation due to right retrosplenial lesion. *Neurology, 49*, 464–469.

Tanridag, O., & Kirshner, H. S. (1985) Aphasia and agraphia in lesions of the posterior internal capsule and putamen. *Neurology, 35*, 1797–1801.

Tranel, D., Biller, J., Damasio, H., Adams, H. P. Jr, & Cornell, S. H. (1987) Global aphasia without hemiparesis. *Archives of Neurology, 44*, 304–308.

Tucker, D. M., Watson, R. T., & Heilman, K. M. (1977) Discrimination and evocation of affectively intoned speech in patients with right parietal disease. *Neurology (NY), 27*, 947–950.

Valenstein, E., & Heilman, K. M. (1981) Unilateral hypokinesia and motor extinction. *Neurology (NY), 31*, 445–448.

Valenstein, E., Van Den Abell, T., Watson, R. T., & Heilman, K. M. (1982) Non-sensory neglect from parietotemporal lesions in monkeys. *Neurology, 32*, 1198–1201.

Von Cramon, D. Y., Hebel, N., & Schuri, U. (1988) Verbal memory and learning in unilateral posterior cerebral infarction. A report on 30 cases. *Brain, 111*, 1061–1077.

Walker-Batson, D., Smith, P., Curtis, S., Unwein, H., & Greenlee, R. (1995) Amphetamine paired with physical therapy accelerates motor recovery after stroke. Further evidence. *Stroke, 26*, 2254–2259.

Wapner, W., Hamby, S., & Gardner, H. (1981) The role of the right hemisphere in the apprehension of complex language materials. *Brain and Language, 14*, 15–33.

Watson, R. T., Miller, B. D., & Heilman, K. M. (1978) Non-sensory neglect. *Ann Neurol, 3*, 505–508.

Watson, R. T., Valenstein, E., & Heilman, K. M. (1981) Thalamic neglect: possible role of the medial thalamus and nucleus reticularis in behavior. *Archives of Neurology, 38*, 501–506.

Weintraub, S., Mesulam, M.-M., & Kramer, L. (1981) Disturbances in prosody: a right hemisphere contribution to language. *Archives of Neurology, 38*, 742–744.

Wertz, R. T., Henschel, C. R., Auther, L., Ashford, J., & Kirshner, H. S. (1998) Affective prosodic disturbance subsequent to right hemisphere stroke. *Journal of Neurolinguistics, 11*, 89–102.

Chapter 4
Cerebral Aneurysms and Subarachnoid Hemorrhage

John DeLuca and Charles J. Prestigiacomo

Introduction/Background

Though a recognized entity since the days preceding Morgagni in the seventeenth century, a clear understanding of why aneurysms form, grow, and rupture as well as the best strategies for treating unruptured and ruptured aneurysms still eludes the neuroscience community (Prestigiacomo 2006). Recent advances in neurosurgical techniques and neuro-intensive care have resulted in progressive improvement in mortality, morbidity, and functional status following subarachnoid hemorrhage (SAH) secondary to the rupture of a cerebral aneurysm (Heros & Morcos, 2000).

Unlike other causes of stroke, SAH occurs in persons in the prime of their working years, with a mean age of onset between 40 and 60 years (Sethi, Moore, Dervin, Clifton, & MacSweeney, 2000). With an estimated incidence of 37,500 in the United States alone, and a lifetime cost of over $230,000 per individual, spontaneous aneurysmal SAH cost the United States over $5.6 billion in 1990 dollars (Taylor et al., 1996). Thus, a critical part of the treatment of patients sustaining SAH is the successful rehabilitation of these individuals to improve quality of life and their reintegration as productive members of society. This chapter will review the pathophysiology, natural history, and treatment of patients sustaining spontaneous aneurysmal SAH, with a particular focus upon the recent advances in rehabilitative efforts for these patients. Though traumatic SAH is indeed the most common form of SAH reported in the literature, it is a separate disease entity with a different epidemiology, etiology, and outcome and as such, it is beyond the scope of this chapter.

Neuropathology/Pathophysiology

Cerebral aneurysms are the fourth leading cause of cerebrovascular accident (behind artherothrombosis, embolism, and intracerebral hemorrhage) and account for 5–10% of all strokes (Dombovy, Drew-Cates, & Serdans, 1998). Saccular or "berry" aneurysms are the most common type and occur primarily at bifurcations or branch-points of the vasculature. Recent estimates of the prevalence of intracranial aneurysms range between 1 and 2% of the general population, although most will never rupture (Winn, Jane, Taylor, Kaiser, & Britz, 2002). Rupture of an aneurysm causes blood to flow into the subarachniod space, resulting in an SAH. Rupture of an intracranial aneurysm is the most

J. DeLuca (✉)
Neuropsychology and Neuroscience Laboratory, Kessler Medical Rehabilitation Research and Education Center, 300 Executive Drive, Suite 10, West Orange, NJ 07052, USA
e-mail: jdeluca@kmrrec.org

J.R. Festa, R.M. Lazar (eds.), *Neurovascular Neuropsychology*, DOI 10.1007/978-0-387-70715-0_4,
© Springer Science+Business Media, LLC 2009

common cause of spontaneous SAH, accounting for approximately 80% of all SAH. SAH can result in a high mortality rate estimated at 10–15% before hospitalization, 40% in the first week, and 50% in the first 6 months (Schievink, 1997). The incidence of non-traumatic SAH in the United States is 6–25 per 100,000 (Clinchot, Bogner, & Kaplan, 1997; Schievink, 1997). Risk factors for formation and rupture of cerebral aneurysms include aneurysm size, female gender, increasing age cigarette smoking, alcohol consumption, and high life stress. (See Weir, 2002 for an extensive review) While hypertension is more frequent among those with an aneurysm, aneurysms occur most frequently among those with normal blood pressure. First-degree relatives of patients with SAH are at increased risk of SAH, which can be up to seven times higher than the general population (Raaymakers & the MARS Study Group, 1999). About 90–95% of saccular aneurysms lie at the anterior portion of the circle of Willis, most commonly around the anterior communicating artery (ACoA), the origin of the posterior communicating artery (PCoA), the first major bifurcation of the middle cerebral artery (MCA) and the bifurcation of the internal carotid into the middle and anterior cerebral arteries (Victor & Ropper, 2001).

Complications after SAH include vasospasm, hydrocephalus, seizure, rebleeding, electrolyte imbalance, and cardiopulmonary dysfunction. Vasospasm typically occurs within 2 weeks of the SAH, angiographically occurring in 50–70% of patients, and can result in cerebral ischemia in up to 46% of patients or death in about 10–30% of patients (Stern, Chang, Odell, & Sperber, 2006). Hydrocephalus after SAH ranges from 6–67%. Though most patients do well with temporary diversion of the cerebral spinal fluid via an external ventricular drain, approximately 10% of patients will require placement of a ventricular-peritoneal shunt (Vale, Bradley, & Fisher, 1997; Sheehan, Polin, Sheehan, Baskaya, & Kassell, 1999).

Diagnostic Criteria

The diagnosis and management of ruptured and unruptured aneurysms are substantially different and should be treated independently since outcomes in these two groups differ. As will be demonstrated, because of its varied presentation, and its relative infrequency, the diagnosis of SAH can be missed in 5–51% of patients (Vermeulen & Schull, 2007), a truly broad range which reflects differences in outpatient versus inpatient screening.

Subarachnoid Hemorrhage

The *sine quo non* of SAH is the presence of blood in the subarachnoid space. Prior to the era of modern imaging, when SAH was suspected clinically, the patient required a lumbar puncture to visually inspect the cerebrospinal fluid (CSF) to determine if blood was present. Careful analysis of the CSF was necessary because in many instances blood could be introduced into the CSF from the puncture itself (a traumatic tap). The distinguishing characteristic of CSF in the setting of SAH is that when blood sits in CSF for an extended period of time (over 2 hours), it undergoes partial metabolism resulting in the presence of bilirubin. This metabolite gives the CSF a xanthochromic appearance, which is not seen in the setting of a traumatic tap. Another important criterion to determining whether blood in the CSF is secondary to SAH is a serial cell count at the time of the lumbar puncture. By analyzing the first and last tubes of CSF during a lumbar puncture, a diminishing red cell count suggests a traumatic tap whereas a relative steady red cell count points to the presence of true subarachnoid blood.

The advent of non-invasive imaging has displaced, though not rendered obsolete, the lumbar puncture. With a sensitivity of over 98% within several hours of the ictus, a non-contrast CT scan of the head has become the initial study of choice for the detection of

SAH. In the setting where the clinical suspicion is high and the CT scan is negative, a lumbar puncture must be performed to definitively rule out SAH.

Once diagnosed with SAH, detection of the aneurysm (accounting for approximately 95% of all spontaneous SAH) is paramount. Though diagnostic, catheter-based cerebral angiography is currently the gold-standard for detecting intracranial aneurysms; CT angiography has been shown to approach a high degree of sensitivity in detecting these lesions (Hoh et al., 2004). Among its many advantages, CT angiography allows for performing the study at the moment the SAH is detected on the initial non-contrast study.

Patients with SAH can present with a wide spectrum of symptoms. The "classic" presentation is that of a sudden-onset, thunderclap headache, usually described as "the worst headache of my life," and is often-times associated with nausea and vomiting. The hemorrhage can be so severe as to cause sudden death in 12% of individuals (Huang & Gelder, 2002). Because the condition at presentation is associated with varied clinical outcomes, several classification schemes have been developed to help describe and categorize how patients present, ranging from a mild-to-moderate headache, to a moribund state (Table 1, Hunt & Hess,1968)

In patients with CT findings consistent with SAH, the amount of blood present at the time of hemorrhage has been correlated with outcome as it relates to the onset of cerebral vasospasm, a potentially debilitating and sometimes lethal complication of SAH (Table 2. Fisher, Kistler, & Davis, 1980).

Table 1 Hunt-Hess Classification for Subarachnoid Hemorrhage

I.	Asymptomatic; mild headache and/or slight nuchal rigidity
II.	Cranial nerve palsy; moderate to severe headache; nuchal rigidity
III.	Mild focal deficit, lethargy or confusion
IV.	Stupor; moderate to severe hemiparesis; early extensor posturing
V.	Rigidity; deep coma; decerebrate rigidity; moribund appearance

Table 2 Fisher Grade (on CT scan)

1.	No blood detected on CT
2.	Diffuse or vertical layers < 1 mm thick
3.	Localized clot and/or vertical layers ≥ 1 mm
4.	Intracerebral or intraventricular clot with diffuse or no subarachnoid hemorrhage

Unruptured Aneurysms

Prevalence of intracranial aneurysms in the general population is estimated at about 0.65–5% of the population, with an estimated yearly rate of rupture of 1–2% (Juvela, Porras, & Poussa, 2000; Winn et al., 2002). Unruptured cerebral aneurysms are usually detected incidentally, though at times focal neurologic findings such as seizures or a third nerve palsy may be the presenting sign that warrants imaging studies. In this setting, an MRI with MRA provides excellent resolution and exquisite sensitivity for aneurysms greater than 2 mm in size. Equivocal studies would then undergo either CTA or catheter-based diagnostic angiography. Decisions for surgical treatment depend on the relative risks of rupture versus the risks of treatment; however, no definite standard of care is currently available (Weir, 2002).

Characteristic Neurobehavioral Syndrome

With the recent increase in survival from surgical repair of cerebral aneurysms, investigators have become more interested in quality of life issues among survivors (Heros & Morcos, 2000). Despite these improvements, mortality following rupture resulting in SAH remains at 40–50%, with about 50% of survivors experiencing significant long-term cognitive deficits (Hackett & Andersen, 2000; Ogden, Levin, & Mee, 1990). A number of outcome studies have demonstrated that cognitive and behavioral impairments are frequent sequelae of such aneurysms, even among patients who show "no neurologic impairments" or who show "good outcome" (DeLuca & Diamond, 1995;

Powell, Kitchen, Heslin, & Greenwood, 2002; Kim, Haney, & Van Ginhoven, 2005).

There is somewhat conflicting data regarding outcome with some studies suggesting that most SAH patients have few long-term sequelae (Hellawell & Pentland, 2001; Hillis, Anderson, Sampath, & Rigamonti, 2000), while others show significant disability (e.g., Dombovy, et al., 1998). For example, some studies report that approximately 50% of SAH patients return to full-time employment 5–7 years post insult (Hellawell & Pentland, 2001), while others report that no patients return to work after 1 year, even among those who receive rehabilitation (Dombovy et al., 1998). However, methodological differences often explain discrepant findings across studies. Thus studies that examine consecutive admissions to an acute hospital (e.g., Hellawell & Pentland, 2001), which include all patients as subjects, lead to different results from studies that are selective in subject inclusion. As such, it is not surprising that none of the SAH subjects in Dombovy et al. (1998) returned to work, since only the more severe SAH patients are referred for rehabilitation services and thus have poorer long-term outcome.

Overall, recent studies of long term outcome generally show that about 50% of SAH patients report significant cognitive difficulties (i.e., at least moderately disabling) and everyday life problems up to 7 years post discharge from the acute hospital, even among patients with presumed "good recovery" (e.g., Hellawell & Pentland, 2001), including a large international population-based study (Hackett & Anderson, 2000). Problems include cognition (mostly memory), mood, fatigue, passivity, speech, language, and self-care issues. In fact, fatigue is a frequent, underappreciated, and not well understood consequence of SAH (Ogden et al., 1990). However, such studies rely primarily on self or family report of functioning. Hillis et al. (2000) conducted neuropsychological assessment both pre- and post surgery, including data up to 1 year post surgery in persons with ruptured and unruptured cerebral aneurysms. They concluded that moderate to severe cognitive impairment was observed in a minority of patients. Further, they showed that such impairments were attributed to a variety of reasons including the SAH itself in some subjects, while cognitive impairment in other cases result from the effects of the brain surgery (e.g., prolonged anesthesia, brain retraction, temporary regional blood flow restriction), and still some may simply reflect reduced premorbid levels. Recent studies suggest that genetic factors can significantly affect cognitive and other neurological sequelae after SAH. Lanterna et al. (2005) reported that aneurysmal SAH patients with the E4 allele of the APoE genotype displayed significantly worse cognitive performance as well as worse overall outcome, and were at higher risk for developing clinical vasospasm and long-term neurologic deficits. The APoE E4 allele is known to be associated with dementia in Alzheimer's disease, stroke, and traumatic brain injury (Slooter, Tang, van Dujin, Hoffman, & van Dujin, 1997; Mayeux et al., 1993).

The relationship between various medical variables and outcome following SAH is unclear. There is no clear consensus on perioperative variables in predicting outcome such as vasospasm, post-operative imaging, clinical severity, or timing of surgery. For example, while some studies demonstrate an effect of variables such as vasospasm, or timing of surgery on outcome (e.g., Saveland, Hillman, Brandt, Edner, Jakobsson, & Algers, 1992), others show no relationship with medical variables such as clinical severity, type of SAH, or timing of surgery (e.g., Ogden et al., 1990; Hackett & Anderson, 2000), effects of subarachnoid blood (Germano, Caruso, Caffo, Cacciola, Belvedere, et al., 1998) on outcome. Clearly, predictors of functional outcome is multifaceted and must take into account a variety of factors, most of which have some impact at the individual level, but overall are too diffuse in nature to have global predictive validity. Indeed, current studies are redefining the outcome measures for subarachnoid hemorrhage and include psychological and neurocognitive outcomes in addition to the more "traditional" neurological outcome measures.

Of the approximately 50% of SAH patients who display more disabling outcome, a wide range of cognitive impairment can be observed, largely due to both severity and location of the SAH. Increased severity of the initial SAH results in more severe and long lasting cognitive difficulties and also leads to a wider range of impaired areas of cognition (see Table 3). Studies that have examined the influence of aneurysm location on severity of neurobehavioral symptoms following SAH have been mixed and largely influenced by design type (i.e., case studies versus group studies). In general, group studies such as population based or those which include consecutive admissions to acute care tend to show little to no consistent findings across aneurysm sites, although there still seems to be a propensity for worse outcome following ACoA

Table 3 Cognitive, physical and psychosocial consequences following SAH

Cognition:
Episodic Memory
Attention/concentration (working memory)
Processing speed (e.g., reaction time)
Psychomotor slowing
Executive dysfunction
Aphasia
Visual perceptual difficulties
Akinesia/Abulia
Lack of initiative
Motor
Hemiparesis
Quadraparesis
Other
Debilitating fatigue
Sleep disturbance (e.g., daytime sleepiness, problems sleeping at night)
Behavioral dyscontrol
Headache
Emotional distress (anxiety, depression, frustration, temperament)
Altered personality
Difficulties returning to premorbid leisure and social activities
Difficulties returning to work
Health-related quality of life

aneurysm (e.g., Bornstein, Weir, Petruk, & Disney, 1987; c.f., DeLuca & Diamond, 1995). In contrast, there are numerous "case report" studies (single or multiple cases) that tend to show that the ACoA is particularly susceptible to neurobehavioral impairments (c.f., DeLuca & Diamond, 1995). Located at the circle of Willis at the ventral portion of the brain, the ACoA is the most common site of aneurysm rupture and cerebral infarct (Weir, Disney & Karrison, 2002). ACoA aneurysm can result in a triad of impairments, which have been collectively referred to as the "ACoA syndrome" (See DeLuca and Diamond, 1995 for a review). This triad consists of a memory deficit often described as "Korsakoff-like" in nature, confabulation, and personality change. While reference to an "ACoA syndrome" is plentiful in the literature, most ACoA subjects do not show this discrete pattern. For instance, some subjects are amnesic but do not confabulate (e.g., Vilkki, 1985), while others may show changes in personality without amnesia (see DeLuca and Diamond, 1995). The most common and disabling neuropsychological deficits among persons with ACoA aneurysm are in episodoc memory and executive functions (DeLuca & Diamond, 1995; Simard, Rouleau, Brosseau, Laframboise, & Bojanowsky, 2003). Nonetheless, despite the fact that neurobehavioral syndromes are seen most often following ACoA aneurysm, it should be noted that up to 85% of cases have been reported to show "good outcome" (e.g., Chalif & Weinberg, 1998) or return to work (c.f., DeLuca & Diamond, 1995). However, as stated above, even patients with "good outcome" or showing "no neurological impairment" often still have significant cognitive, emotional, psychosocial, and everyday life difficulties.

The psychosocial outcomes following SAH can be devastating, even among those with "good neurological outcome." Numerous studies show that despite overwhelming positive recovery in most individuals, many continue to display psychosocial challenges up to 7 years post onset. Examining a consecutive series of 83 patients with SAH, Vilkki, Holst, Ohman, Servo, & Heiskanen (1990) found that the degree of cognitive and neurologic deficit was associated with social competence 1 year after surgery, but not with anxiety and depression. Powell et al. (2002) reported that SAH patients with "good recovery" showed significant psychosocial distress 3–6 months post onset, including post-traumatic stress symptoms (60% and 30% for 3 and 6 months, respectively), independence in activities of daily living (about 50% and 33%, respectively), and decreased level of productive employment. Ogden, Utley, & Mee (1997) found that while most survivors interviewed reported good psychosocial recovery, a subset continue to report emotional distress, sleep disturbances (up to 35%), decreased ability to work (about 20%), serious and long-term family disruption (although rare), and personality change (48%) 4–7 years post SAH. Clinchot et al. (1997) examined rehabilitation outcomes in SAH who were admitted to rehabilitation. Since this sample consists of SAH patients who required continued inpatient care, this time at a rehabilitation facility, they likely represent a more severely impaired sample than the studies above. Right-sided lesions and more severe motor impairment was associated with increased length hospital of stay. In contrast to the studies mentioned earlier, which examined patients with "good outcome," 85% of SAH patients in the Clinchot study required supervision at discharge, most requiring constant supervision, despite most of these patients being discharged to home. There was a trend for those with better motor scores and functional level at admission to be less likely to require supervision at discharge.

Relatively Rare Neurobehavioral Syndromes Following Aneurysmal SAH

There are a number of cognitive and behavioral disorders that are relatively rare but do occur after SAH. Alien Hand Syndrome is a rare condition whereby the left hand interferes

with the actions of the right hand, resulting in intermanual conflict. It is an involuntary and autonomous, but apparently purposeful, behavior of the affected limb, which is perceived by the patient to be controlled by an external force. When caused by stroke, it can be observed by either ischemic or hemorrhagic, and is often associated with ACoA aneurysm (e.g., Diamond and DeLuca, 1995; Kikkert, Ribbers, & Koudstall, 2006).

Reduplicative paramanesia is a delusion regarding location in which the patient insists that a particular location (e.g., hospital, home, etc.) exists in two or more places simultaneously. Although rare following SAH, Hinkebein, Callahan, and Gelber (2001) reported a case of reduplicative paramnesia in a patient with SAH from a right MCA aneurysm rupture and clipping.

Akinesia, or absence of movement, has been observed following rupture of the ACoA, and was presumably mediated by damage to the dopamine system or its projections (Tanaka Bachman, & Miyazaki, 1991). A few reports of paresis are also present in the literature (e.g., Ohno, Masaoka, Suzuki, Monma, & Matsushima, 1991). Hemiparesis or other motor impairments are more typically observed following SAH from sites other than the ACoA, such as the MCA or aneurysms of the posterior circulation. Loss of sense of taste or smell can occur, even following treatment for unruptured intracranial aneurysm patients (Togwood, Ogden, & Mee, 2005).

Hanlon, Clontz, Bradly, & Milton (1993) reported a patient with severe behavioral dyscontrol following SAH secondary to right MCA aneurysm. This patient developed an unusual neurobehavioral syndrome characterized by "persistent, repetitive, involuntary, forceful oral exhalations; repetitive involuntary vocalizations; and oral-facial dyskinesia, involving facial grimacing, tongue protrusion, lip smacking, and eye closure." Three months of conventional rehabilitation as well as several medication trials proved ineffective in decreasing the uncontrollable vocal and motor behaviors. In contrast, a target behavioral intervention significantly decreased these involuntary behaviors, which was maintained at 3 months post inpatient discharge. Decreased behavioral dyscontrol was also associated with improved cognition and daily functioning. Although rare, unilateral spatial neglect has been seen after SAH (Wilson, Manly, Coyle, & Robertson, 2000).

Unruptured Aneurysms

Published reviews suggest that overall outcome is generally good following treatment for unruptured cerebral aneurysms. Estimated mortality rates are between 0 and 7% and morbidity between 5 and 25%, although morbidity is typically limited to gross neurological impairment (Towgood, Ogden, & Mee, 2004). While outcome is generally better for patients with unruptured versus ruptured aneurysms (Wiebers, Whisnant, Huston, Meissner, Brown, Piepgras et al., 2003), few studies have examined cognitive status, psychosocial functioning, and quality of life as part of the outcomes examined for unruptuted aneurysms (Towgood et al., 2004). A recent study measuring neuropsychological functioning using a reliability of change analysis revealed mild to moderate cognitive impairment at 6 months post treatment (Towgood, Ogden, & Mee, 2005). Like ruptured aneurysms, there is evidence that neuropsychological outcome is worse in persons with unruptured ACoA aneurysm relative to other aneurysm sites (Fukunaga, Uchida, Hashimoto, & Kawase, 1999). ACoA subjects in this study also showed reduced cerebral blood flow using SPECT following surgery.

Supporting Laboratory Studies Following SAH

In addition to the initial CT scan that is critical in the diagnosis of SAH and the subsequent CT angiogram or catheter-based angiogram to determine the location, size, and configuration of the aneurysm, the patient undergoes numerous additional studies over the course of the patient's 10- to 12-day stay in the intensive care unit. Patients sustaining spontaneous SAH have a high incidence of hyponatremia secondary to excessive antidiuretic hormone secretion of cerebral salt-wasting syndrome (Harrigan, 1996). Because the sodium fluctuations can be quite significant and may result in mental status changes, daily (or more frequent) assessment of sodium and all electrolytes is performed.

In addition to the potential electrolyte abnormalities that can ensue, daily transcranial Doppler (TCD) evaluation is often performed to monitor for the potential onset of cerebral vasospasm (Lysakowski, Walder, Costanza, & Tramer, 2001). At present, though cerebral vasospasm remains primarily a clinical diagnosis of exclusion (ruling out hyponatremia, fever, and hydrocephalus as other potential causes for mental status changes in the days following subarachnoid hemorrhage), TCD and other methods of determining blood flow (such as CT perfusion studies or SPECT scans) are useful adjuncts to the diagnosis of cerebral vasospasm.

Treatment and Prognosis

The outcomes for patients suffering from a subarachnoid hemorrhage secondary to aneurysmal rupture, despite the many years of clinical and bench-top research, are still quite unsatisfactory with a combined morbidity and mortality of approximately 75% (Prestigiacomo, 1996). Current research suggests that a substantial portion of the long-term poor outcomes is associated with neuropsychological and cognitive dysfunction, which had not been previously detected. Thus recent research in subarachnoid hemorrhage now is beginning to address management algorithms in the acute phase that may in fact alter the long-term neurocognitive as well as overall neurological outcome in this population of patients.

Currently, invasive treatment for cerebral aneurysm includes a craniotomy with microsurgical clipping of the aneurysm at its neck and endovascular coiling. Endovascular coiling, also termed embolization, represents one of the more significant recent advances in the treatment of cerebral aneurysms. It is particularly useful for medically fragile patients or aneurysms with a narrow neck (Heros & Morcos, 2000).

Coiling carries a high risk that the aneurysm may not be completely occluded with one review showing complete occlusion in only 54% of cases (Brilstra, Rinkel, van der Graaf, van Rooij, & Algra, 1999), let alone the unknown long-term risks of coiling. Despite these findings, current studies suggest that endovascular coiling is safer to perform in certain settings with good overall outcomes (Johnston, 2002).

Molyneux, Kerr, Yu, Clarke, Sneade, Yarnold, & Sandercock (2005) completed a multicenter trial of 2,143 intracranial aneurysm patients who were randomly assigned to neurosurgical clipping or endovascular coiling. They found that the survival at 1 year was significantly better in the endovascular coiling group, a benefit that continued for at least 7 years. However, while the risk for rebleeding was low overall, it was more common after coiling versus clipping. Hadjivassiliou, Tooth, Romanowski, Byrne, Battersby, et al. (2001) presented preliminary evidence that endovascular coiling caused less structural brain damage than surgical clipping, and more favorable cognitive outcome, although cognitive impairment was observed after both procedures. While similar findings have been observed by others (e.g., Bellebaum, Schafers, Schoch, Wanke, Stolke et al., 2004; Chan, Ho, & Poon, 2002), not all studies have found a clear benefit from endovascular coiling (e.g., Koivisto et al., 2000). Interestingly, patients with ACoA aneurysm may show particular benefit from the endovascular coiling procedure, where significant fewer and less severe cognitive impairment was observed relative to surgical coiling (Bellebaum et al., 2004) likely due to the less invasive nature of the procedure.

Although SAH is a subtype of stroke, its rehabilitation and treatment differs significantly from ischemic or embolic stroke (Stern et al., 2006). Regarding rehabilitation, SAH survivors make significant functional gains in rehabilitation, but the rate of gain is less than that observed in TBI or stroke (Dombovy et al., 1998). For example, SAH tend to have longer length of stays in rehabilitation compared to TBI or stroke, but no significant difference in overall outcome (Westerkam, Cifu, & Keyser, 1997). Longer rehabilitation stays have been associated with right-sided lesions and significant motor impairments (Clinchot et al., 1997). Overall, there are very few studies closely examining rehabilitation outcome after SAH. One significant problem with examining functional outcome is that graded scales such as the Glasgow Outcome Scale (GOS) and Functional Independence Measure (FIM) correlate poorly with actual everyday life outcome. Scales with improved ecological validity are clearly required in order to more closely examine rehabilitation effectiveness (Stern et al., 2006).

References

Bellebaum, C., Schafers, L., Schoch, B., Wanke, I., Stolke, D., et al. (2004) Clipping vs coiling: Neuropsychological follow up after aneurismal subarachnoid haemorrhage (SAH). *Journal Clinical Experimental Neuropsychology, 26,* 1081–1092.

Bornstein, R. A., Weir, B. K. A., Petruk, K. C., & Disney, L. B. (1987) Neuropsychological function in patients after subarachnoid hemorrhage. *Neurosurgery, 21,* 651–654.

Brilstra, E. H., Rinkel, G. J. E., van der Graff, Y., van Rooij, W. J. J., & Algra, A. (1999) Treatment of intracranial aneurysms by embolization with coils: A systematic review. *Stroke, 30,* 470–476.

Chalif, D. J., & Weinberg, J. S. (1998) Surgical treatment of aneurysm of the anterior cerebral artery. *Neurosurgery Clinicas of North America, 9,* 797–821.

Chan, A., Ho, S., & Poon, W. S. (2002) Neuropsychological sequelae of patients treated with microsurgical clipping or endovascular embolization for anterior communicating artery aneurysm. *European Neurology, 47,* 37–44.

Clinchot, D. M., Bogner, J. A., & Kaplan, P. E. (1997) Cerebral aneurysms: Analysis of rehabilitation outcomes. *Archives of Physical Medicine and Rehabilitation, 78,* 346–349.

DeLuca, J., & Diamond, B. J. (1995) Aneurysm of the anterior communicating artery: A review of neuroanatomical and neuropsychological sequelae. *Journal of Clinical and Experimental Neuropsychology, 17,* 100–121.

Dombovy, M., Drew-Cates, J., & Serdans, R. (1998) Recovery and rehabilitation following subarachnoid haemorrhage: Part II long-term follow-up. *Brain Injury, 12,* 887–894.

Fisher, C. M., Kistler, J. P., & Davis, J. M. (1980) Relation of cerebral vasospasm to subarachnoid hemorrhage visualized by CT scanning. *Neurosurgery 6,* 1–9.

Fukunaga, A. Uchida, K., Hashimoto, J., & Kawase, T. (1999) Neuropsychological evaluation and cerebral blood flow study of 30 patients with unruptured cerebral aneurysms before and after surgery. *Surgical Neurology, 51,* 132–139.

Germano, A., Caruso, G., Caffo, M., Cacciola, F., Belvedere, A. et al. (1998) Does subarachnoid blood extravasation per se induce long-term neuropsychological and cognitive alteration? *Acta Neurochirurgica, 140,* 805–812.

Hackett, M. L., & Anderson, C. S. (2000) Health outcomes 1 year after subarachnoid hemorrhage: An international population-based study. *Neurology, 55,* 658–662.

Hadjivassiliou, M., Tooth, C. L., Romanowski, C. A. J., Byrne, J., Battersby, R. D. E., et al. (2001) Aneurysmal SAH: Cognitive outcome and structural damage after clipping or coiling. *Neurology, 56,* 1672–1677.

Hanlon, R., Clontz, B., & Thomas, M. (1993) Management of severe behavioral dyscontrol following subarachnoid haemorrhage. *Neuropsychological Rehabilitation. 3(1),* 63–76.

Harrigan M. R. (1996) Cerebral salt wasting syndrome: A review. *Neurosurgery, 38,* 152–160.

Hellawell, D., & Pentland, B. (2001) Relatives' reports of long term problems following traumatic brain injury or subarachnoid haemorrhage. *Disability and Rehabilitation, 23,* 300–305.

Heros, R., & Morcos, J. (2000) Cerebrovascular surgery: Past, present, and future. *Neurosurgery, 47,* 1007–1033.

Hillis, A. E., Anderson, N., Sampath, P., & Rigamonti, D. (2000) Cognitive impairments after surgical repair of ruptured and unruptured aneurysms. *Journal of Neurology, Neurosurgery and Psychiatry, 69,* 608–615.

Hinkebein, H., Callahan, C. D., & Gelber, D. (2001) Reduplicative paramnesia: Rehabilitation of content-specific delusion after brain injury. *Rehabilitation Psychology, 46,* 75–81.

Hoh, B. L., Cheung, A. C., Rabinov, J. D., Pryor, J. C., Carter, B. S., & Ogilvy, C. S. (2004) Results of a prospective protocol of computed tomographic angiography in place of catheter angiography as the only diagnostic and pretreatment planning study for cerebral aneurysms by a combined neurovascular team. *Neurosurgery, 54,* 1329–1340.

Huang, J., & van Gelder, J. M. (2002) The probability of sudden death from rupture of intracranial aneurysms: a meta-analysis. *Neurosurgery, 51,* 1101–1105.

Hunt, W. E., & Hess, R. M. (1968) Surgical risk as related to time of intervention in the repair of intracranial aneurysms *Journal of Neurosurgery, 28,* 14–20.

Johnston, S. C. (2002) Effect of endovascular services and hospital volume on cerebral aneurysm treatment outcomes. *Stroke, 31,* 111–117.

Juvela, S., Porras, M., & Poussa, K. (2000) Natural history of unruptured intracranial anueurysms: A long-term follow-up study. *Journal of Neurosurgery, 93,* 379–387.

Kikkert, M. A., Ribbers, G. M., & Koudstall, P. J. (2006) Alien Hands Syndrome in stroke: A report of 2 cases and review of the literature. *Archives of Physical Medicine & Rehabilitation, 87,* 728–732.

Kim, D., Haney, C., & Van Ginhoven, G. (2005) Utility of outcome measures after treatment for intracranial aneurysms: A prospective trial involving 520 patients. *Stroke, 36,* 792–796.

Koivisto, T., Vanninen, R., Hurskainen, H., Saari, T., Hernesniemi, J., & Vapalahti, M. (2000) Outcomes of early endovascular vs surgical treatment of ruptured cerebral aneurysms. A prospective randomized study. *Strike, 31,* 2369–2377.

Lanterna, L. A., Rigoldi, M., Biroli, F., Cesana, C., Gaini, S. M., & Dalpra, L. (2005) APOE influences vasospasm and cognition of noncomatose patients with subarachnoid hemorrhage. *Neurology, 64,* 1238–1244.

Lysakowski, C., Walder, B., Costanza, M. C., & Tramer, M. R. (2001) Transcranial *Doppler* versus angiography in patients with vasospasm due to a ruptured cerebral aneurysm: A systematic review. *Stroke, 32,* 2292–2298.

Molyneux, A. J., Kerr, R. S. C., Yu, L-M., Clarke, M., Sneade, J. A., Yarnold, J. A., & Sandercock, P. (2005) International subarachnoid aneurysm trial (ISAT) of neurosurgical clipping versus endovascular coiling in 2143 patients with ruptured intracranial aneurysms: A randomized comparison of effects on survival, dependency, seizures, rebleeding, subgroups, and aneurysm occlusion. *Lancet, 366,* 809–817.

Mayeux, R. Ottman, R., Tang, M. X., Noboa-Bauza, L., Marder, K., Gurland, B., et al. (1993) Genetic susceptibility and heaed injury as risk factors for Alzheimer's disease among community-dwelling elserly persons and their first-degree relatives. *Annals of Neurology ,33,* 494–501.

Ogden, J. A., Levin, P. L., & Mee, E. W. (1990) Long-tern neuropsychological and psychological effects of subarachnoid hemorrhage. *Neuropsychiatry, Neuropsychology, and Behavioral Neurology, 3,* 260–274.

Ogden, J. A., Utley, T., & Mee, E. W. (1997) Neurological and psychosocial outcome 4 to 7 years after subarachnoid hemorrhage. *Neurosurgery*, *41*, 25–34.

Ohno, K., Masaoka, H., Suzuki, R., Monma, S., & Matsushima, Y. (1991) Symptomatic cerebral vasospasm of unusually late onset after aneurysm rupture. *Acta Neurochirurgica*, *108*(3–4), 163–166.

Powell, J., Kitchen, N., Heslin, J., & Greenwood, R. (2002) Psychosocial outcomes at three and nine months after good neurological recovery from aneurismal subarachnoid haemorrhage: Predictors and prognosis. *Journal of Neurology, Neurosurgery and Psychiatry*, *72*, 772–781.

Prestigiacomo, C. J. (2006) Historical perspectives: The surgical and endovascular treatment of intracranial aneurysms. *Neurosurgery 59*, S39–S47.

Prestigiacomo, C. J., Connolly, E. S. Jr, & Quest, D. O. (1996) Use of carotid ultrasound as a preoperative assessment of extracranial carotid artery blood flow and vascular anatomy. *Neurosurgery Clinics of North America*, *7*, 577–587.

Raaymakers, T. W. M., & the MARS Study Group, (1999) Aneurysms in relatives of patients with subarachnoid hemorrhage: Frequency and risk factors. *Neurology*, *53*, 982–988.

Rhoton, A. (2002) Aneurysms. *Neurosurgery*, *51*, S121–S158.

Saveland, H., Hillman, J., Brandt, L., Edner, G., Jakobsson, K-E., & Algers, G. (1992) Overall outcome in aneurysmal subarachnoid hemorrhage. A prospective study from neurosurgical units in Sweden during a 1-year period. *Journal of Neurosurgery*, *6*, 729–734.

Sethi, H., Moore, A., Dervin, J., Clifton, A., & MacSweeney, J. E. (2000) Hydrocephalus: comparison of clipping and embolization in aneurysm treatment. *Journal of Neurosurgery*, *92*, 991–994.

Schievink, W. I. (1997) Intracranial aneurysms. *New England Journal of Medicine*, *336*, 28–40.

Sheehan, J. P., Polin, R. S., Sheehan, J. M., Baskaya, M. K., & Kassell, N. F. (1999) Factors associated with hydrocephalus after aneurismal subarachnoid hemorrhage. *Neurosurgery*, *45*, 1120–1127.

Slooter, A. J., Tang, M. X., van Dujin, C. M., Hoffman A., van Dujin C. M., (1997) Apolipoprotein E polymorphism and neuropsychological outcome following subarachnoid haemorrhage. *Journal of the American Medical Association*, *277*, 818–821.

Simard, S., Rouleau, I., Brosseau, J., Laframboise, M., & Bojanowsky, M. (2003) Impact of executive dysfunctions on episodic memory abilities in patients with ruptured aneurysm of the anterior communicating artery. *Brain and Cognition*, *53*, 354–358.

Stern, M., Chang, D., Odell, M., & Sperber, K. (2006) Rehabilitation implications of non-traumatic subarachnoid haemorrhage. *Brain Injury*, *20*, 679–685.

Tanaka, Y., Bachman, D. L., & Miyazaki, M. (1991) Pharmacotheraoy for akinesia following anterior communicating artery aneurysm hemorrhage. *Japanese Journal of Medicine*, *30*, 542–544.

Taylor, T. N., Davis, P. H., Torner, J. C., Holmes, J., Meyer, J. W., & Jacobson, M. F. (1996) Lifetime cost of stroke in the United States. *Stroke*, *27*, 1459–1466.

Towgood, K., Ogden, J. A., & Mee, E. (2004) Neurological, neuropsychological and psychosocial outcome following treatment for unruptured intracranial aneurysms: A review and commentary. *Journal of the International Neuropsychological Society*, *10*, 114–134.

Towgood, K., Ogden, J. A., & Mee, E. (2005) Neurological, neuropsychological and functional outcome following treatment for unruptured intracranial aneurysms. *Journal of the International Neuropsychological Society*, *11*, 522–534.

Vale, F. L. Bradley, E. L., & Fisher, W. S. III. (1997) The relationship of subarachnoid hemorrhage and the need for postoperative shunting. *Journal of Neurosurgery*, *86*, 462–466

Vermeulen, M. J., & Schull, M. J. (2007) Missed diagnosis of subarachnoid hemorrhage in the emergency department. *Stroke*, *38*, 1216-1221.

Victor, M., & Ropper, A. H. (2001) Cerebrovascular diseases. In Adams, R. D. & Victor, M., (Eds.), *Principles of neurology* (pp 821–924). New York: McGraw-Hill.

Vilkki, J., Holst, P., Ohman, J., Servo, A., & Heiskanen, O. (1990) Social outcome related to cognitive performance and computed tomographic findings after surgery for a ruptured intracranial aneurysm. *Neurosurgery*, *26*, 579–584.

Wiebers, D. O., Whisnant, J. P., Huston, J., III., Meissner, I., Brown, R. D. Jr., Piepgras, D. G. et al. (2003) International Study of Unruptured Intracranial Aneurysms Investigators. Unruptured intracranial aneurysms: natural history, clinical outcome, and risks of surgical and endovascular treatment. *Lancet*, *362*(9378), 103–1010.

Weir, B. (2002) Unruptured intracranial aneurysm: A review. *Journal of Neurosurgery*, *96*, 3–42.

Weir, B., Disney, L., & Karrison, T. (2002) Sizes of ruptured and unruptured aneurysms in relation to their sites and the ages of patients. *Journal of Neurosurgery*, *96*, 64–70.

Westerkam, R., Cifu, D. X., & Keyser, L. (1997) Functional outcome after inpatient rehabilitation following aneurismal subarachnoid hemorrhage: A prospective analysis. *Top Stroke Rehabilitation*, *4*, 20–37.

Wilson, F. C., Manly, T., Coyle, D., & Robertson, I. H. (2000) The effect of contralesional limb activation training and sustained attention training for self-care programmes in unilateral spatial neglect. *Restorative Neurology and Neuroscience*. *16*, 1–4.

Winn, H. R., Jane, J. A., Sr., Taylor, J., Kaiser, D., & Britz, G. W. (2002) Prevalence of asymptomatic incidental aneurysms: Review of 4568 arteriograms. *Journal of Neurosurgery*, *96*, 43–49.

Chapter 5
Neuropsychological Effects of Brain Arteriovenous Malformations

Emily R. Lantz and Ronald M. Lazar

Introduction

Brain arteriovenous malformations (AVMs) are congenital vascular malformations, which can be located in any part of the brain (cortical, sub-cortical, dural, or brain stem). They are vascular anomalies which are made up of a complex tangle of abnormal veins and arteries that are missing a capillary bed (AVM Study Group, 1999; Stapf, Mohr, Pile-Spellman et al., 2001) and instead, artery and vein are connected by fistulas and characterized by "shunting" of blood from artery to vein (Bambakidis et al., 2001; Klimo, Rao, & Brockmeyer, 2007; O'Brien, Neyastani, Buckley, Chang, & Legiehn, 2006). This shunting mechanism causes hypertension within the AVM and in the draining vein (AVM Study Group, 1999; Iwama, Hayashida, Takahashi, Nagata, & Hashimoto, 2002; Loring, 1999) and hypotension in the surrounding and feeding vessels (AVM Study Group, 1999). The feeding arteries have high volume flow with low pressure, creating hypoperfusion in surrounding normal brain tissue with little apparent clinical effect (Diehl, Henkes, Nahser, Kuhne, & Berlit, 1994; Fogarty-Mack et al., 1996; Mast, Mohr

E.R. Lantz (✉)
Neurological Institute, 710 West 168th Street, New York, NY 10032, USA
e-mail: elantz@neuro.columbia.edu

Supported in part by the Salvatore P. Marra Foundation.

et al., 1995; Murphy, 1954). AVMs are often found in the borderzone region and thus share anterior cerebral artery (ACA), middle cerebral artery (MCA), and/or posterior cerebral artery (PCA) circulation (Stapf, Mohr, Pile-Spellman, et al., 2001) (Fig. 1).

Often, AVMs are asymptomatic and go undetected unless there is a clinical event (such as hemorrhage or seizure). Unlike other brain lesions, the AVM itself often does not cause cognitive dysfunction. This phenomenon has been explained by Lazar, Marshall, Pile-Spellman, Hacein-Bey et al. (1997) and Lazar, Marshall, Pile-Spellman, Duong et al. (2000), who suggested that brain reorganization could be due to the chronic nature of the AVM. Rather, it is usually a hemorrhage that is responsible for functional/cognitive changes seen in patients with AVM. Pathological data have shown that approximately 12% of AVMs are symptomatic and the others are captured either inadvertently or on autopsy (Hashimoto, Iida, Kawaguchi, & Sakaki, 2004; McCormick, 1978).

Neuropathology and Pathophysiology

The central point of abnormal development in the AVM is the nidus (Loring, 1999), which is a tangle of arteries and veins in which there are feeding arteries and draining veins. The

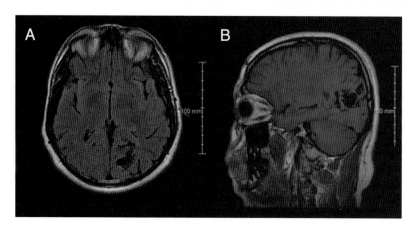

Fig. 1 MRI T_1-weighted images of a brain arteriovenous malformation (AVM) in the left occipitoparietal region. (A) Coronal view; (B) Axial view

feeding artery can include branches off the main cerebral arteries (e.g., MCA, PCA, ACA), carotid or vertebral arteries, or the choroidal arteries from the subcortical regions (AVM Study Group,1999). The feeding arteries can have multiple destinations. They may terminate at the nidus or continue beyond the AVM to feed healthy brain tissue (Choi & Mohr, 2005).

Arteriovenous malformations can be in the parenchyma (located in essential neural tissue) or dural (located in dura). Both parenchymal and dural AVMs have the potential to cause a more focal deficit (similar to that seen in stroke), while dural AVM had also been shown to cause a more global dementia-like syndrome (Festa et al., 2004; Hurst et al., 1998; Ito, Sonokawa, Mishina, & Sato, 1995; Matsuda et al., 1999; Tanaka, Morooka, Nakagawa, & Shimizu, 1999). Subcortical (deep) AVMs have been associated with deficits such as neglect and memory disturbance (Buklina, 2001, 2002). AVMs are equally common in all parts of the brain and are proportionally represented (i.e., frontal lobe is 30% of the brain, and frontal AVMs represent 30% of all AVMs) (Mohr, 2004).

Research has demonstrated significant structural changes in the vessels of an AVM as compared to normal vessels (McCormick, 1966;

Mohr, 2004; Yamada, Liwnicz, Lonser, & Knierim, 1999). Pathology has demonstrated that the neurons within the AVM are non-functional and devoid of any normal brain tissue (Mohr, 2004). At the molecular level, brain AVMs have been shown to demonstrate genetic abnormalities when compared with normal tissue (Hashimoto, Lawton et al., 2004; Pawlikowska et al., 2004; Takemori, 1992).

Hemodynamic changes are well documented in brains with AVM. Van Roost and Schramm (2001) found abnormal regional cerebral blood flow in AVM territory (distal from the nidus). In general, regional cerebral blood flow (rCBF) was reduced (20% less than the contralateral side) and impaired (<10.0 ml per 100 g per min) in vessels that supply the AVM (Van Roost & Schramm). In addition, increased cerebral blood volume (rCBV) has been found in both the ipsilateral and contralateral hemispheres (Tyler et al., 1989).

Demographics and Epidemiology

Arteriovenous malformations are an uncommon vascular phenomenon occurring in approximately 4.3% of the population based on 4,530 consecutive autopsies (McCormick &

Rosenfield, 1973). Pathology data have shown that approximately 12% of AVMs are symptomatic (Hashimoto, Iida et al., 2004; McCormick, 1978) and researchers report that approximately 0.1–1% of the population will have a symptomatic AVM annually (Brown, Wiebers, Torner, & O'Fallon, 1996; Group, 1999; Hofmeister et al., 2000; Mohr, 2004; Redekop, TerBrugge, Montanera, & Willinsky, 1998). Females account for 45–51% of AVM cases (Hofmeister, et al.). The mean age of diagnosis is 31.2 years, with significant variability in reporting across clinical sites. Sixty-nine to seventy-four percent of patients had AVM location in eloquent (functional) brain regions and the majority (52–59%) showed deep venous drainage (Hofmeister, et al.). As for AVM size, 38% were small (<3 cm), 55% were medium AVMs (3–6 cm), and 7% were large AVMs (>6 cm) (Hofmeister, et al.).

Natural History

While AVMs are considered to be congenital or developmental, there are currently no in utero reports of AVM, suggesting that it may not be due to embryonic vessel development as once theorized (Stapf, Mohr, Pile-Spellman et al., 2001). Rather, they are likely formed during the late fetal or immediate postpartum periods (Stapf, Mohr, Pile-Spellman et al., 2001), although the mechanism is still unknown. Most researchers classify AVM clinical presentation into two major categories, hemorrhagic and non-hemorrhagic, which can present with identical symptoms (e.g., headache, seizure, or neurological deficit) with one significant differentiation: a bleed (Stapf, Mast et al., 2006a).

Hemorrhage

Hemorrhage related to AVMs account for approximately 1–2% of all strokes (Furlan, Whisnant, & Elveback, 1979; Gross, Kase,

Mohr, Cunningham, & Baker, 1984; Hashimoto, Iida et al., 2004; Perret & Nishioka, 1966). Intracranial hemorrhage (ICH) is the most frequent symptom of AVM, occurring annually in 2–4% of the AVM population (Brown, Wiebers, & Forbes, 1990; Graf, Perret, & Torner, 1983; Ondra, Troupp, George, & Schwab, 1990). Other authors have proposed a higher probability by using a formula for calculating hemorrhage risk ($1-0.97^{\text{expected years of remaining life}}$) and they have estimated approximately a 60% life-time risk (Kondziolka, McLaughlin, & Kestle, 1995). Overall lifetime risk for initial ICH is 35–50% (Choi & Mohr, 2005). Re-hemorrhage was found in 18% of the population, suggesting that initial hemorrhage was a significant predictor of repeat hemorrhage (Mast, Young et al., 1997; Mohr, 2004). Other researchers have found that previous hemorrhage does not predict future hemorrhage (Ondra et al., 1990). Arteriovenous malformation is implicated in subarachnoid hemorrhage only 9% of the time as compared to ICH in which AVM is more often the culprit, especially in younger adults (4–33% of first time ICH) (Furlan et al., 1979; Kloster, 1997; Ruiz-Sandoval, Cantu, & Barinagarrementeria, 1999).

Multiple factors have been associated with increased risk of hemorrhage, such as AVM size, venous drainage characteristics (i.e., deep drainage), and high intranidal pressure (Duong et al., 1998; Spetzler et al., 1992). Additionally, location, cerebellar hypertension, size, and deep venous drainage may be related to increased risk of hemorrhage (Langer et al., 1998). AVMs fed by dural arteries demonstrate a decreased risk of hemorrhage (Langer et al., 1998). More recently, Stapf, Mast et al. (2006a) analyzed a prospective database (Columbia AVM Databank) and found that hemorrhagic AVM presentation in combination with additional significant risk factors (increased age, deep AVM location, and exclusive deep venous drainage) were the only factors that were associated with increased hemorrhage risk. They created a risk model in which 0.9% of AVM patients with no risk factors bled, while bleeding occurs in up to 34.4% of patients with three risk factors. These data alter the previous estimated hemorrhage risk of 2–4% and help guide treatment decisions based on a modified risk factor model.

Seizure

Non-hemorrhagic seizures co-occur in 16–53% of the AVM population (AVM Study Group, 1999; Hofmeister et al., 2000) and are the second most common presentation. The AVM Data Bank of the Columbia-Presbyterian Medical Center demonstrated 49% of AVM-related seizure activity is generalized tonic-clonic, 22% are focal, 22% are focal with secondary generalization, 4% are complex partial, and 4% were not classified (Choi & Mohr, 2005).

Temporal lobe AVMs frequently cause seizures. Temporal lobe AVMs account for 12–16% of all AVMs (Brown, Wiebers, Forbes, O'Fallon et al., 1988; Drake, 1979; Malik, Seyfried, & Morgan, 1996) and 46% of patients with temporal lobe AVMs report seizures, as compared to the 24% in non-temporal lobe AVMs (Kumar, Malik, & Demeria, 2002; Nagata, Morioka, Matsukado, Natori, & Sasaki, 2006). Factors significantly associated with seizure occurrence were male sex, age below 62 years, AVM size (>3 cm) and temporal lobe location (Hoh, Chapman, Loeffler, Carter, & Ogilvy, 2002). In general, seizures are associated with cerebral location and not with sub-cortical/deep AVM's (Garrido & Stein, 1978; Graeb & Dolman, 1986; Hoh et al., 2002; Perret & Nishioka, 1966; Turjman et al., 1995). Hoh et al. found a minority (22%) of seizures occurred in deep AVM, although deep location and posterior fossa were statistically unrelated to seizure occurrence. Most epileptogenic AVMs are superficial and supratentorial, and are fed by the MCA (Turjman et al., 1995).

Treatment outcomes of AVM-related seizures are mixed, but generally surgical obliteration of the AVM is associated with improved seizure outcome (Hoh et al., 2002; Piepgras, Sundt, Ragoowansi, & Stevens, 1993). Other factors such as short seizure history, hemorrhage-related seizures, generalized tonic clonic seizure type, and deep and posterior fossa location are associated with positive outcome (Hoh et al.). Piepgras et al. (1993) found 83% of patients with AVM-related seizures were seizure free after surgery, however, the majority (52%) still required anticonvulsant medications following AVM resection. Another factor that has been associated with seizure control in AVM patients is age of onset. Yeh, Tew, and Gartner et al. (1993) demonstrated that older age was associated with better treatment outcome (60% seizure control age 30 and under, 83.3% seizure control age 31 and older).

Headache

Arteriovenous malformations is occasionally associated with headache. Within the AVM population approximately 14–16% of the population reported headaches (Ghossoub et al., 2001; Hofmeister et al., 2000). In a sample of 700 AVM patients, headaches that were unrelated to hemorrhage or seizure occurred in only 6% (Ghossoub et al.). Arteriovenous malformation-related headaches were mostly non-pulsating and ipsilateral to the AVM, and they were found to correspond with the AVM location in the brain of 80–97.4% of patients (Ghossoub et al., 2001) Frishberg reported that only 0.3% of headache patients harbored cerebral AVMs (Frishberg, 1994). Even less frequent were migraines, only 0.07% were found to be related to AVM incidence (Frishberg, 1997).

Neurological/Neuropsychological Deficits

Neurological deficit associated with brain AVMs are reported with varying frequency

(1.3% to 48%), with reversible deficits significantly more common (8%) than persistent deficits (7%) (Hofmeister et al., 2000; Mast, Mohr et al., 1995; Wenz et al., 1998). Some researchers have demonstrated significant deficits in neuropsychological functioning of patients, some of which unfortunately combined the outcomes of ruptured and unruptured AVMs (Baker, McCarter, & Porter, 2004; Mahalick, Ruff, Heary, & U, 1993; Marshall, Jonker, Morgan, & Taylor, 2003; Steinvorth et al., 2002; Wenz et al., 1998). Wenz et al. found that AVM patients (both with and without hemorrhage) demonstrated below normal performance on tests of general IQ (24% of patients), attention (34% of patients), and memory (48% of patients). However, this study did not differentiate between ruptured and un-ruptured AVMs so the actual occurrence of cognitive deficit in AVM, per se, cannot be determined. Mahalick et al. also demonstrated significantly lower performance on tests of neuropsychological functioning for AVM patients as compared to "normals," but they also did not control for prior hemorrhage. In another study combining ruptured and unruptured AVM, it was found that AVM patients were again significantly below normals on test of intelligence, memory, and attention (Steinvorth et al., 2002).

In contrast, when only patients with unruptured AVMs were included, researchers have found a much lower incidence of neurological deficit. Mast, Mohr et al. (1995) studied patients from their prospective database (AVM Data Bank of the Columbia-Presbyterian Medical Center) with unruptured AVMs and found that only 1.3% of AVM patients met criteria for progressive functional neurological deficit, while 7.2% met criteria for non-progressive functional neurological deficits. The difference in incidence of neurological deficits in these studies (1.3% up to 48%) can be explained by hemorrhage status, rather than the AVM itself. Hemorrhage is likely accounting for the vast difference in neurological deficit seen among these AVM patients.

Researchers have demonstrated improvement in neuropsychological functioning post-surgery (Malik et al., 1996; Wenz et al., 1998). Cognitive improvements after AVM treatment have been attributed to improved cerebral blood flow and reduction of the "steal effect" (Malik et al., 1996; Steinvorth et al., 2002; Wenz et al., 1998). The steal effect refers to the assumption that shunting and hypertension through the AVM decreases cerebral perfusion in the region surrounding the AVM, thus causing cerebral ischemia and ultimately neurological deficits (Mast, Mohr et al., 1995). Iwama et al. (2000) demonstrated that intracranial steal and venus hypertension, and not decreased neurological activity or mass effect, are responsible for the hemodynamic changes seen in high-flow AVMs.

Other researchers disagree with the "steal" hypotheses (Mast, Mohr et al., 1995; Stabell & Nornes, 1994). Stabell and Nornes reported that AVM patients performed the same as normal controls on presurigcal cognitive assessment. While some significant improvement was observed, Stabell and Nornes dispute the "steal" hypothesis as an explanation for cognitive improvement after AVM surgery. Mast, Mohr et al. (1995) were unable to replicate the "steal effect" using their prospective database. They demonstrated that an AVM patient with chronic cerebral hypotension did not have any functional cognitive impairment. In addition, they used positron emission tomography (PET) to study 14 AVM patients and demonstrated that while these patients did have hypoperfusion in surrounding tissue, they did not have any parenchymal volume loss and metabolism was normal (Mast, Mohr et al., 1995). Kumar, Fox, Vinuela, and Rosenbaum (1984) found that the mass effect (space-taking effect of the AVM nidus itself or edema surrounding the AVM) was present in 55% of AVMs on computed tomography (Kumar et al.). Mast, Mohr et al. (1995) commented on this study and proposed that it is mass effect rather than "steal" effect that may help to explain functional neurological deficits seen in unruptured AVM patients.

More recent studies have focused on postsurgical cognitive functioning associated with AVM. A case series that included three pre-adolescents (age 10 and 11) and two adolescents (age 15), considered to be cognitively intact before AVM discovery, showed that regardless of the AVM location, mild to moderate executive dysfunction was evident after surgical excision of the AVM (Whigham & O'Toole, 2007). Whigham and O'Toole suggested that perhaps the age of their adolescent patients (executive functions thought to develop at this point in development) help explain the vulnerability toward executive dysfunction after AVM treatment. In contrast, a study on neurocognition and radiosurgery in adults ($N = 34$) demonstrated that AVM patients improved significantly ($p < 0.001$) on the Wisconsin Card Sorting Test (WCST) after radiosurgical treatment (Guo, Lee, Chang, & Pan, 2006).

In addition, developmental learning disorders have been found in 66% of adults with AVMs (Lazar, Connaire et al., 1999). In this study, AVM patients reported four times the rate of learning disability than the normal population (17%). Lazar et al. reported that perhaps these disorders of higher intellectual functioning (e.g., learning) may serve as a marker for subtle developmental cerebral dysfunction in AVM patients.

Related Vascular Anomalies

Dural arteriovenous fistulas consist of shunts that are located within the dural layer. They make up approximately 10–15% of cerebrovascular malformations and account for 1% of all strokes (Festa et al., 2004; Hurst et al., 1998; Kurl, Saari, Vanninen, & Hernesniemi, 1996; Newton & Cronqvist, 1969). Dural AV fistulas (while located in the dura and not directly associated with eloquent cortex) have been found to cause focal deficits, such as Wernicke's aphasia and transient right hemiparesis, identical to symptoms caused by a focal stoke (Festa et al., 2004). Unlike AVMs located within the parenchyma, which are not likely to cause global neuropsychological dysfunction, dural AV fistulas have been demonstrated to cause a dementia syndrome, which presents like encephalopathy (Hurst et al., 1998; Matsuda et al., 1999; Tanaka et al., 1999). These authors reported patients with angiographically confirmed dural AV fistulas who presented with global cognitive dysfunction including progressive memory decline, slowed mentation, low initiation, and almost all patients reported focal headaches. This dementia-like syndrome may be reversible, since multiple case reports have presented data on patients with dural AVM dementia that was reversed after treatment of the fistula (Hurst et al., 1998; Tanaka et al., 1999; Zeidman et al., 1995).

Aneurysms have also been associated (approximately 10–20%) with AVMs (Redekop et al., 1998). One study reported 46% of AVM patients presented with aneurysms (Meisel et al., 2000). Another author reported a prevalence rate of 15.3% of AVM patients who presented with aneurysm (Redekop et al., 1998). Aneurysms associated with AVM are considered "weak points" and are associated with greater risk for hemorrhage (Meisel et al., 2000). Brown et al. reported the risk of hemorrhage was 7% for the first year in patients with AVM and aneurysms and 3% per year with AVM alone. While the risk decreased to 1.7% with AVM alone, AVM and aneurysm remained at 7% risk of hemorrhage at 5 years (Brown et al., 1990).

Imaging Studies

Multiple imaging techniques are currently used to diagnose brain AVM. With the availability of technology such as computerized tomography (CT), magnetic resonance imaging (MRI), and angiography, AVMs are often detected before they rupture allowing treatment options to be explored. While CT scan and MRI are often the first and least invasive methods for detecting AVM in the brain, angiography is the "gold standard" for formal diagnosis, mapping the vascular anatomy of the AVM, and subsequent treatment planning (Ogilvy et al., 2001).

catheterized angiography is now the most reliable and considered to be the standard procedure for diagnosis and assessment of brain AVM. Researchers have demonstrated a significantly lower risk for angiography-related morbidity with AVM (0.3–0.8%) than with stroke (3.0–3.7%) (Cloft, Joseph, & Dion, 1999) (Fig. 2).

Angiography

An angiogram is an radiograph of the vascular system designed to show detailed anatomy of the arteries and veins by injecting a contrast agent through a microcatheter. In the past, catheters were placed into very large vessels such as the internal carotid artery in order to map AVMs supplied by the middle or anterior cerebral arteries. With the recent development of microcatheters, it became possible to selectively inject vessels distal to the circle of Willis for a more detailed view of the neurovascular geography of vascular malformations such as AVMs. Superselective

CT and MR

Although catheter angiography is standard and has the highest spatial resolution (approximately 0.2 mm), researchers continue to look for less invasive techniques (Warren et al., 2001). CT, CT-angiography, CT-perfusion, MRI, MR angiography (MR-A), and MR perfusion (MR-P) are important diagnostic tools used to evaluate patients with AVMs. In the future, these tests may supplant some of the diagnostic need for catheter cerebral angiography.

A CT scan is used to assess gross changes in the brain due to AVM. It can determine

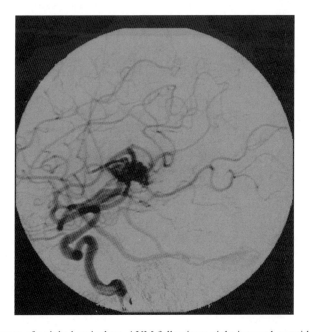

Fig. 2 Cerebral angiogram of a right hemisphere AVM following a right internal carotid artery injection

current and past hemorrhage, as well as the presence of draining veins (Riina & Gobin, 2001). While it has low sensitivity, calcification and hypointensity can still be seen demonstrating the mass effect of the AVM (Ogilvy et al., 2001).

An MRI is used to determine size, localization, and topography (Ogilvy et al., 2001; Riina & Gobin, 2001). Functional MRI (fMRI) is also used with AVM patients. fMRI measures regional cerebral blood flow and has been used with AVM patients to study brain reorganization and help with presurgical planning (Cannestra et al., 2004). Cannestra et al. found that fMRI testing was sensitive when identifying eloquent language regions in patients with left perisylvian AVMs. They were able to categorize the patients into three surgical risk groups from fMRI alone and predicted surgical outcomes from their classification system. They reported that 75% of patients avoided awake, invasive brain mapping by using fMRI. However, in 25% of patients, they were not able to be successfully determine operative risk, and electrocortical stimulation mapping (ESM) was required. In addition, ESM suggested nidus eloquence in some patients, which was not initially detected on fMRI.

The utility of fMRI in studying AVMs remains controversial. Hemodynamic abnormalities in AVMs make measuring regional cerebral blood flow on fMRI problematic (Alkadhi et al., 2000; Cannestra et al., 2004; Lehericy et al., 2002). Therefore, it has been proposed that fMRI should be followed up with superselective Wada testing or EMS for AVMs with significant blood flow disruptions or when eloquent cortex is thought to be bordering the AVM (Cannestra et al., 2004; Lehericy et al., 2002).

Magnetic resonance angiography (MRA), a variant of MRI, shows the anatomical structure of feeding arteries, draining veins, and the nidus in three-dimensional detail. Contrast-enhanced MRA, for example, provides significantly better morphological information about the vessels and correlates with angiography at 95% sensitivity (Unla et al., 2006; Warren et al., 2001). One advantage of contrast-enhanced MRA in AVM studies is that it is less vulnerable than fMRI to signal loss due to slow-flowing blood (Ogilvy et al., 2001), which is a general problem with imaging AVM due to abnormal blood flow. Most authors agree, however, that MRA should be used only as an adjunct to standard diagnostic angiography because it cannot provide the necessary vascular detail, information which can be obtained from angiography (St George, Butler, & Plowman, 2002; Unla et al., 2006; Warren et al., 2001).

Disease Course

People with brain AVMs can live their entire life without symptoms. As previously stated, AVMs rarely cause cognitive or neurological deficits in the absence of hemorrhage or seizures. It is suspected that the brain reorganizes early in development, thus compensating for mass effect of the AVM nidus. Because AVM is often not associated with cognitive decline and the natural history for risk of hemorrhage is relatively low, some authors argue that treatment of unruptured AVMs (those that have not caused hemorrhage) may not be justified (Stapf, Mast et al., 2006a).

Treatment and Prognosis

Because only 0.1–1% of the population will have a symptomatic AVM, there is extensive research and discussion within the field regarding whether to perform preemptive surgery on unruptured AVMs (Stapf, Mohr, Choi et al., 2006b). Natural history risk must be weighed with surgical risks in order to determine the risk-to-benefit ratio of treating unruptured AVMs. Because the risk of re-bleeding after initial ICH is significant, most researchers agree that treating a ruptured AVM is worth the risk. Whether treating an unruptured AVMs is worth the risk, however, is more controversial. A randomized multicenter clinical trial of unruptured AVMs is currently underway (ARUBA, funded by NINDS) to potentially understand the natural history risk of medical management versus the treatment risk for appropriate surgical intervention. Meanwhile, individual AVM patients are provided with current data of natural history risk versus risk of surgery and are left to decide whether to treat their AVM. To date, however, there are no specific neuropsychological outcomes.

Treatment decisions are determined by appearance (size, location, etc.) of the AVM (AMCS, 2005). The Spetzler-Martin grading system has been adopted as a standardized system to rate AVMs according to their size, location (functional importance, often referred to as eloquence, of surrounding brain tissue), and venous drainage (Riina & Gobin, 2001). AVM can be graded from I to V. Research has demonstrated that higher grades have increased risk of negative outcomes during and after surgery. Spetzler and Martin (1986) found that 98% of grade I and II AVMs were successfully removed in one stage procedure, while grade III and IV AVM required additional treatment stages. Similarly, other researchers confirmed the reliability of the grading system and have demonstrated that grade I and II AVMs have a 100% to 94.3% chance of good outcome, while III and IV AVMs have a 88.6% to 28.6% chance of full removal with positive outcome (Heros, Korosue, & Diebold, 1990).

The current treatments for AVM are embolization, radiosurgery (gamma knife), and craniotomy. Each treatment can be given on its own, but are more often administered in combination. One goal of embolization and radiosurgery is to minimize the size of the AVM, thereby lowering the grade and improving treatment outcome after craniotomy. The ultimate goal of treatment is complete obliteration of the AVM nidus allowing for a return to normal hymodynamics

and preservation of neurological functioning (Lunsford et al., 1991).

Embolization

Embolization is a procedure in which a micro-catheter guided by superselective angiography is used to locate the feeding vessels and a thrombotic substance is injected into the vessel with the goal of reducing blood flow to the AVM. The microcatheter is pulled by blood flow and can be guided by the interventional neuroradiologist with precision to almost any vessel in the brain (Richling et al., 2006). The embolizing substance consists of acrylic glue (e.g., NBCA, Glubran-2, Neuroacryl) and oily dye (Lipiodol), so the injection is visible under X-ray (Richling et al., 2006). While embolization sometimes can be used as a stand-alone treatment, it is often used as a pre-surgical staged treatment for larger and more difficult AVMs. Patients who undergo staged embolizations have better treatment outcome because their brain has time to slowly adjust to the change in hemodynamics, making surgical excision less risky (Spetzler, Martin, Carter et al., 1987). Embolization is also used for surgically inaccessible, deep, or dural feeding AVMs (Fig. 3).

Neurosurgery

Complete removal of the AVM through craniotomy has been suggested when the risk of neurosurgery is less than that of the natural history risk of hemorrhage (Lunsford et al., 1991; Spetzler & Martin, 1986). The biggest advantage of complete surgical excision is that the chance of re-bleeding is eliminated (Heros et al., 1990). The chance of developing post-operative seizures is 7.4%, and approximately 58% of patients with pre-operative seizures had no recurrence of seizures (Heros et al.). One downfall of neurosurgery is that if

AVM   Catheter Tip

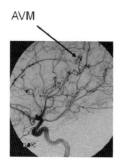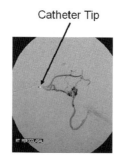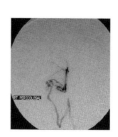

Fig. 3 Left panel: a lateral view of a cerebral angiogram following injection of the right internal carotid artery; middle panel: a lateral view of the same AVM following superselective injection in the right peri-collosal artery, a segment of the anterior cerebral artery; right panel: an anterior–posterior view of the same right peri-callosal segment after injection

the lesion is not fully removed then re-bleeding remains a risk (Spetzler & Martin, 1986). One population-based study found that neurosurgery is the ideal form of treatment for low grade AVMs with the goal of total obliteration (Hillman, 2001). Mahalick et al. (1993) reported that surgical excision of the AVM resulted in significant improvements in tasks involving short and long-term verbal memory, long-term visual-spatial memory, verbal learning, and verbal and non-verbal intelligence. Overall, they found 60% of AVM patients performed in the normal range on neuropsychological examination post-surgery (Mahalick, et al.).

Radiosurgery

When an AVM is inoperable due to size and/or location or a patient chooses not to undergo surgery given the natural history risk of bleeding, stereotactic gamma-knife radiosurgery is the treatment of choice. Gamma-knife (radiation therapy) is most effective in smaller lesions, but unlike neurosurgery, complete removal is not always possible, leading to future risk of re-bleeding. The complete obliteration of the AVM takes two to three years after the treatment and possible risk for hemorrhage during this time remains. Some

researchers reported the incidence of hemorrhage after radiosurgery is 2–4%, which is almost equivalent to the rate from natural history (Lunsford et al., 1991; Ogilvy, 1990; Steiner & Lindquist, 1987). If the AVM is fully obliterated, radiosurgery provides the same level of protection against hemorrhage as neurosurgical excision. Approximately 80% of patients who received radiosurgery have full obliteration of the AVM.

Wenz et al. (1998) found that radiosurgery improved attention by 14% and memory functioning by 12%. Similarly, they found statistically significant improvements in cognitive functioning after radiosurgery, which is an unanticipated finding since the authors were initially investigating the neurotoxic side effects of radiosurgery. In addition, Steinvorth et al. (2002) compared patients with and without presurgical ICH. They found that presurgical ICH status was not related to cognitive improvement after radiosurgery.

Other researchers have looked at seizure morbidity after radiosurgery. Lundsford et al. found that 51% reported decline in seizure activity while Steiner et al. reported a 69.4% improvement rate. In addition, Lundsford et al. reported a 75% improvement in headaches and Steiner et al. also demonstrated a significant decline in headaches (66.3% headaches disappeared, 9.2% some improvement).

Superselective Wada testing and Electrocortical Stimulation Mapping

Superselective Wada testing and ESM are in vivo procedures used to help interventional neuroradiologists and neurosurgeons to identify eloquent cortex that may be surrounding the AVM and helps to predict neurological and cognitive changes that would occur as an adverse effect of treatment. Currently, the Spetzler-Martin grading system aids surgeons by establishing a risk model to assess the size and location of the AVM. The treating physician must assume eloquence from the location of the AVM (i.e., if the AVM is located in Broca's area, the surgeon will assume this area is crucial for expressive language). However, because brain reorganization has been widely associated with AVM (Lazar, Marshall, Pile-Spellman, Hacein-Bey et al., 1997; Lazar, Marshall, Pile-Spellman, Duong et al., 2000), the grading system without empirical data from in vivo testing of eloquence cannot establish true treatment risk.

Superselective Wada testing is a clinical procedure that is used to help the interventional neuroradiologist determine prior to embolization whether a feeding artery to an AVM also supplies blood necessary for eloquent function in nearby brain areas. With the microcatheter in place for embolization (See Fig. 3), the neuroradiologist injects a short acting anesthetic (usually amobarbital, or a combination of amobarbital and lidocaine) that lasts for approximately 3–5 min. During this brief testing period a neuropsychologist (who has previously collected baseline neurocognitive data for this particular patient) performs tests of cognitive functioning typically associated with brain region supplied by the feeding vessel. For example, if the neuroradiologist is embolizing a vessel in the left MCA territory, tests of language will be performed. The neuroradiologist will use the results of Wada testing to help determine course of treatment. If a deficit is apparent during Wada testing, the radiologist may choose to embolize closer to the AVM nidus to diminish neurocognitive damage or perhaps decide not to embolize at all. A negative Wada test result allows the neuroradiologist to embolize the feeding vessel with diminished risk for significant neurological damage. Most evaluations during superselective Wada testing are typically adapted from well-known neuropsychological tests (i.e., Boston Diagnostic Aphasia Tests, Wechsler Memory Scale) with well established norms (Fitzsimmons, Marshall, Pile-Spellman, & Lazar, 2003; Goodglass & Kaplan, 1983; Wechsler, 1987).

While amobarbital and lidocaine can be used in combination as they are at our center, they can be administered separately for superselective Wada testing. Amobarbital is a GABA inhibitor that acts only on gray matter, while lidocaine is an anesthetic that acts on both gray and white matter (Fitzsimmons et al., 2003). Based on four case studies, Fitzsimmons et al. (2003) found that lidocaine alone can cause clinical deficits while amabarbital alone did not. They theorized that the use of lidocaine was more sensitive to white matter changes and therefore helped to determine eloquent brain structures that may be affected from embolization. They concluded that lidocaine should be included in combination with amobarbitol as part of preembolization Wada testing.

Another in vivo procedure that can be used to determine eloquence of surrounding cortex is ESM. ESM is performed intraoperatively, during an awake craniotomy. While the patient performs different tasks, the brain is stimulated and essential versus non-essential cortical sites can be mapped out (Cannestra et al., 2004).

Cannestra et al. (2004) compared fMRI, superselective Wada testing, and EMS for efficacy as pre-surgical tools to identify eloquent cortex surrounding the AVM. They reported that superselective Wada testing was not sensitive in identifying eloquent cortex and that fMRI in combination with EMS were required to adequately predict surgical risk.

AVM and Cerebral Reorganization

Because AVMs are developmental, chronic lesions they have been able to provide unique information about the brain. Researchers have demonstrated brain reorganization of language function using superselective Wada testing, MRI, and fMRI studies (Lazar, Marshall, Pile-Spellman, Duong et al., 2000; Lazar, Marshall, Pile-Spellman, Hacein-Bey et al., 1997; Maldjian et al., 1996). Lazar et al. reported on three cases (all with left frontal AVMs) in which expressive language function was at least partially controlled by the right hemisphere and had also been transferred to ispilesional territory not typically associated with language.

Some authors propose functional displacement simply due to the fact that brain tissue located within the AVM is non-functional (Alkadhi et al., 2000; Burchiel, Clarke, Ojemann, Dacey, & Winn, 1989; Choi & Mohr, 2005). Further, Lazar, Marshall, Pile-Spellman, Duong et al. (2000) demonstrated that the left frontal region, which is normally responsible for expressive language, was no longer responsible for that function. They did so by using superselective Wada testing in which the target region (left frontal AVM feeder) was anesthetized and language function was not disrupted. Receptive language, as expected, was controlled by the left temporoparietal region. Lazar, Marshall, Pile-Spellman, Duong et al. (2000) hypothesized that expressive language had been reorganized to the right hemisphere of these AVM patients. Using fMRI, they determined that in fact these AVM patients did show activation in the right hemisphere where normal controls do not show activation for such language functions. In another study, Lazar, Marshall, Pile-Spellman, Hacein-Bey et al. (1997) found that patients with left posterior AVMs in the receptive language region had receptive language deficits when the frontal lobe (typically expressive language regions) was anesthetized. This finding again suggested the presence of language reorganization in brains of AVM patients. Lazar, Marshall, Pile-Spellman, Hacein-Bey et al. (1997) and Lazar, Marshall, Pile-Spellman, Duong et al. (2000) concluded that brain reorganization was likely a function of the chronic AVM lesion and suggested that there is a pre-existing language network that is malleable to change with structural reorganization due to chronic neuronal lesions.

Other researchers have demonstrated similar structural reorganization involving the motor cortex (Alkadhi et al., 2000). They examined six cases of AVMs located within the motor cortex with fMRI studies and found functional displacement of motor control in all six patients. For example, one patient with a right hemisphere AVM (located in the foot representation region of primary motor cortex, M1) showed activation in the ipsilateral M1 region, supplementary motor area (SMA), cingulate motor area (CMA), and in bilateral dorsal premotor and parietal areas (Alkadhi et al., 2000). They concluded that AVMs located in primary motor cortex were related to reorganization of motor function to primary and non-primary motor regions.

Conclusions

Arteriovenous malformations continue to provide researchers with information about reorganization and hemodynamics of the human brain. When an AVM has ruptured, the isolated, functional effect of AVM can no longer be studied. Therefore, future studies that wish to explain neurological/cognitive deficits associated with AVM must exclude ruptured AVMs. Future studies comparing the incidence of cognitive deficits associated with unruptured versus ruptured AVMs would also help neurologists, neuroradiologists, and surgeons to better assess the natural history risk to their AVM patients.

References

Alkadhi, H., Kollias, S. S., Crelier, G. R., Golay, X., Hepp-Reymond, M. C., & Valavanis, A. (2000). Plasticity of the human motor cortex in patients with arteriovenous malformations: a functional MR imaging study. *AJNR American Journal of Neuroradiology, 21*(8), 1423–1433.

AVM Study Group (1999). Arteriovenous malformations of the brain in adults. *The New England Journal of Medicine, 340*(23), 1812.

Baker, R. P., McCarter, R. J., & Porter, D. G. (2004). Improvement in cognitive function after right temporal arteriovenous malformation excision. *British Journal of Neurosurgery, 18*(5), 541–544.

Bambakidis, N. C., Sunshine, J. L., Faulhaber, P. F., Tarr, R. W., Selman, W. R., & Ratcheson, R. A. (2001). Functional evaluation of arteriovenous malformations. *Neurosurgical Focus, 11*(5), e2.

Brown, R. D., Jr., Wiebers, D. O., Forbes, G., O'Fallon, W. M., Piepgras, D. G., Marsh, W. R., et al. (1988). The natural history of unruptured intracranial arteriovenous malformations. *Journal of Neurosurgery, 68*(3), 352–357.

Brown, R. D., Jr., Wiebers, D. O., & Forbes, G. S. (1990). Unruptured intracranial aneurysms and arteriovenous malformations: frequency of intracranial hemorrhage and relationship of lesions. *Journal of Neurosurgery, 73*(6), 859–863.

Brown, R. D., Jr., Wiebers, D. O., Torner, J. C., & O'Fallon, W. M. (1996). Frequency of intracranial hemorrhage as a presenting symptom and subtype analysis: a population-based study of intracranial vascular malformations in Olmsted Country, Minnesota. *Journal of Neurosurgery, 85*(1), 29–32.

Buklina, S. B. (2001). Memory impairment and deep brain structures. *Neuroscience and Behavioral Physiology, 31*(2), 171–177.

Buklina, S. B. (2002). The unilateral spatial neglect phenomenon in patients with arteriovenous malformations of deep brain structures. *Neuroscience and Behavioral Physiology, 32*(6), 555–560.

Burchiel, K. J., Clarke, H., Ojemann, G. A., Dacey, R. G., & Winn, H. R. (1989). Use of stimulation mapping and corticography in the excision of arteriovenous malformations in sensorimotor and language-related neocortex. *Neurosurgery, 24*(3), 322–327.

Cannestra, A. F., Pouratian, N., Forage, J., Bookheimer, S. Y., Martin, N. A., & Toga, A. W. (2004). Functional magnetic resonance imaging and optical imaging for dominant-hemisphere perisylvian arteriovenous malformations. *Neurosurgery, 55*(4), 804–812; discussion 812–804.

Choi, J. H., & Mohr, J. P. (2005). Brain arteriovenous malformations in adults. *Lancet Neurology, 4*(5), 299–308.

Cloft, H. J., Joseph, G. J., & Dion, J. E. (1999). Risk of cerebral angiography in patients with subarachnoid hemorrhage, cerebral aneurysm, and arteriovenous malformation: a meta-analysis. *Stroke, 30*(2), 317–320.

Diehl, R. R., Henkes, H., Nahser, H. C., Kuhne, D., & Berlit, P. (1994). Blood flow velocity and vasomotor reactivity in patients with arteriovenous malformations. A transcranial Doppler study. *Stroke, 25*(8), 1574–1580.

Drake, C. G. (1979). Cerebral arteriovenous malformations: considerations for and experience with surgical treatment in 166 cases. *Clinical Neurosurgery, 26*, 145–208.

Duong, D. H., Young, W. L., Vang, M. C., Sciacca, R. R., Mast, H., Koennecke, H. C., et al. (1998). Feeding artery pressure and venous drainage pattern are primary determinants of hemorrhage from cerebral arteriovenous malformations. *Stroke, 29*(6), 1167–1176.

Festa, J. R., Lazar, R. M., Marshall, R. S., Pile-Spellman, J., Chong, J. Y., & Duong, H. (2004). Dural arteriovenous fistula presents like an ischemic stroke. *Cognitive and Behavioral Neurology, 17*(1), 50–53.

Fitzsimmons, B. F., Marshall, R. S., Pile-Spellman, J., & Lazar, R. M. (2003). Neurobehavioral differences in superselective Wada testing with amobarbital versus lidocaine. *AJNR American Journal of Neuroradiology, 24*(7), 1456–1460.

Fogarty-Mack, P., Pile-Spellman, J., Hacein-Bey, L., Osipov, A., DeMeritt, J., Jackson, E. C., et al. (1996). The effect of arteriovenous malformations on the distribution of intracerebral arterial pressures. *AJNR American Journal of Neuroradiology, 17*(8), 1443–1449.

Frishberg, B. M. (1994). The utility of neuroimaging in the evaluation of headache in patients with normal neurologic examinations. *Neurology, 44*(7), 1191–1197.

Frishberg, B. M. (1997). Neuroimaging in presumed primary headache disorders. *Seminars in Neurology, 17*(4), 373–382.

Furlan, A. J., Whisnant, J. P., & Elveback, L. R. (1979). The decreasing incidence of primary intracerebral hemorrhage: a population study. *Annals of Neurology, 5*(4), 367–373.

Garrido, E., & Stein, B. (1978). Removal of an arteriovenous malformation from the basal ganglion. *Journal of Neurology, Neurosurgery, and Psychiatry, 41*(11), 992–995.

Ghossoub, M., Nataf, F., Merienne, L., Devaux, B., Turak, B., & Roux, F. X. (2001). Characteristics of headache associated with cerebral arteriovenous malformations. *Neurochirurgie, 47*(2–3 Pt 2), 177–183.

Goodglass, H., & Kaplan, E. (1983). *Boston Diagnostic Aphasia Examination (BDAE)*. Philidelphia: Lea & Febiger.

Graeb, D. A., & Dolman, C. L. (1986). Radiological and pathological aspects of dural arteriovenous fistulas. Case report. *Journal of Neurosurgery, 64*(6), 962–967.

Graf, C. J., Perret, G. E., & Torner, J. C. (1983). Bleeding from cerebral arteriovenous malformations as part of their natural history. *Journal of Neurosurgery, 58*(3), 331–337.

Gross, C. R., Kase, C. S., Mohr, J. P., Cunningham, S. C., & Baker, W. E. (1984). Stroke in south Alabama: incidence and diagnostic features – a population based study. *Stroke, 15*(2), 249–255.

Guo, W. Y., Lee, S. M., Chang, Y. C., & Pan, H. C. (2006). The impact of arteriovenous malformation radiosurgery on the brain: From morphology and perfusion to neurocognition. *Stereotactic and Functional Neurosurgery, 84*(4), 162–169.

Hashimoto, H., Iida, J., Kawaguchi, S., & Sakaki, T. (2004). Clinical features and management of brain arteriovenous malformations in elderly patients. *Acta Neurochirurgica (Wien), 146*(10), 1091–1098; discussion 1098.

Hashimoto, T., Lawton, M. T., Wen, G., Yang, G. Y., Chaly, T., Jr., Stewart, C. L., et al. (2004). Gene microarray analysis of human brain arteriovenous malformations. *Neurosurgery, 54*(2), 410–423; discussion 423–415.

Heros, R. C., Korosue, K., & Diebold, P. M. (1990). Surgical excision of cerebral arteriovenous malformations: late results. *Neurosurgery, 26*(4), 570–577; discussion 577–578.

Hillman, J. (2001) Population-based analysis of arteriovenous malformation treatment. *Journal of Neurosurgery, 95*(4), 633–637.

Hofmeister, C., Stapf, C., Hartmann, A., Sciacca, R. R., Mansmann, U., terBrugge, K., et al. (2000). Demographic, morphological, and clinical characteristics of 1289 patients with brain arteriovenous malformation. *Stroke, 31*(6), 1307–1310.

Hoh, B. L., Chapman, P. H., Loeffler, J. S., Carter, B. S., & Ogilvy, C. S. (2002). Results of multimodality treatment for 141 patients with brain arteriovenous malformations and seizures: factors associated with seizure incidence and seizure outcomes. *Neurosurgery, 51*(2), 303–309; discussion 309–311.

Hurst, R. W., Bagley, L. J., Galetta, S., Glosser, G., Lieberman, A. P., Trojanowski, J., et al. (1998). Dementia resulting from dural arteriovenous fistulas: the pathologic findings of venous hypertensive encephalopathy. *AJNR American Journal of Neuroradiology, 19*(7), 1267–1273.

Ito, M., Sonokawa, T., Mishina, H., & Sato, K. (1995). Reversible dural arteriovenous malformation-induced venous ischemia as a cause of dementia: treatment by surgical occlusion of draining dural sinus: case report. *Neurosurgery, 37*(6), 1187–1191; discussion 1191–1182.

Iwama, T., Hayashida, K., Takahashi, J. C., Nagata, I., & Hashimoto, N. (2002). Cerebral hemodynamics and metabolism in patients with cerebral arteriovenous malformations: an evaluation using positron emission tomography scanning. *Journal of Neurosurgery, 97*(6), 1314–1321.

Klimo, P. Jr., Rao, G., & Brockmeyer, D. (2007). Pediatric arteriovenous malformations: a 15-year experience with an emphasis on residual and recurrent lesions. *Child's Nervous System, 23*(1), 31–37.

Kloster, R. (1997). Subarachnoid hemorrhage in Vestfold county. Occurrence and prognosis. *Tidsskr Nor Laegeforen, 117*(13), 1879–1882.

Kondziolka, D., McLaughlin, M.R. & Kestle, J.R. (1995). Simple risk predictions for arteriovenous malformation hemorrhage. *Neurosurgery, 37*(5), 851–855.

Kumar, A. J., Fox, A. J., Vinuela, F., & Rosenbaum, A. E. (1984). Revisited old and new CT findings in unruptured larger arteriovenous malformations of the brain. *Journal of Computer Assisted Tomography, 8*(4), 648–655.

Kumar, K., Malik, S., & Demeria, D. (2002). Treatment of chronic pain with spinal cord stimulation versus alternative therapies: cost-effectiveness analysis. *Neurosurgery, 51*(1), 106–115; discussion 115–106.

Kurl, S., Saari, T., Vanninen, R., & Hernesniemi, J. (1996). Dural arteriovenous fistulas of superior sagittal sinus: case report and review of literature. *Surgical Neurology, 45*(3), 250–255.

Langer, D. J., Lasner, T. M., Hurst, R. W., Flamm, E. S., Zager, E. L., & King, J. T., Jr. (1998). Hypertension, small size, and deep venous drainage are associated with risk of hemorrhagic presentation of cerebral arteriovenous malformations. *Neurosurgery, 42*(3), 481–486; discussion 487–489.

Lazar, R. M., Connaire, K., Marshall, R. S., Pile-Spellman, J., Hacein-Bey, L., Solomon, R. A., et al. (1999). Developmental deficits in adult patients with arteriovenous malformations. *Archives of Neurology, 56*(1), 103–106.

Lazar, R. M., Marshall, R. S., Pile-Spellman, J., Duong, H. C., Mohr, J. P., Young, W. L., et al. (2000). Interhemispheric transfer of language in patients with left frontal cerebral arteriovenous malformation. *Neuropsychologia, 38*(10), 1325–1332.

Lazar, R. M., Marshall, R. S., Pile-Spellman, J., Hacein-Bey, L., Young, W. L., Mohr, J. P., et al. (1997). Anterior translocation of language in patients with left cerebral arteriovenous malformation. *Neurology, 49*(3), 802–808.

Lehericy, S., Biondi, A., Sourour, N., Vlaicu, M., du Montcel, S. T., Cohen, L., et al. (2002). Arteriovenous brain malformations: is functional MR imaging reliable for studying language reorganization in patients? Initial observations. *Radiology, 223*(3), 672–682.

Loring, D. W. (1999). *INS dictionary of neuropsychology*. New York, Oxford: Oxford University Press.

Lunsford, L. D., Kondziolka, D., Flickinger, J. C., Bissonette, D. J., Jungreis, C. A., Maitz, A. H., et al. (1991). Stereotactic radiosurgery for arteriovenous malformations of the brain. *Journal of Neurosurgery, 75*(4), 512–524.

Mahalick, D. M., Ruff, R. M., Heary, R. F., & U, H. S. (1993). Preoperative versus postoperative neuropsychological sequelae of arteriovenous malformations. *Neurosurgery, 33*(4), 563–570; discussion 570–561.

Maldjian, J., Atlas, S. W., Howard, R. S., II, Greenstein, E., Alsop, D., Detre, J. A., et al. (1996). Functional magnetic resonance imaging of regional brain activity in patients with intracerebral arteriovenous malformations before surgical or endovascular therapy. *Journal of Neurosurgery, 84*(3), 477–483.

Malik, G. M., Seyfried, D. M., & Morgan, J. K. (1996). Temporal lobe arteriovenous malformations: surgical management and outcome. *Surgical Neurology, 46*(2), 106–114; discussion 114–105.

Marshall, G. A., Jonker, B. P., Morgan, M. K., & Taylor, A. J. (2003). Prospective study of neuropsychological and psychosocial outcome following surgical excision of intracerebral arteriovenous malformations. *J Clin Neurosci, 10*(1), 42-47.

Mast, H., Mohr, J. P., Osipov, A., Pile-Spellman, J., Marshall, R. S., Lazar, R. M., et al. (1995). 'Steal' is an unestablished mechanism for the clinical presentation of cerebral arteriovenous malformations. *Stroke, 26*(7), 1215–1220.

Mast, H., Young, W. L., Koennecke, H. C., Sciacca, R. R., Osipov, A., Pile-Spellman, J., et al. (1997). Risk of spontaneous haemorrhage after diagnosis of cerebral arteriovenous malformation. *Lancet, 350*(9084), 1065–1068.

Matsuda, S., Waragai, M., Shinotoh, H., Takahashi, N., Takagi, K., & Hattori, T. (1999). Intracranial dural arteriovenous fistula (DAVF) presenting progressive dementia and parkinsonism. *Journal of the Neurological Sciences, 165*(1), 43–47.

McCormick, W. (1978). Classification, pathology, and natural history of the central nervous system. *Neurological Neurosurgery,* 14, 2–7.

McCormick, W. F. (1966). The pathology of vascular ("arteriovenous") malformations. *Journal of Neurosurgery, 24*(4), 807–816.

McCormick, W. F., & Rosenfield, D. B. (1973). Massive brain hemorrhage: a review of 144 cases and an examination of their causes. *Stroke, 4*(6), 946–954.

Meisel, H. J., Mansmann, U., Alvarez, H., Rodesch, G., Brock, M., & Lasjaunias, P. (2000). Cerebral arteriovenous malformations and associated aneurysms: analysis of 305 cases from a series of 662 patients. *Neurosurgery, 46*(4), 793–800; discussion 800–792.

Mohr, J. H., A., Mast, H., Pile-Spellman, J., Schumacher, H. C. & Stapf, C. (2004). Anteriovenous malformations and other vascular anomalies. In J. P. C. Mohr, D.W.; Grotta J.C.; Weir B., & Wolf P.A. (Eds.), *Stroke pathophysiology, diagnosis and management* (pp. 397–421). Philidelphia: Churchill Livingstone.

Murphy, J. (1954). Vascular tumors: Arteriovenous malformations of the brain. In Mohr J. P (Ed.), *Cerebrovascular Disease* (pp. 242–262). Chicago: Yearbook Medical Publishers.

Nagata, S., Morioka, T., Matsukado, K., Natori, Y., & Sasaki, T. (2006). Retrospective analysis of the surgically treated temporal lobe arteriovenous malformations with focus on the visual field defects and epilepsy. *Surgical Neurology, 66*(1), 50–55; discussion 55.

Newton, T. H., & Cronqvist, S. (1969). Involvement of dural arteries in intracranial arteriovenous malformations. *Radiology, 93*(5), 1071–1078.

O'Brien, P., Neyastani, A., Buckley, A. R., Chang, S. D., & Legiehn, G. M. (2006). Uterine arteriovenous malformations: from diagnosis to treatment. *Journal of Ultrasound in Medicine, 25*(11), 1387–1392.

Ogilvy, C. S. (1990). Radiation therapy for arteriovenous malformations: a review. *Neurosurgery, 26*(5), 725–735.

Ogilvy, C. S., Stieg, P. E., Awad, I., Brown, R. D., Jr., Kondziolka, D., Rosenwasser, R., et al. (2001). AHA Scientific Statement: Recommendations for the management of intracranial arteriovenous malformations: a statement for healthcare professionals from a special writing group of the Stroke Council, American Stroke Association. *Stroke, 32*(6), 1458–1471.

Ondra, S. L., Troupp, H., George, E. D., & Schwab, K. (1990). The natural history of symptomatic arteriovenous malformations of the brain: a 24-year follow-up assessment. *Journal of Neurosurgery, 73*(3), 387–391.

Pawlikowska, L., Tran, M. N., Achrol, A. S., McCulloch, C. E., Ha, C., Lind, D. L., et al. (2004). Polymorphisms in genes involved in inflammatory and angiogenic pathways and the risk of hemorrhagic presentation of brain arteriovenous malformations. *Stroke, 35*(10), 2294–2300.

Perret, G., & Nishioka, H. (1966). Report on the cooperative study of intracranial aneurysms and subarachnoid hemorrhage. Section VI. Arteriovenous malformations. An analysis of 545 cases of craniocerebral arteriovenous malformations and fistulae reported to the cooperative study. *Journal of Neurosurgery, 25*(4), 467–490.

Piepgras, D. G., Sundt, T. M., Jr., Ragoowansi, A. T., & Stevens, L. (1993). Seizure outcome in patients with surgically treated cerebral arteriovenous malformations. *Journal of Neurosurgery, 78*(1), 5–11.

Redekop, G., TerBrugge, K., Montanera, W., & Willinsky, R. (1998). Arterial aneurysms associated with cerebral arteriovenous malformations: classification, incidence, and risk of hemorrhage. *Journal of Neurosurgery, 89*(4), 539–546.

Richling, B., Killer, M., Al-Schameri, A. R., Ritter, L., Agic, R., & Krenn, M. (2006). Therapy of brain arteriovenous malformations: multimodality treatment from a balanced standpoint. *Neurosurgery, 59*(5 Suppl 3), S148–S157.

Riina, H. A., & Gobin, Y. P. (2001). Grading and surgical planning for intracranial arteriovenous malformations. *Neurosurgical Focus, 11*(5), e3.

Ruiz-Sandoval, J. L., Cantu, C., & Barinagarrementeria, F. (1999). Intracerebral hemorrhage in young people: analysis of risk factors, location, causes, and prognosis. *Stroke*, *30*(3), 537-541.

Spetzler, R. F., Hargraves, R. W., McCormick, P. W., Zabramski, J. M., Flom, R. A., & Zimmerman, R. S. (1992). Relationship of perfusion pressure and size to risk of hemorrhage from arteriovenous malformations. *Journal of Neurosurgery*, *76*(6), 918–923.

Spetzler, R. F., Martin, N. A., Carter L. P., Flom, R. A., Raudzens, P. A., & Wilkinson, E. (1987). Surgical management of large AVM's by staged embolization and operative excision. *Journal of Neurosurgery*, *67*(1), 17–28.

Spetzler, R. F., & Martin, N. A. (1986). A proposed grading system for arteriovenous malformations. *Journal of Neurosurgery*, *65*(4), 476–483.

St George, E. J., Butler, P., & Plowman, P. N. (2002). Can magnetic resonance imaging alone accurately define the arteriovenous nidus for gamma knife radiosurgery? *Journal of Neurosurgery*, *97*(5 Suppl), 464–470.

Stabell, K. E., & Nornes, H. (1994). Prospective neuropsychological investigation of patients with supratentorial arteriovenous malformations. *Acta Neurochirurgica (Wien)*, *131*(1–2), 32–44.

Stapf, C., Mast, H., Sciacca, R. R., Choi, J. H., Khaw, A. V., Connolly, E. S., et al. (2006a). Predictors of hemorrhage in patients with untreated brain arteriovenous malformation. *Neurology*, *66*(9), 1350–1355.

Stapf, C., Mohr, J. P., Choi, J. H., Hartmann, A., & Mast, H. (2006b). Invasive treatment of unruptured brain arteriovenous malformations is experimental therapy. *Current Opinion in Neurology*, *19*(1), 63–68.

Stapf, C., Mohr, J. P., Pile-Spellman, J., Solomon, R. A., Sacco, R. L., & Connolly, E. S., Jr. (2001). Epidemiology and natural history of arteriovenous malformations. *Neurosurgery Focus*, *11*(5), e1.

Steiner, L., & Lindquist, C. (1987). *Radiosurgery in cerebral arteriovenous malformation*. Philidelphia: Hanley and Belfus, Inc.

Steinvorth, S., Wenz, F., Wildermuth, S., Essig, M., Fuss, M., Lohr, F., et al. (2002). Cognitive function in patients with cerebral arteriovenous malformations after radiosurgery: prospective long-term follow-up. *International Journal of Radiation Oncology, Biology, Physics*, *54*(5), 1430–1437.

Takemori, A. E. (1992). Opioid pharmacology a'la mode. *NIDA Research Monograph*, *119*, 21–26.

Tanaka, K., Morooka, Y., Nakagawa, Y., & Shimizu, S. (1999). Dural arteriovenous malformation manifesting as dementia due to ischemia in bilateral thalami. A case report. *Surgical Neurology*, *51*(5), 489–493; discussion 493-484.

Turjman, F., Massoud, T. F., Sayre, J. W., Vinuela, F., Guglielmi, G., & Duckwiler, G. (1995). Epilepsy associated with cerebral arteriovenous malformations: a multivariate analysis of angioarchitectural characteristics. *AJNR American Journal of Neuroradiology*, *16*(2), 345–350.

Tyler, J. L., Leblanc, R., Meyer, E., Dagher, A., Yamamoto, Y. L., Diksic, M., & Hakim, A. (1989). Hemodynamic and metabolic effects of cerebral arteriovenous malformations studied by positron emission tomography. *Stroke*, *20*(7), 890–898.

Unla, E., Teminzoz, O., Abayram, S., Genchellac, H., Hamamcioglu, M. K., Kurt, I., et al. (2006). Contrast-enhanced MR 3D angiography in the assessment of brain AVMs. *European Journal of Radiology*, *60* (3), 367–378.

Van Roost, D., & Schramm, J. (2001). What factors are related to impairment of cerebrovascular reserve before and after arteriovenous malformation resection? A cerebral blood flow study using xenon-enhanced computed tomography. *Neurosurgery*, *48*(4), 709–716; discussion 716–707.

Warren, D. J., Hoggard, N., Walton, L., Radatz, M. W., Kemeny, A. A., Forster, D. M., et al. (2001). Cerebral arteriovenous malformations: comparison of novel magnetic resonance angiographic techniques and conventional catheter angiography. *Neurosurgery*, *48*(5), 973–982; discussion 982–973.

Wechsler, D. (1987). *Weschler Memory Scale: revised manual*. San Antonio: Psychological Corporation/ Harcourt Brace Jovanovich.

Wenz, F., Steinvorth, S., Wildermuth, S., Lohr, F., Fuss, M., Debus, J., et al. (1998). Assessment of neuropsychological changes in patients with arteriovenous malformation (AVM) after radiosurgery. *International Journal of Radiation Oncology, Biology, Physics*, *42*(5), 995–999.

Whigham, K. B., & O'Toole, K. (2007). Understanding the neuropsychologic outcome of pediatric AVM within a neurodevelopmental framework. *Cognitive and Behavioral Neurology*, *20*(4), 244–257.

Yamada, S., Liwnicz, B., Lonser, R. R., & Knierim, D. (1999). Scanning electron microscopy of arteriovenous malformations. *Neurology Research*, *21*(6), 541–544.

Yeh, H. S., Tew, J. M. & Gartner, M. (1993). Seizure control after surgery on arteriovenous malformations. *Journal of Neurosurgery*, *78*(1), 12–18.

Zeidman, S. M., Monsein, L. H., Arosarena, O., Aletich, V., Biafore, J. A., Dawson, R. C., et al. (1995). Reversibility of white matter changes and dementia after treatment of dural fistulas. *AJNR American Journal of Neuroradiology*, *16*(5), 1080–1083.

Chapter 6
Vascular Cognitive Impairment

David J. Libon, Catherine C. Price, Rodney A. Swenson, Dana Penney, Bret Haake, and Alfio Pennisi

Introduction

Vascular Cognitive Impairment or VCI can be compared to the proverbial blind men palpating the elephant. Sometimes the "parts" appear to be diverse and disparate. Thus, VCI tends to mean different things to different people. Despite this diversity of opinions, the study of vascular brain disease has a long and quite distinguished history in neurology.

A fundamental issue regarding mild cognitive impairment associated with vascular disease is the ultimate relationship of VCI to vascular dementia (VaD). Here is when a simple palpation of the "parts" may cause confusion. In this chapter we do not necessarily draw a definitive line that separates VCI from VaD. The exact relationship between these entities is a work in progress. Nonetheless, it is very clear that VCI and VaD are opposite sides of the same coin.

This chapter will be divided into five parts. First, we present a short historical perspective of vascular disease as related to VCI. The second part of this chapter will review some of the epidemiological studies that have identified and followed patients with mild cognitive disability, but without dementia. Next, we review the neuropsychological literature as it relates

to VCI. This is followed by a discussion of recent findings associating biomarkers with VCI. Finally, the last part of this chapter will address public health and treatment issues.

Vascular Cognitive Impairment: Historical and Modern Perspectives

During the 19th century and until the middle of the 20th century, problems related to vascular disease were the focus of considerable interest in clinical neurology. Dementia associated with vascular disease versus syphilis was a major diagnostic problem and considerable effort was devoted toward the description of a variety of vascular syndromes (see Libon, Price, Heilman, & Grossman, 2006 for a review). For example, as early as the 1830s, Durand-Fardel (Hauw, 1995) described a number of vascular syndromes including lacunar infarcts, etat crible, and atrophe interstitelle du cerveau. Durand-Fardel's purpose was to show how these vascular syndromes were different from vascular lesions associated with haemorrhages and large infarcts. For Durand-Fardel (Hauw, 1995), a lacune represented a small cavity in the brain and he believed these lesions were healed infarcts. Durand-Fardel's used the etat crible or "sieve-like state" to describe sections of the subcortical white matter that "were riddled with a number of little holes, with sharp edges, usually surrounded by

D.J. Libon (✉)
Department of Neurology, Drexel Medical College
MS 423, 245 N. 15th St Phil, PA 19102
e-mail: dlibon@drexelmed.edu

J.R. Festa, R.M. Lazar (eds.), *Neurovascular Neuropsychology*, DOI 10.1007/978-0-387-70715-0_6,
© Springer Science+Business Media, LLC 2009

a quite normal white matter, without any change in color or consistency" (Hauw, 1995). Finally, the term atrophe interstitelle du cerveau or interstitial atrophy of the brain represented, "alterations of the cerebral pulp different from infarctions not due to a change in the consistency of the brain but a rarefaction of the pulp." It has been pointed out (Hauw, 1995) that Durand-Fardel's atrophe interstitelle du cerveau is similar to the modern description of leukoaraiosis (Hachinski, Meresky, & Potter, 1987).

The work of early French neurologists stressed macroscopic, as well as histological phenomena, rather than the clinical observations that might be associated with vascular syndromes. Nonetheless, our current experience suggests mild cognitive and functional deficits are often seen in conjunction with all three of these vascular syndromes. In this sense the work done in the 19th and early 20th centuries can be viewed as part of the foundation for the concept of VCI.

It is a little known fact that Alzheimer wrote many more papers on VaD than on pre-senile dementia (Libon et al., 2006). Several of these papers have been translated. In a report published in 1895, Alzheimer demonstrated how arteriosclerotic degeneration of the brain can be distinguished from general paresis. In this paper many of the clinical features we now commonly associate with multi-infarct dementia (MID) were discussed. In 1898, Alzheimer described a variety of vascular syndromes. Included in this nosology was Alzheimer's description of arteriosclerotic brain atrophy. For Alzheimer this syndrome included "a step-wise deterioration with shorter or longer intervals." Alterations in personality, the appearance of depression, and the presence of focal neurological signs were emphasized. Alzheimer's 1902 paper entitled "Mental Disturbances of Arteriosclerotic Origin" is interesting in that not only did he describe dementia associated with subcortical white matter disease, he anticipated the more modern differentiation between cortical and subcortical dementia. For example, Alzheimer described

memory impairment associated with subcortical white matter disease as a retrieval deficit, i.e., "difficulty in retrieving certain ideas, and not a true deficit." Alzheimer also associated "prolonged reaction times" (i.e., bradyphrenia) with subcortical white matter dementia. Alzheimer's clinical observations regarding vascular disease continue to be relevant today.

The modern history of VCI dates from the work of Hachinski and colleagues (Bowler 2004; Bowler, 2005; Bowler & Hachinski, 1995; Devasenapathy & Hachinski, 2000; Hachinski, 1994). Hachinski et al. do not use the term VCI to identify a prodromal state of what might evolve into a VaD. Rather, VCI is used to describe a broad continuum of alterations in cognition and functional abilities including mild and/or prodromal states to frank dementia associated with vascular disease or vascular risk factors. Several reasons define Hachinski's rationale for the introduction of the term VCI. First, the clinical presentation of vascular states as related to putative alterations in cognition and functional disabilities is quite heterogeneous. For this reason, existing nomenclature associated with current diagnostic criteria for VaD does not necessarily capture the rich and diverse clinical presentation of vascular states. Second, Hachinski noted that cerebrovascular and cardiovascular risk factors can, in many cases, be easily identified. As an extension to the identification of cerebrovascular and cardiovascular risk factors, treatment that may have a meaningful effect on the course of an illness can be instituted. Third, Hachinski and colleagues reject the *"Alzheimerization"* of dementia. This speaks to the notions that most cases of dementia must present with evidence of a primary (encoding) memory disorder and are associated with histopathological evidence of a neurodegenerative illness. Vascular disease, when identified, is marginalized as an epiphenomenon. At present, Hachinski and colleagues have not defined specific criteria for the diagnosis of VCI.

Recently the term VCI has come to mean different things to different people. Drawing on data from the Consortium to Investigate Vascular Impairment of Cognition, Rockwood et al. (2003) echo all of the points raised by Hachinski and colleagues. Using a statistical modeling method, Song et al. (2005) were able to identify and measure a variety of risk factors associating VCI with individual and separate clinical characteristics. This methodology has been developed into a paradigm that has been able to separate patients presenting with AD versus a mixed AD/VaD profile versus VCI (Rockwood, Black et al., 2006). Roman (2004) and Roman, Sachdev et al. (2004) tend to agree with many of the points originally put forth by Hachinski et al. However, they substitute the term "vascular cognitive disorder" (VCD) to describe the continuum of mild or prodromal to frank dementia as associated with vascular disease. Roman suggest reserving the term VCI to describe situations when vascular disease is only associated with mild changes in cognition do not meet criteria for dementia. This perspective is echoed by Erkinjuntti and Rockwood (2003).

The current lack of consensus whether the term VCI should be utilized to describe either mild or prodromal clinical states or used to describe the entire continuum of alterations in cognitive and functional abilities associated with vascular disease needs to be resolved.

Empirical Support for the Construct of VCI

Data supporting the validity of VCI as a construct may be derived from several sources: (1) research demonstrating differences in the rate and presentation of mild/prodromal cognitive impairment to the emergence of VaD versus conversion to Alzheimer's disease (AD); (2) research associating vascular risk factors with the eventual emergence of dementia; and (3) research demonstrating a unique cognitive profile associated with mild/prodromal vascular states.

Conversion from Mild Cognitive Disability to Dementia

A number of studies have attempted to identify and separate individuals presenting with a prodromal VaD versus AD and document differential rates of conversion to an actual dementia syndrome. For example, several studies have found that the annual conversion rate for AD was higher when compared to the rate for VaD (Huang et al., 2005; Zhang et al., 2005). Similar findings were reported by Luis and colleagues (2004) and Meyer and colleagues (2002). Both studies reported an almost two to one higher rate of conversion to AD versus VaD. Solfrizzi and colleagues (2004) analyzed data from the Italian Longitudinal Study on Aging. They also found that conversion from a state of mild cognitive dysfunction to dementia was almost three times greater for AD versus VaD.

By contrast, Xu and colleagues (2004) studied individuals in China and the United States with mild cognitive deficits. Participants from China were more likely to develop VaD than AD. However, the reverse was found for people in the United States. Zanetti and colleagues (2006) conducted a population study and identified individuals with amnesic versus vascular mild cognitive impairment. The amnesic group was characterized by poor performance on tests of memory while the vascular group was characterized by slower time to completion on tests of information processing speed (Trail Making Test—Part B) and reduced output on tests of letter fluency. Upon follow-up most patients in the amnesic and vascular groups went on to develop AD and VaD, respectively.

In sum, these studies suggest that the course that ultimately leads to a clinical diagnosis of AD versus VaD differ. The pathway that ultimately leads to AD is likely more homogenous than VaD. A wide variety of medical risk factors may underlie the eventual evolution of a mild cognitive or functional disability into VaD. From a statistical perspective the differential conversion of mild cognitive disabilities to VaD may be associated with greater variability.

Mild Cognitive Disabilities and Vascular Risk Factors

Several studies have attempted to evaluate the relationship between risk factors for stroke and the evolution to dementia. Prencipe and colleagues (2003) studied a group from a rural Italian community with mild cognitive deficits but no dementia and found that 20% of this population had a history of prior stroke and hypertension which were associated with VCI. This suggests that VCI may be more common that generally appreciated. In another Italian study, Di Carlo and colleagues (2000) reported similar results demonstrating a history of prior stroke and heart failure was associated with the eventual presentation of dementia. Echoing the sentiments of Hachinski and colleagues, these authors note the early identification of individuals with potential VCI may offer an opportunity for treatment.

Cognitive Tests Predicting Conversion of VCI to VaD

Some of the original research documenting conversion to AD suggests that before actual dementia develops, isolated memory impairment can be present (Albert et al., 2002). However, more recent research regarding this issue demonstrates notably variable results. For example, Jones and colleagues (2004) found MMSE delayed memory test performance was equally associated with conversion to both AD and VaD. However, in a population-based study conducted in Gottenborg, Sweden, designed to address this issue, Sacuiu and colleagues (2005) did not find any association between specific memory impairment and conversion to either VaD or AD. Rather, prelude to both dementia syndromes was associated with low scores on multiple areas of cognitive functioning. In another population-based study, van den Heuvel and colleagues (2006) found that MRI evidence of periventricular white matter alterations and reduced scores on tests of information processing speed, including a Digit Symbol Substitution Test were associated with the eventual diagnosis of VaD. Data from the Sydney Older Persons Study presented by Waite and colleagues (2005) found persons initially presenting with a gait disorder and motor slowing were more likely to eventually develop dementia. Ingles, Wentzel, Fisk, & Rockwood (2002) identified a group of individuals believed to be presenting with vascular cognitive impairment but no dementia. They found low baseline performance on tests of category fluency and memory predicted the eventual emergence of dementia. However, these authors also noted they were unable to find any differential neuropsychological test performance that predicted the eventual emergence of VaD versus AD.

The variability reported in these studies is likely due to multiple factors. First, there is over reliance on the MMSE. The MMSE was never intended to be used in this kind of research and is a poor choice as an outcome measure. Second, the plethora of neuropsychological tests used from study to study places some limits on the external validity of these studies. Tests that assess working memory and information processing speed have consistently been shown to differentiate patients with AD from VaD (Lamar, Price, Davis, Kaplan, & Libon, et al., 2002; Lamar, Price, Libon et al., 2007). It is likely that such neuropsychological tests might also be useful in identifying persons with VCI.

Neuropsychology of VCI

One consistent finding that has emerged over the last several years is the dissociation between VaD and AD such that patients with VaD tend to present with greater impairment on tests of executive control, visuoconstruction, and information processing speed, whereas AD patients present with worse performance on tests of declarative memory and certain tests related to lexical retrieval (Libon, Bogdanoff, et al., 1998; Libon, Price, Garrett, & Giovannetti 2004; Price et al., 2005; Desmond, 2004). Findings reported by Wolfe, Linn, Babikian, Knoefel, and Albert (1990) and Ishii, Nishihara, & Imamura (1986) also associated greater impairment on executive control tests with patients presenting with subcortical lacunes. However, it is likely many of these patients were, in fact, demented. The issue at hand is whether this dissociation regarding executive control and related cognitive functions versus memory and lexical retrieval can also distinguish persons with mild cognitive disabilities who go on to develop either VaD or AD.

VCI and Post-Stroke Cognitive Disabilities

Similar to findings reported by Wolfe and colleagues (1990) and Ishii and colleagues (1986), patients who present with evidence of prior stroke, but who do not fulfill criteria for an actual dementia, appear to be disadvantaged on tests related to executive control. Kramer, Reed, Mungas, Weiner, & Chui (2002) examined a group of patients who had suffered one or more strokes. Compared to a control group, patients with prior stroke obtained low scores on tests of processing speed and inhibition (Stroop Test), concept formation (California Card Sort Test), and the initiation-perseveration portion of the Mattis Dementia Rating Scale. No differences were noted on tests of language or memory. Poor performance on these executive control measures were also positively correlated with periventricular and deep white matter alterations. In a follow-up study this same research group (Reed et al., 2004) found that subcortical lacunes correlated with reduced activity in the dorsolateral prefrontal cortex. Reduced dorsolateral prefrontal activity was also selectively correlated with poorer performance on executive tests.

Stephens and colleagues (2004) also studied a non-demented post-stroke group and found that patients who had suffered stroke were differentially impaired on tests of executive control and serial reaction time. However, the post-stroke group also displayed impairment on tests of memory and expressive language functioning. Stephens and colleagues also found that activities of daily living (ADL) were reduced among patients with post-stroke VCI. Nyenhuis and colleagues (2004) used logistic regression analysis and were able to show that non-demented post-stroke patients could also be classified on the basis of slower performance on tests related to information processing speed and memory. Jokinen and colleagues (2006) also found a combination of reduced performance on tests of executive control and delayed memory best characterized their sample of non-demented post-stroke patients. Few studies have addressed the association between post-stroke VCI and ADL.

VCI and Subcortical White Matter Disease

A variety of studies have examined patients with mild cognitive deficits associated with MRI evidence of subcortical white matter disease. Consistent with studies that have looked at dementia patients with significant white matter disease, differential impairment on a wide number of executive control tests have been reported in non-demented patients presenting with subcortical white matter hyperintensities. For example, Garrett and colleagues (2004) found that poor performances on tests of cognitive flexibility, lexical retrieval, and delayed recognition memory were associated with non-demented patients presenting with subcortical white matter disease. Sachdev and colleagues (2004) assessed many VCI patients with evidence of prior stroke or TIAs. These patients obtained lower scores on tests of abstraction, mental flexibility, working memory, and information processing speed when compared to controls. There was a higher correlation between impairment on executive control tests and MRI deep white matter hyperintensities as defined by the number or volume of infarcts. De Jager and colleagues (2003) also found that performance on tests of attention and information processing speed best discriminated non-demented patients with cerebrovascular disease from control participants.

Past research has demonstrated that patients with VaD associated with subcortical white matter disease performed worse on tests of letter fluency versus tests of semantic fluency such as the "animal" fluency tasks (see Carew, Lamar, Cloud, & Libon, 1997 for a review). Caninng and colleagues (2004) also reported that patients with VCI associated with subcortical white matter disease generated fewer exemplars to the letter "F" versus output when as generating animal exemplars. Frisoni and colleagues (2002) studied patients with both mild amnesic and vascular cognitive deficits. Patients with VCI presented with reduced output on tests of letter fluency tests. Interestingly, of those patients followed for more than three years, many patients with VCI died, whereas no patients with amnesic cognitive impairment died. Galluzzi, Sheu, Zanetti, and Frisoni (2005) also found that reduced output on tests of letter fluency characterized a dysexecutive syndrome of non-demented patients presenting with subcortical white matter disease. Electrophysiological measures are a novel way to assess the effects of subcortical white matter disease. van Harten and colleagues (2006) found that N2 latencies were significantly slower in their sample of non-dementia patients with subcortical white matter disease. No differences were found regarding the P3 or N1 latencies. Electrophysiological measures were not correlated with neuropsychological performances. Unfortunately the authors did not address how their findings relate to earlier work reporting greater working memory and executive deficits among patients with vascular disease (Libon, Price, Garrett et al., 2004; Lamar, Price, Libon et al., in press).

In sum, the literature on profiles of neuropsychological deficits associated with suspected VCI generally supports the notion of differential impairment on tests of executive control for patients with subcortical CVA and subcortical white matter disease. However, the neuropsychological tests employed in these studies are quite variable. The exact relationship between performance on executive tests and performance on neuropsychological tests measuring other domains of cognition are lacking. Finally, virtually all prior studies have been empirical in nature. Thus, an explanation of the cognitive constructs or mechanisms that underlie or explain why subcortical vascular disease results in differential executive impairment is lacking. In this regard the imaging and electrophysiological literature cited above offer some intriguing possibilities.

Biomarkers for Vascular Cognitive Impairment

Recently there has been interest in a variety of physiological biomarkers and their ability to identify individuals who may be either clinically diagnosed with VCI and/or predict the eventual onset of dementia. In this section, we will review some of the recent literature related to the assessment of arterial integrity as well as a number of blood or fluid biomarkers.

Arterial Integrity and VCI

There has been recent interest in measuring intima-media thickness to obtain a measure of carotid stenosis. Johnston and colleagues (2004) studied patients without any history of stroke, TIA, or prior carotid endarterectomy and found an association between left but not right-sided carotid stenosis and decline in cognitive functioning. The authors argued that their finding suggests a direct link between carotid stenosis and cognitive functioning rather than carotid stenosis as a marker for vascular disease. The authors suggested the agency by which carotid disease is associated with a decline in cognitive function may be generalized atherosclerosis.

Talelli and colleagues (2004) conducted a similar study focusing on non-demented patients with prior stroke to see if carotid artery intima-media thickness could be associated with a decline in cognitive functioning 1 year after stroke. Their cognitive outcome measure was the MMSE. These authors found a significant association between intima-media thickness and lower scores on the MMSE. This association remained even after adjusting for vascular risk factors. The results of both of these studies suggest an evaluation of carotid-intima-media thickness may be helpful in screening patients at risk for VCI and stroke.

Carotid-femoral pulse wave velocity (PWV) is another technique used to assess arterial integrity. Several research groups have used PWV as a measure of arterial "stiffness." Scuteri, Brancati, Gianni, Assisi, & Volpe (2005) evaluated patients seen in an outpatient memory clinic with no prior history of stroke. They found inverse relationships between increased PWV or compromised arterial integrity and lower scores on the MMSE as well as reduced scores on the Lawton and Brody (1969) Instrumental Activities of daily Living (IADL) Scale. A similar study was conducted by Hanon and colleagues (2005), who studied patients with AD, VaD, and mild cognitive deficits associated with either memory or executive dysfunction. Arterial stiffness was measured by carotid-femoral PWV. PWV was higher (suggesting greater arterial stiffness) in non-demented patients with mild cognitive deficits compared to a control group. An inverse relationship between PWV and the lower scores on the MMSE was also reported. Nagai and colleagues (2004) reported a negative correlation between brachial ankle PMV and the MMSE among VCI participants.

These types of biomarkers are relatively inexpensive and non-invasive. Combining information derived from these techniques with comprehensive neuropsychological assessment and information derived from MRI studies could offer more insight into the interaction between vascular anatomy and cognitive functioning. Also, longitudinal studies using these techniques have yet to be carried out. Nonetheless, these research paradigms show promise that an analysis of arterial integrity might be an effective biomarker for VCI and/VaD.

Blood Biomarkers and VCI

There has been increasing interest in role of impaired antioxidant enzymatic activity as a factor associated with mild or prodromal cognitive dysfunction as well as dementia (Guidi et al., 2006). Quadri and colleagues (2004) reported an association between hyperhomocysteinemia (tHcy) and VCI. Specifically, they found for patients with mild cognitive deficits (i.e., clinical dementia rating = 0.5), reduced scores on the MMSE were associated with elevated tHcy levels. Ravaglia and colleagues (2004) studied a group of healthy community dwelling participants and also found an association between elevated tHcy levels and reduced scores on the MMSE as well as lower output on tests of letter fluency. These studies suggest that elevations in tHcy may be a marker for VCI/VaD under some circumstances.

The presence of the APOE epsilon4 allele has traditionally been viewed as risk factor for AD. However, data from the Rotterdam Study has associated the presence of the APOE 4 allele and atherosclerosis in AD (Hofman et al., 1997). de Leeuw and colleagues (2004) also studied a cohort of participants from the Rotterdam Study. They found an association between MRI subcortical white matter disease and the presence of both APOE 4 alleles. Participants with both hypertension and at least one APOE 4 allele presented with significantly greater MRI subcortical as well as deep white matter disease. These authors postulated a complex interaction between the presence of the APOE 4, hypertension, and increased subcortical vascular disease. Tervo and colleagues (2004) found the presence of at least one APOE 4 allele and treated hypertension was a risk factor for the eventual development of mild cognitive dysfunction.

Yip and colleagues (2005) autopsied the brains of patients with confirmed AD to assess the relationship between the APOE allele and the presence of cerebrovascular lesions. Brains positive for the E4 allele also had a greater amount of small vessel arteriolosclerosis. Specifically, the E4 allele was associated with greater thickness in the walls of blood vessels. The E4 allele was also associated with micro infarcts in the deep gray matter nuclei. This type of vasculopathy could very well be a factor contributing to the cognitive impairment seen in VCI.

Treatment and Public Health Issues

Less studied, but equally important as identifying the constituent components of VCI, is research documenting the societal costs associated with VCI. Estimates from the Canadian Study of Health and Aging suggest medical and other costs associated with VCI are over $14,000 per year (Rockwood, Brown et al., 2002). This figure increases with disease severity. A similar study conducted in Europe (Sicras et al., 2005) found annual costs were greater for VaD versus AD. VaD was also associated with greater caregiver burden on the part of families of dementia patients. Hill and colleagues (2005) found that greater healthcare utilization and costs associated with vascular disease compared to AD. Therefore, to the extent VCI represents a prodromal dementia; this study underscores the economic and societal benefits for early identification and treatment.

Several studies have investigated the treatment of patients with VaD with anticholinesterase inhibitors. The results of these studies tend to show modest improvement such that medication lessened caregiver burden and improved psychiatric functioning. In one study, Thomas and colleagues (2005) studied a group of patients with mild dementia but divided patients into groups on the basis of the severity of MRI periventricular and deep white matter alterations. Patients were treated with Donepezil. Patients who initially presented with moderate to severe MRI white matter alterations demonstrated significant improvement on tests of executive function. In addition to improvement on tests of executive function, there was also improvement on tests of delayed recognition memory as measured by a verbal serial list learning test. Research designed to offer treatment for VCI is just getting underway. Pedelty and Nyenhuis (2006) suggest that anticholinesterase inhibitors agents and N-methyl-D-aspartate antagonists may result in clinical improvement. To treat VCI, these researchers stress the need for the early identification and prevention of risk factors associated with vascular disease.

There also has been interest in the possible beneficial role of vitamin antioxidants in the treatment of VCI. Maxwell and colleagues (2005) followed participants for 5 years. They reported that participants using any antioxidant vitamin use at baseline also showed a significantly lower risk for incident VCI. Certain modifications to diet and the use of alcohol have also been linked to a reduction in VCI/VaD. In a study conducted in southern Italy, the use of the so-called "Mediterranean diet," which includes high energy intake of monounsaturated fatty acids and moderate amounts of red wine, was associated with less future cognitive impairment (Panza et al., 2004). The "Mediterranean diet" includes modest alcohol consumption. Data from the Rotterdam Study (Lancet, 2002) found that light-to-moderate drinking (one to three drinks per day) was associated with a lower risk of any dementia (hazard ratio 0.58 [95% CI 0.38–0.90]) including VaD. Whether one needs to drink the wine or merely eat the grapes is an empirical question that needs to be addressed.

Summary

It was the introduction of MRI technology that rekindled our interest in vascular disease as a major cause of dementia. During the late 1980s and 1990s, there was the tendency to view AD and VaD as separate and distinct entities. We now understand that the separation of AD from VaD is more nuanced and more complex than previously appreciated. VCI research provides an excellent platform with which to study brain-behavior relationships and is the latest chapter in the evolving study of the interaction between AD and VaD.

The population and clinic studies reviewed above suggest individuals at risk for the future development of VaD can be identified. The most common methods to identify persons with suspected VCI have been with a combination of neuropsychological tests and close attention to medical risk factors for stroke. Differential impairment on neuropsychological tests of executive control appears to be associated with VCI. It is very likely neuropsychological tests that assess working memory and information processing speed may prove most sensitive to identifying VCI. Emerging assessment techniques such as measuring carotid intima-media thickness and arterial PWV might eventually become tools that can help identify and operationally define VCI. An analysis of blood biomarkers also holds promise in future our understanding of prodromal dementia states.

We feel that there has been sufficient research on the various "parts" of VCI such that these "parts" can and should be integrated into provisional operational criteria design to diagnosis or characterize VCI. In the United States the impeding retirement of the baby boomer generation has sharpened our interest in identifying prodromal dementia states as early as possible. However, dementia is worldwide public health problem. The manner in which dementia presents in various parts of the world is quite diverse. Because many of the vascular risks associated with VCI/VaD can be treated, there is some urgency to operationally define, characterize, and diagnosis VCI. For all of these reasons, greater sophistication is needed in order to operationally define VCI. Combining statistical modeling procedures using the assessment techniques discussed earlier, along with the longitudinal assessment of participants drawn from both the community and memory clinic may ultimately lead to appropriate diagnostic criteria. Such research has the potential alleviate suffering throughout the world.

References

Bowler, J. V. (2004). Vascular cognitive impairment. *Stroke*, 35, 386–388.

Bowler, J. V. (2005). Vascular cognitive impairment. *Journal of Neurology, Neurosurgery, and Psychiatry, 76*, 35–44.

Bowler, J. V., & Hachinski, V. (1995). Vascular cognitive impairment: A new approach to vascular dementia. In *Bailliere's clinical neurology, 4*, 357–376.

Canning, S. J., Leach, L., Stuss, D., Ngo, L., & Black, S. E. (2004). Diagnostic utility of abbreviated fluency measures in Alzheimer disease and vascular dementia. *Neurology, 62*, 556–562.

Carew, T. G., Lamar, M., Cloud, B. S., & Libon, D. J. (1997).Impairment in category fluency in ischaemic vascular dementia. *Neuropsychology, 11*, 400–412.

Davis, H.S., & Rockwood, K. (2004). Conceptualization of mild cognitive impairment: a review. *International Journal of Geriatric Psychiatry, 19,* 313–319.

de Leeuw, F., Richard, F., de Groot, J. C, van Duijn, C. M., Hofman, A., van Gijn, J., et al. (2004). Interaction between hypertension, apoE, and cerebral white matter lesions. *Stroke, 35*, 1057–1060.

De Jager, C. A., Hogervorst, E., Combrinck, M., & Budge, M. M. (2003). Sensitivity and specificity of neuropsychological tests for mild cognitive impairment, vascular cognitive impairment, and Alzheimer's disease. *Psychological Medicine, 33,*1039–1050.

Devasenapathy, A., & Hachinski, V. C. (2000).Vascular cognitive impairment. *Current Treatment Options in Neurology, 2,*61–71.

Di Carlo, A., Baldereschi, M., Amaducci, L., Maggi, S., Grigoletto, F., Scarlato, G., et al. (2000). Cognitive impairment without dementia in older people: prevalence, vascular risk factors, impact on disability. The Italian longitudinal study on aging.Journal *of the American Geriatrics Society, 48,* 775–782.

Erkinjuntti, T., & Rockwood, K. (2003). Vascular dementia.*Seminars in Clinical Neuropsychiatry, 8,* 37–45.

Frisoni, G. B., Galluzzi, S., Bresciani, L., Zanetti, O., & Geroldi, C. (2002). Mild cognitive impairment with subcoritcal vascular features: clinical characteristics and outcome.*Journal of Neurology, 249,* 1423–1432.

Galluzzi, S., Sheu, C. F., Zanetti, O., & Frisoni, G. B. (2005). Distinctive clinical features of mild cognitive impairment with subcortical cerebrovascular disease. *Dementia and Geriatric Cognitive Disorders, 19,* 196–203.

Garrett K. D., Browndyke J. N., Whelihan W., Paul R. H., DiCarlo M., Moser D. J., et al. (2004). The neuropsychological profile of vascular cognitive impairment – no dementia: Comparisons to patients at risk for cerebrovascular disease and vascular dementia. *Archives of Clinical Neuropsychology, 19,* 745–757.

Guidi, I., Galimberti, D., Lonati, S., Novembrino, C., Bamonti, F., Tiriticco, M., et al. (2006). Oxidative imbalance in patients with mild cognitive impairment and Alzheimer's disease.*Neurobiology of Aging, 27,* 262–269.

Hachinski, V. C. (1994). Vascular dementia: a radical definition.*Dementia, 5,* 130–132.

Hachinski, V. C., Potter, P., & Merskey, H. (1987). Leuko-araiosis.*Archives of Neurology, 44,* 21–23.

Hanon, O., Haulon, S., Lenoir, H., Seux, M. L., Rigaud, A. S., Safar, M., et al. (2005). Relationship between arterial stiffness and cognitive function in elderly subjects with complaints of memory loss. *Stroke, 36,* 2193–2197.

Hauw, J. J. (1995). The history of lacunes. In G. A. Donnan, B. Norrving, J. M. Bamford, & J. Bogousslavsky (Eds.), *Lacunar and other subcortical infarctions* (pp.3–15).New York, NY: Oxford University Press.

Hill, J., Fillit, H., Shah, S. N., del Valle, M. C., & Futterman, R. (2005). Patterns of healthcare utilization costs for vascular dementia in a community-dwelling population.*Journal of Alzheimer's Disease, 8,* 43–50.

Hofman, A., Ott, A., Breteler, M. M. B., Bots, M. L., Slooter, A. J. C., van Harskamp, F., et al. (1997). Atherosclerosis, apolipoprotein E and the prevalence of dementia and Alzheimer's disease in a population based study: The Rotterdam Study. *The Lancet, 349,* 151–154.

Huang, J., Meyer, J. S., Zhang, Z., Wei, J., Hong, X., Wang, J., et al. (2005). Progression of mild cognitive impairment to Alzheimer's or vascular dementia versus normative aging among elderly Chinese. *Current Alzheimer Research, 2,* 571–578.

Ingles, J. L., Wentzel, C., Fisk, J. D., & Rockwood, K. (2002). Neuropsychological predictors of incident dementia in patients with vascular cognitive impairment, without dementia. *Stroke, 33,* 1999–2002.

Ishii, N., Nishihara, Y., & Imamura, T. (1986). Why do frontal lobe symptoms predominate in vascular dementia with lacunes? *Neurology, 36,* 340–345.

Johnston, S. C., O'Meara, E. S., Manolio, T. A., Lefkowitz, D., O'Leary, D. H., Goldstein, S., et al. (2004). Cognitive impairment and decline are associated with carotid artery disease in patients without clinically evident cerebrovascular disease. *Annals of Internal Medicine, 140,* 237–247.

Jokinen, H., Kalska, H., Mantyla, R., Pohjasvaara, T., Ylikoski, R., Hietanen, M., et al. (2006). Cognitive profile of subcortical ischaemic vascular disease. *Journal of Neurology, Neurosurgery, and Psychiatry, 77,* 28–33.

Jones, S., Jonsson Laukka, E., Small, B. J., Fratiglioni, L., & Backman, L. (2004). A preclinical phase in vascular dementia: cognitive impairment three years before diagnosis. *Dementia and Geriatric Cognitive Disorders, 18,* 233–239.

Kramer, J. H., Reed, B. R., Mungas, D., Weiner, M. W., & Chui, H. C. (2002).Executive dysfunction in subcortical ischaemic vascular disease.*Journal of Neurology, Neurosurgery, and Psychiatry, 72,* 217–220.

Lamar, M., Price, C. C., Libon, D. J., Penney, D. L., Kaplan, E., Grossman, M. et al. (2007). Alterations in working memory as a function of leukoaraiosis in dementia. *Neuropsychologia, 45,* 245–254.

Lamar, M., Price, C. C., Davis, K. L., Kaplan, E., & Libon, D. J. (2002). Capacity to maintain a mental set in dementia.*Neuropsychologia, 40,* 435–445.

Lawton, M. P., & Brody, E. M. (1969).Assessment of older people: self-maintaining and instrumental activities of daily living. *The Gerontologist, 9,* 179–186.

Libon, D. J., Price, C. C., Heilman, K. M., & Grossman, M. (2006).Alzheimer's "other dementia". *Cog Behav Neurol, 19,* 112–116.

Libon, D. J., Price, C. C., Garrett, K. D., & Giovannetti, T. (2004). From Binswanger's disease to Leukoaraiosis: What we have learned about subcortical vascular dementia.*The Clinical Neuropsychologist, 18,* 83–100.

Libon, D. J., Bogdanoff, B., Cloud, B. S., Skalina, S., Carew, T. G., Gitlin, H. L. et al. (1998). Motor learning and qualitative measures of the hippocampus and subcortical white alterations in Alzheimer's disease and ischemic vascular dementia. *Journal of Clinical and Experimental Neuropsychology, 20,* 30–41.

Luis, C. A., Barker, W. W., Loewenstein, D. A., Crum, T. A, Rogaeva, E., Kawarai, T., et al. (2004). Conversion to dementia among two groups with cognitive impairment. *Dementia and Geriatric Cognitive Disorders, 18,* 307–313.

Maxwell, C. J., Hicks, M. S., Hogan, D. B., Basran, J., & Elby, E. M. (2005) Supplemental use of antioxidant vitamins and subsequent risk of cognitive decline and dementia.*Dementia and Geriatric Cognitive Disorders, 20,* 45–51.

Meyer, J., Xu, G., Thomby, J., Chowdhury, M., & Quach, M. (2002). Longitudinal analysis of abnormal domains comprising mild cognitive impairment (MCI) during aging. *Journal of Neuroscience, 201,* 19–25.

Nagai, K., Akishita, M., Machida, A., Sonohara, K., Ohni, M., & Toba, K. (2004).Correlation between pulse wave velocity and cognitive function in nonvascular dementia.*Journal of the American Geriatric Society,* 52, 1037–1038.

Nyenhuis, D. L., Gorelick, P. B., Geenen, E. J., Smith, C. A., Gencheva, E., Freels, S. et al. (2004). The pattern of neuropsychological deficits in vascular cognitive impairment – no dementia (vascular CIND). *The Clinical Neuropsychologist,* 18, 41–49.

Panza, F., Solfrizzi, V., Colacicco, A. M., D'Intorno, A., Capurso, C., Torres, F., et al. (2004). Mediterranean diet and cognitive decline.*Public Health Nutrition,* 7, 959–963.

Pedelty, L., & Nyenhuis, D. L. (2006).Vascular cognitive impairment.*Current Treatment Options in Cardiovascular Medicine,* 8, 243–250.

Prencipe, M., Santini, M., Casini, A. R., Pezzella, F. R., Scaldaferri, N., & Culasso, F. (2003). Prevalence of non-dementing cognitive disturbances and their association with vascular risk factors in an elderly population. *Journal of Neurology,* 250, 907–912.

Price, C. C., Jefferson, A. L., Merino, J., Heilman, K., & Libon, D.J. (2005). Towards an operational definition of the *'Research Criteria for Subcortical Vascular Dementia':* integrating neuroradiological and neuropsychological data. *Neurology,* 65, 376–382.

Quadri, P., Fragiacomo, C., Pezzati, R., Zanda, E., Forloni, G., Tettemanti, M. et al. (2004). Homocysteine, folate, and vitamin B-12 in mild cognitive impairment, Alzheimer disease, and vascular dementia. *American Journal of Clinical Nutrition,* 80, 114–122.

Ravaglia, G., Forti, P., Maioli, F., Scali, R. C., Saccheitti, L., Talerico, T., et al. (2004). Homocysteine and cognitive performance in healthy elderly subjects. *Arch Gerontol Geriatr,* 9, 349–357.

Reed, B. R., Eberling, J. L., Mungas, D., Weiner, M., Kramer, J. H., & Jagust, W. J. (2004).Effects of white matter lesions and lacunes on cortical function.*Archives of Neurology,* 61, 1545–1550.

Rockwood, K., Black, S. E., Song, X., Hogan, D. B., Gauthier, S., MacKnight, C., et al. (2006). Clinical and radiographic subtypes of vascular cognitive impairment in a clinic-based cohort study. *Journal of Neurological of the Sciences,* 240, 7–14.

Rockwood, K., Davis, H., MacKnight, C., Vandorpe, R., Gauthier, S., Guzman, A., et al. (2004). The consortium to investigate vascular impairment of cognition: methods and first findings. *Canadian Journal of Neurological Sciences,* 30, 237–243.

Rockwood, K., Brown, M., Merry, H., Sketris, I., Fisk, J., & Wolfson C.(2002). Societal Costs of Vascular Cognitive Impairment in Older Adults. *Stroke,* 33, 1605–1609.

Roman, G. C. (2004).Vascular dementia: advances in nosology, diagnosis, treatment and prevention. *Panminerva Medical,* 46, 207–215.

Roman, G. C., Sachdev, P., Royall, D. R., Bullock, R. A., Orgogozo, J. M., Lopez-Pousa, S., et al. (2004). Vascular cognitive disorder: a new diagnostic category updating vascular cognitive impairment and vascular dementia.*Journal of the Neurological Sciences,* 226, 81–87.

Sachdev, P. S., Brodaty, H., Valenzuela, M. J., Lorentz, L., Looi, J. C., Wen, W. et al. (2004).The neuropsychological profile of vascular cognitive impairment in stroke and TIA patients.*Neurology,* 62, 912–919.

Sacuiu, S. Sjogren, M., Johansson, B., Gustafson, D., & Skoog, I. (2005). Prodromal cognitive signs of dementia in 85-year-olds using four sources of information. *Neurology,* 65, 1894–1900.

Scuteri, A., Brancati, A. M., Gianni, W., Assisi, A., & Volpe, M. (2005). Arterial stiffness is an independent risk factor for cognitive impairment in the elderly: a pilot study. *Journal of Hypertension,* 23, 1211–1216.

Sicras, A, Rejas, J., Arco, S., Flores, E., Ortega, G., Esparcia, A., et al. (2005). Prevalence, resource utilization and costs of vascular dementia compared to Alzheimer's disease in a population setting. *Dementia and Geriatric Cognitive Disorders,* 19, 305–315.

Solfrizzi, V., Panza, F., Colacicco, A. M., D'Introno, A., Capurso, C., Torres, F., et al. (2004). Vascular risk factors, incidence of MCI, and rates of progression to dementia.*Neurology,* 63, 1882–1891.

Song, X., Mitnitski, A., & Rockwood, K. (2005).Index variables for studying outcomes in vascular cognitive impairment.*Neuroepidemiology,* 25, 196–204.

Stephens, S., Kenny, R. A., Rowan, E., Allan, L., Kalaria, R. N., Bradbury, M., et al. (2004). Neuropsychological characteristics of mild vascular cognitive impairment and dementia after stroke. *International Journal of Geriatric Psychiatry,* 19, 1053–1057.

Stephens, S., Kenny, R. A., Rowan, E., Kalaria, R. N., Bradbury, M., Pearce, R., et al. (2005). Association between mild vascular cognitive impairment and impaired activities of daily living in older stroke survivors without dementia. *Journal of the American Geriatric Society,* 53, 103–107.

Talelli, P., Ellul, J., Terzis, G., Lekka, N. P., Gioldasis, G., Chrysanthopoulou, A. et al. (2004). Common carotid artery intima media thickness and poststroke cognitive impairment. *Journal of the Neurological Sciences,* 223, 129–134.

Tervo, S., Kivipelto, M., Hanninen, T., Vanhanen, M., Hallikainen, M., Mannermaa, A. et al. (2004). Incidence and risk factors for mild cognitive impairment: a population-based three-year follow-up study of cognitively healthy elderly subjects. *Dementia and Geriatric Cognitive Disorders,* 17, 196–203.

Thomas, D. A., Libon, D. J., & Ledakis, G. (2005). Treating dementia patients with vascular lesions with donepezil: a preliminary analysis. *Applied Neuropsychology*, 12, 12–18.

van Harten, B., Laman, D. M., van Duijn, H., Knol, D. L., Stam, C. J., Scheltens, P. et al. (2006). The auditory oddball paradigm in patients with vascular cognitive impairment: a prolonged latency of the N2 complex. *Dementia and Geriatric Cognitive Disorders*, 21, 322–327.

van den Heuvel, D. M. J., ten Dam, V. H., de Craen, A. J. M., Admiraal-Behloul, F., Olofsen, H., Bollen, E. L. E. M., et al. (2006). Increase in periventricular white matter hyperintensities parallels decline in mental processing speed in a non-demented elderly population. *Journal of Neurology, Neurosurgery, and Psychiatry*, 77, 149–153.

Waite, L. M., Grayson, D. A., Piguet, O., Creasey, H., Bennett, H. P., & Broe, G. A. (2005). Gait slowing as a predictor of incident dementia: 6-year longitudinal data from the Sydney Older Persons Study. *Journal of the Neurological Sciences*, 229–230, 89–93.

Wolfe, N., Linn, R., Babikian, V. L., Knoefel, J. E., & Albert, M. (1990). Frontal systems impairment following multiple lacunar infarcts. *Archives of Neurology*, 47, 129–132,

Xu, G., Meyer, J. S., Huang, Y., Chen, G., Chowdhury, M., & Quach, M. (2004). Cross-cultural comparison of mild cognitive impairment between China and USA. *Current Alzheimer Research*, 1, 55–61.

Yip, A. G., McKee, A. C., Green, R. C., Wells, J., Young, H., Cupples, L. A.et al. (2005). APOE, vascular pathology, and the AD brain. *Neurology*, 65, 259–265.

Zanetti, M., Ballabio, C., Abbate, C., Cutaia, C., Vergani, C., & Bergamaschini, L. (2006).Mild cognitive impairment subtypes and vascular dementia in community-dwelling elderly people: a 3-year follow-up study. *Journal of the American Geriatric Society*, 54, 580–586.

Zhang, Z., Zahner, G. E. P., Roman, G. C., Lui, J., Hong, Z., Qu, Q., et al. (2005). Dementia subtypes in China: prevalence in Beijing, Xian, Shanghai, and Chengdu. *Archives of Neurology*, 62, 447–453.

Chapter 7
Vascular Dementia

Joel H. Kramer and Margaret E. Wetzel

Dementia is one of the major health risks facing elderly individuals. Prevalence of dementia in the United States is currently around seven million individuals with the number of cases expected to increase by 25% over the next 20 years.

As currently defined, dementia represents cognitive impairment that is severe enough to significantly interfere with occupational, social, or functional abilities. The causes of dementia are varied and accurate differential diagnosis is critical for identifying treatable disorders and ameliorating the impact of disorders for which there are no treatments. In the vast majority of patients over the age of 50, the most disabling and progressive conditions are either neurodegenerative (Alzheimer's disease, frontotemporal lobar degeneration, parkinsonian syndromes) or vascular in origin. In this chapter, we will review several features of vascular dementia (VaD), including diagnostic criteria, prevalence, underlying mechanisms and subtypes, comorbidity with other disorders, and neuropsychological and neurobehavioral characteristics.

Vascular dementia is considered one of the most common types of dementia in the elderly (Rabinstein, Romano, Forteza, & Koch, 2004). Beyond this somewhat general concept,

however, there is much less agreement about the frequency with which VaD occurs and the mechanisms by which cerebrovascular disease produces a dementia syndrome (Black, 2005; Erkinjuntti, 2002; O'Brien et al., 2003). Given the heterogeneity of cerebrovascular disorders, it is not surprising that no clear consensus has emerged regarding their causal factors, underlying neuropathology, clinical symptoms, characteristic neuropsychological profiles, and developmental course.

Risk of cerebrovascular disease increases with age and thus plays an increasing role in dementia in older cohorts. By the age of 70, 70% of the population has white matter lesions (WMLs) on MRI brain scans (O'Brien et al., 2003), and it is estimated that 11 million Americans may have a silent stroke every year without showing symptoms (de la Torre, 2002). According to population-based studies, silent lacunes are found in 11–24% of the population, with WMLs appearing in 62–95% of the elderly on imaging (Roman, Erkinjuntti, Wallin, Pantoni, & Chui, 2002). Age is the single strongest risk factor for cerebrovascular disease and stroke (Gorelick, 2004; Roman, 2005). Importantly, several risk factors for cerebrovascular disease, including atrial fibrillation, hypertension, cardiac disease, diabetes mellitus, smoking, alcoholism, and hyperlipidemia are potentially modifiable, highlighting the need for accurate diagnosis of VaD (Sacco, 1994; Schoenberg, 1988; Tell, Crouse, & Furberg, 1988; Wolf, D'Agostino, Belanger, & Kannel, 1991).

J.H. Kramer (✉)
Department of Neurology, University of California, San Francisco, Box 1207, San Francisco, CA, 94143-1207, USA
e-mail: jkramer@memory.ucsf.edu

J.R. Festa, R.M. Lazar (eds.), *Neurovascular Neuropsychology*, DOI 10.1007/978-0-387-70715-0_7,
© Springer Science+Business Media, LLC 2009

Subtypes of Vascular Dementia

Cerebrovascular disease can cause significant cognitive and functional impairment in a variety of ways. Acute injury secondary to cerebrovascular disease can result from hemorrhages or ischemia. Though not as common as ischemia, hemorrhage can have both profound and subtle affects on cognition, and makes up roughly 20% of all strokes. Hemorrhages are typically either intraparenchymal or subarachnoid. Nontraumatic subarachnoid hemorrhage usually occurs from a ruptured cerebral aneurysm or arteriovenous malformation. Morbidity rates are high and survivors are often left with significant cognitive deficits, particularly impairments in memory and executive function (Bjeljac, Keller, Regard, & Yonekawa, 2002; D'Esposito, Alexander, Fischer, McGlinchey-Berroth, & O'Connor, 1996; Jimbo et al., 2000).

Hemorrhages can also occur from cerebral amyloid angiopathy (CAA). In CAA, β-amyloid accumulates in the cerebral blood vessels, compromising their structural integrity and leaving them prone to rupture, causing intracranial hemorrhage. Although CAA is particularly common in patients with Alzheimer's disease, it can also lead to hemorrhages and associated cognitive deficits in patients without Alzheimer's disease.

Roughly 80% of strokes are ischemic, and the relationship between ischemic injury and dementia will be the primary focus of this chapter. Under the rubric of ischemic stroke, there are four main subtypes that produce dementia syndromes: white matter injury, strategic infarcts, large vessel disease, and small vessel disease.

In 1894, Otto Binswanger described eight patients with slowly progressive mental deterioration and pronounced white matter changes, with secondary dilatation of the ventricles. In Binswanger's disease, also known as subcortical arteriosclerotic encephalopathy, there is typically a history of persistent hypertension or systemic vascular disease. While relatively uncommon, its clinical course may be insidious, with long plateaus and the accumulation of focal neurologic signs (Babikan & Ropper, 1987; Roman, 1987). Neuropathological features include extensive demyelination and destruction of subcortical white matter, with relative sparing of the cortical U fibers. Pathology is typically more pronounced in the temporal and occipital lobes. Criteria for clinical diagnosis have been offered by Caplan and Schoene (1978) and include the presence of vascular risk factors, focal ischemic lacunar lesions in the white matter that are confluent on neuroimaging, age of onset between 55 and 75, subacute onset of focal neurological signs, and extensive white matter attenuation on T1 and hyperintensity on T2 weighted MR images. The resulting dementia syndrome has a decidedly prefrontal flavor, including apathy, lack of drive, mild depression, alterations of mood, and slowed information processing (Libon, Price, Davis Garrett, & Giovannetti, 2004; Loeb, 2000).

A strategically placed infarct, typically in the thalamus, frontal white matter, basal ganglia, or angular gyrus can also result in dementia. For example, in some individuals, a single paramedian branch supplies both anteromedial thalamic regions. Occlusion of the paramedian artery in these cases will lead to bilateral infarction of the dorsomedial nucleus and the mammillothalamic tracts (Bogousslavsky, Regli, & Uske, 1988), disconnecting the prefrontal executive and limbic-diencephalic memory systems. Similarly, an infarct in the inferior genu of the internal capsule may strategically disrupt the inferior and medial thalamic peduncles carrying thalamo-cortical fibers related to cognition and memory (Tatemichi, Desmond, Paik, & al, 1993; Tatemichi et al., 1992). Kooistra and Heilman (1988) also reported on a lacune in the posterior limb of the left internal capsule resulting in a persistent verbal memory disorder.

Multi-infarct dementia is a term that was previously used broadly to refer to all types of VaD, though it now refers more specifically to large vessel disease, usually occlusions of main branches of the anterior, middle, and posterior cerebral arteries that produce cortical lesions. These infarcts are typically caused by either atherosclerotic plaques within the arterial walls or from emboli of cardiac origin. In an autopsy series of 175 cases of dementia, large vessel disease made up roughly 15% of all VaD cases (Brun, 1994). Large vessel disease is more characteristically associated with step-wise progression and does not occur in concordance with AD as often as other ischemic dementias. The sudden onset and step-wise progression traditionally thought to be associated with cerebrovascular disease is probably specific to large vessel disease and is less characteristic of the other vascular syndromes. Neurobehavioral symptoms vary greatly as a function of where and how large the cortical lesions are, but can include aphasia, apraxia, agnosia, and inattention syndromes. Some ambiguity between lesion location and cognitive symptoms also exists; Henon (2002) has suggested that no clear association between stroke location and size has yet been identified, and that more diffuse pathology such as cerebral atrophy and white matter disease may be better predictors of post-stroke dementia.

Atherosclerosis and small vessel disease are the main causes of brain infarction. Cummings (1995) suggested that anywhere between 13 and 51% of patients with VaD have subcortical lacunes, while Fein et al. (2000) reported that small vessel disease accounts for 36–50% of all VaDs. This condition is typically the result of occlusions of the deep penetrating arterioles and arteries that feed the basal ganglia, thalamus, white matter, and internal capsule. The lesions are small and are often referred to as lacunes or lacunar infarcts; the syndrome is sometimes known as lacunar state dementia or etat lacunaire. Lacunes average 2 mm in volume, but can range from 0.2 to 15 mm (Capizzano et al., 2000; Cummings, 1995). Advances in neuroimaging during the past two decades have enabled researchers and clinicians to more accurately and reliably determine when small vessel ischemic vascular disease is present. The relationship between small vessel disease and dementia is complex,

however, with considerable controversy regarding prevalence rates and comorbidity with neurodegenerative diseases. The neuropsychology of dementia due to small vessel disease also remains controversial and will be the primary focus of this chapter. Many investigators refer to this condition as subcortical ischemic vascular dementia (SIVD), although in light of recent studies suggesting more widespread microvascular changes, the terms SIVD and small vessel VaD will be used interchangeably.

While SIVD is typically associated with age and hypertension, there is also a variant of SIVD called cerebral autosomal dominant arteriopathy with subcortical infarcts and leukoencephalopathy (CADASIL). CADASIL is a genetic disorder linked to a mutation in the Notch 3 gene of chromosome 19 (Davous, 1998; Markus et al., 2002). Although patients are typically free of classical vascular risk factors like hypertension and diabetes, the disorder effects the small vessels of the brain and results in extensive subcortical infarcts and leukoencephalopathy and can affect cognition. Moreover, it has been suggested (Charlton, Morris, Nitkunan, & Markus, 2006; Peters et al., 2005) that CADASIL may offer insight into a "pure" cognitive profile for subjects with VaD, as patients with CADASIL tend to display cognitive decline at an early age, thereby ruling out the likelihood of a concomitant neurodegenerative dementia process.

The Challenge of Diagnosis

If there is a neuropsychological presentation characteristic of VaD, issues related to comorbidity with other disorders, different diagnostic criteria, and variable methodology have made elucidation of such a presentation difficult to ascertain. These issues have also made it difficult to determine the prevalence of VaD. Although cerebrovascular disease is common in the elderly, the presence of cerebrovascular disease in a dementia patient is not sufficient to imply a causal relationship between the two, or in which direction the causal relationship runs. Prevalent rates of VaD in autopsy series also vary dramatically, in part because of referral bias. Perhaps the lowest prevalence rates come from dementia centers, since they are less likely to see patients with strokes. A review of seven clinical series of patients with dementia ($n = 689$) showed the most common diagnosis by far to be Alzheimer's disease (47%); a diagnosis of VaD was made in only 9% (Chui, 1989). VaD rates appear to be highest in Asian patient samples. In an autopsy case of 78 patients with dementia in China, for example, VaD alone was found in 38.5%, while Alzheimer's dementia accounted for 14% (Wang, Zhu, Gui, & Li, 2003). In Japan, pure VaD has been reported in 22–35% of patients at autopsy, as compared to 7–10% in the west (Jellinger, 2002). Even in AD samples, however, cerebrovascular disease is common. In a series of 50 autopsied cases of dementia, Tomlinson et al. (1970) observed that "at least one third of all patients with dementia have a significant vascular component," and Knopman, DeKosky et al. (2001) noted that between 30 and 40% of dementia cases have a degree of CVD pathology at autopsy. Among the first 106 autopsies of patients enrolled in the Consortium to Establish a Registry for Alzheimer Disease (CERAD) with a clinical diagnosis of AD, 87% showed histological changes confirming a diagnosis of AD, but vascular lesions of varying nature and size were also present in 21% (Gearing et al., 1995). De la Torre (2002) also reports that 30% of Alzheimer disease brains at autopsy also show some form of cerebrovascular pathology.

Several different diagnostic criteria for VaD have been proposed over the years and are summarized in Table 1. The DSM-IV requires the presence of multiple cognitive deficits, and at minimum includes memory impairment and either aphasia, apraxia, agnosia, or executive impairment. DSM-IV also requires that there be either focal neurological signs and symptoms or laboratory evidence indicative of cerebrovascular disease.

Although widely applied, the emphasis on memory and cortical dementia symptoms like aphasia and apraxia in DSM-IV may be less appropriate for predominately subcortical syndromes. In addition, clinicians must judge the cerebrovascular disease to be etiologically related to the dementia, a connection that is difficult to make in cases where the infarcts are small and localized in subcortical regions. Reed et al. (2004) also reported little correlation between clinical signs and cerebrovascular pathology evident on autopsy, suggesting that criteria requiring focal neurological signs or symptoms could potentially miss up to half of the patients with significant amounts of pathology-confirmed cerebrovascular disease.

The International Classification of Diseases (10th revision [ICD-10]) (WHO, 1993) uses different criteria than DSM, and low rates of agreement between ICD-10 and DSM-IV have been reported (Erkinjuntti, 1997). Introduced in 1993, the ICD-10 allows classification for different VaD subtypes and requires at minimum an unequal distribution of deficits in higher cognitive functions, clinical evidence of focal brain damage, and significant cerebrovascular disease. Relatively new, these criteria have not been widely used and have been criticized for their low accuracy in diagnosing VaD (Cosentino et al., 2004; Wetterling, Kanitz, & Borgis, 1993).

The National Institute of Neurological Disorders and Stroke in conjunction with the Association Internationale pour la Recherche et l'Enseignement en neurosciences published the NINDS-AIREN consensus criteria in 1993 (Roman, Tatemichi, & Erkinjuntii, 1993). In the NINDS-AIREN system, dementia is defined by cognitive decline manifested by impairment of memory and of two or more cognitive domains. Cerebrovascular disease is defined by the presence of focal signs on neurological examination and evidence of relevant cerebrovascular disease on neuroimaging. The cerebrovascular disease can be a large cortical infarct, a single strategically placed infarct, or multiple subcortical or WMLs. The relationship between the dementia syndrome and the cerebrovascular disease is more sharply

Table 1 Diagnostic criteria for vascular dementia

Modified HIS	<ul><li>Abrupt onset (2 pts.)</li><li>Stepwise deterioration (2 pts.)</li><li>Somatic complaints (1 pt.)</li><li>Emotional incontinence (1 pt.)</li><li>History of hypertension (1 pt.)</li><li>History of stroke (1 pt.)</li><li>Focal neurologic symptoms (2 pts.)</li><li>Focal neurologic signs (2 pts.)</li></ul>	Pros:<ul><li>Widely used</li><li>Distinguishes between mixed and pure VaD</li><li>Good specificity</li></ul>Cons:<ul><li>Low sensitivity</li><li>Less appropriate for subcortical ischemic VaD</li></ul>
ICD-10	<ul><li>Unequal distribution of higher cognitive functions</li><li>Decline in memory</li><li>Decline in social functioning</li><li>Clinical evidence of focal brain damage: unilateral spastic weakness of the limbs, unilaterally increased tendon reflexes, an extensor plantar response, pseudobulbar palsy</li><li>Evidence of cerebrovascular disease</li></ul>	Pros:<ul><li>Good specificity</li><li>Allows classification of different VaD subtypes</li></ul>Cons:<ul><li>Low sensitivity</li><li>Emphasis on memory decline</li></ul>
DSM-IV	<ul><li>Multiple cognitive deficits, at minimum includes memory impairment and either aphasia, apraxia, agnosia, or executive impairment</li><li>Focal neurological signs and symptoms (unilateral spastic weakness of the limbs, unilaterally increased tendon reflexes, an extensor plantar response, pseudobulbar palsy)</li><li>Laboratory evidence and symptoms of cerebrovascular disease</li><li>Decreased executive functioning</li><li>Temporal relationship of stroke and dementia</li></ul>	Pros:<ul><li>Better sensitivity (0.50)</li><li>Excludes mixed dementias well</li></ul>Cons:<ul><li>Lower specificity (0.84)</li><li>Reliance on memory deficit</li><li>Low correlation between neurological signs and pathology</li><li>Requires judgment of etiology</li></ul>
NINDS-AIREN	<ul><li>Dementia: memory impairment and cognitive decline in two or more cognitive domains (orientation, attention, language, visuospatial functions, executive functions, motor control, and praxis)</li><li>Relevant cerebrovascular disease on brain imaging (large cortical infarct, single strategically placed infarct, or multiple subcortical or white matter lesion)</li><li>Temporal relationship between cerebrovascular disease and onset of dementia; with dementia occurring within three months of a stroke, abrupt onset of cognitive decline or fluctuating, stepwise progression</li><li>Focal neurological signs on neurological examination</li><li>Post-mortem neuropathological criteria (for probably VaD and possible VaD)</li></ul>	Pros:<ul><li>Good specificity (0.93) for probable VaD</li><li>Good sensitivity (0.55) for possible VaD</li><li>Excludes mixed dementias well</li><li>Widely used</li></ul>Cons:<ul><li>Poor sensitivity (0.20) for probable VaD</li><li>Reliance on memory deficit to establish dementia</li><li>Temporal relationship cutoff arbitrary and less appropriate for subcortical ischemic VaD</li></ul>
ADDTC	<ul><li>Evidence of two or more ischemic strokes by history, neurological signs, and/or neuroimaging studies</li><li>OR a single stroke with a clearly documented temporal relationship to the onset of dementia</li></ul>	Pros:<ul><li>Good sensitivity (0.70) for possible VaD</li><li>Good specificity for probable VaD (0.91)</li><li>Memory impairment not needed</li></ul>Cons:<ul><li>Poor sensitivity (0.25) for probable VaD</li><li>Poor exclusion of mixed dementias</li></ul>

HIS = Hachinski Ischemia Score; ICD-10 = International Classification of Diseases, 10th revision; DSM-IV = Diagnostic and Statistical Manual of Mental Disorders – Fourth Edition; NINDS-AIREN = National Institute of Neurological Disorders and Stroke-Association Internationale pour la Recherche et l'Enseignement en Neuosciences; ADDTC = Alzheimer's Disease Diagnostic and Treatment Centers defined than in the DSM-IV, and is inferred by the dementia occurring within 3 months of a stroke, abrupt onset of cognitive impairment, or fluctuating, stepwise progression. NINDS-AIREN further establishes criteria for probable VaD and possible VaD that is confirmed using post-mortem neuropathological criteria. The emphasis on a clear temporal relationship between stroke and cognitive impairment, however, make these criteria less sensitive to subcortical ischemic VaD that can have insidious onset and gradual progression.

Chui, Victoroff et al. (1992) proposed a different diagnostic system based on the experience of the State of California Alzheimer's Disease Diagnostic and Treatment Centers (ADDTC). The ADDTC criteria focus are unique in that memory impairment is not necessary for making the diagnosis of dementia. The key criterion for dementia is a deterioration from prior levels in two or more areas of intellectual functioning sufficient to interfere with the patient's customary affairs of life. A diagnosis of probable VaD is made when there is evidence of two or more ischemic strokes by history, neurological signs, and/or neuroimaging studies, or a single stroke with a clearly documented temporal relationship to the onset of dementia.

To assess the role that vascular risk factors may have in a dementia syndrome, Hachinski et al. (1975) proposed the Hachinski Ischemia Score (HIS) in 1975. The HIS is structured as a one- and two-point checklist, including focal neurological signs, depression, and history of stroke and hypertension. The HIS was introduced before modern imaging techniques like CT and MRI were available, and several modified ischemia scales have since been established. The most widely used include the Rosen Modified Hachinski Ischemia Score (Rosen, Terry, Fuld, Katzman, & Peck, 1980) in 1980 and the Loeb and Gandolfo's Modified Ischemic Score (Loeb & Gandolfo, 1983) in 1983. Loeb and Gandolfo's criteria, in particular, have provided a more useful modified scale which incorporates focal abnormality on CT imaging. While these do not serve as

diagnostic criteria, they can aid in the diagnosis of a vascular syndrome, and many studies of VaD require a minimum value for the HIS for inclusion in their VaD group.

Unfortunately, these different diagnostic criteria do not overlap sufficiently and generate confusion for clinicians and researchers alike. The concomitant use of NINDS-AIREN, DSM-IV, and ICD-10 criteria in selected series have shown that they overlap in less than 50% of the cases (Wetterling, Kanitz, & Borgis, 1996). Chui, Mack et al. (2000) compared four of these five criteria (DSM-IV, HIS, NINDS-AIREN, and ADDTC) to determine interrater reliability and prevalence of diagnosis. Twenty-five case vignettes were reviewed by clinical teams at seven centers; vignettes included a narrative of the chief complaint, history of present illness, medical history, family history of dementia, results of physical and neurologic examination, MMSE, Blessed Memory Information Concentration Test, laboratory test results, neuroimaging results, and neuropsychological data. The most frequently diagnosed VaD cases came from using modified HIS or DSM-IV criteria, while the NINDS-AIREN criteria resulted in the smallest amount of cases. The original HIS and ADDTC diagnosed cases at a moderate frequency. Interrater reliability was highest for the HIS and lowest for a diagnosis of probable VaD with the ADDTC, but none of the criteria yielded acceptable levels of interrater reliability. They also conclude that the clinical criteria for VaD were not interchangeable. Thus, depending on the clinical criteria used, the prevalence and clinical characteristics of VaD can vary significantly. Gold et al. (2002) reached a similar conclusion when they compared the clinical with the neuropathological diagnosis of 89 autopsied patients. They found that the ADDTC criteria for possible VaD were the most sensitive (0.70) for the detection of VaD, although the DSM-IV and NINDS-AIREN criteria might be more effective in excluding mixed dementia.

The Neuropsychology of Dementia Secondary to Small Vessel Disease: Differentiation From AD

Despite the many methodological challenges to studying dementia secondary to small vessel disease, several attempts have been made at defining the neuropsychological features and suggesting ways to address the clinically relevant need to differentiate between SIVD and AD. An almost universal underlying assumption is that the patterns of neuropsychological deficits in SIVD and AD would vary as a function of differences in their underlying neuropathology (Mendez & Ashla-Mendez, 1991). AD involves neurofibrillary tangles and neuritic plaques in temporal limbic structures and posterior association cortex, and commonly presents with impairment in memory, language, and conceptual abilities. In SIVD, the presence of multiple subcortical lacunes and white matter hyperintensities are thought to affect subcortical-frontal circuits that mediate cognitive, motivational and emotional processes (Cummings, 1995). In particular, the dorsolateral prefrontal circuit plays a prominent role mediating executive functioning, including response inhibition, fluency, and working memory. A subcortical-frontal deficit model for SIVD predicts that executive functioning and motor programming abnormalities would be disproportionately affected in SIVD, while memory and language would be disproportionately affected in AD.

Considerable evidence in support of this divergence has been reported. Kertesz and Clydesdale (1994) found that patients clinically diagnosed with SIVD performed worse on tests that are influenced by frontal and subcortical structures. For example, SIVD patients had greater difficulty on the MDRS-derived scale of motor performance, which measures motor perseveration and bimanual coordination. SIVD patients also showed greater impairment on the WAIS-R Picture Arrangement subtest. In comparison to the SIVD group, patients with AD were found to perform poorly on measures of memory

(WMS-R immediate story recall) and language (Western Aphasia Battery repetition subtest).

Kemenoff et al. (1999) compared 27 patients with SIVD to 34 patients without lacunes on a broad range of neuropsychological measures. All patients with SIVD met ADDTC criteria for VaD and had MRI evidence for one or more subcortical lacunes (Chui, Victoroff et al., 1992). No group differences were found on age, education, and total Mattis DRS score. Patients with SIVD performed relatively better on the memory versus the conceptualization subscale of the DRS, while AD patients demonstrated the opposite pattern. Patients with SIVD showed greater impairment on phonemic fluency relative to category fluency, while AD patients provided more intrusions and exhibited poorer visual memory. After entering the discriminating neuropsychological variables into a logistic regression, SIVD and AD patients were categorized with 84% accuracy. Results support the view that a subcortical-frontal pattern of neuropsychological performance is present in SIVD and may be useful for clinical diagnosis.

Lending further support for a subcortical-frontal deficit model, Wolfe et al. (1990) tested the hypothesis that patients with multiple subcortical lacunes were selectively impaired on neuropsychological tests susceptible to frontal lobe impairment. Executive abilities including verbal fluency, semantic clustering, shifting of mental set, and response inhibition were all compromised in patients with multiple subcortical lacunes on CT.

Tei et al. (1997) found that patients with early-stage AD had significantly lower scores on a test of visuospatial memory, while patients with multiple subcortical infarction with mild cognitive impairment demonstrated significantly worse performance on an executive function test sensitive to frontal lobe dysfunction (Wisconsin Card Sorting Test). Padovani et al. (1995) found that VaD patients were more impaired on measures of frontal lobe functioning such as Controlled Oral Word Association and Wisconsin Card Sorting Test perseverative errors, whereas AD patients were more impaired on measures of memory functioning (e.g., CVLT-Total Recall and Delayed Recall, Spatial Recall Test) and on a measure of language comprehension.

In one of the more methodologically robust studies, Lafosse et al. (1997) individually matched 32 patients with SIVD and 32 patients with AD on the basis of age, dementia severity, years of education, and gender. They hypothesized that patients with SIVD would demonstrate better confrontation naming, worse verbal fluency (COWAT), and better memory performance than patients with AD. While notable differences in confrontation naming were not found, patients with SIVD had poorer verbal fluency, but better free recall, fewer intrusions, and better recognition memory than patients with AD. Based on their marked relative impairment in verbal fluency, Lafosse et al. (1997) suggested that the unifying feature of the SIVD patients' neuropsychological deficits was related to a failure of executive functions mediated by the frontal lobes. The pattern of deficit on verbal fluency tasks may also have utility in differential diagnosis. Carew et al. (Carew, Lamar, Cloud, Grossman, & Libon, 1997) reported that SIVD patients and normal elderly controls performed better on category than letter fluency tasks, whereas the opposite was observed among patients with AD. In addition, patients with SIVD produced fewer responses than AD participants on letter fluency tasks, but there was no difference between AD and SIVD patients on category fluency.

Other studies have emphasized differences in memory functioning in AD and SIVD. Erker, Searight, and Peterson (1995) compared Alzheimer's and VaD patients on both global and specific indices of cognitive and neuropsychological functioning. The AD and VaD patients were equivalent in their global level of neuropsychological impairment. However, a significant interaction was found between diagnosis and cognitive deficit; compared to the AD group, patients with VaD showed relative preservation of memory in the context of deterioration in global cognitive functioning.

Hassing and Beckman (1997) also found greater memory impairment among Alzheimer's versus VaD patients. They compared the two dementia groups on a series of episodic memory tasks, assessing face recognition, word recall, and object recall. While no group differences were found on face recognition and object recall, VaD patients showed an advantage over Alzheimer's patients in word recall. Hassing and Backman suggest that this selective word recall deficit may also be interpreted in terms of greater impairment of language related functions in AD compared with VaD.

Libon et al. (1998) demonstrated that patients with AD and SIVD can be dissociated on the basis of differing patterns of impairment on tests of declarative and procedural memory. The California Verbal Learning Tests (CVLT) was used to measure declarative memory, while a pursuit rotor learning task was used as a measure of procedural memory. The SIVD group performed as poorly as the AD group on the CVLT List-A immediate free recall test trials. By contrast, patients with SIVD showed a greater capacity to retain information as evidenced by their significantly higher score on the CVLT recognition discriminability index. An opposite pattern of performance was demonstrated on the pursuit rotor task, with AD subjects exhibiting greater learning than SIVD subjects. These results are consistent with other reports of subcortical dementia patients (e.g., Huntington's disease) exhibiting deficits in procedural memory (Knopman & Nissen, 1991).

Mechanisms of Injury

Subcortical ischemic vascular dementia is a complex and multi-faceted disorder and the ways in which it produces a dementia syndrome are only just beginning to be understood. Several different components of SIVD could potentially disrupt cognition, including lacunar infarction, injury to underlying white matter, hippocampal sclerosis, and more diffuse brain dysfunction extending beyond the specific regions of infarction. In addition, clinicians must always entertain the possibility other conditions, particularly AD, are co-occuring with the vascular changes and may be playing a role in the observed cognitive deficits.

Several studies have linked specific parameters of subcortical pathology to dementia severity. Lafosse et al. (1997) reported that the amount of white-matter disease in an SIVD sample was associated with reduced fluency and poorer spontaneous recall, whereas increasing number of infarcts was associated with poorer recognition memory. Furthermore, ventricular enlargement was related to poorer delayed cued recall.

Tomlinson et al. (1970) initially proposed that dementia would occur when the volume of infarcted tissue exceeded 100 ml, although Loeb and Meyer noted that dementia can occur with only 20–30 ml of infarcted brain tissue (Loeb & Meyer, 1996). However, strong correlations between lacunar volume and cognitive functioning have not been routinely found (Mungas et al., 2001).

Functional imaging studies tend to show that brain regions surrounding or even remote from the infarction are hypometabolic, indicating that brain dysfunction in SIVD is more widespread. These remote effects are thought to be related to disconnections within subcortical-cortical circuits. In light of the neuropsychological evidence supporting a sub-cortical-frontal model of dysfunction, it would be reasonable to hypothesize that the frontal lobes are particularly vulnerable to these disconnections. Using positron emission tomography (PET), Sultzer et al. (1995) found the metabolic rate in the frontal cortex was lower in patients with a lacunar infarct of the basal ganglia or thalamus than in those without. Both Tullberg et al. (Tullberg et al., 2004) and Kwan and colleagues (Kwan et al., 1999) also showed that SIVD patients had lower whole brain regional cerebral metabolic rates of glucose than controls or cognitively normal subjects with lacunes. Structural imaging

studies have also described widespread cortical changes in SIVD. Cortical gray matter (cGM) is reduced in cognitively impaired and demented patients with lacunes compared to controls (Fein et al., 2000). The extent of cGM reduction in patients with SIVD was similar to that of patients with AD, although the patients with SIVD had greater ventricular size and more WMLs. Fein et al. (2000) further reported that eight subjects in their cohort had a pathologically confirmed absence of AD pathology, indicating that comorbidity cannot explain the cortical grey matter reductions. Lafosse et al. (1997) reported that cortical atrophy in their SIVD subjects was related to poorer performance on most of the neuropsychological measures. They argued that the pattern of correlations with cortical atrophy and their findings of greater cortical atrophy in the SIVD group than AD group suggest that a degenerative cortical process may be involved in SIVD as well. These researchers concluded that characteristic deficits in SIVD may result from a combination of diminished executive functions based on direct ischemic damage to subcortical-frontal circuits and diffuse cortical dysfunction based on transsynaptic degeneration. Alternately, the diffuse cortical atrophy may be associated with microvascular ischemic changes in the cortex.

The Comorbidity Dilemma

Many demented patients have neuroimaging and clinical evidence for cerebrovascular disease. However, this does not imply that the cerebrovascular disease is the source of the cognitive impairment. Several studies have suggested that a high proportion of well-functioning community-dwelling elderly has had a lacunar infarct without obvious clinical impact (Kobayashi, Okada, Koide, Bokura, & Yamaguchi, 1997; Longstreth et al., 1998; Price et al., 1997). In fact, some investigators argue that lacunes do not cause dementia. Nolan et al. (1998), for example, studied 87 consecutive dementia patients at autopsy and concluded that dementia could not be attributed to the effects of cerebrovascular disease alone. There is also uncertainty as to whether lacunes pose a risk factor for developing neurodegenerative disease. Loeb, Gandolfo, Croce, and Conti (1992) reported that 23% of patients who initially presented with a single lacunar infarct who were followed for 4 years ultimately developed dementia. In contrast, DeCarli et al. (2004) studied 52 patients with mild cognitive impairment and concluded that while vascular risk factors, including lacunes and white matter disease, can cause cognitive decline, they are not predictive of a progression to dementia.

These findings highlight the major methodological challenge to SIVD research: ruling out the possibility that the patients have a concomitant neurodegenerative disease, most typically AD, and that the neurodegenerative disorder is the primary contributor to the dementia syndrome.

This issue is highlighted in a recent study by Chui, Zarow, and colleagues (2006), who studied a large series of patients with pathologically confirmed diagnoses. Subjects were recruited from several dementia centers that specifically targeted subjects with subcortical lacunes, thus providing a sample relatively biased toward cerebrovascular disease. Subjects were followed to autopsy. One of the first challenges faced by this study was how to operationalize pathological evidence of cerebrovascular disease. While senile plaques and neurofibrillary tangles are agreed upon markers of AD, and widely accepted systems for quantifying these markers exist (e.g., CERAD; Braak and Braak staging), there is no consensus on how to quantify cerebrovascular injury. Chui et al. developed a CVD score that quantifies ischemic disease that enabled them, along with a Braak and Braak score, to assign pathological diagnosis of AD, SIVD, or mixed. They defined probable AD as a Braak and Braak score of greater or equal to 4 and a CVD score of less than 20, probable SIVD as a Braak and

Braak score of less than 4 and a CVD score of greater or equal to 20, and mixed dementia when the CVD and Braak and Braak scores were both high.

The study yielded two important findings. In their initial series of 79 cases, 43 cases had been clinically diagnosed with a dementia syndrome before death. Of these, seven cases, or 16.3% of the dementia sample, had a pathological diagnosis of SIVD. This finding indicates that while not rare, the prevalence of SIVD without significant concomitant AD pathology is relatively low, even in a sample biased toward the presence of cerebrovascular disease. The second important finding concerns the accuracy of the clinical diagnosis. Accuracy rates for AD were relatively high. Of the 20 cases with a clinical diagnosis of AD, 18 had pathologically confirmed AD, one case was mixed AD and SIVD, and one had no clear evidence for either AD or SIVD. Accuracy rates were much lower for patients clinically diagnosed with SIVD. Of the 11 clinically diagnosed cases of SIVD, only four (36%) met pathological criteria; five had AD, one had mixed dementia, and one had no clear evidence for either AD or SIVD. The main point here is that even with clinicians with relative expertise in SIVD, clinical diagnoses of SIVD were typically wrong, with more than half of the cases having significant AD pathology. Clinical diagnoses of mixed dementia were also only marginally accurate. Only 7 of the 22 clinically diagnosed mixed dementia cases were pathologically confirmed; eight cases were pathologically diagnosed as AD and three were pathologically diagnosed as SIVD.

The Neuropsychology of Dementia Secondary to Small Vessel Disease: More Recent Studies

The take-home point of studies like Chui, Zarow et al. (2006) is that until there are readily available methods for ruling out comorbid neurodegenerative disease, a clinical diagnosis of SIVD is inherently unreliable. Therefore, studies that categorize clinical patients into SIVD and AD groups are unlikely to yield easily interpretable data. Nonetheless, there is a wealth of data that convincingly argues that SIVD contributes to cognitive decline, and this line of research remains very clinically relevant. Two scientific approaches reasonably circumvent the conundrum of clinical diagnosis: (1) treating cerebrovascular disease as a continuous variable, and (2) carrying out prospective research and studying pathologically confirmed cases.

Several investigators have used structural MRI to quantify cerebrovascular disease and treated these measures as continuous variables when studying cognition. Mungas et al. (2001), for example, studied 157 subjects with a range of cognitive impairment and MRI evidence of cerebrovascular disease. Dependent variables were neuropsychological tests of global cognitive function, memory, language, and executive function. Independent variables were quantitative MRI measures of volume of lacunar infarcts in specific subcortical structures, volume of WML, volume of cGM, and total hippocampal volume (HV). Multiple regression analyses were used to identify MRI predictors of cognition. One key finding was that subcortical lacunes were not related to cognitive measures independent of effects of other MRI variables. The other cerebrovascular marker, WML, was independently related only to selected, timed measures. In contrast, HV and cGM were strong and independent predictors of cognitive variables, with effects that did not differ in subjects with and without subcortical lacunes. These data suggest that cognitive impairment associated with subcortical ischemic vascular disease is primarily a result of associated hippocampal and cortical changes, consistent with the notion that much of the cognitive impairment may be driven by AD pathology.

Similarly, Kramer et al. (2004) studied a heterogeneous group of 62 dementia patients, 35 of whom had subcortical lacunes, and 27 of whom did not. Their goal was to understand the impact of subcortical ischemic vascular disease on memory performance. Despite comparable levels of initial acquisition, patients without lacunes showed more rapid forgetting than patients with lacunes, consistent with the hypothesis that dementia patients without lacunes are likely to have AD. Further analysis indicated that memory patterns within the lacune group were heterogeneous, with some participants exhibiting rapid forgetting and some exhibiting good retention. Lacune patients with good retention showed a trend for greater executive impairments relative to lacune patients with rapid forgetting and patients without lacunes. These results suggest that rapid forgetting in dementia patients with lacunes may imply concomitant AD, whereas the dementia in patients with good retention may be purely vascular in origin.

Ultimately, autopsy-confirmed cases of SIVD provide the best way to understand the nature of cognitive impairment in patients without significant AD pathology. Recently, Reed et al. (2007) described individual patterns of memory and executive dysfunction in autopsy confirmed AD, SIVD, and mixed dementia. One significant methodological strength of the study was the application of psychometrically matched scales of memory and executive functioning that were derived using item response theory (Mungas, Reed, & Kramer, 2003). Three neuropsychological profiles were defined: Low Memory (relative to Executive), Low Executive (relative to Memory), and Other (comparable Memory and Executive scores). Each subject was characterized by one of these three profiles. Groups defined by these profiles were closely matched on age and education and did not differ on overall severity of cognitive impairment as measured by the DRS total score. As expected, pathologically confirmed AD subjects mostly (71%) had the Low Memory profile while only 10% showed a Low Executive profile. In contrast, patients with only vascular disease on autopsy had a less consistent neuropsychological pattern. Although Low Executive was the most common profile, Low Executive described less than half (45%) the cases, 36% fit neither pattern, and 18% had Low Memory. When only the subset of cases with MCI or dementia at the time of baseline examination was examined, however, the cognitive patterns were more distinct. Of those patients with only cerebrovascular disease, 67% had Low Executive and none had Low Memory. However, the diagnostic sensitivity of the Low Executive profile as a test for the presence of vascular cognitive impairment/VaD was modest at best; among patients with cognitive impairment or dementia only, the sensitivity of the Low Executive profile was 0.67 (CI = 0.24–0.94), specificity was 0.86 (CI = 0.69–0.95), and the positive likelihood ratio was 4.7 (CI = 1.7–12.5).

In summary, there is an extensive literature suggesting that SIVD and AD patients differ in their pattern of performance on specific measures of cognitive functioning, with SIVD having disproportional involvement in subcortical-frontal executive functions, and AD having relatively more memory impairment. Much of this literature, however, has been based on clinical diagnoses of AD and SIVD, but our ability to accurately classify dementia patients into SIVD and AD groups is poor. Prospectively studied patients with cognitive impairment and dementia that are followed to autopsy have relatively low rates of pure SIVD, and careful studies of the relationships between structural brain changes and cognition suggest that MRI changes most typically associated with AD (i.e., HVs and cortical atrophy) are the major predictors of cognitive decline. Finally, although there is some autopsy confirmed support for cerebrovascular pathology to be more strongly associated with executive dysfunction than with memory impairment, these cognitive markers do not offer sufficient sensitivity for widespread clinical application.

Areas for Future Research

Predicting the underlying pathology in elderly patients with cognitive decline continues to be a vexing problem. Cognitive and behavioral symptoms generally reflect the location of the underlying pathology and not the specific pathological mechanisms. Several converging lines of evidence highlight the neuroanatomical overlap and possibly interactions between cerebrovascular disease and Alzheimer's disease, making inferences about the relative contributions of different disease states unreliable. Clinicians should always consider the possibility of concomitant neurodegenerative disease even in patients with unambiguous cerebrovascular injury, particularly since treatments for Alzheimer's disease are available. Nonetheless, studying cognitive sequelae of subcortical ischemic vascular disease remains highly relevant. Subcortical ischemic changes are present in a large proportion of nondemented elderly, and understanding their associations with dementia has significant public health ramifications. Our current base of knowledge about SIVD is hindered by the lack of uniformity in how SIVD is defined and how well comorbid neurodegenerative disease can be ruled out. There remains a considerable need for better in vivo markers of both AD and cerebrovascular disease beyond the current measures of lacune counts and white matter signal hyperintensity. One potentially exciting development is amyloid imaging using the Pittsburgh-B and other compounds that offer the possibility of identifying AD related pathology. Cerebrospinal fluid markers of either AD or cerebrovascular injury also hold some promise.

Much of the clinical research on SIVD has focused on neuropsychological changes. While this research continues to be relevant, the emphasis going forward needs to be on pathology proven cases. Increasing attention might also be paid to neuropsychiatric features of dementia syndromes. We know from studies of depression that psychiatric symptoms are associated with subcortical hyperintensities, particularly in the elderly (Firbank, Lloyd, Ferrier, & O'Brien, 2004; Simpson, Jackson, Baldwin, & Burns, 1997; Tupler et al., 2002). Anxiety, depression, and the overall severity of neuropsychiatric symptoms in VaD patients have also been associated with the extent of white matter ischemia (Sultzer et al., 1995). Greater awareness of the neuropsychiatric features of SIVD can simultaneously improve patient care and guide our understanding of brain-behavior relationships.

Finally, treatment aimed at primary prevention, secondary prevention, and tertiary care is needed. Primary intervention should dovetail with efforts aimed at reducing the prevalence of vascular disease in general. However, there are a large number of the normal elderly with so-called silent lacunes, who are at greater risk than their peers for developing a dementia. For those patients with SIVD, more clinical trials are needed to assess the viability of anticholinesterases and other medications that may improve cognitive functioning in other dementing disorders.

References

Babikan, V., & Ropper, A. H. (1987). Binswanger's disease: a review. *Stroke*, *18*, 2–12.

Bjeljac, M., Keller, E., Regard, M., & Yonekawa, Y. (2002). Neurological and neuropsychological outcome after SAH. *Acta Neurochirurgica. Supplement*, *82*, 83–85.

Black, S. E. (2005). Vascular dementia. Stroke risk and sequelae define therapeutic approaches. *Postgraduate Medicine*, *117*(1), 15–16, 19–25.

Bogousslavsky, J., Regli, F., & Uske, A. (1988). Thalamic infarcts: clinical syndromes, etiology, and prognosis. *Neurology*, *38*(6), 837–848.

Brun, A. (1994). Pathology and pathophysiology of cerebrovascular dementia: pure subgroups of obstructive and hypoperfusive etiology. *Dementia*, *5*(3–4), 145–147.

Capizzano, A. A., Schuff, N., Amend, D. L., Tanabe, J. L., Norman, D., Maudsley, A. A., et al. (2000). Subcortical ischemic vascular dementia: assessment with quantitative MR imaging and 1H MR spectroscopy. *AJNR American Journal of Neuroradiology*, *21*(4), 621–630.

Caplan, L. R., & Schoene, W. C. (1978). Clinical features of subcortical arteriosclerotic encephalopathy (Binswanger disease). *Neurology*, *28*(12), 1206–1215.

Carew, T. G., Lamar, M., Cloud, B. S., Grossman, M., & Libon, D. J. (1997). Impairment in category fluency in ischemic vascular dementia. *Neuropsychology*, *11*(3), 400–412.

Charlton, R. A., Morris, R. G., Nitkunan, A., & Markus, H. S. (2006). The cognitive profiles of CADASIL and sporadic small vessel disease. *Neurology*, *66*(10), 1523–1526.

Chui, H. C. (1989). Dementia. A review emphasizing clinicopathologic correlation and brain-behavior relationships. *Archives of Neurology*, *46*(7), 806–814.

Chui, H. C., Mack, W., Jackson, J. E., Mungas, D., Reed, B. R., Tinklenberg, J., et al. (2000). Clinical criteria for the diagnosis of vascular dementia: a multicenter study of comparability and interrater reliability. *Archives of Neurology*, *57*(191–6).

Chui, H. C., Victoroff, J. I., Margolin, D., Jagust, W., Shankle, R., & Katzman, R. (1992). Criteria for the diagnosis of ischemic vascular dementia proposed by the State of California Alzheimer's Disease Diagnostic and Treatment Centers. *Neurology*, *42*(3 Pt 1), 473–480.

Chui, H. C., Zarow, C., Mack, W. J., Ellis, W. G., Zheng, L., Jagust, W. J., et al. (2006). Cognitive impact of subcortical vascular and Alzheimer's disease pathology. *Annals of Neurology*, *60*(6), 677–687.

Cosentino, S. A., Jefferson, A. L., Carey, M., Price, C. C., Davis-Garrett, K., Swenson, R., et al. (2004). The clinical diagnosis of vascular dementia: A comparison among four classification systems and a proposal for a new paradigm. *Clinical Neuropsychologist*, *18*(1), 6–21.

Cummings, J. L. (1995). Anatomic and behavioral aspects of frontal-subcortical circuits. *Annals of the New York Academy of Sciences*, *769*, 1–13.

Davous, P. (1998). CADASIL: a review with proposed diagnostic criteria. *European Journal of Neurology*, *5*(3), 219–233.

de la Torre, J. C. (2002). Alzheimer disease as a vascular disorder: nosological evidence. *Stroke*, *33*(4), 1152–1162.

DeCarli, C., Mungas, D., Harvey, D., Reed, B., Weiner, M., Chui, H., et al. (2004). Memory impairment, but not cerebrovascular disease, predicts progression of MCI to dementia. *Neurology*, *63*(2), 220–227.

D'Esposito, M., Alexander, M. P., Fischer, R., McGlinchey-Berroth, R., & O'Connor, M. (1996). Recovery of memory and executive function following anterior communicating artery aneurysm rupture. *Journal of the International Neuropsychological Society*, *2*(6), 565–570.

Erker, G. J., Searight, H. R., & Peterson, P. (1995). Patterns of neuropsychological functioning among patients with multi-infarct and Alzheimer's dementia: a comparative analysis. *International Psychogeriatrics*, *7*(3), 393–406.

Erkinjuntti, T. (1997). Vascular dementia: challenge of clinical diagnosis. *International Psychogeriatrics, 9* Suppl 1, 51–58; discussion 77–83.

Erkinjuntti, T. (2002). Diagnosis and management of vascular cognitive impairment and dementia. *Journal of Neural Transmission. Supplementum*, (63), 91–109.

Fein, G., Di Sclafani, V., Tanabe, J., Cardenas, V., Weiner, M. W., Jagust, W. J., et al. (2000). Hippocampal and cortical atrophy predict dementia in subcortical ischemic vascular disease. *Neurology*, 55(11), 1626–1635.

Firbank, M. J., Lloyd, A. J., Ferrier, N., & O'Brien, J. T. (2004). A volumetric study of MRI signal hyperintensities in late-life depression. *American Journal of Geriatric Psychiatry*, 12(6), 606–612.

Gearing, M., Mirra, S. S., Hedreen, J. C., Sumi, S. M., Hansen, L. A., & Heyman, A. (1995). The Consortium to Establish a Registry for Alzheimer's Disease (CERAD). Part X. Neuropathology confirmation of the clinical diagnosis of Alzheimer's disease. *Neurology*, 45(3 Pt 1), 461–466.

Gold, G., Bouras, C., Canuto, A., Bergallo, M. F., Herrmann, F. R., Hof, P. R., et al. (2002). Clinicopathological validation study of four sets of clinical criteria for vascular dementia. *American Journal of Psychiatry*, 159(1), 82–87.

Gorelick, P. B. (2004). Risk factors for vascular dementia and Alzheimer disease. *Stroke*, 35(11 Suppl 1), 2620–2622.

Hachinski, V. C., Illiff, L. D., Zilhka, E., du Boulay, G. H., McAllister, V. L., & Marchall, J. (1975). Cerebral blood flow in dementia. *Archives of Neurology*, 32, 632–637.

Hassing, L., & Backman, L. (1997). Episodic memory functioning in population-based samples of very old adults with Alzheimer's disease and vascular dementia. *Dementia and Geriatric Cognitive Disorders*, 8(6), 376–383.

Henon, H. (2002). Neuroimaging predictors of dementia in stroke patients. *Clinical and Experimental Hypertension*, 24(7–8), 677–686.

Jellinger, K. A. (2002). The pathology of ischemic-vascular dementia: an update. *Journal of the Neurological Sciences*, 203–204, 153–157.

Jimbo, H., Hanakawa, K., Ozawa, H., Dohi, K., Sawabe, Y., Matsumoto, K., et al. (2000). Neuropsychological changes after surgery for anterior communicating artery aneurysm. *Neurologia Medico-Chirurgica (Tokyo)*, 40(2), 83–86; discussion 86–87.

Kemenoff, L. A., Kramer, J.H., Mungas, D., Reed, B., Willis, L., Weiner, M., and Chui, H. (1999). Neuropsychological differentiation of vascular and Alzheimer's dementia. Poster session presented at the 107th Annual Convention of the American Psychological Association, Boston.

Kertesz, A., & Clydesdale, S. (1994). Neuropsychological deficits in vascular dementia vs Alzheimer's disease: frontal lobe deficits prominent in vascular dementia. *Archives of Neurology*, 51, 1226–1231.

Knopman, D. S., DeKosky, S. T., Cummings, J. L., Chui, H., Corey-Bloom, J., Relkin, N., et al. (2001). Practice parameter: diagnosis of dementia (an evidence-based review). Report of the Quality Standards Subcommittee of the American Academy of Neurology. *Neurology*, 56(9), 1143–1153.

Knopman, D. S., & Nissen, M. J. (1991). Procedural learning is impaired in Huntington's disease: evidence from the serial reaction time task. *Neuropsychologia*, 29, 245–254.

Kobayashi, S., Okada, K., Koide, H., Bokura, H., & Yamaguchi, S. (1997). Subcortical silent brain infarction as a risk factor for clinical stroke. *Stroke*, 28(10), 1932–1939.

Kooistra, C. A., & Heilman, K. M. (1988). Memory loss from a subcortical white matter infarct. *Journal of Neurology, Neurosurgery, and Psychiatry*, 51(6), 866–869.

Kramer, J. H., Mungas, D., Reed, B. R., Schuff, N., Weiner, M. W., Miller, B. L., et al. (2004). Forgetting in dementia with and without subcortical lacunes. *Clinical Neuropsychologist*, 18(1), 32–40.

Kwan, L. T., Reed, B. R., Eberling, J. L., Schuff, N., Tanabe, J., Norman, D., et al. (1999). Effects of subcortical cerebral infarction on cortical glucose metabolism and cognitive function. *Archives of Neurology*, 56(7), 809–814.

Lafosse, J. M., Reed, B. R., Mungas, D., Sterling, S. B., Wahbeh, H., & Jagust, W. J. (1997). Fluency and memory differences between ischemic vascular dementia and Alzheimer's disease. *Neuropsychology*, 11(4), 514–522.

Libon, D. J., Bogdanoff, B., Cloud, B. S., Skalina, S., Giovannetti, T., Gitlin, H. L., et al. (1998). Declarative and procedural learning, quantitative measures of the hippocampus, and subcortical white alterations in Alzheimer's disease and ischaemic vascular dementia. *Journal of Clinical and Experimental Neuropsychology*, 20(1), 30–41.

Libon, D. J., Price, C. C., Davis Garrett, K., & Giovannetti, T. (2004). From Binswanger's disease to leuokoaraiosis: what we have learned about subcortical vascular dementia. *Clinical Neuropsychologist*, 18(1), 83–100.

Loeb, C. (2000). Binswanger's disease is not a single entity. *Neurological Sciences*, 21(6), 343–348.

Loeb, C., & Gandolfo, C. (1983). Diagnostic evaluation of degenerative and vascular dementia. *Stroke*, 14(3), 399–401.

Loeb, C., Gandolfo, C., Croce, R., & Conti, M. (1992). Dementia associated with lacunar infarction. *Stroke*, 23(9), 1225–1229.

Loeb, C., & Meyer, J. S. (1996). Vascular dementia: still a debatable entity? *Journal of Neurological Sciences*, 143(1–2), 31–40.

Longstreth, W. T., Jr., Bernick, C., Manolio, T. A., Bryan, N., Jungreis, C. A., & Price, T. R. (1998). Lacunar infarcts defined by magnetic resonance imaging of 3660 elderly people: the Cardiovascular Health Study. *Archives of Neurology*, 55(9), 1217–1225.

Markus, H. S., Martin, R. J., Simpson, M. A., Dong, Y. B., Ali, N., Crosby, A. H., et al. (2002). Diagnostic strategies in CADASIL. *Neurology*, 59(8), 1134–1138.

Mendez, M. F., & Ashla-Mendez, M. (1991). Differences between multi-infarct dementia and Alzheimer's disease on unstructured neuropsychological tasks. *Journal of Clinical and Experimental Neuropsychology, 13*(6), 923–932.

Mungas, D., Jagust, W. J., Reed, B. R., Kramer, J. H., Weiner, M. W., Schuff, N., et al. (2001). MRI predictors of cognition in subcortical ischemic vascular disease and Alzheimer's disease. *Neurology, 57*(12), 2229–2235.

Mungas, D., Reed, B. R., & Kramer, J. H. (2003). Psychometrically matched measures of global cognition, memory, and executive function for assessment of cognitive decline in older persons. *Neuropsychology, 17*(3), 380–392.

Nolan, K. A., Lino, M. M., Seligmann, A. W., & Blass, J. P. (1998). Absence of vascular dementia in an autopsy series from a dementia clinic. *Journal of the American Geriatrics Society, 46*(5), 597–604.

O'Brien, J. T., Erkinjuntti, T., Reisberg, B., Roman, G., Sawada, T., Pantoni, L., et al. (2003). Vascular cognitive impairment. *Lancet Neurology, 2*(2), 89–98.

Padovani, A., Di Piero, V., Bragoni, M., Iacoboni, M., Gualdi, G. F., & Lenzi, G. L. (1995). Patterns of neuropsychological impairment in mild dementia: a comparison between Alzheimer's disease and multi-infarct dementia. *Acta Neurologica Scandinavica, 92*(6), 433–442.

Peters, N., Opherk, C., Danek, A., Ballard, C., Herzog, J., & Dichgans, M. (2005). The Pattern of Cognitive Performance in CADASIL: A Monogenic Condition Leading to Subcortical Ischemic Vascular Dementia. *American Journal of Psychiatry, 162*(11), 2078–2085.

Price, T. R., Manolio, T. A., Kronmal, R. A., Kittner, S. J., Yue, N. C., Robbins, J., et al. (1997). Silent brain infarction on magnetic resonance imaging and neurological abnormalities in community-dwelling older adults. The Cardiovascular Health Study. CHS Collaborative Research Group. *Stroke, 28*(6), 1158–1164.

Rabinstein, A. A., Romano, J. G., Forteza, A. M., & Koch, S. (2004). Rapidly Progressive Dementia Due to Bilateral Internal Carotid Artery Occlusion with Infarction of the Total Length of the Corpus Callosum. *Journal of Neuroimaging, 14*(2), 176–179.

Reed, B. R., Mungas, D. M., Kramer, J. H., Betz, B. P., Ellis, W., Vinters, H. V., et al. (2004). Clinical and neuropsychological features in autopsy-defined vascular dementia. *Clinical Neuropsychologist, 18*(1), 63–74.

Reed, B. R., Mungas, D. M., Kramer, J. H., Ellis, W., Vinters, H. V., Zarow, C., et al. (2007). Profiles of neuropsychological impairment in autopsy-defined Alzheimer's disease and cerebrovascular disease. *Brain, 130*(Pt 3), 731–739.

Roman, G. C. (1987). Senile dementia of the Binswanger type. A vascular form of dementia in the elderly. *JAMA, 258*(13), 1782–1788.

Roman, G. C. (2005). Vascular dementia prevention: a risk factor analysis. *Cerebrovascular Diseases, 20 Suppl 2*, 91–100.

Roman, G. C., Erkinjuntti, T., Wallin, A., Pantoni, L., & Chui, H. C. (2002). Subcortical ischaemic vascular dementia. *Lancet Neurology, 1*(7), 426–436.

Roman, G. C., Tatemichi, T. K., & Erkinjuntii, T. (1993). Vascular Dementia: Diagnostic criteria for research studies. *Neurology, 43*, 250–260.

Rosen, W. G., Terry, R. D., Fuld, P. A., Katzman, R., & Peck, A. (1980). Pathological verification of ischaemic score in differentiation of the dementias. *Annals of Neurology, 7*, 486–488.

Sacco, R. L. (1994). Ischemic Stroke. In P. B. Gorelick, M. Alter (Ed.), *Handbook of Neuroepidemiology* (pp. 77–119). New York: Marcel Decker, Inc.

Schoenberg, B. S., & Shulte, B.P.M. (1988). Cerebrovascular disease: epidemiology and geopathology. In P. J. Vinkin, G.W. Bruyn, H.L. Klawans, (Ed.), *Handbook of Clinical Neurology, Vascular Diseases* (Vol. Part 1, Volume 53, pp. 1–26).

Simpson, S. W., Jackson, A., Baldwin, R. C., & Burns, A. (1997). 1997 IPA/Bayer Research Awards in Psychogeriatrics. Subcortical hyperintensities in late-life depression: acute response to treatment and neuropsychological impairment. *International Psychogeriatrics, 9*(3), 257–275.

Sultzer, D. L., Mahler, M. E., Cummings, J. L., Van Gorp, W. G., Hinkin, C. H., & Brown, C. (1995). Cortical abnormalities associated with subcortical lesions in vascular dementia. Clinical and position emission tomographic findings. *Archives of Neurology, 52*(8), 773–780.

Tatemichi, T. K., Desmond, D. W., Paik, M., & et al. (1993). Clinical determinants of dementia related to stroke. *Annals of Neurology, 33*, 568–575.

Tatemichi, T. K., Desmond, D. W., Prohovnik, I., Cross, D. T., Gropen, T. I., Mohr, J. P., et al. (1992). Confusion and memory loss from capsular genu infarction: a thalamocortical disconnection syndrome? *Neurology, 42*, 1966–1979.

Tei, H., Miyazaki, A., Iwata, M., Osawa, M., Nagata, Y., & Maruyama, S. (1997). Early-stage Alzheimer's disease and multiple subcortical infarction with mild cognitive impairment: neuropsychological comparison using an easily applicable test battery. *Dementia and Geriatric Cognitive Disorders, 8*(6), 355–358.

Tell, G. S., Crouse, J. R., & Furberg, C. D. (1988). Relation between blood lipids, lipoproteins, and cerebrovascular atherosclerosis. A review. *Stroke, 19*(4), 423–430.

Tomlinson, B. E., Blessed, G., & Roth, M. (1970). Observations on the brains of demented old people. *Journal of the Neurological Sciences, 11*(3), 205–242.

Tullberg, M., Fletcher, E., DeCarli, C., Mungas, D., Reed, B. R., Harvey, D. J., et al. (2004). White matter lesions impair frontal lobe function regardless of their location. *Neurology, 63*(2), 246–253.

Tupler, L. A., Krishnan, K. R., McDonald, W. M., Dombeck, C. B., D'Souza, S., & Steffens, D. C. (2002). Anatomic location and laterality of MRI signal hyperintensities in late-life depression. *Journal of Psychosomatic Research*, *53*(2), 665–676.

Wang, L. N., Zhu, M. W., Gui, Q. P., & Li, X. H. (2003). An analysis of the causes of dementia in 383 elderly autopsied cases. *Zhonghua Nei Ke Za Zhi*, *42*(11), 789–792.

Wetterling, T., Kanitz, R. D., & Borgis, K. J. (1993). Clinical evaluation of the ICD-10 criteria for vascular dementia. *European Archives of Psychiatry and Clinical Neuroscience*, *243*(1), 33–40.

Wetterling, T., Kanitz, R. D., & Borgis, K. J. (1996). Comparison of different diagnostic criteria for vascular dementia (ADDTC, DSM-IV, ICD-10, NINDS-AIREN). *Stroke*, *27*(1), 30–36.

WHO. (1993). *The ICD-10 classification of mental and behavioural disorders: diagnostic criteria for research*. Geneva: Author.

Wolf, P. A., D'Agostino, R. B., Belanger, A. J., & Kannel, W. B. (1991). Probability of stroke: a risk profile from the Framingham Study. *Stroke*, *22*(3), 312–318.

Wolfe, N., Linn, R., Babikian, V. L., Knoefel, J. E., & Albert, M. L. (1990). Frontal systems impairment following multiple lacunar infarcts. *Archives of Neurology*, *47*(2), 129–132.

Chapter 8
Cerebral Autosomal Dominant Arteriopathy with Subcortical Infarcts and Leukoencephalopathy (CADASIL) and Mitochondrial Encephalomyopathy Lactic Acidosis and Stroke-like Episodes (MELAS)

Sarah Benisty and Hugues Chabriat

CADASIL

Definition and Genetic and Pathological Aspects

Cerebral Autosomal Dominant Arteriopathy with Subcortical Infarcts and Leukoencephalopathy (CADASIL) (Tournier-Lasserve, Joutel et al., 1993) is an inherited small artery disease of the brain caused by mutations of the *NOTCH3* gene on chromosome 19 (Joutel, Corpechot, Ducros et al., 1996). It is considered as a model of "pure" vascular dementia related to a small vessel disease and as an archetype of the so-called "subcortical ischemic vascular dementia" (Charlton, Morris, Nitkunan, & Markus, 2006). CADASIL is not limited to Caucasians families, although the disorder was initially recognized in European pedigrees. It has now been diagnosed in Asian, African, American as well as in Australian and European families. In France, Germany, and United Kingdom, several hundreds of CADASIL families have been identified (Dichgans, Mayer et al., 1998). Though the exact frequency of CADASIL remains unknown, it is now considered as one of the most frequent hereditary neurological disorders.

S. Benisty (✉)
Department of Geriatric medicine and Department of Neurology, Hopital Lariboisiere-Fernand-Widal, Université Paris VII, France
e-mail: sarah.benisty@lrb.aphp.fr

CADASIL is caused by stereotyped mutations of the *NOTCH3* gene (Joutel, Corpechot, Ducros et al., 1996). Unlike other members of the Notch gene family whose expression is ubiquitous, the *NOTCH3* gene is expressed only in vascular smooth muscle cells of arterial vessels. Domenga et al. recently showed that *NOTCH3* is required specifically to generate functional arteries in mice by regulating arterial differentiation and maturation of vascular smooth muscle cells (Domenga et al., 2004). The stereotyped mis-sense mutations (Joutel, Corpechot, Ducros et al., 1996) or deletions (Joutel, Francois et al., 2000) responsible for CADASIL are within epidermal-growth-factor-like (EGF-like) repeats and only located in the extracellular domain of the *NOTCH3* protein (Dotti, Federico, Mazzei et al., 2005; Joutel, Corpechot, Ducros et al., 1997; Peters et al., 2005a, 2005b). All mutations responsible for the disease lead to an uneven number of cystein residues. The *NOTCH3* protein usually undergoes complex proteolytic cleavages, leading to an extracellular and a transmembrane fragment (Blaumueller, Qi, Zagouras, & Artavanis-Tsakonas 1997). After cleavage, these two fragments form a heterodimer at the cell surface of smooth muscle cells. In CADASIL, the ectodomain of the *NOTCH3* receptor accumulates within the vessel wall of affected subjects (Joutel, Andreux et al., 2000). This accumulation is found near but not within the characteristic granular osmiophilic material seen on electron microscopy. It is observed in all vascular smooth muscle cells and in pericytes within all organs (brain, heart, muscles, lungs, skin). An abnormal clearance of the *NOTCH3* ectodomain from the smooth muscle cell surface is presumed to cause this accumulation (Joutel, Andreux, et al.; Joutel, Francois et al., 2000; Joutel & Tournier-Lasserve 2002).

Macroscopic examination of the brain shows a diffuse myelin pallor and rarefaction of the hemispheric white-matter, sparing the U fibres (Baudrimont, Dubas, Joutel, Tournier-Lasserve, & Bousser 1993). Lesions predominate in the periventricular areas and centrum semiovale. They are associated with lacunar infarcts located in the white-matter and basal ganglia (lentiform nucleus, thalamus, caudate) (Ruchoux, Brulin et al., 2002; Ruchoux & Maurage, 1997). The most severe hemispheric lesions are the most profound (Baudrimont, et al.). In the brainstem, the lesions are more marked in the pons and are similar to the pontine ischemic rarefaction of myelin described by Pullicino, Ostrow, Miller, Snyder, and Munschauer (1995). Small, deep infarcts and dilated Virchow-Robin spaces are also associated with the white-matter lesions. The vessels close to these lesions do not appear occluded. Microscopic investigations show that the wall of cerebral and leptomeningeal arterioles is thickened, with a significant reduction of the lumen (Baudrimont, et al.), thus, penetrating arteries in the cortex and white-matter appear stenosed (Miao et al., 2004; Okeda, Arima, & Kawai, 2002). Some inconstant features are similar to those reported in patients with hypertensive encephalopathy (Zhang et al., 1994): duplication and splitting of internal elastic lamina, adventitial hyalinosis and fibrosis, and hypertrophy of the media. However, a distinctive feature is the presence of a granular material within the media extending into the adventitia (Baudrimont, et al.; Bergmann, Ebke, Yuan, Brück, Mugler, & Schwendemann, 1996; Desmond et al., 1999; Mikol et al., 2001; Ruchoux, Guerouaou et al., 1995). On electron-microscopy, the smooth muscle cells appear swollen and often degenerated, some of them with multiple nuclei. There is a granular osmiophilic material (GOM) within

the media (Gutierrez-Molina et al., 1994). This material consists of granules of about 10–15 nm in diameter. It is localized close to the cell membrane of the smooth muscle cells where it appears very dense. The smooth muscle cells are separated by large amounts of this unidentified material. Rafalowska made the observation that this material can be also be detected in capillaries deprived of smooth muscle cells and that it is sometimes associated with perivascular inflammatory infiltrates or with eosinophilic fibrinoid necrosis (Rafalowska et al., 2003).

Ruchoux et al. made the crucial observation that the vascular abnormalities observed in the brain were also detectable in other organs or territories (Ruchoux, Guerouaou et al., 1995). These vascular lesions can be detected by nerve or muscle biopsy. The presence of the granular osmiophilic material in the skin vessels now allows the intra vitam diagnosis of CADASIL using punch skin biopsies (Chabriat, Joutel et al., 1997; Ebke et al., 1997; Ruchoux, Guerouaou, et al.), although the sensitivity and specificity of this method have not yet been completely established. In some cases, the vessel changes may be focal requiring a thorough evaluation of the biopsy specimen (Schultz, Santoianni, Hewan-Lowe, 1999). Joutel et al. proposed to use anti-*NOTCH3* antibodies to reveal the accumulation of *NOTCH3* products within the vessel wall in CADASIL patients as an alternative diagnostic method (Joutel, Favrole et al., 2001). This method appears highly sensitive (96%) and specific (100%).

The diagnosis of CADASIL is made by genetic testing or skin biopsy. Genetic tests are initially focused on exons where the mutations are most frequent (Joutel, Corpechot, Ducros et al., 1997). Peters et al. found 90% of mutations within exons 2–6 (Peters et al., 2005a, 2005b). Diagnostic testing with immunostaining using anti-*NOTCH3* antibodies is an alternative method that seems easier than electron microscopy and useful before initiating a complete screening of the gene in difficult cases (Joutel, Favrole et al., 2001).

Main Clinical Features and Neurobehavioral Symptoms

The main clinical manifestations of CADASIL are as follows: (1) attacks of migraine with aura, occurring between age 20 and 40 years; (2) ischemic episodes such as transient ischemic attacks or completed subcortical ischemic strokes, occurring from age 40 years and reported in 60–80% of patients, (3) mood disturbances; and (4) cognitive alterations (Chabriat, Joutel et al., 1997).

Cognitive impairment represents the second most common clinical manifestation in CADASIL, and may be observed in the absence of any other clinical symptoms (Buffon et al., 2006). Its degree may vary with the course of disease, the age of the patient, and the occurrence of stroke (Amberla et al., 2004; Buffon, et al.). In most cases, it is mild for several decades, but by the age of 65, two thirds of the patients have dementia (Dichgans, Mayer et al., 1998).

The onset of cognitive deficits is usually mild and insidious, and the exact time is difficult to ascertain. Cross-sectional studies (Taillia et al., 1998; Amberla et al., 2004; Peters et al., 2005a, 2005b; Buffon, et al., 2006) have shown that early in the disease cognitive functions, most frequently attention and executive functions, may be impaired. In a recent series of 42 patients, attention and executive functions were affected in nearly 90% of patients of age between 35 and 50 (Buffon et al.). In contrast, other functions such as verbal episodic memory and visuospatial abilities are usually preserved and may remain spared until late stages of the disease.

Some tests are particularly sensitive to the detection of early cognitive changes. They include the digit span backward and forward, the Trail Making Test B, the Stroop Test, and the Wisconsin Card Sorting Test (Taillia et al.,

1998). The errors of CADASIL patients may predominantly affect latency measures in timed tasks (Stroop, Trail Making Test, Symbol Digit, Digit cancellation), though errors in monitoring are also observed to a lesser extent (Peters et al., 2005a, 2005b). Patients may also show poor strategy and planning when completing tasks such as the Wisconsin Card Sorting Test and the Rey-Osterreith memory test. The memory deficit may be associated with executive dysfunction, but its profile is usually distinct from dementias primarily involving the mesiotemporal cortex such as Alzheimer's disease. This is well illustrated by procedures used in the Grober and Buschke test. This test allows the differentiation of phases of memory processes and is likely to show the preservation of the encoding process even though the retrieval is impaired. It is composed of the following: (1) an encoding phase in which 16 words belonging to 16 different semantic categories have to be retrieved; (2) three phases of free recall and cued recall (the last being delayed); and (3) a recognition test. In CADASIL, this test distinguishes a pattern characterized by low scores in immediate and delayed free recall, improving with cues and associated with relatively intact recognition. Intrusions may occur in the free recall task. This profile supports preservation of the encoding process and, anatomically, of the mesiotemporal cortex. It is observed in about two thirds of the CADASIL patients with dementia (Buffon et al., 2006).

Global cognitive scales may also be used in the assessment of cognitive functions. The Mini Mental State Examination (MMSE) is not sensitive to executive dysfunction, and so is not a good screening test for cognitive impairment in CADASIL. In contrast, scales designed for assessment of vascular cognitive impairment, such as the VADAS-Cog may be of particular interest (Madureira et al., 2006).

A similar pattern of cognitive impairment, with prominent early executive dysfunction, has been observed in patients with sporadic small vessel disease (Charlton et al., 2006).

Together with aging and the evolution of the disease, two thirds of the patients in their sixties and older have dementia (Dichgans, Mayer et al., 1998) and more than 80% of the deceased subjects were reported to have dementia before death (Chabriat, Vahedi et al., 1995). When dementia is present, the cognitive declines become more homogenous with significant alterations in most cognitive domains. Still, executive functions and attention remain predominantly affected and the encoding process appears preserved even at late stages of the disease. Dementia often occurs in association with motor and urinary disturbances and pseudobulbar palsy.

The development of cognitive impairment appears associated with the occurrence of stroke. Nevertheless, a cognitive deficit and even a dementia state may also occur in patients without any clinical history of stroke. The cognitive profile of CADASIL patients was analyzed before and after the occurrence of strokes in two cross-sectional studies and showed some discrepant results. Amberla et al. (2004) reported that executive functions were more widely affected with a significant mental slowing in CADASIL patients with a positive history of stroke. Conversely, Buffon et al. (2006) observed that visuospatial abilities were mostly impaired in patients with stroke.

The temporal progression of cognitive symptoms varies among subjects, from rapid and marked deterioration to stable or even slightly improving performances (Peters, Herzog, Opherk, & Dichgans, 2004). Two patterns of deterioration can be distinguished, although they often coexist in a same patient. The evolution may be mainly stepwise and the worsening mostly associated with repeated acute ischemic events associated with an accumulation of lesions within strategic regions such as the thalamus, which is critically involved in cognition. The cognitive performances can also deteriorate progressively with dementia developing parallel to the accumulation of new cognitive deficits. This pattern is detected in about 10% of the patients. (Chabriat, Joutel et al., 1997)

The occurrence of psychiatric symptoms is estimated to affect about 30% of the cases (Dichgans, Mayer et al., 1998). They may be inaugural or dominate the clinical course of the disease and thus lead to misdiagnosis. Patients with a long period of psychiatric symptoms before the onset of dementia have indeed been reported (Filley et al., 1999) Depression, sometimes severe, is the most common manifestation and is inconstantly improved by antidepressant drugs (Chabriat, Vahedi et al., 1995). In a few patients, severe depression of the melancholic type alternates with mania episodes suggesting bipolar mood disorder (Kumar and Mahr 1997). Panic disorder, delusional episodes, and a picture of schizophrenia have also been observed in CADASIL (Lagas and Juvonen 2001).

Among behavioral symptoms, apathy and irritability are often present independently of the occurrence of a depressive state. Finally, behavioral disturbances and their interactions with the cognitive performances remain poorly investigated in CADASIL.

Cerebral Tissue Lesions and Cognitive Dysfunction in CADASIL

MRI is crucial for the diagnosis of CADASIL and is much more sensitive than a CT-scan. It is always abnormal in patients with neurological symptoms other than migraine attacks (Chabriat, Joutel et al., 1997; Tournier-Lasserve, Joutel, et al., 1993). MRI signal abnormalities can also be detected during a presymptomatic period of variable duration, observed as early as 20 years of age. After age 35, all subjects having the affected gene have an abnormal MRI (Tournier-Lasserve, Joutel, et al.; Tournier-Lasserve, Iba-Zizen, Romero, & Bousser, 1991). The frequency of asymptomatic subjects with abnormal MRI decreases progressively with aging and becomes less than 5% after 60 years (Chabriat, Levy et al., 1998).

On T2-weighted images, MRI shows widespread areas of increased signal in the white-matter associated with focal hyperintensities in

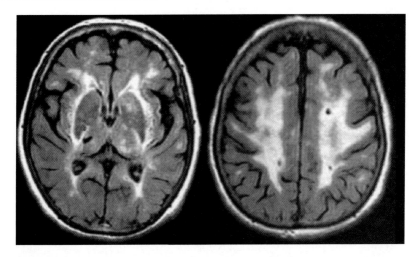

Fig. 1 T2-weighted MRI (FLAIR images) showing widespread and symmetrical hyperintensities in the white-matter and small deep infarcts (hypointensities) located in the thalamus and within the centrum semi-ovale. Note the involvement of the external capsules observed in two thirds of CADASIL patients

basal ganglia, thalamus, and brainstem (Fig. 1) (Chabriat, Levy et al., 1998; Desmond et al., 1999). The extent of white-matter signal abnormalities is highly variable, increasing dramatically with age. In subjects under 40 years of age, T2 hypersignals are usually punctuate or nodular with a symmetrical distribution, and predominate in periventricular areas and within the centrum semi-ovale. Later in life, white-matter lesions are diffuse and can involve the whole of white-matter including the U fibers under the cortex (Chabriat, Mrissa et al., 1999; Coulthard, Blank, Bushby, Kalaria, & Burn 2000; Dichgans, Filippi et al., 1999). Scores of severity based on semi-quantitative rating scales increase significantly with age not only in the white-matter but also in basal ganglia and brainstem. Frontal and occipital periventricular lesions are invariably present when MRI is abnormal. The frequency of signal abnormalities in the external capsule (two-thirds of the cases) and in the anterior part of the temporal lobes (60%) is noteworthy and particularly useful for differential diagnosis with other small-vessel diseases (Auer et al., 2001; Markus et al., 2002; O'Sullivan, Jarosz et al., 2001). T2 hyperintensities can also be detected in the corpus callosum (Coulthard, et al.). Brainstem lesions predominate in the

pons in areas irrigated by perforating arteries and can involve the mesencephalon (Chabriat, Mrissa, et al.). In contrast, the medulla is usually spared.

On T1-weighted images, punctiform or larger focal hypointensities are frequent in the same areas and detected in about two thirds of individuals with T2 hyperintensities (Chabriat, Levy et al., 1998) (identical to hypointense lesions as seen on FLAIR images as in Fig. 2). They are observed both in the white-matter and basal ganglia, but also in the brainstem and correspond mostly to lacunar infarctions. Numerous hypointensities on T1-weighted images may also correspond to Virchow-Robin spaces, which are more frequent and extensive in CADASIL than in healthy subjects (Cumurciuc et al., 2006). MRI signal abnormalities within the temporal white-matter in CADASIL, and particularly within the subcortical white-matter, are considered as a characteristic feature of the disease (Fig. 2). They are also caused by a distension of the perivascular space of perforating arteries at the level of the junction of gray and white matter, and by spongiosis in the surrounding parenchyma (van Den Boom et al., 2002).

Cognitive dysfunction in CADASIL is presumably related to cerebral tissue lesions,

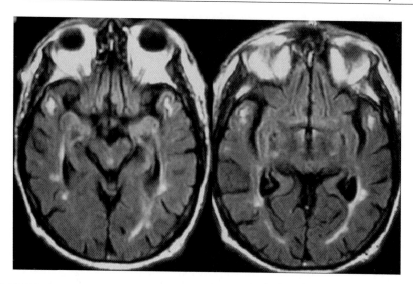

Fig. 2 MRI (FLAIR images) showing the characteristic bilateral signal changes in the subcortical white-matter of CADASIL patients within the anterior part of temporal lobes; note the linear hyposignal between the cortical rim and the hyperintense white-matter corresponding to the accumulation of multiple dilated perivascular spaces

mainly represented by lacunar infarcts and microstructural tissues changes detected within the white and grey matter. However, the contribution of these lesions to the cognitive status may be extremely variable. Dementia and disability are better correlated with the load of T1 lesions within the white matter than with the extent of white-matter hyperintensities (Holtmannspotter et al., 2005). Besides the degree of tissue destruction reflected by the T1 lesions load, the location of tissue lesions—mainly lacunar infarcts—may play also a key role in the occurrence of cognitive deficit and dementia. Lacunar infarcts are frequent in basal ganglia, especially in the thalamus, which is considered as a "strategic" area involved in cognition. This is supported by the findings of a positron emission tomography (PET) study performed in two CADASIL-affected brothers—one demented and the other asymptomatic. A severe cortical metabolic depression was found in the affected subject, who only had infarcts within basal ganglia and thalamus (Chabriat, Bousser, & Pappata. 1995). This is also in line with MRI data obtained in sporadic small-vessel diseases in the general population (Vermeer et al., 2003).

Diffusion tensor imaging (DTI) allows white matter tracts to be imaged in vivo and provides measures of diffusivity reflecting the severity of microstructural tissue alterations. This technique provides a more powerful marker of the severity of subcortical damage than the classical T2- and FLAIR-weighed images. An increase in diffusion is indeed detected in white matter and grey matter (thalamus, putamen, globus pallidum) while appearing unaffected on conventional MRI (Chabriat, Vahedi et al., 1995; O'Sullivan, Singhal, Charlton, & Markus, 2004) sequences and this increase is better correlated with cognitive function than the load of T2 lesions. Thus, Chabriat et al. (Chabriat, Pappata et al., 1999, #81) demonstrated that global DTI measures over the whole brain were strongly correlated with the MMSE. O'Sullivan et al. also reported that diffusion changes at the subcortical level was correlated with performances in executive functions (O'Sullivan, Singhal, et al.).

The exact mechanisms of cognitive dysfunction in CADASIL remain unknown. The main hypothesis is that accumulation of subcortical lesions may damage particularly the striato-cortical circuits linking basal ganglia to frontal cortical areas with possible secondary cortical degeneration (Molko et al., 2001). This hypothesis is supported by evidence of strong correlations between cortical atrophy and the cognitive decline in the disease in both imaging and neuropathological studies. As described previously, severe cortical metabolic depression has indeed been observed by PET study in association with basal ganglia and thalamic infarcts in a patient with dementia (Chabriat, Bousser et al., 1995). The post-mortem brain examination of a CADASIL case previously showed evidence of a diffuse loss of cortical neurons associated with cholinergic denervation (Mesulam, Siddique, & Cohen, 2003). In a recent neuropathological study, Viswanathan et al. reported the presence of widespread neuronal apoptosis in the cerebral cortex of four CADASIL patients. Semiquantitative analysis suggested that the degree of cortical neuronal apoptosis was related to the extent of white matter lesions and to the intensity of axonal damage in subcortical areas (Viswanathan, Gray, Bousser, Baudrimont, & Chabriat, 2006) and was associated with the severity of cognitive impairment. Therefore, subcortical axonal damage may induce cortical apoptosis through deafferentation and/or retrograde neuronal degeneration in CADASIL.

Disruption of cortical connections may affect striato-cortical circuits, relaying in the thalamus and basal ganglia as well as cortical networks. This is supported by recent DTI findings from O'Sullivan et al. who observed (1) a strong correlation between mean diffusivity measured in the thalamus (which could reflect either direct pathological damage or secondary degeneration due to disruption of white matter tracts relaying in this structure) and executive dysfunction (O'Sullivan, Singhal et al., 2004) and (2) executive performances also correlated with mean diffusivity in the anteroposterior fasciculus of the cingulum bundle, which connects the dorsolateral prefrontal lobe with more posterior cortical regions including the hippocampal formation (O'Sullivan, Barrick, Morris, Clark, & Markus, 2005).

Noteworthily, if cognitive dysfunction is associated with cortical lesions and cholinergic denervation, their distribution with a relative sparing of the hippocampal areas appears distinct from the pattern of lesions observed in Alzheimer's disease (Mesulam et al., 2003). There are very few anecdotal cases showing the association of lesions typical of Alzheimer's disease with ischemic cerebral lesions caused by CADASIL (Gray, Robert, Labrecques, 1994; Filley et al., 1999; Thijs, Robberecht, De Vos, & Sciot, 2003). This association is probably only fortuitous.

Treatment

To date, there are no treatment options for CADASIL. Since evidence of cholinergic denervation has been reported (Mesulam et al., 2003), an international multicenter study was recently performed to examine the efficacy of the cholinesterase inhibitor donepezil in the disorder. The results of this study are not yet available.

Because CADASIL is a vascular disorder responsible for cerebral ischemic events, different authors prescribe aspirin for secondary prevention, but its benefit in the disease has not been demonstrated. The occurrence of intracerebral hemorrhage in two anecdotal cases (Maclean, Woods et al., 2005 #62; Ragoschke-Schumm et al., 2005) and in one patient at time of death (Baudrimont et al., 1993) suggests that anticoagulant therapy may be dangerous in CADASIL.

Some drugs are useful in relieving specific symptoms during the course of CADASIL. However, for migraine, all vasoconstrictive drugs such as ergot derivatives and triptans are not recommended during the course of the disease. Cortical oligemia has been reported in asymptomatic patients (Chabriat, Vahedi et al., 1995). Also, the blood-brain barrier is possibly altered because of the vascular lesions (Ruchoux, Brulin et al., 2002). Therefore, we cannot exclude some deleterious effects of triptans on the cerebral circulation.

As a result, treatment of migraine should be restricted to analgesic agents and non-steroidal anti-inflammatory drugs.

As reported for other ischemic diseases, rehabilitation procedures are crucial, particularly when a new ischemic event occurs. If stroke occurs at an early stage of the disease, recovery is often complete.

Psychological support for the patient and family is finally of the upmost importance. Not only the psychological consequences of the neurological deficits but also those related to the hereditary nature of the disease should be considered. The diagnosis of this familial disorder may have major consequences within the family and modify relationships among close relatives. Genetic testing raises important ethical problems similar to those encountered in families with Huntington disease, particularly for asymptomatic members at risk for having the deleterious mutation. Therefore, genetic counseling and testing should be performed only at specialized centers that have the necessary experience.

MELAS

Mitochondrial Encephalomyopathy Lactic Acidosis and Stroke-like episodes (MELAS) are one of the most important encephalomyopathies related to mitochondrial dysfunction and is another inherited disease leading to vascular lesions. The acronym refers to a particular clinical syndrome described in 1984 by Pavlakis et al. that may be associated with different mutations in the mitochondrial DNA. In most cases of MELAS, the enzymatic defect is a complex I respiratory chain deficiency, and to a lesser degree, a complex IV deficiency. The enzyme abnormality is associated with a point mutation at np3243 in the tRNA Leu (UUR) region, which accounts for 80% of the patients with MELAS (Goto, Nonaka, Horai 1990). About 20% of the patients positive for this "MELAS mutation" present with a different clinical syndrome.

In the MELAS syndrome, the onset of symptoms usually occurs before the age of 40. The main symptoms (as summarized by the acronym) include stroke, seizures, lactic acidosis, and exercise intolerance. Additional clinical manifestations include dementia, limb weakness, short stature, recurrent migraine-like headaches, hearing loss, and diabetes (Goto, Horai et al., 1992). Psychiatric symptoms such as a schizophrenia-like clinical picture have been reported (Thomeer, Verhoeven, Klompenhouwer, 1998). The clinical expression is highly variable. It ranges from asymptomatic to severe disability and may overlap with others mitochondrial syndromes such as progressive external ophthalmoplegia (Damian et al., 1995) and a syndrome associating diabetes mellitus and deafness (Maassen et al., 1996).

The characteristics of the cognitive profile associated with MELAS have been poorly described in the literature. There is no specific pattern of cognitive impairment in the MELAS that can involve both cortical and subcortical regions. When it occurs in childhood, it may lead to mental retardation.

The commonest radiological finding of subjects carrying the MELAS mutation is basal ganglia calcification, which is progressive and symmetric. Other abnormalities include focal lesions most commonly involving cerebellum and grey matter of the parietal and occipital lobes. Cortical and cerebellar atrophy are present in severe cases (Sue, Crimmins et al., 1998).

The stroke-like episodes are characteristic of the MELAS syndrome and are not observed in the other main mitochondrial cytopathy, the MERRF syndrome (Myoclonic Epilepsy with Ragged Red Fibers). These episodes are often associated with headache, nausea, and followed by visual symptoms such as hemianopia or cortical blindness, aphasia, and psychosis. Their pathogenesis is not fully understood. Morphologic evidence of mitochondrial dysfunction has been demonstrated in the capillary endothelium of the small cerebral blood vessels in autopsies of patients with MELAS

(Ohama et al., 1987), suggesting that the neurological manifestations are related to a "mictochondrial angiopathy."

In 2003, Iuzuka et al. described the MRI features of stroke-like lesions in four patients with MELAS. In all patients, diffusion weighted MRI demonstrated a slow progression of stroke-like lesions with a moderate decrease of diffusion and involvement of different cortical regions distinct from ischemic stroke. Moreover, they observed that clinical and electrophysiological epileptic activities were associated with these events. These authors suggested that stroke-like episodes may be non-ischemic, neurovascular events characterized by focal neuronal hyperexcitability related to the "mitochondrial angiopathy." Another characteristic of these stroke-like lesions is their preferential localization to the occipital and parietal lobes, but exact mechanism of this posterior predilection remains to be elucidated.

Current approaches to the treatment are based on the use of antioxydants, respiratory chain substrates, and cofactors in the form of vitamins. However, no consistent benefits have been observed using these treatments (Scaglia & Northrop 2006).

References

Amberla, K., Waljas M., Tuominen S., Almkvist, O., Pöyhönen, M., & Tuisku, S., et al. (2004). Insidious cognitive decline in CADASIL. Stroke, 35(7), 1598–1602.

Auer, D. P., Putz B., Gössl C, Elbel G-K, Gasser T, & Dichgans, M (2001). Differential lesion patterns in CADASIL and sporadic subcortical arteriosclerotic encephalopathy: MR imaging study with statistical parametric group comparison. Radiology, 218(2), 443–451.

Baudrimont, M., Dubas F., Joutel A, Tournier-Lasserve E, & Bousser, M. G. (1993). Autosomal dominant leukoencephalopathy and subcortical ischemic stroke. A clinicopathological study. Stroke, 24(1), 122–125.

Bergmann, M., Ebke, M., Yuan, Y., Brück, W., Mugler, M., & Schwendemann, G. (1996). Cerebral autosomal dominant arteriopathy with subcortical infarcts and leukoencephalopathy (CADASIL): a morphological study of a German family. Acta Neuropathologica (Berl), 92(4), 341–350.

Blaumueller, C. M., Qi, H., Zagouras, P., & Artavanis-Tsakonas S. (1997). Intracellular cleavage of Notch leads to a heterodimeric receptor on the plasma membrane. Cell, 90(2), 281–291.

Buffon, F., Porcher R., Hernandez K., Kurtz A., Pointeau S., & Vahedi K., et al. (2006). Cognitive profile in CADASIL. Journal of Neurology, Neurosurgery, and Psychiatry, 77(2), 175–180.

Chabriat, H., Bousser, M. G., & Pappata, S. (1995). Cerebral autosomal dominant arteriopathy with subcortical infarcts and leukoencephalopathy: a positron emission tomography study in two affected family members. Stroke, 26(9), 1729–1730.

Chabriat, H., Joutel, A., Vahedi, K., Iba-Zizen, M. T., Tournier-Lasserve, E., Bousser, M. G. (1997). CADASIS. Cerebral Autosomal Dominant Arteriopathy with Subcortical Infarcts and Leukoencephalophathy. Revista de Neurologia (Paris), 153(6–7), 376–385.

Chabriat, H., Levy, C., Taillia, H., Iba-Zizen, M.-T., Vahedi, K., & Joutel, A., et al. (1998). Patterns of MRI lesions in CADASIL. Neurology, 51(2), 452–457.

Chabriat, H., Mrissa, R., Vahedi, K., Taillia, H., Iba-Zizen, M. T., & Joutel, A., et al. (1999). Brain stem MRI signal abnormalities in CADASIL. Stroke, 30(2), 457–459.

Chabriat, H., Pappata, S., Poupon, C., Clark, C. A., Vahedi, K., & Poupon, F., et al. (1999). Clinical severity in CADASIL related to ultrastructural damage in white matter: in vivo study with diffusion tensor MRI. Stroke, 30(12), 2637–2643.

Chabriat, H., Vahedi, K., Iba-Zizen, M.-T., Joutel, A., Nibbio, A., & Nagy, T. G., et al. (1995). Clinical spectrum of CADASIL: a study of 7 families. Cerebral autosomal dominant arteriopathy with subcortical infarcts and leukoencephalopathy. Lancet, 346(8980), 934–939.

Charlton, R. A., Morris R. G., Nitkunan A., & Markus H. S. (2006). The cognitive profiles of CADASIL and sporadic small vessel disease. Neurology, 66(10), 1523–1526.

Coulthard, A., Blank, S. C., Bushby, K., Kalaria, R. N., & Burn, D. J. (2000). Distribution of cranial MRI abnormalities in patients with symptomatic and subclinical CADASIL. The British Journal of Radiology, 73(867), 256–265.

Cumurciuc, R., Guichard, J. P. Reizine, D., Gray, F., Bousser, M. G., & Chabriat, H. (2006). Dilation of Virchow-Robin spaces in CADASIL. European Journal of Neurology, 13(2), 187–190.

Damian, M. S., Seibel, P., Reichmann, H., Schachenmayr, W., Laube, H., & Bachmann, G., et al. (1995). Clinical spectrum of the MELAS mutation in a large pedigree. Acta Neurologica Scandinavica, 92(5), 409–415.

Desmond, D. W., Moroney, J. T., Lynch, T., Chan, S., Chin, S. S., & Mohr, J. P. et al. (1999). The natural history of CADASIL: a pooled analysis of previously published cases. *Stroke*, *30*(6), 1230–1233.

Dichgans, M., Filippi, M., Bruning, R., Iannucci, G., Berchtenbreiter, C. , & Minicucci, L., et al. (1999). Quantitative MRI in CADASIL: correlation with disability and cognitive performance. *Neurology*, *52*(7), 1361–1367.

Dichgans, M., Mayer, M., Uttner, I., Brüning, R., Müller-Höcker, J., & Rungger, G., et al. (1998). The phenotypic spectrum of CADASIL: clinical findings in 102 cases. Annals of Neurology, *44*(5), 731–739.

Domenga, V., Fardoux, P., Lacombe, P., Monet, M., Maciazek, J., & Krebs, L.T., et al. (2004). Notch3 is required for arterial identity and maturation of vascular smooth muscle cells. *Genes and Development*, *18*(22), 2730–2735.

Dotti, M. T., Federico, A., Mazzei, R., Bianchi, S., Scali, O., & Conforti, F. L., et al. (2005). The spectrum of Notch3 mutations in 28 Italian CADASIL families. *Journal of Neurology, Neurosurgery, and Psychiatry*, *76*(5), 736–738.

Ebke, M., Dichgans, M., Bergmann, M., Voelter, H. U., Rieger, P., & Gasser, T., et al. (1997). CADASIL: skin biopsy allows diagnosis in early stages. *Acta Neurologica Scandinavica*, *95*(6), 351–357.

Filley, C. M., Thompson, L. L., Sze, C.-I., Simon, J. S., Paskavitz, J. F., & Kleinschmidt-DeMasters, B. K. et al. (1999). White matter dementia in CADASIL. *Journal of the Neurological Sciences*, *163*(2): 163–167.

Goto, Y., Horai, S., Matsuoka, T., Koga, Y., Nihei, K., & Kobayashi, M., et al. (1992). Mitochondrial myopathy, encephalopathy, lactic acidosis, and stroke-like episodes (MELAS): a correlative study of the clinical features and mitochondrial DNA mutation. *Neurology*, *42*(3 Pt 1), 545–550.

Goto, Y., Nonaka, I., & Horai, S., (1990). A mutation in the tRNA (Leu)(UUR) gene associated with the MELAS subgroup of mitochondrial encephalomyopathies. *Nature*, *348*(6302), 651–653.

Gray, F., Robert, F., & Labrecques, R. (1994). Autosomal dominant arteriopathic leuko-encephalopathy and Alzheimer's disease. *Neuropathology and Applied Neurobiology*, *20*(1), 22–30.

Gutierrez-Molina, M., Caminero Rodriguez, A., Martinez Garcia, C., Arpa Gutierrez, J., Morales Bastos, C., & Amer, G. (1994). Small arterial granular degeneration in familial Binswanger's syndrome. *Acta Neuropathologica (Berl)*, *87*(1), 98–105.

Holtmannspotter, M., Peters, N., Opherk, C., Martin, D. Herzog, J., & Bruckmann, H., et al. (2005). Diffusion magnetic resonance histograms as a surrogate marker and predictor of disease progression in CADASIL: a two-year follow-up study. *Stroke*, *36*(12), 2559–2565.

Iizuka, T., Sakai, F., Kan, S., & Suzuki, N. (2003). Slowly progressive spread of the stroke-like lesions in MELAS. *Neurology*, *61*(9), 1238–1244.

Joutel, A., Andreux, F., Gaulis, S., Domenga, V. Cecillon, M., & Battail, N., et al. (2000). The ectodomain of the Notch3 receptor accumulates within the cerebrovasculature of CADASIL patients. *The Journal of Clinical Investigation*, *105*(5), 597–605.

Joutel, A., Corpechot, C., Ducros, A., Vahedi, K., Chabriat, H., & Mouton, P., et al. (1996). Notch3 mutations in CADASIL, a hereditary adult-onset condition causing stroke and dementia. *Nature*, *383*(6602), 707–710.

Joutel, A., Corpechot, C., Ducros, A., Vahedi, K., Chabriat, H., & Mouton, P., et al. (1997). Notch3 mutations in cerebral autosomal dominant arteriopathy with subcortical infarcts and leukoencephalopathy (CADASIL), a mendelian condition causing stroke and vascular dementia. *Annals of the New York Academy of Sciences*, *826*, 213–217.

Joutel, A., Favrole, P., Labauge, H., Chabriat, C., Lescoat, F., & Andreux, V., et al. (2001). Skin biopsy immunostaining with a Notch3 monoclonal antibody for CADASIL diagnosis. *Lancet*, *358*(9298), 2049–2051.

Joutel, A., A. Francois, Chabriat, H., Vahedi, K., Andreux, F., & Domenga, V., et al. (2000). CADASIL: genetics and physiopathology. *Bulletin de l'Académie Nationale de Medicine*, *184*(7), 1535–1542; discussion 1542–1544.

Joutel, A., & Tournier-Lasserve, E. (2002). Molecular basis and physiopathogenic mechanisms of CADASIL: a model of small vessel diseases of the brain. *Journal de la Société de Biologie 196* (1), 109–115.

Kumar, S. K., & Mahr, G. (1997). CADASIL presenting as bipolar disorder. *Psychosomatics*, *38*(4), 397–398.

Lagas, P. A., & Juvonen, V. (2001). Schizophrenia in a patient with cerebral autosomally dominant arteriopathy with subcortical infarcts and leucoencephalopathy (CADASIL disease). *Nordic Journal of Psychiatry*, *55*(1), 41–42.

Maassen, J. A., Jansen, J. J., Kadowaki, T., Van Den Ouweland, J. M. W., Thart, L. M., & Lemkes, H. H. P. J. (1996). The molecular basis and clinical characteristics of Maternally Inherited Diabetes and Deafness (MIDD), a recently recognized diabetic subtype. *Experimental and Clinical Endocrinology & Diabetes*, *104*(3), 205–211.

Maclean, A. V., Woods, R., Alderson, L. M., Salloway, S. P., Correai, S., Cortez, s., & Stopa, E. G. (2005). Spontaneous lobar haemorrhage in CADASIL. J Neurol Neurosurg Psychiatry, 76(3), 456–457.

Madureira, S., Verdelho, A., Ferro, J., Basile, A.-M., Chabriat, H., & Erkinjuntti, T. (2006). Development of a neuropsychological battery for the Leukoaraiosis and Disability in the Elderly Study (LADIS): experience and baseline data. *Neuroepidemiology*, *27*(2), 101–116.

Markus, H. S., Martin, R. J., Simpson, M. A., Dong, Y. B., Ali, N., & Crosby, A. H., et al. (2002). Diagnostic strategies in CADASIL. *Neurology, 59*(8), 1134–1138.

Mesulam, M., Siddique, T., & Cohen B. (2003). Cholinergic denervation in a pure multi-infarct state: observations on CADASIL. *Neurology, 60*(7), 1183–1185.

Miao, Q., Paloneva, T., Tuominen, S., Poyhonen, M., Tuisku, S., & Viitanen, M., et al. (2004). Fibrosis and stenosis of the long penetrating cerebral arteries: the cause of the white matter pathology in cerebral autosomal dominant arteriopathy with subcortical infarcts and leukoencephalopathy. *Brain Pathology, 14*(4), 358–364.

Mikol, J., Henin, D., Baudrimont, M., Gaulier, A., Bacri, D., & Tillier, J. N., et al. (2001). Atypical CADASIL phenotypes and pathological findings in two new French families. *Revue Neurologique, 157*(6–7), 655–667.

Molko, N., Pappata, S., Mangin, J. F., Poupon, C., Vahedi, K., & Jobert, A., et al. (2001). Diffusion tensor imaging study of subcortical gray matter in cadasil. *Stroke, 32*(9), 2049–2054.

Ohama, E., Ohara, S. Ikuta, F., Tanaka, K., Nishizawa, K., & Nishizawa, M., et al. (1987). Mitochondrial angiopathy in cerebral blood vessels of mitochondrial encephalomyopathy. *Acta Neuropathologica (Berl), 74*(3), 226–233.

Okeda, R., Arima, K., & Kawai, M. (2002). Arterial changes in cerebral autosomal dominant arteriopathy with subcortical infarcts and leukoencephalopathy (CADASIL) in relation to pathogenesis of diffuse myelin loss of cerebral white matter: examination of cerebral medullary arteries by reconstruction of serial sections of an autopsy case. *Stroke, 33*(11), 2565–2569.

O'Sullivan, M., Barrick, T. R., Morris, R. G. Clark, C. A. & Markus, H. S. (2005). Damage within a network of white matter regions underlies executive dysfunction in CADASIL. *Neurology, 65*(10), 1584–1590.

O'Sullivan, M., Jarosz, J. M., Martin, R. J., Deasy, N., Powell, J. F., & Markus, H. S. (2001). MRI hyperintensities of the temporal lobe and external capsule in patients with CADASIL. *Neurology, 56*(5), 628–634.

O'Sullivan, M., Singhal, S., Charlton, R. & Markus, H. S. (2004). Diffusion tensor imaging of thalamus correlates with cognition in CADASIL without dementia. *Neurology, 62*(5), 702–707.

Pavlakis, S. G., Phillips, P. C., DiMauro, S., De Vivo, D. C., & Rowland, L. P. (1984). Mitochondrial myopathy, encephalopathy, lactic acidosis, and strokelike episodes: a distinctive clinical syndrome. *Annals of Neurology, 16*(4), 481–488.

Peters, N., Herzog, J., Opherk, C., & Dichgans, M. (2004). A two-year clinical follow-up study in 80 CADASIL subjects: progression patterns and implications for clinical trials. *Stroke, 35*(7), 1603–1608.

Peters, N., Opherk, C., Danek, A. Ballard, C., Herzog, J., & Dichgans M., (2005a). Spectrum of mutations in biopsy-proven CADASIL: implications for diagnostic strategies. *Archives of Neurology, 62*(7), 1091–1094.

Peters, N., Opherk, C., Danek, A., Ballard, C., Herzog, J., & Dichgans, M. (2005b). The pattern of cognitive performance in CADASIL: a monogenic condition leading to subcortical ischemic vascular dementia. *The American Journal of Psychiatry 162*(11): 2078–2085.

Pullicino, P., Ostrow, P., Miller, L., Snyder, W., & Munschauer, F. (1995). Pontine ischemic rarefaction. *Annals of Neurology 37*(4): 460–466.

Rafalowska, J., Fidzianska, A., Dziewulska, D., Podlecka, A., Szpak, G. M.,& Kwieciński, H. (2003). CADASIL: new cases and new questions. *Acta Neuropathologica (Berl), 106*(6), 569–574.

Ragoschke-Schumm, A., Axer, H., Witte, O. W., Isenmann, S., Fitzek, C., & Dichgans, M. et al. (2005). Intracerebral haemorrhage in CADASIL. *Journal of Neurology, Neurosurgery, and Psychiatry, 76*(11), 1606–1607.

Ruchoux, M. M., Brulin, P., Brillault, J., Dehouck, M. P., Cecchelli, R., & Bataillard, M. (2002). Lessons from CADASIL. *Annals of the New York Academy of Sciences 977*, 224–231.

Ruchoux, M. M., Guerouaou, D., Vandenhaute, B., Pruvo, J. P., Vermersch, P., & Leys, D. (1995). Systemic vascular smooth muscle cell impairment in cerebral autosomal dominant arteriopathy with subcortical infarcts and leukoencephalopathy. *Acta Neuropatholgica (Berl)* 89(6): 500–512.

Ruchoux, M. M., & Maurage, C. A. (1997). CADASIL: Cerebral autosomal dominant arteriopathy with subcortical infarcts and leukoencephalopathy. *J Neuropathol Exp Neurol 56*(9), 947–964.

Santa, Y., Uyama, E., Chui, D. H., Arima, M., Kotorii, S., & Takahashi, K., et al. (2003). Genetic, clinical and pathological studies of CADASIL in Japan: a partial contribution of Notch3 mutations and implications of smooth muscle cell degeneration for the pathogenesis. *Journal of the Neurological Sciences, 212*(1–2), 79–84.

Scaglia, F., & Northrop, J. L. (2006). The mitochondrial myopathy encephalopathy, lactic acidosis with stroke-like episodes (MELAS) syndrome: a review of treatment options. *CNS Drugs, 20*(6), 443–464.

Schultz, A., Santoianni, R., & Hewan-Lowe, K. (1999). Vasculopathic changes of CADASIL can be focal in skin biopsies. *Ultrastructural Pathology* 23(4): 241–247.

Sue, C. M., Crimmins, D. S., Soo, Y. S., Pamphlett, R., Presgrave, C. M., & Kotsimbos, N., et al. (1998). Neuroradiological features of six kindreds with MELAS tRNALeu A3243G point mutation: implications for pathogenesis. *Journal of Neurology, Neurosurgery, and Psychiatry, 65*(2), 233–240.

Taillia, H., Chabriat, H., Kurtz, A., Verin, M., Levy, C., & Vahedi, K., et al. (1998). Cognitive alterations in non-demented CADASIL patients. *Cerebrovascular Diseases*, 8(2), 97–101.

Thijs, V., Robberecht, W., De Vos, R., & Sciot, R. (2003). Coexistence of CADASIL and Alzheimer's disease. *Journal of Neurology, Neurosurgery, and Psychiatry*, 74(6), 790–792.

Thomeer, E. C., Verhoeven, W. M., & Klompenhouwer, J. L. (1998). Psychiatric symptoms in MELAS; a case report. *Journal of Neurology, Neurosurgery, and Psychiatry* 64(5), 692–693.

Tournier-Lasserve, E., Iba-Zizen, M. T., Romero, N., & Bousser, M. G. (1991). Autosomal dominant syndrome with strokelike episodes and leukoencephalopathy. *Stroke*, 22(10), 1297–1302.

Tournier-Lasserve, E., Joutel, A., Melki J., Weissenbach, J., Lathrop, G. M., & Chabriat, H., et al. (1993). Cerebral autosomal dominant arteriopathy with subcortical infarcts and leukoencephalopathy maps to chromosome 19q12. *Nature Genetics*, 3(3), 256–259.

van Den Boom, R., Lesnik Oberstein, S. A., van Duinen, S. G., Bornebroek, M., Ferrari, M. D., & Haan, J. et al. (2002). Subcortical lacunar lesions: an MR imaging finding in patients with cerebral autosomal dominant arteriopathy with subcortical infarcts and leukoencephalopathy. *Radiology*, 224(3): 791–796.

Vermeer, S. E., Prins, N. D. den Heijer, T., Hofman, A., Koudstaal, P. J., & Breteler, M. M. B. (2003). Silent brain infarcts and the risk of dementia and cognitive decline. *The New England Journal of Medicine*, 348(13), 1215–1222.

Viswanathan, A., Gray, F., Bousser, M.-G., Baudrimont, M., & Chabriat, H. (2006). Cortical Neuronal Apoptosis in CADASIL. *Stroke, 37*(11), 2690–2695.

Zhang, W. W., Ma, K. C., Andersen, O., Sourander, P., Tollesson, P. O., & Olsson, Y., (1994). The microvascular changes in cases of hereditary multi-infarct disease of the brain. *Acta Neuropathologica (Berl)*, 87(3), 317–324.

Chapter 9
Carotid Artery Occlusion and Stenosis

Mohamad Chmayssani and Joanne Festa

Introduction

C. Miller Fischer's clinical observations that led to a further understanding of carotid artery disease, in addition to angiography advancements in the 1930s, brought a new focus to the prevalence of carotid disease and led to an increased interest in stroke and its co-morbidities. Symptomatic carotid artery disease, by some estimates, accounts for 25% of all ischemic strokes (Hanel, Levy, Guterman, & Hopkins, 2005). The media played an essential role in promoting awareness of carotid disease and encouraging patients to seek medical care even if they are asymptomatic. New medical advancements in recent decades have increased life expectancy substantially, leading to an increased incidence of carotid disease, since the prevalence of symptomatic carotid stenosis increases steeply with advanced age (Fairhead & Rothwell, 2006). Moreover, physicians are more aware of the seriousness of carotid disease, since it frequently complicates existing CNS pathology in the ageing population (de la Torre, 2000), increasing the pressure to diagnose and treat. Finally the advent of new imaging modalities such as computed tomography angiography (CTA), magnetic

resonance angiography (MRA), cerebral angiography, and carotid Doppler ultrasound (CDUS) made it possible to diagnose patients with carotid disease prior to the onset of symptoms. In a large population-based study, the prevalence of carotid stenosis 35% or greater was found in 3.8% of men and in 2.7% of women: prevalence increased with age in both genders (Mathiesen et al., 2001). Others have reported the prevalence of asymptomatic carotid stenosis of 50% or greater detected by ultrasonography to be 6.4% among people aged 50–79 (Mineva et al., 2002). Rates of internal carotid artery stenosis > 40% are higher among Type II diabetics and increase with advancing age from 5.0% at 50–59 years to 7.3% at 60–69 years and 9.5% at 70–79 years (Park et al., 2006).

The possible causative relationship between carotid disease and cognitive impairment suggests that restoration of blood supply could restore cognitive functions. This hypothesis kindled the first carotid reconstruction (Carrea, Molins, & Murphy, 1955) and carotid endarterectomies (CEAs) (DeBakey, 1975; Eastcott, Pickering, & Rob, 1954) on patients with stroke and internal carotid artery stenosis. Studies aiming to characterize the neurobehavioral syndrome of carotid disease soon followed, providing the basis for strategies to prevent and eliminate morbidities of carotid disease. The aim of this chapter is to review the current state of knowledge about the nature, severity, and course of cognitive deficits as

J. Festa (✉)
Stroke and Critical Care Division, Department of Neurology, Neurological Institute, New York Presbyterian Hospital, Columbia University, College of Physicians and Surgeons, New York, NY, USA
e-mail: jf2128@columbia.edu

J.R. Festa, R.M. Lazar (eds.), *Neurovascular Neuropsychology*, DOI 10.1007/978-0-387-70715-0_9,
© Springer Science+Business Media, LLC 2009

well as the surgical means for reversing dysfunction in patients with stenosis or occlusion of the carotid arteries.

Pathophysiology

Carotid disease was primarily associated with stroke and TIA through embolism of thrombotic material and hypoperfusion secondary to stenosis with insufficient collateral compensation (Fischer & Weber, 1983; Kistler, Ropper, & Heros, 1984a, 1984b; Mohr, 1978). Similarly, in stroke-free patients, hypoperfusion (de la Torre, 2000; Tatemichi, Desmond, Prohovnik, & Eidelberg, 1995) and showering of atheroemboli (Klijn, Kappelle, Tulleken, & van Gijn, 1997) are the main factors implicated in cognitive decline in patients with carotid artery stenosis or occlusion. Miller Fischer's classic papers, regarded as the earliest evidence proposing hypoperfusion-mediated cognitive impairment, were the groundwork from which investigators developed this field of research. (See Fig. 1).

Major evidence highlighting the effects of chronic cerebral hypoperfusion on cognitive functioning stems from the cardiac literature. End stage heart failure constitutes a state of global ischemia of the brain where 35–50% of patients have suboptimal cognitive functioning (Almeida & Flicker, 2001; Zuccala et al., 2001; Zuccala et al., 2003) Recent studies illustrated that cardiac recipients suffered a significant reduction in cerebral blood flow (CBF) prior to transplantation (Georgiadis et al., 2000; Gruhn et al., 2001; Kamishirado et al., 1997; Rajagopalan, Raine, Cooper, & Ledingham, 1984). Following transplantation, patients experienced neuropsychological improvement (Deshields, McDonough, Mannen, & Miller, 1996; Grimm et al., 1996; Gruhn et al., 2001; Roman et al., 1997) that was coupled with significant increases in CBF (Gruhn et al., 2001) and middle cerebral artery (MCA) mean flow velocity (Georgiadis et al., 2000). The enhanced cerebral perfusion offers a physiological explanation for the neuropsychological improvements commonly noted in cardiac recipients (Deshields et al., 1996; Grimm et al., 1996; Jones et al., 1988; Kugler et al., 1994; Roman et al., 1997).

In a manner analogous to congestive heart failure, hypoperfusion due to carotid stenosis/occlusion may result in cognitive dysfunction. With the refinement of new imaging techniques, PET and SPECT, it became possible to demonstrate the impact of hypoperfusion on

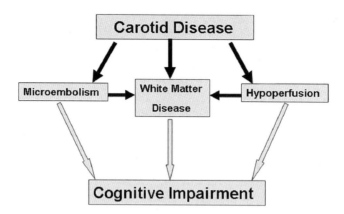

Fig. 1 Carotid disease is implicated in cognitive impairment through three direct mechanisms: (1) Microembolism (2) White Matter Disease and (3) Hypoperfusion. Microembolism and hypoperfusion have a further contribution to cognitive impairment by increasing the burden of white matter disease. Reprinted from Neuroimaging Clinics of North America, 17/3, Chmayssani, Festa, & Marshall, Chronic Ischemia and Neurocognition, pg 317, August 2007, with permission from Elsevier

neuronal metabolism and cognitive derangement. Tatemichi et al. (1995) reported a case of a 55-year-old man with bilateral internal carotid artery (ICA) and unilateral vertebral artery occlusions presenting subacutely with significant behavioral and cognitive changes marking frontal lobe deficits. A baseline PET scan showed a 40–50% reduction in blood flow and metabolism; however, following a revascularization procedure, the patient had a prominent improvement on neuropsychological testing, particularly executive functioning, that was coupled with increases in CBF and metabolism. Similarly, by means of SPECT, Tsuda et al. (1994) reported a case of a patient with generalized cognitive dysfunction in the left hemisphere attributed to extensive hypoperfusion in the left anterior-parietal and parieto-temporal cortex secondary to left ICA occlusion.

Episodic embolization by platelet or cholesterol material stemming from a thrombus with subsequent microinfarction of cerebral tissue is a potential mechanism of brain damage in the setting of carotid disease (Klijn et al., 1997). Atherosclerotic disruption is often the precipitating event of embolization and is the basis for the development of clinical ischemia and cognitive decline (Carr, Farb, Pearce, Virmani, & Yao, 1996; Fisher, Blumenfeld, & Smith, 1987; Milei et al., 1998). Instability of plaques is highly dependent on their composition. Unstable plaques are more prone to result in intraplaque hemorrhage, ulceration, or rupture. Homogenous fibrous rich carotid plaques are fairly stable and have fewer tendencies to break and shower emboli (Fuster, Moreno, Fayad, Corti, & Badimon, 2005; Stary, 2000; Stary et al., 1995); whereas an increase in lipid core (Bassiouny et al., 1997; Falk, 1992; Kilpatrick et al., 2001), thinning of fibrous cap (Bassiouny et al., 1997; Kilpatrick et al., 2001), ulceration (Bassiouny et al., 1997; Fisher et al., 2005; Kilpatrick et al., 2001), and intraplaque hemorrhage (Avril et al., 1991) render plaque unstable. Intra carotid plaque hemorrhages and ulcerations are more frequently identified in patients with ipsilateral

hemispheral infarcts (Avril et al., 1991; Golledge, Greenhalgh, & Davies, 2000; Pedro et al., 2000).

By means of random transcranial Doppler (TCD) monitoring, spontaneous microemboli can be detected in 21–60% of patients with documented carotid disease (Babikian et al., 1997; Del Sette, Angeli, Stara, Finocchi, & Gandolfo, 1997; Droste et al., 1997; Grosset, Georgiadis, Abdullah, Bone, & Lees, 1994; Wijman et al., 1998). Emboli targeting one hemisphere or retina commonly originate from the ispilateral carotid artery, specifically from the distal or proximal stump or from atherosclerotic plaques in the common carotid artery (Barnett, 1978; Barnett, Peerless, & Kaufmann, 1978; Finklestein, Kleinman, Cuneo, & Baringer, 1980). However, medical and surgical evidence have shown that ischemic events may result from transhemispheric emboli, i.e., microemboli originating from carotid artery on one side resulting in microinfarction in the opposite hemisphere. Ischemic events were reduced following clipping of the proximal base of the stenosed ICA (Barnett et al., 1978), endarterectomy in the contralateral ICA stenosis (Georgiadis, Grosset, & Lees, 1993), or usage of antithrombotic agents (Barnett et al., 1978) by decreasing the microemboli occurring in the cerebral hemisphere ipsilateral to the occluded ICA.

The clinical impact of microembolism due to carotid disease remains unclear. Although Droste and colleagues (1997) reported up to 142 embolic signals per hour in patients with carotid stenosis and recent transient attacks, symptoms manifested at a surprisingly low rate (Crawley et al., 1997; Heyer et al., 2006; Pugsley et al., 1994). Furthermore, several studies found no correlation between T2-weighted MRI examinations and induced microemboli when intraprocedural TCD were implemented during carotid artery stenting (CAS) procedures (Poppert et al., 2004; van Heesewijk et al., 2002). Investigators attempted to attribute specific infarcts to silent areas of the brain but no firm conclusion was reached (Calandre, Gomara, Bermejo,

Millan, & del Pozo, 1984; Norris & Zhu, 1992). Therefore, several explanations have been suggested to explain why microemboli occur without overt clinical manifestation or MRI evidence: (1) the human cortex contains extensive collateral vasculature that wash out the emboli; (2) there is a size threshold for acute ischemic events such that the likelihood of an emboli causing symptoms is proportionally related to the size of the emboli (Rapp et al., 2000); and (3) mild transient symptoms are not appreciable when patients experience microembolization during sleep or sedation. Finally, the sequelae of microemboli may be more prominent over the long term if embolic fragments induce an inflammatory process that results in cellular infiltration and fibrosis leading ultimately to neuronal death and development of scar tissue (Gore, McCombs, & Lindquist, 1964; Kassirer, 1969). The latter could explain the late worsening in cognition that is commonly witnessed in patients following carotid artery bypass (Newman et al., 2001).

Characteristic Neurobehavioral Syndrome

Cognitive dysfunction resulting from large infarctions in cortical areas supplied by carotid disease is well established (Pohjasvaara, Erkinjuntti, Vataja, & Kaste, 1997; Tatemichi et al., 1994). The unsettled component is the unclear causative relationship between carotid disease and cognitive impairment in the absence of stroke (Rao, 2002). The question as to whether carotid atherosclerosis is the cause of cognitive impairment or is a marker for underlying risk factors and vascular disease that are themselves the cause, stems from several cross-sectional population based studies demonstrating a positive correlation between carotid plaques, intima media thickness (IMT), and neuropsychological dysfunction (Bakker, Klijn, Jennekens-Schinkel, & Kappelle, 2000; Gold & Lauritzen, 2002). IMT reflects the burden of atherosclerosis and generalized

vascular disease without requiring stenosis of the carotid vasculature. However, a subsequent 6-year prospective study conducted by the Atherosclerosis Risk in Communities (ARIC) study investigators (Knopman et al., 2001) did not replicate the correlation between IMT and cognitive decline. The relationship was examined again in a well-designed study by Johnston et al. (2004). For 5 years they prospectively followed 4,006 patients from the Cardiovascular Health Study of whom 29 participants had high-grade (>75%) right ICA stenosis and 32 subjects had high-grade left ICA stenosis. Using a Modified Mini Mental State examination (MMSE) that tests primarily left hemisphere functions, they hypothesized that if carotid stenosis is simply a marker for vascular disease, then a similar cognitive performance should be detected in patients with either left-sided or right-sided carotid disease. After adjusting for other vascular risk factors, their results were compatible with the view that carotid stenosis is the direct culprit for hemispheral cognitive dysfunction, whereas IMT is a marker for underlying risk factors and does not mediate cognitive dysfunction.

Bakker et al. (2000) conducted a comprehensive review of the literature evaluating the impact of carotid occlusive disease on cognitive functioning. In patients with carotid disease, cognitive impairment was apparent even in the absence (Benke, Neussl, & Aichner, 1991; Hamster & Diener, 1984; Naugle, Bridgers, & Delaney, 1986) or recovery of neurological deficits (TIA) (Baird et al., 1984; Hamster & Diener, 1984; Hemmingsen, Mejsholm, Boysen, & Engell, 1982; Hemmingsen et al., 1986; Nielsen, Hojer-Pedersen, Gulliksen, Haase, & Enevoldsen, 1985; Younkin et al., 1985). Among those studies, two noted a generalized cognitive impairment (Benke, et al.; Hemmingsen et al., 1982), three documented focal deficits for memory (Hamster & Diener, 1984; Nielsen et al., 1985), learning (Nielsen et al., 1985), psychomotor speed (Hamster & Diener, 1984), and problem solving (Naugle et al., 1986; Nielsen et al., 1985), and two did not specify the nature of cognitive deficits

(Baird et al., 1984; Hemmingsen et al., 1986). Several studies failed to demonstrate a direct relationship between carotid stenosis and cognitive dysfunction (Boeke, 1981; Heilmann, Lickert, & Hauger, 1975; Kelly, Garron, & Javid, 1980; van den Burg et al., 1985). However, these studies did not include long-term follow-up and there was a selection bias among the patient population, given that 67% of the studies were designed to evaluate the outcome after surgery (CEA and bypass); therefore, only surgical candidates were enrolled. A further limitation of these studies is that they often included both patients with carotid occlusion and carotid stenosis, precluding the exact characterization of distinct neurobehavioral syndromes. As a result, the available information on the natural course of cognitive functioning in patients who did not undergo surgery is too limited to draw conclusions.

A more recent study conducted by the same group (Bakker et al., 2003) enrolled 39 consecutive patients, not necessarily surgical candidates, with carotid occlusion, who had ipsilateral cerebral and retinal TIA but no stroke on MRI. Cognitive impairment was demonstrated in 44% of the patients and was even manifested in patients with isolated retinal symptoms. Cognitive deficits were mild and nonspecific in nature. A more recent investigation prospectively followed up 73 consecutive patients with TIA or minor stroke who had an occlusion of the ICA (Bakker, Klijn, van der Grond, Kappelle, & Jennekens-Schinkel, 2004). As a part of the assessment, H-MR spectroscopy (^{1}H-MRS) was implemented to study cerebral metabolic changes since these are indicative of cerebral hypoperfusion (van der Grond, van Everdingen, Eikelboom, Kenez, & Mali, 1999). Among patients with carotid occlusion and a history of TIAs, high lactate levels in noninfarcted white matter correlated with a decline in several cognitive functions including nonverbal intelligence, executive functioning, reaction time, motor speed, as well as verbal learning and memory (Bakker et al., 2003). Evaluating the same cognitive tasks, they showed that at baseline, 70% of

patients with strokes and 40% of patients with TIAs were cognitively impaired. At 1-year follow-up, improvement in cognitive functioning was witnessed in patients who had no lactate at baseline and who did not experience recurrence of transient or permanent neurological deficit.

A few studies have evaluated the impact of carotid stenosis on cognitive functioning in stroke-free patients, and even fewer studies have addressed this relationship in nonsurgical candidates. Mathiesen et al. (2004) used a cross-sectional population-based study to evaluate neuropsychological performance in 189 asymptomatic carotid stenosis patients. They demonstrated a significantly lower performance on tests of attention, memory, psychomotor speed, and motor functioning as compared with 202 healthy controls.

Conflicting results were reported in several studies evaluating cognition in asymptomatic carotid stenosis patients. Using tests of set shifting, verbal memory, visual memory, verbal fluency, and the MMSE Iddon et al. (1997) failed to demonstrate impairment in cognitive functions as compared to controls. Similar findings were also observed by King et al. (1977) when testing verbal IQ. Alternatively, Benke et al. (1991) noted significant impairment when testing mental speed, learning, visuospatial abilities, verbal processing, and deductive reasoning. Similarly, frontal lobe dysfunction as measured by verbal fluency and the Behavioral Dyscontrol score (BDCS) was illustrated by Rao (2002). A recent investigation conducted by Boessema et al. (2005) showed reduced cognition in various functions in asymptomatic surgical candidates including attention, planning of motor behavior, psychomotor skills, executive function, and verbal and visual memory.

Supporting Laboratory Studies

Multiple imaging techniques have been used in efforts to prevent the adverse outcome of carotid disease through monitoring for carotid atherosclerosis that might predispose patients to cerebral ischemia and irreversible injury. Four diagnostic modalities, now widely available, are used to directly image the ICA: cerebral angiography, carotid duplex ultrasound (CDUS), MRA, and CTA. Although the severity of stenosis is the parameter used to determine the extent of carotid disease, there is not a standard criterion for calculating the degree of angiographic stenosis. At present, the three internationally used criterions are NASCET (North American Symptomatic Carotid Endarterectomy Trial), ECST (European Carotid Surgery Trial), and CC (Common Carotid) methods. Although all three approaches were initially devised for use with conventional contrast angiography, their application has been extended to cover magnetic resonance angiography and CTA. Despite the differences among the three methods, studies have found that the results of all three methods have a linear relationship to each other and provide data of similar prognostic value (Rothwell, Eliasziw et al., 2003; Rothwell, Gibson, Slattery, Sellar, & Warlow, 1994).

Carotid Stenosis

Angiography

Cerebral Angiography is an X-ray of the cerebrovasculature. Normally, arteries are not visible in an X-ray, for this reason a contrast dye is injected via a sizeable catheter placed into a large artery. Cerebral angiography is the gold standard for imaging the carotid arteries (Rothwell, 2003). Currently, it constitutes the "reference standard" for evaluating patency and degree of stenosis in intracranial vessels. It permits classification of carotid lesions into one of the three groups: (1) nonsignificant stenosis (<50%) that does not impede blood flow, (2) severe hypoperfusion inducing stenosis (70–99%), and (3) complete vascular occlusion (Wilterdink & Feldmann, 1996). Furthermore, the use of angiography allows the visualization of the entire carotid system

extending beyond the stenosis. It provides information about tandem atherosclerotic disease, plaque morphology, and collateral circulation, which is of great value for management decisions (Wilterdink & Feldmann, 1996). For instance, the coexistence of intracranial atherosclerotic disease in patients with moderate carotid stenosis of 50–70% may identify a subgroup of patients that are more susceptible to hypoperfusion and hence, more likely to benefit from a revascularization procedure such as CEA or CAS (Rothwell, 2003).

Cerebral angiography is a resource intensive diagnostic and its use for assessment of the cerebral vasculature has to be considered in the context of its high cost, invasive nature, and most importantly, its small but definite risk of neurological complications (Heiserman et al., 1994; Waugh & Sacharias, 1992). These limitations render angiography ill suited for screening purposes. A review of eight prospective and seven retrospective studies using cerebral angiography showed the likelihood of inducing a disabling stroke is 1% (Hankey, Warlow, & Sellar, 1990). The risk is not limited to overt neurological deficits since some evidence shows increased silent embolism following diagnostic cerebral angiography (Bendszus et al., 1999).

CTA and MRA

CT Angiography (CTA) requires specially designed X-rays and intravenous contrast to evaluate the detailed anatomy of the blood vessels whereas MRA is a type of magnetic resonance imaging (MRI) scan that uses a magnetic field and pulses of radio wave energy to image the structure of blood vessels. Both techniques image flowing blood noninvasively and provide 3D anatomic information on the entire carotid system that is essential for diagnosis and surgical strategy planning. However, they do not permit the evaluation of the hemodynamic status of the vascular network, which is possible only via cerebral angiography. The reliability of MRA and CTA have been evaluated in a meta analysis showing the sensitivity and specificity of MRA to cerebral angiography for evaluation of carotid stenosis were 88% and 84% (Wardlaw, Chappell, Best, Wartolowska, & Berry, 2006) and CTA to cerebral angiography were 77% and 95%, respectively (Wardlaw et al., 2006). (See Fig. 2).

Carotid Duplex Ultrasound

Carotid duplex is a noninvasive diagnostic tool that uses ultrasound to view plaques, thrombus, or other blood flow abnormalities in the carotid artery. Currently, carotid duplex ultrasound (CDUS) is the primary screening test for carotid artery imaging because it is noninvasive and accurate, as well as relatively low in cost. Many clinicians are now using carotid duplex as the single preoperative evaluation diagnostic test, essentially avoiding the risk and the cost of preoperative carotid angiography (Dawson, Zierler, Strandness, Clowes, & Kohler, 1993; Gelabert & Moore, 1990). Peak blood flow velocity is the parameter used to

measure the severity of stenosis. Increases in blood flow velocity detected in the narrowed portion of the carotid lumen is directly proportional to the severity of obstruction (Hunink, Polak, Barlan, & O'Leary, 1993; Huston et al., 2000).

Carotid duplex ultrasound is unique among other imaging modalities for its ability to evaluate the surface and the composition of the atherosclerotic plaque. Substantial evidence demonstrates that the internal structure of plaque is associated with increased stroke risk. Areas of intraplaque hemorrhage (Houser, Sundt, Holman, Sandok, & Burton, 1974) and increased fat deposition (Caplan & Wolpert, 1991; Ringelstein, Zeumer, & Angelou, 1983) show up as hypoechoic areas on CDUS and represent areas of plaque vulnerability rendering patients at higher risk of suffering a stroke (Gronholdt, Nordestgaard, Schroeder, Vorstrup, & Sillesen, 2001; Polak et al., 1998). Furthermore, recent evidence showed that plaque irregularity increased the risk of stroke 3-fold in a population-based cohort (Prabhakaran et al., 2006). (See duplex

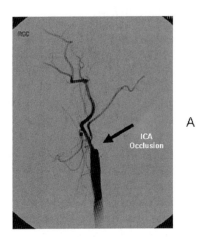

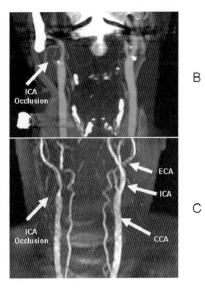

Fig. 2 Angiogram, magnetic resonance angiography (MRA), and computed tomography angiography (CTA) from a patient with right internal carotid artery (ICA) occlusion. A. Cervical angiogram with arrow pointing to ICA occlusion at the carotid bifurcation; B. CTA of the arteries in the neck with arrow pointing to ICA occlusion; C. MRA with arrows pointing to right ICA occlusion and patent CCA, external carotid artery (ECA), and ICA vessels on the left

ultrasonography Figure 7 in Chapter 2, Neurovascular Geography of the Brain.)

A meta analysis comparing CDUS with intraarterial cerebral angiography for the diagnosis of high grade carotid stenosis (70–99%) showed that CDUS had a sensitivity of 89% and specificity of 84% (Wardlaw et al., 2006). Although CDUS is a highly accurate diagnostic tool, it carries some limitation. CDUS is not capable of providing a global perspective of cerebral vasculature since only the cervical portion of the carotid and vertebral arteries can be examined in detail. Furthermore, it has limited use in patients with calcified carotid lesions or tortuous carotid arteries. Another serious draw back, the diagnostic accuracy of CDUS relies heavily upon the technical skills and expertise of the operator (Criswell, Langsfeld, Tullis, & Marek, 1998). Other sources of variability include the difference in equipment, and measurement threshold properties (Criswell et al., 1998; Jahromi, Cina, Liu, & Clase, 2005). Since these variations are clinically significant, physicians will often repeat TCD studies performed elsewhere and rely on data obtained from a trusted ultrasound laboratory.

Transcranial Doppler (TCD)

As an adjunct to CDUS, TCD measures blood flow velocity and direction in the major intracerebral arteries distal to the carotid arteries (Babikian et al., 2000). Principally, TCD is used in conjunction with CDUS to evaluate the intracranial hemodynamic consequence of high grade carotid stenosis. Several TCD findings have been highly associated with critical carotid stenosis, for example, absence of ophthalmic artery and carotid siphon TCD signals (Wilterdink, Feldmann, Bragoni, Brooks, & Benavides, 1994). Other hemodynamic changes in the ipsilateral MCA have been linked to severe ipsilateral ICA stenosis: reduced MCA flow velocity, decreased pulsatility index, and diminished flow acceleration (Kelley, Namon, Juang, Lee, & Chang, 1990; Kelley, Namon, Mantelle, & Chang, 1993; Lindegaard et al., 1985; Molina et al., 2001; Schneider, Rossman, Bernstein, Ringelstein, & Otis, 1991; Wilterdink, Feldmann, Furie, Bragoni, & Benavides, 1997). Furthermore, development of collateral flow patterns is a common finding in the setting of severe carotid stenosis. For instance, reversed flow in the ipsilateral anterior cerebral artery (ACA) or augmented flow velocity in the contralateral ACA suggests collateral flow from the contralateral ICA (Schneider et al., 1991). Also, reversed flow in the ipsilateral ophthalmic artery implies collateral flow from the external carotid artery (ECA) to the ICA (Schneider et al., 1991). The use of TCD can also be extended to detect MCA micro emboli stemming from the heart or carotid artery (MRC European Carotid Surgery Trial: interim results for symptomatic patients with severe (70–99%) or with mild (0–29%) carotid stenosis. European Carotid Surgery Trialists' Collaborative Group, 1991).

Carotid Occlusion

It is essential to adequately differentiate between highly stenosed vessels and completely occluded carotid arteries since the latter are not amenable to interventions such as carotid endarterectomy (CEA) and CAS. The noninvasive imaging modalities previously discussed are reliable means for detection of severe carotid artery stenosis, particularly for detection of carotid occlusion. Earlier studies found that when compared with cerebral angiography for diagnosing complete carotid occlusion, the sensitivity and specificity for CDUS were 97% and 100% (Nederkoorn, van der Graaf, & Hunink, 2003), for CTA were 97% and 99% (Chen et al., 2004; Koelemay, Nederkoorn, Reitsma, & Majoie, 2004), and for MRA were 98% and 100% (Nederkoorn et al., 2003), respectively.

Cognition and Revascularization

Given that carotid disease is associated with cognitive dysfunction, an emerging hypothesis is that revascularization procedures could potentially improve or preserve cognitive functioning. Though the prophylactic effect of revascularization procedures against neurological deficits has been indisputably established in large randomized trials, the impact of vascular reconstruction on brain function, as evidenced by measures of behavioral and cognitive performance, remains inconclusive (Irvine, Gardner, Davies, & Lamont, 1998; Lehrner et al., 2005; Lunn, Crawley, Harrison, Brown, & Newman, 1999). On the basis of what has been previously discussed, the underlying mechanisms for anticipated cognitive improvement are the cessation of repeated embolic episodes and restoration of blood flow. However, the incidence of cognitive decline following CEA varied between 12 and 30% (Irvine et al., 1998; Lunn et al., 1999). This implies the presence of several mechanisms in cognitive dysfunction following revascularization, some patient specific and others procedure specific. (See Fig. 3) The former include plaque morphology (Fuster et al., 2005; Stary, 2000; Stary et al., 1995), severity and extent of cerebral ischemia, (Chmayssani, Festa, & Marshall, 2007), baseline neuronal injury, and the presence of *APOE*-ε4 allele, which is associated with a worse outcome following CEA (Heyer et al., 2005). The procedure specific mechanisms include the perioperative complications: new cerebral infarction (Jansen et al., 1994), intraoperative ischemia (Heyer et al., 1998; Heyer et al., 2006), and postoperative hyperperfusion (Ogasawara et al., 2005). The net outcome of cognition following revascularization procedures and bypass is a result of both patient- and procedure-related mechanisms. The present section sets out to review the studies

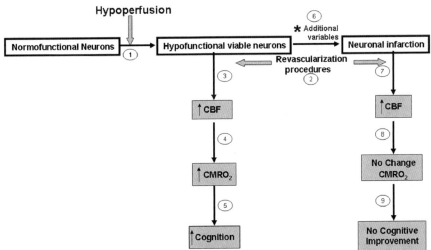

*Microembolism, white matter disease, prolonged hypoperfusion, increased severity of hypoperfusion, increased volume of ischemia

Reprinted from Neuroimaging Clinics of North America, 17/3, Chmayssani, Festa, & Marshall, Chronic Ischemia and Neurocognition, pg 317, August 2007, with permission from Elsevier.

Fig. 3 The scheme illustrates the natural history of neurons subjected to chronic ischemia. A mild hypoperfusion (1) shifts cells into a hypofunctional but viable state. If a revascularization procedure (2) is performed at that point, a resultant increase in CBF (3) leads to a concomitant increase in neuronal metabolism (4), and this manifests in improved cognitive performance (5). Alternatively, if the hypoperfusion state is prolonged, increased in severity or volume, or coexists with either microemboli or white matter disease, infarction occurs and revascularization (2) will result in CBF restoration (6) that does produce increased neuronal metabolism (7) or consequently cognitive improvement (8)

that have evaluated the extent and nature of cognitive changes that occur post-operatively.

Carotid Endarterectomy and Cognition

Carotid endarterectomy (CEA) is in widespread use to treat carotid stenosis; between 80,000 and 100,000 CEAs have been performed for Medicare patients per year in the United States since 1995 (Hsia, Moscoe, & Krushat, 1998). Frequent studies spanning several decades have explored the impact of CEA on cognitive functioning. The first formal study was conducted in 1964 (Williams & McGee, 1964). In reviews by Irvine et al. (1998) and Lunn et al. (1999) in the late 1990s, 16 of 28 (57%) studies reported cognitive improvement following CEA, others showed no change (39%), and still others demonstrated cognitive deterioration (4%). The inconsistent findings were attributed to the fact that the vast majority of these publications suffered poor methodology (Irvine et al., 1998; Lunn et al., 1999). Most studies lack appropriate controls and therefore, cannot account for several potential confounds such as practice effects, preoperative heightened anxiety and depression, and perioperative effects. Another limitation of these studies is the wide variation in retest intervals (3 days to 8 months). Without long-term follow-up, it is impossible to account for the effects of surgery and anesthesia and to monitor any long-term benefit on cognitive performance. An additional complicating factor is the wide range of patient characteristics that can affect cognitive functioning including age, education, IQ, and presence of co-morbid cerebrovascular disease. Inclusion of patients suffering major strokes makes firm conclusions about cause and effect more difficult. For instance, cognitive improvement witnessed in those patients might be confounded by the natural recovery of stroke (Duke, Bloor, Nugent, & Majzoub, 1968; Goldstein, Kleinknecht, & Gallo, 1970);

alternatively, an absence of improvement can be attributed to the presence of permanent neurological damage, hindering any improvement (Haynes, King, & Dempsey, 1975; Horne & Royle, 1974). The CEA literature also includes outcomes from a broad range of neurocognitive tests rendering results and conclusion among studies less comparable.

In designing subsequent studies, the design limitations of previous studies were addressed. Several studies have included surgical controls with unrelated disease yet highly similar demographics to correct for the influences of anesthesia, surgery, and practice effects on cognition (Fearn et al., 2003; Heyer et al., 2002; Sinforiani et al., 2001). However, Bossema et al. (2005) and Aleksic et al. (2006) included patients with severe atherosclerotic disease undergoing peripheral vascular surgery. Vascular risk factors have been implicated in the gradual cognitive decline, equivalent to about 4 or 5 years of additional age based on a large cohort of 1,500 men (Elwood, Pickering, Bayer, & Gallacher, 2002). Sinforiani et al. (2001) and Fearn et al. (2003) were able to demonstrate a benefit of CEA on cognitive functioning in verbal memory and attention. In contrast, Heyer et al. (2002) reported a decline in visuospatial organization found on the Rey Complex Figure copy task 1 month after CEA. In addition, Boessema et al. (2005) and Aleksic et al. (2006) reported no restorative effect on cognitive functioning.

Only a few studies have evaluated both CBF and cognition following CEA. Fukunaga et al. (Fukunaga, Okada, Inoue, Hattori, & Hirata, 2006) reported improvement in frontal lobe functions as reflected in improved categories achieved as well as reductions in loss of set and perseverations on the Wisconsin Card Sorting Test, particularly for those with severe stenosis or reduced cerebral perfusion prior to surgery. When compared to controls, Kishikawa (2003) found improved performance on a block design test in patients with the highest degree of stenosis and impaired vasomotor reactivity pre-operatively.

Some studies investigated the influence of surgical laterality on cognitive functioning, based on the premise that hemodynamic impairment would be more beneficial to cognitive functions associated with the hypoperfused hemisphere. This argument is supported by pre- and post-operative MRI studies showing that carotid stenosis induces ipsilateral white matter changes, which were shown to regress following CEA (Soinne et al., 2003). No solid results were reached with respect to side-specific benefits of CEA on cognitive functioning (Brand, Bossema, Ommen Mv, Moll, & Ackerstaff, 2004; Fearn et al., 2003; Fukunaga et al., 2006; Heyer et al., 2002; Kishikawa et al., 2003). However, Sinforiani (2001) showed a significant improvement in spatial memory and copying drawing in right stenosis patients as compared to left stenosis patients.

As a result of the review conducted by Irvine et al. (1998) concluding that the inconsistent results reported in the literature are explained by poor methodological designs, the majority of subsequent studies have addressed those limitations; however, they yielded conflicting results. Therefore in the absence of large trials, the impact of ICA stenosis and subsequent CEA on cognitive function will remain a matter of debate.

Carotid Artery Stenting

Carotid artery stenting is a newly emerging technique that offers patients a less invasive approach to treating carotid stenosis. Over the last few years, CAS has more often been promoted to treat carotid stenosis as an alternative to the gold standard, CEA. However, long-term results of CAS are still not available: several controlled trials comparing CAS and CEA are currently underway such as the NIH funded Carotid Revascularization Endarterectomy vs. Stenting Trial (CREST). For this reason, the impact of CAS on cognitive functioning has not been elucidated, but

it is presumed to improve cognition in a manner similar to CEA by restoring cerebral hypoperfusion.

Carotid artery stenting represents a rapidly evolving technique, therefore special attention should be given to reviewing studies addressing stroke and cognitive outcomes following CAS procedures, as the published outcomes often lag behind current advancement in the field. The first reported study compared cognitive outcome in 20 patients randomized to carotid angioplasty without stenting to 26 patients undergoing CEA (Crawley et al., 2000). At the two postoperative follow-ups, 6 weeks and 6 months, five patients in each group suffered equivalent decline in cognitive performance. Lehner et al. (2005) reported no significant cognitive changes in 20 stroke free patients—nine symptomatic with TIA and eleven asymptomatic—undergoing unilateral carotid stenting. Another study aimed to test cognitive changes after CAS with concurrent use of a proximal protection device to reduce thromboembolic events. Ten patients assessed 48 hours post-op demonstrated trends toward improvement in several cognitive functions, including word fluency, delayed recall, and cognitive speed as measured by the Number Connection Test (Grunwald et al., 2006). It is premature to draw final conclusions on the impact of CAS procedures on cognition based on these few case series.

EC-IC Bypass

Cerebral hypoperfusion in the setting of ICA occlusion has been implicated in intellectual decline, with revascularization as a possible therapeutic option. EC-IC bypass provides an opportunity to study the behavioral parameters of surgical therapy for cerebral ischemia. It should be noted that CEA carries a significant advantage over EC-IC bypass, since EC-IC bypass restores blood flow across the carotid bifurcation without reducing the incidence of showering of

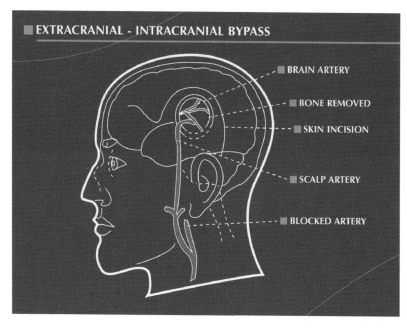

Fig. 4 Reprinted with permission from William J. Powers, MD Principle Investigator, Carotid Occlusion Surgery Study

atheremboli leaving the distal end of the carotid artery as a continued potential source of emboli. (See Fig. 4).

In a manner similar to CEA, the efficacy of EC-IC bypass was pursued initially in the form of sporadic case studies that suffered major design limitations and yielded an array of conflicting results. For example, Nieslon et al. (1986) found that among 33 patients undergoing EC-IC bypass, only the 23 with left carotid occlusive disease had a pre-surgical performance that was significantly worse than controls on mental sequencing (Trail Making Part B, Digit Span) and word learning and memory. Postoperatively, the left-occlusive patients' performance was not significantly worse than controls. However, two other controlled studies have yielded less promising results of the EC-IC bypass procedure (Binder, Tanabe, Waller, & Wooster, 1982; Drinkwater, Thompson, & Lumley, 1984). Binder et al. (1982) compared 12 EC-IC bypass surgery patients to seven patients with ICA occlusion treated medically. Although limited by a small sample size and better pre-operative

cognitive functioning in the medically treated patients, both surgical and medical group had improved on comprehension and verbal memory at the 2-month follow-up. There was no statistical additional benefit ascribed to surgical intervention. In a similar case series of 38 patients undergoing EC-IC bypass, Drinkwater et al. (1984) reported minor improvement in aspects of memory and processing speed but not prominent global improvement. This study can be criticized for evaluating young controls, administering lengthy testing, and more importantly lacking post-operative control angiography to ensure bypass patency. Other investigators evaluated CBF with a ^{133}Xe inhalation technique in a series of 44 patients undergoing EC-IC bypass (Younkin et al., 1985). Despite generalized improvement in cognitive functioning at 3- and 9-month follow-up, the authors proposed that the clinical improvements were due to natural recovery from stroke deficits, since there was no concomitant increase in CBF measures and those with the greatest improvements had a recent CVA (Younkin et al.,

1985). Reports of chronic CBF changes following EC-IC bypass using the old imaging tools conflict: Hasely et al. (1982) reported a significant increase in CBF values at 6 months, but Yonekura et al. (1982) found no change at 6 months and decreased CBF at 2 years. Since these case series suffer major design limitations and provide inconclusive data on post-operative CBF values, it is premature to draw final conclusions on the efficacy of EC-IC bypass on mental functions.

With refinement of more advanced imaging techniques, SPECT and PET, it became possible to decipher the physiological interactions among EC-IC bypass, subsequent hemodynamic changes, and cognitive functioning. By means of SPECT, Tsuda et al. (1994) reported a case of a patient with occlusion of left ICA siphon, where the improvement in CBF and neuronal metabolism was associated with general cognitive improvement. CBF was restored over a period of 3–9 months, whereas cognitive improvement on a dementia rating scale was manifested in the first 2 postoperative months and was sustained over a 3-year follow-up. In a more recent investigation, Sasoh et al. (2003) used PET to perform pre- and post-bypass CBF and metabolism assessment in 25 patients with chronic cerebral ischemia due to internal carotid occlusion. They showed that elevated OEF (oxygen extraction fraction) and reduced $CMRO_2$ (cellular metabolism) is related to cognitive dysfunction. Post-operatively, there was normalization in hemodynamic factors: OEF, CMRO2, CBF, and CVR (cerebrovascular reactivity) and improvement in WAIS-R IQ scores. Unfortunately specific subtest performances were not reported.

These valuable contributions to the literature highlighted the efficacy of EC-IC bypass in patients with stage II hemodynamic failure and were the basis for initiating the randomized clinical trial, Randomized Evaluation of Carotid Occlusion, and Neurocognition (RECON). RECON is an ancillary study of the Carotid Occlusion Surgery Study, a randomized trial intended to test the question of whether EC-IC bypass when added to the best medical therapy can reduce subsequent ipsilateral ischemic stroke at 2 years in patients with symptomatic ICA occlusion and stage II hemodynamic failure. In designing RECON, researchers addressed many of the design limitations of previous studies; thus RECON offers a unique opportunity to assess the impact of EC-IC bypass on cognitive functioning in the context of a randomized trial.

Conclusion

In an individual with carotid stenosis and cognitive impairment, alternative explanations should be sought before assuming that carotid disease causes or contributes to cognitive dysfunction (Barnett, 2004). Since the early days of C. Miller Fischer, investigators have provided solid evidence of an association between carotid disease and the development of cognitive impairment. However, cognitive dysfunction has been reported in a wide spectrum of clinical studies in patients with carotid disease but more frequently in global terms rather than by specific cognitive functions. In addition, major methodological shortcomings have limited research on this topic. The majority of studies that have addressed the reversal of pre-operative deficits with revascularization have yielded conflicting results; however, the separate question about possible long-term prevention of carotid disease induced cognitive deterioration, requiring a large number of patients followed for several years, has not been addressed.

At the present time, the endpoints in the assessment of patients with carotid disease have been neurological morbidity and death. There is general but not unanimous consensus that the evaluation of patients with carotid disease should include quality of life, which necessitates adequate cognitive functioning. Several randomized trials are currently underway in an attempt to demonstrate the influence that preserved cognition following revascularization can have on the ability of an elderly patient to live independently. A positive finding will offer a firm argument for including cognitive functioning in the algorithm for the management of carotid artery disease.

References

Almeida, O. P., & Flicker, L. (2001). The mind of a failing heart: a systematic review of the association between congestive heart failure and cognitive functioning. *Internal Medicine Journal, 31*(5), 290–295.

Avril, G., Batt, M., Guidoin, R., Marois, M., Hassen-Khodja, R., Daune, B., et al. (1991). Carotid endarterectomy plaques: correlations of clinical and anatomic findings. *Annals of Vascular Surgery, 5*(1), 50–54.

Babikian, V. L., Feldmann, E., Wechsler, L. R., Newell, D. W., Gomez, C. R., Bogdahn, U., et al. (2000). Transcranial Doppler ultrasonography: year 2000 update. *Journal of Neuroimaging, 10*(2), 101–115.

Babikian, V. L., Wijman, C. A., Hyde, C., Cantelmo, N. L., Winter, M. R., Baker, E., et al. (1997). Cerebral microembolism and early recurrent cerebral or retinal ischemic events. *Stroke, 28*(7), 1314–1318.

Baird, A. D., Adams, K. M., Shatz, M. W., Brown, G. G., Diaz, F., & Ausman, J. I. (1984). Can neuropsychological tests detect the sites of cerebrovascular stenoses and occlusions? *Neurosurgery, 14*(4), 416–423.

Bakker, F. C., Klijn, C. J., Jennekens-Schinkel, A., & Kappelle, L. J. (2000). Cognitive disorders in patients with occlusive disease of the carotid artery: a systematic review of the literature. *Journal of Neurology, 247*(9), 669–676.

Bakker, F. C., Klijn, C. J., Jennekens-Schinkel, A., van der Tweel, I., van der Grond, J., van Huffelen, A. C., et al. (2003). Cognitive impairment is related to cerebral lactate in patients with carotid artery occlusion and ipsilateral transient ischemic attacks. *Stroke, 34*(6), 1419–1424.

Bakker, F. C., Klijn, C. J., van der Grond, J., Kappelle, L. J., & Jennekens-Schinkel, A. (2004). Cognition and quality of life in patients with carotid artery occlusion: a follow-up study. *Neurology, 62*(12), 2230–2235.

Barnett, H. J. (1978). Delayed cerebral ischemic episodes distal to occlusion of major cerebral arteries. *Neurology, 28*(8), 769–774.

Barnett, H. J. (2004). Carotid disease and cognitive dysfunction. *Annals of Internal Medicine, 140*(4), 303–304.

Barnett, H. J., Peerless, S. J., & Kaufmann, J. C. (1978). "Stump" on internal carotid artery – a

source for further cerebral embolic ischemia. *Stroke, 9*(5), 448–456.

Bassiouny, H. S., Sakaguchi, Y., Mikucki, S. A., McKinsey, J. F., Piano, G., Gewertz, B. L., et al. (1997). Juxtalumenal location of plaque necrosis and neoformation in symptomatic carotid stenosis. *Journal of Vascular Surgery, 26*(4), 585–594.

Bendszus, M., Koltzenburg, M., Burger, R., Warmuth-Metz, M., Hofmann, E., & Solymosi, L. (1999). Silent embolism in diagnostic cerebral angiography and neurointerventional procedures: a prospective study. *Lancet, 354*(9190), 1594–1597.

Benke, T., Neussl, D., & Aichner, F. (1991). Neuropsychological deficits in asymptomatic carotid artery stenosis. *Acta Neurologica Scandinavica, 83*(6), 378–381.

Binder, L. M., Tanabe, C. T., Waller, F. T., & Wooster, N. E. (1982). Behavioral effects of superficial temporal artery to middle cerebral artery bypass surgery: preliminary report. *Neurology, 32*(4), 422–424.

Boeke, S. (1981). The effect of carotid endarterectomy on mental functioning. *Clinical Neurology and Neurosurgery, 83*(4), 209–217.

Brand, N., Bossema, E. R., Ommen Mv, M., Moll, F. L., & Ackerstaff, R. G. (2004). Left or right carotid endarterectomy in patients with atherosclerotic disease: ipsilateral effects on cognition? *Brain and Cognition, 54*(2), 117–123.

Calandre, L., Gomara, S., Bermejo, F., Millan, J. M., & del Pozo, G. (1984). Clinical-CT correlations in TIA, RIND, and strokes with minimum residuum. *Stroke, 15*(4), 663–666.

Caplan, L. R., & Wolpert, S. M. (1991). Angiography in patients with occlusive cerebrovascular disease: views of a stroke neurologist and neuroradiologist. *AJNR American Journal of Neuroradiology, 12*(4), 593–601.

Carr, S., Farb, A., Pearce, W. H., Virmani, R., & Yao, J. S. (1996). Atherosclerotic plaque rupture in symptomatic carotid artery stenosis. *Journal of Vascular Surgery, 23*(5), 755–765; discussion 765–756.

Carrea, R., Molins, M., & Murphy, G. (1955). Surgery of spontaneous thrombosis of the internal carotid in the neck; carotido-carotid anastomosis; case report and analysis of the literature on surgical cases. *Medicina (B Aires), 15*(1), 20–29.

Chen, C. J., Lee, T. H., Hsu, H. L., Tseng, Y. C., Lin, S. K., Wang, L. J., et al. (2004). Multi-Slice CT angiography in diagnosing total versus near occlusions of the internal carotid artery: comparison with catheter angiography. *Stroke, 35*(1), 83–85.

Crawley, F., Clifton, A., Buckenham, T., Loosemore, T., Taylor, R. S., & Brown, M. M. (1997). Comparison of hemodynamic cerebral ischemia and microembolic signals detected during carotid endarterectomy and carotid angioplasty. *Stroke, 28*(12), 2460–2464.

Crawley, F., Stygall, J., Lunn, S., Harrison, M., Brown, M. M., & Newman, S. (2000). Comparison of microembolism detected by transcranial Doppler and neuropsychological sequelae of carotid surgery and percutaneous transluminal angioplasty. *Stroke*, *31*(6), 1329–1334.

Criswell, B. K., Langsfeld, M., Tullis, M. J., & Marek, J. (1998). Evaluating institutional variability of duplex scanning in the detection of carotid artery stenosis. *American Journal of Surgery*, *176*(6), 591–597.

Dawson, D. L., Zierler, R. E., Strandness, D. E., Jr., Clowes, A. W., & Kohler, T. R. (1993). The role of duplex scanning and arteriography before carotid endarterectomy: a prospective study. *Journal of Vascular Surgery*, *18*(4), 673–680; discussion 680–673.

de la Torre, J. C. (2000). Critically attained threshold of cerebral hypoperfusion: can it cause Alzheimer's disease? *Annals of the New York Academy of Sciences*, *903*, 424–436.

DeBakey, M. E. (1975). Successful carotid endarterectomy for cerebrovascular insufficiency. Nineteen-year follow-up. *JAMA*, *233*(10), 1083–1085.

Del Sette, M., Angeli, S., Stara, I., Finocchi, C., & Gandolfo, C. (1997). Microembolic signals with serial transcranial Doppler monitoring in acute focal ischemic deficit. A local phenomenon? *Stroke*, *28*(7), 1311–1313.

Deshields, T. L., McDonough, E. M., Mannen, R. K., & Miller, L. W. (1996). Psychological and cognitive status before and after heart transplantation. *General Hospital Psychiatry*, *18*(6 Suppl), 62S-69S.

Drinkwater, J. E., Thompson, S. K., & Lumley, J. S. (1984). Cerebral function before and after extra-intracranial carotid bypass. *Journal of Neurology Neurosurgery and Psychiatry*, *47*(9), 1041–1043.

Droste, D. W., Hansberg, T., Kemeny, V., Hammel, D., Schulte-Altedorneburg, G., Nabavi, D. G., et al. (1997). Oxygen inhalation can differentiate gaseous from nongaseous microemboli detected by transcranial Doppler ultrasound. *Stroke*, *28*(12), 2453–2456.

Duke, R. B., Bloor, B. M., Nugent, G. R., & Majzoub, H. S. (1968). Changes in performance on WAIS, trail making test and finger tapping test associated with carotid artery surgery. *Perceptual & Motor Skills*, *26*(2), 399–404.

Eastcott, H. H., Pickering, G. W., & Rob, C. G. (1954). Reconstruction of internal carotid artery in a patient with intermittent attacks of hemiplegia. *Lancet*, *267*(6846), 994–996.

Elwood, P. C., Pickering, J., Bayer, A., & Gallacher, J. E. (2002). Vascular disease and cognitive function in older men in the Caerphilly cohort. *Age Ageing*, *31*(1), 43–48.

Fairhead, J. F., & Rothwell, P. M. (2006). Underinvestigation and undertreatment of carotid disease in elderly patients with transient ischaemic attack and stroke: comparative population based study. *Brithish Medical Journal*, *333*(7567), 525–527.

Falk, E. (1992). Why do plaques rupture? *Circulation*, *86*(6 Suppl), III30–III42.

Fearn, S. J., Hutchinson, S., Riding, G., Hill-Wilson, G., Wesnes, K., & McCollum, C. N. (2003). Carotid endarterectomy improves cognitive function in patients with exhausted cerebrovascular reserve. *European Journal of Vascular and Endovascular Surgery*, *26*(5), 529–536.

Finklestein, S., Kleinman, G. M., Cuneo, R., & Baringer, J. R. (1980). Delayed stroke following carotid occlusion. *Neurology*, *30*(1), 84–88.

Fischer, S., & Weber, P. C. (1983). Thromboxane A3 (TXA3) is formed in human platelets after dietary eicosapentaenoic acid (C20:5 omega 3). Biochemistry and Biophysics *Research Communication*, *116*(3), 1091–1099.

Fisher, M., Blumenfeld, A. M., & Smith, T. W. (1987). The importance of carotid artery plaque disruption and hemorrhage. *Archives of Neurology*, *44*(10), 1086–1089.

Fisher, M., Paganini-Hill, A., Martin, A., Cosgrove, M., Toole, J. F., Barnett, H. J., et al. (2005). Carotid plaque pathology: thrombosis, ulceration, and stroke pathogenesis. *Stroke*, *36*(2), 253–257.

Fukunaga, S., Okada, Y., Inoue, T., Hattori, F., & Hirata, K. (2006). Neuropsychological changes in patients with carotid stenosis after carotid endarterectomy. *European Neurology*, *55*(3), 145–150.

Fuster, V., Moreno, P. R., Fayad, Z. A., Corti, R., & Badimon, J. J. (2005). Atherothrombosis and high-risk plaque: part I: evolving concepts. *Journal of the American College of Cardiology*, *46*(6), 937–954.

Gelabert, H. A., & Moore, W. S. (1990). Carotid endarterectomy without angiography. *Surgical Clinics of North America*, *70*(1), 213–223.

Georgiadis, D., Grosset, D. G., & Lees, K. R. (1993). Transhemispheric passage of microemboli in patients with unilateral internal carotid artery occlusion. *Stroke*, *24*(11), 1664–1666.

Georgiadis, D., Sievert, M., Cencetti, S., Uhlmann, F., Krivokuca, M., Zierz, S., et al. (2000). Cerebrovascular reactivity is impaired in patients with cardiac failure. *European Heart Journal*, *21*(5), 407–413.

Gold, L., & Lauritzen, M. (2002). Neuronal deactivation explains decreased cerebellar blood flow in response to focal cerebral ischemia or suppressed neocortical function. *Proceedings of the National Academy of Sciences of the United States of America*, *99*(11), 7699–7704.

Goldstein, S. G., Kleinknecht, R. A., & Gallo, A. E., Jr. (1970). Neuropsychological changes associated with carotid endarterectomy. *Cortex*, *6*(3), 308–322.

Golledge, J., Greenhalgh, R. M., & Davies, A. H. (2000). The symptomatic carotid plaque. *Stroke*, *31*(3), 774–781.

Gore, I., McCombs, H. L., & Lindquist, R. L. (1964). Observations on the Fate of Cholesterol Emboli. *Jounal of* Atherosclerosis *Research, 4*, 527–535.

Grimm, M., Yeganehfar, W., Laufer, G., Madl, C., Kramer, L., Eisenhuber, E., et al. (1996). Cyclosporine may affect improvement of cognitive brain function after successful cardiac transplantation. *Circulation, 94*(6), 1339–1345.

Gronholdt, M. L., Nordestgaard, B. G., Schroeder, T. V., Vorstrup, S., & Sillesen, H. (2001). Ultrasonic echolucent carotid plaques predict future strokes. *Circulation, 104*(1), 68–73.

Grosset, D. G., Georgiadis, D., Abdullah, I., Bone, I., & Lees, K. R. (1994). Doppler emboli signals vary according to stroke subtype. *Stroke, 25*(2), 382–384.

Gruhn, N., Larsen, F. S., Boesgaard, S., Knudsen, G. M., Mortensen, S. A., Thomsen, G., et al. (2001). Cerebral blood flow in patients with chronic heart failure before and after heart transplantation. *Stroke, 32*(11), 2530–2533.

Grunwald, I. Q., Supprian, T., Politi, M., Struffert, T., Falkai, P., Krick, C., et al. (2006). Cognitive changes after carotid artery stenting. *Neuroradiology, 48*(5), 319–323.

Hamster, W., & Diener, H. C. (1984). Neuropsychological changes associated with stenoses or occlusions of the carotid arteries. A comparative psychometric study. *European Archives of Psychiatry and Clinical Neuroscience, 234*(1), 69–73.

Hanel, R. A., Levy, E. I., Guterman, L. R., & Hopkins, L. N. (2005). Cervical carotid revascularization: the role of angioplasty with stenting. *Neurosurgery Clinics of North America, 16*(2), 263–278, 8.

Hankey, G. J., Warlow, C. P., & Sellar, R. J. (1990). Cerebral angiographic risk in mild cerebrovascular disease. *Stroke, 21*(2), 209–222.

Haynes, C. D., King, G. D., & Dempsey, R. L. (1975). Improvement of cognitive and personality changes after carotid endarterectomy. *Surgical Forum, 26*, 288–289.

Heilmann, H. P., Lickert, H., & Hauger, W. (1975). RODOC – a system for the documentation of radiographic diagnoses with electronic data processing (author's transl). *Rofo, 123*(1), 79–83.

Heiserman, J. E., Dean, B. L., Hodak, J. A., Flom, R. A., Bird, C. R., Drayer, B. P., et al. (1994). Neurologic complications of cerebral angiography. *AJNR American Journal of Neuroradiology, 15*(8), 1401–1407; discussion 1408–1411.

Hemmingsen, R., Mejsholm, B., Boysen, G., & Engell, H. C. (1982). Intellectual function in patients with transient ischaemic attacks (TIA) or minor stroke. Long-term improvement after carotid endarterectomy. *Acta Neurologica Scandinavica, 66*(2), 145–159.

Hemmingsen, R., Mejsholm, B., Vorstrup, S., Lester, J., Engell, H. C., & Boysen, G. (1986). Carotid surgery, cognitive function, and cerebral blood flow in patients with transient ischemic attacks. *Annals of Neurology, 20*(1), 13–19.

Heyer, E. J., Adams, D. C., Solomon, R. A., Todd, G. J., Quest, D. O., McMahon, D. J., et al. (1998). Neuropsychometric changes in patients after carotid endarterectomy. *Stroke, 29*(6), 1110–1115.

Heyer, E. J., DeLaPaz, R., Halazun, H. J., Rampersad, A., Sciacca, R., Zurica, J., et al. (2006). Neuropsychological dysfunction in the absence of structural evidence for cerebral ischemia after uncomplicated carotid endarterectomy. *Neurosurgery, 58*(3), 474–480; discussion 474–480.

Heyer, E. J., Sharma, R., Rampersad, A., Winfree, C. J., Mack, W. J., Solomon, R. A., et al. (2002). A controlled prospective study of neuropsychological dysfunction following carotid endarterectomy. *Archives of Neurology, 59*(2), 217–222.

Heyer, E. J., Wilson, D. A., Sahlein, D. H., Mocco, J., Williams, S. C., Sciacca, R., et al. (2005). APOE-epsilon4 predisposes to cognitive dysfunction following uncomplicated carotid endarterectomy. *Neurology, 65*(11), 1759–1763.

Horne, D. J., & Royle, J. P. (1974). Cognitive changes after carotid endarterectomy. *Medical Journal of Australia, 1*(9), 316–317.

Houser, O. W., Sundt, T. M., Jr., Holman, C. B., Sandok, B. A., & Burton, R. C. (1974). Atheromatous disease of the carotid artery. Correlation of angiographic, clinical, and surgical findings. *Journal of Neurosurgery, 41*(3), 321–331.

Hsia, D. C., Moscoe, L. M., & Krushat, W. M. (1998). Epidemiology of carotid endarterectomy among Medicare beneficiaries: 1985–1996 update. *Stroke, 29*(2), 346–350.

Hunink, M. G., Polak, J. F., Barlan, M. M., & O'Leary, D. H. (1993). Detection and quantification of carotid artery stenosis: efficacy of various Doppler velocity parameters. *AJR American Journal of Roentgenology, 160*(3), 619–625.

Huston, J., III, James, E. M., Brown, R. D., Jr., Lefsrud, R. D., Ilstrup, D. M., Robertson, E. F., et al. (2000). Redefined duplex ultrasonographic criteria for diagnosis of carotid artery stenosis. *Mayo Clinic Proceedings, 75*(11), 1133–1140.

Iddon, J. L., Sahakian, B. J., & Kirkpatrick, P. J. (1997). Uncomplicated carotid endarterectomy is not associated with neuropsychological impairment. *Pharmacol Biochem Behav, 56*(4), 781–787.

Irvine, C. D., Gardner, F. V., Davies, A. H., & Lamont, P. M. (1998). Cognitive testing in patients undergoing carotid endarterectomy. *European Journal of Vascular and Endovascular Surgery, 15*(3), 195–204.

Jahromi, A. S., Cina, C. S., Liu, Y., & Clase, C. M. (2005). Sensitivity and specificity of color duplex ultrasound measurement in the estimation of internal carotid artery stenosis: a systematic review and meta-analysis. *Journal of Vascular Surgery, 41*(6), 962–972.

Jansen, C., Sprengers, A. M., Moll, F. L., Vermeulen, F. E., Hamerlijnck, R. P., van Gijn, J., et al. (1994). Prediction of intracerebral haemorrhage after carotid endarterectomy by clinical criteria and intraoperative transcranial Doppler monitoring: results of 233 operations. *European Journal of Vascular Surgery, 8*(2), 220–225.

Jones, B. M., Chang, V. P., Esmore, D., Spratt, P., Shanahan, M. X., Farnsworth, A. E., et al. (1988). Psychological adjustment after cardiac transplantation. *Medical Journal of Australia, 149*(3), 118–122.

Kamishirado, H., Inoue, T., Fujito, T., Kase, M., Shimizu, M., Sakai, Y., et al. (1997). Effect of enalapril maleate on cerebral blood flow in patients with chronic heart failure. *Angiology, 48*(8), 707–713.

Kassirer, J. P. (1969). Atheroembolic renal disease. *New England Journal of Medicine, 280*(15), 812–818.

Kelley, R. E., Namon, R. A., Juang, S. H., Lee, S. C., & Chang, J. Y. (1990). Transcranial Doppler ultrasonography of the middle cerebral artery in the hemodynamic assessment of internal carotid artery stenosis. *Archives of Neurology, 47*(9), 960–964.

Kelley, R. E., Namon, R. A., Mantelle, L. L., & Chang, J. Y. (1993). Sensitivity and specificity of transcranial Doppler ultrasonography in the detection of high-grade carotid stenosis. *Neurology, 43*(6), 1187–1191.

Kelly, M. P., Garron, D. C., & Javid, H. (1980). Carotid artery disease, carotid endarterectomy, and behavior. *Archives of Neurology, 37*(12), 743–748.

Kilpatrick, D., Goudet, C., Sakaguchi, Y., Bassiouny, H. S., Glagov, S., & Vito, R. (2001). Effect of plaque composition on fibrous cap stress in carotid endarterectomy specimens. *Journal of Biomechanical Engineering, 123*(6), 635–638.

King, G. K., Gideon, D. A., Haynes, C. D., Dempsey, R. L., & Jenkins, C. W. (1977). Intellectual and personality changes associated with carotid endarterectomy. *J Clin Psychol, 33*(1), 215–220.

Kishikawa, K., Kamouchi, M., Okada, Y., Inoue, T., Ibayashi, S., & Iida, M. (2003). Effects of carotid endarterectomy on cerebral blood flow and neuropsychological test performance in patients with high-grade carotid stenosis. *Journal of Neurological Sciences, 213*(1–2), 19–24.

Kistler, J. P., Ropper, A. H., & Heros, R. C. (1984a). Therapy of ischemic cerebral vascular disease due to atherothrombosis (1). *New England Journal of Medicine, 311*(1), 27–34.

Kistler, J. P., Ropper, A. H., & Heros, R. C. (1984b). Therapy of ischemic cerebral vascular disease due to atherothrombosis. (2). *New England Journal of Medicine, 311*(2), 100–105.

Klijn, C. J., Kappelle, L. J., Tulleken, C. A., & van Gijn, J. (1997). Symptomatic carotid artery occlusion. A reappraisal of hemodynamic factors. *Stroke, 28*(10), 2084–2093.

Knopman, D., Boland, L. L., Mosley, T., Howard, G., Liao, D., Szklo, M., et al. (2001). Cardiovascular risk factors and cognitive decline in middle-aged adults. *Neurology, 56*(1), 42–48.

Koelemay, M. J., Nederkoorn, P. J., Reitsma, J. B., & Majoie, C. B. (2004). Systematic review of computed tomographic angiography for assessment of carotid artery disease. *Stroke, 35*(10), 2306–2312.

Kugler, J., Tenderich, G., Stahlhut, P., Posival, H., Korner, M. M., Korfer, R., et al. (1994). Emotional adjustment and perceived locus of control in heart transplant patients. *Journal of Psychosomatic Research, 38*(5), 403–408.

Lehrner, J., Willfort, A., Mlekusch, I., Guttmann, G., Minar, E., Ahmadi, R., et al. (2005). Neuropsychological outcome 6 months after unilateral carotid stenting. *Journal of Clinical and Experimental Neuropsychology, 27*(7), 859–866.

Lindegaard, K. F., Bakke, S. J., Grolimund, P., Aaslid, R., Huber, P., & Nornes, H. (1985). Assessment of intracranial hemodynamics in carotid artery disease by transcranial Doppler ultrasound. *Journal of Neurosurgery, 63*(6), 890–898.

Lunn, S., Crawley, F., Harrison, M. J., Brown, M. M., & Newman, S. P. (1999). Impact of carotid endarterectomy upon cognitive functioning. A systematic review of the literature. *Cerebrovascular Diseases, 9*(2), 74–81.

Mathiesen, E. B., Joakimsen, O., Bonaa, K. H., Mathiesen, E. B., Joakimsen, O., & Bonaa, K. H. (2001). Prevalence of and risk factors associated with carotid artery stenosis: the Tromso Study. *Cerebrovascular Diseases, 12*(1), 44–51.

Mathiesen, E. B., Waterloo, Kl, Joakimsen, O., Bakke, S. J., Jacobsen, E. A., & Bonaa, K. H. (2004). Reduced neuropsychological test performance in asymptomatic carotid stenosis: The Tromso Study. *Neurology, 62*(5), 695–701.

Milei, J., Parodi, J. C., Alonso, G. F., Barone, A., Grana, D., & Matturri, L. (1998). Carotid rupture and intraplaque hemorrhage: immunophenotype and role of cells involved. *American Heart Journal, 136*(6), 1096–1105.

Mineva, P. P., Manchev, I. C., Hadjiev, D. I., Mineva, P. P., Manchev, I. C., & Hadjiev, D. I. (2002). Prevalence and outcome of asymptomatic carotid stenosis: a population-based ultrasonographic study. *European Journal of Neurology, 9*(4), 383–388.

Mohr, J. P. (1978). Transient ischemic attacks and the prevention of strokes. *New England Journal of Medicine, 299*(2), 93–95.

Molina, C. A., Montaner, J., Abilleira, S., Ibarra, B., Romero, F., Arenillas, J. F., et al. (2001). Timing of spontaneous recanalization and risk of hemorrhagic transformation in acute cardioembolic stroke. *Stroke, 32*(5), 1079–1084.

MRC European Carotid Surgery Trial: interim results for symptomatic patients with severe (70–99%) or with mild (0–29%) carotid stenosis. European Carotid Surgery Trialists' Collaborative Group. (1991). *Lancet*, *337*(8752), 1235–1243.

Naugle, R. I., Bridgers, S. L., & Delaney, R. C. (1986). Neuropsychological signs of asymptomatic carotid stenosis. *Archives of Clinical Neuropsychology*, *1*(1), 25–30.

Nederkoorn, P. J., van der Graaf, Y., & Hunink, M. G. (2003). Duplex ultrasound and magnetic resonance angiography compared with digital subtraction angiography in carotid artery stenosis: a systematic review. *Stroke*, *34*(5), 1324–1332.

Newman, M. F., Kirchner, J. L., Phillips-Bute, B., Gaver, V., Grocott, H., Jones, R. H., et al. (2001). Longitudinal assessment of neurocognitive function after coronary-artery bypass surgery. *New England Journal of Medicine*, *344*(6), 395–402.

Nielsen, H., Hojer-Pedersen, E., Gulliksen, G., Haase, J., & Enevoldsen, E. (1985). A neuropsychological study of 12 patients with transient ischemic attacks before and after EC/IC bypass surgery. *Acta Neurologica Scandinavica*, *71*(4), 317–320.

Norris, J. W., & Zhu, C. Z. (1992). Silent stroke and carotid stenosis. *Stroke*, *23*(4), 483–485.

Ogasawara, K., Yamadate, K., Kobayashi, M., Endo, H., Fukuda, T., Yoshida, K., et al. (2005). Postoperative cerebral hyperperfusion associated with impaired cognitive function in patients undergoing carotid endarterectomy. *Journal of Neurosurgery*, *102*(1), 38–44.

Park, J. H., Kim, W. H., Kim, J. H., Park, T. S., Baek, H. S., Park, J. H., et al. (2006). Prevalence of and risk factors for extracranial internal carotid artery stenosis in Korean Type 2 diabetic patients. *Diabetic Medicine*, *23*(12), 1377–1380.

Pedro, L. M., Pedro, M. M., Goncalves, I., Carneiro, T. F., Balsinha, C., Fernandes e Fernandes, R., et al. (2000). Computer-assisted carotid plaque analysis: characteristics of plaques associated with cerebrovascular symptoms and cerebral infarction. *European Journal of Vascular and Endovascular Surgery*, *19*(2), 118–123.

Pohjasvaara, T., Erkinjuntti, T., Vataja, R., & Kaste, M. (1997). Dementia three months after stroke. Baseline frequency and effect of different definitions of dementia in the Helsinki Stroke Aging Memory Study (SAM) cohort. *Stroke*, *28*(4), 785–792.

Polak, J. F., Shemanski, L., O'Leary, D. H., Lefkowitz, D., Price, T. R., Savage, P. J., et al. (1998). Hypoechoic plaque at US of the carotid artery: an independent risk factor for incident stroke in adults aged 65 years or older. Cardiovascular Health Study. *Radiology*, *208*(3), 649–654.

Poppert, H., Wolf, O., Resch, M., Theiss, W., Schmidt-Thieme, T., Graefin von Einsiedel, H., et al. (2004). Differences in number, size and location of intracranial microembolic lesions after surgical versus endovascular treatment without protection device of carotid artery stenosis. *Journal of Neurology*, *251*(10), 1198–1203.

Prabhakaran, S., Rundek, T., Ramas, R., Elkind, M. S., Paik, M. C., Boden-Albala, B., et al. (2006). Carotid plaque surface irregularity predicts ischemic stroke: the northern Manhattan study. *Stroke*, *37*(11), 2696–2701.

Pugsley, W., Klinger, L., Paschalis, C., Treasure, T., Harrison, M., & Newman, S. (1994). The impact of microemboli during cardiopulmonary bypass on neuropsychological functioning. *Stroke*, *25*(7), 1393–1399.

Rajagopalan, B., Raine, A. E., Cooper, R., & Ledingham, J. G. (1984). Changes in cerebral blood flow in patients with severe congestive cardiac failure before and after captopril treatment. *American Journal of Medicine*, *76*(5B), 86–90.

Rao, R. (2002). The role of carotid stenosis in vascular cognitive impairment. *Journal of the Neurological Sciences*, *203–204*, 103–107.

Rapp, J. H., Pan, X. M., Sharp, F. R., Shah, D. M., Wille, G. A., Velez, P. M., et al. (2000). Atheroemboli to the brain: size threshold for causing acute neuronal cell death. *Journal of Vascular Surgery*, *32*(1), 68–76.

Ringelstein, E. B., Zeumer, H., & Angelou, D. (1983). The pathogenesis of strokes from internal carotid artery occlusion. Diagnostic and therapeutical implications. *Stroke*, *14*(6), 867–875.

Roman, D. D., Kubo, S. H., Ormaza, S., Francis, G. S., Bank, A. J., & Shumway, S. J. (1997). Memory improvement following cardiac transplantation. *Journal of Clinical and Experimental Neuropsychology*, *19*(5), 692–697.

Rothwell, P. M. (2003). For severe carotid stenosis found on ultrasound, further arterial evaluation prior to carotid endarterectomy is unnecessary: the argument against. *Stroke*, *34*(7), 1817–1819; discussion 1819.

Rothwell, P. M., Eliasziw, M., Gutnikov, S. A., Fox, A. J., Taylor, D. W., Mayberg, M. R., et al. (2003). Analysis of pooled data from the randomised controlled trials of endarterectomy for symptomatic carotid stenosis. *Lancet*, *361*(9352), 107–116.

Rothwell, P. M., Gibson, R. J., Slattery, J., Sellar, R. J., & Warlow, C. P. (1994). Equivalence of measurements of carotid stenosis. A comparison of three methods on 1001 angiograms. European Carotid Surgery Trialists' Collaborative Group. *Stroke*, *25*(12), 2435–2439.

Schneider, P. A., Rossman, M. E., Bernstein, E. F., Ringelstein, E. B., & Otis, S. M. (1991). Noninvasive assessment of cerebral collateral blood supply through the ophthalmic artery. *Stroke*, *22*(1), 31–36.

Sinforiani, E., Curci, R., Fancellu, R., Facchinetti, P., Mille, T., & Bono, G. (2001). Neuropsychological changes after carotid endarterectomy. *Functional Neurology*, *16*(4), 329–336.

Soinne, L., Helenius, J., Saimanen, E., Salonen, O., Lindsberg, P. J., Kaste, M., et al. (2003). Brain diffusion changes in carotid occlusive disease treated with endarterectomy. *Neurology*, *61*(8), 1061–1065.

Stary, H. C. (2000). Natural history and histological classification of atherosclerotic lesions: an update. *Arteriosclerosis Thrombosis and Vascular Biology*, *20*(5), 1177–1178.

Stary, H. C., Chandler, A. B., Dinsmore, R. E., Fuster, V., Glagov, S., Insull, W., Jr., et al. (1995). A definition of advanced types of atherosclerotic lesions and a histological classification of atherosclerosis. A report from the Committee on Vascular Lesions of the Council on Arteriosclerosis, American Heart Association. *Arteriosclerosis Thrombosis and Vascular Biology*, *15*(9), 1512–1531.

Tatemichi, T. K., Desmond, D. W., Prohovnik, I., & Eidelberg, D. (1995). Dementia associated with bilateral carotid occlusions: neuropsychological and haemodynamic course after extracranial to intracranial bypass surgery. *Journal of Neurology Neurosurgery and Psychiatry*, *58*(5), 633–636.

Tatemichi, T. K., Desmond, D. W., Stern, Y., Paik, M., Sano, M., & Bagiella, E. (1994). Cognitive impairment after stroke: frequency, patterns, and relationship to functional abilities. *Journal of Neurology Neurosurgery and Psychiatry*, *57*(2), 202–207.

Tsuda, Y., Yamada, K., Hayakawa, T., Ayada, Y., Kawasaki, S., Matsuo, H., et al. (1994). Cortical blood flow and cognition after extracranial-intracranial bypass in a patient with severe carotid occlusive lesions. A three-year follow-up study. *Acta Neurochirurgica*, *129*(3–4), 198–204.

van den Burg, W., Saan, R. J., Van Zomeren, A. H., Boontje, A. H., Haaxma, R., & Wichmann, T. E. (1985). Carotid endarterectomy: does it improve cognitive or motor functioning? *Psychology Medicine*, *15*(2), 341–346.

van der Grond, J., van Everdingen, K. J., Eikelboom, B. C., Kenez, J., & Mali, W. P. (1999). Assessment of borderzone ischemia with a combined MR imaging-MR angiography-MR spectroscopy protocol. *Journal of Magnetic Resonance Imaging*, *9*(1), 1–9.

van Heesewijk, H. P., Vos, J. A., Louwerse, E. S., Van Den Berg, J. C., Overtoom, T. T., Ernst, S. M., et al. (2002). New brain lesions at MR imaging after carotid angioplasty and stent placement. *Radiology*, *224*(2), 361–365.

Wardlaw, J. M., Chappell, F. M., Best, J. J., Wartolowska, K., & Berry, E. (2006). Non-invasive imaging compared with intra-arterial angiography in the diagnosis of symptomatic carotid stenosis: a meta-analysis. *Lancet*, *367*(9521), 1503–1512.

Waugh, J. R., & Sacharias, N. (1992). Arteriographic complications in the DSA era. *Radiology*, *182*(1), 243–246.

Wijman, C. A., Babikian, V. L., Matjucha, I. C., Koleini, B., Hyde, C., Winter, M. R., et al. (1998). Cerebral microembolism in patients with retinal ischemia. *Stroke*, *29*(6), 1139–1143.

Williams, M., & McGee, T. F. (1964). Psychological Study of Carotid Occlusion and Endarterectomy. *Archives of Neurology*, *10*, 293–297.

Wilterdink, J. L., & Feldmann, E. (1996). Carotid stenosis. A neurologist's perspective. *Neuroimaging Clinics of North America*, *6*(4), 831–841.

Wilterdink, J. L., Feldmann, E., Bragoni, M., Brooks, J. M., & Benavides, J. G. (1994). An absent ophthalmic artery or carotid siphon signal on transcranial Doppler confirms the presence of severe ipsilateral internal carotid artery disease. *Journal of Neuroimaging*, *4*(4), 196–199.

Wilterdink, J. L., Feldmann, E., Furie, K. L., Bragoni, M., & Benavides, J. G. (1997). Transcranial Doppler ultrasound battery reliably identifies severe internal carotid artery stenosis. *Stroke*, *28*(1), 133–136.

Younkin, D., Hungerbuhler, J. P., O'Connor, M., Goldberg, H., Burke, A., Kushner, M., et al. (1985). Superficial temporal-middle cerebral artery anastomosis: effects on vascular, neurologic, and neuropsychological functions. *Neurology*, *35*(4), 462–469.

Zuccala, G., Onder, G., Pedone, C., Carosella, L., Pahor, M., Bernabei, R., et al. (2001). Hypotension and cognitive impairment: Selective association in patients with heart failure. *Neurology*, *57*(11), 1986–1992.

Zuccala, G., Pedone, C., Cesari, M., Onder, G., Pahor, M., Marzetti, E., et al. (2003). The effects of cognitive impairment on mortality among hospitalized patients with heart failure. *American Journal of Medicine*, *115*(2), 97–103.

Chapter 10
Cardiac Arrest

Chun Lim and Michael Alexander

Introduction

The human brain is dependent upon the delivery of oxygen and glucose and the removal of waste products for normal activity with interruption of this cycle resulting in tissue injury. A reduction of oxygen content within the brain parenchyma is the state of anoxia, while the cessation of blood flow is ischemia. There are many different etiologies of anoxia including a reduction in blood flow—stagnant anoxia; lack of oxygenation—hypoxic anoxia; insufficient oxygen transport—anemic anoxia; and a disturbance in the intracellular oxygen transport—histotoxic anoxia. In adults the most common cause is a combined hypoxic and ischemic injury caused by cardiac arrest.

For a neurological disease state with such high prevalence, surprisingly little is understood about precise patterns of impairment or about the natural history of recovery. There are robust early predictors of outcome of anoxic-ischemic coma (Wijdicks, Hijdra, Young, Bassetti, & Wiebe, 2006), but outcome has rarely been specified beyond good, poor, and death.

This chapter is designed to examine the etiology, pathology, neurological sequelae, treatment, and outcome of patients that survive a cardiac arrest.

Epidemiology and Clinical Burden

Cardiac disease has been the leading cause of death in the United States since 1921, currently accounting for 30% of all deaths (Minino & Smith, 2001). In 1998 in the United States, 456,076 deaths or 63% of all cardiac disease deaths were caused by cardiac arrest (Zheng, Croft, Giles, & Mensah, 2001)—a 7% increase over the previous 10 years. The average age of the cardiac arrest patients is approximately 65 years (Eisenburger et al., 1998; Kuilman, Bleeker, Hartman, & Simoons, 1999). Estimates of short-term survival from large population surveys of patients who have undergone resuscitation for cardiac arrest vary from 1.4% (Becker, Ostrander, Barrett, & Kondos, 1991; Lombardi, Gallagher, & Gennis, 1994) up to 20% (Fischer, Fisher, & Schuttler, 1997; Kuisma & Maata, 1996; Sedgwick, Dalzeil, Watson, Carrington, & Cobbe, 1993; Waalewijn, de Vos, & Koster, 1988). The best survival rate in the United States of about 15–20% comes from a suburban community in Washington State (Cummins, Ornato, Thies, & Pepe, 1991). With a mean survival rate of 5%, there would be 24,000 survivors of cardiac arrest every year in the United States alone. The long-term survival of these patients has been reported as 70–85% at 1 year (Fischer et al., 1997; Graves et al., 1997; Kuilman et al., 1999; Sedgwick et al., 1993), 66% between 2 and 5 years (Ladwig et al., 1997), 52% at 3.5 years (Earnest, Yarnell, Merrill, & Knapp, 1980), 44–77% at 5 years (Graves et al., 1997;

C. Lim (✉)
Behavioral Neurology Unit, Beth Israel Deaconess Medical Center, Boston, MA, USA
e-mail: clim@bidmc.harvard.edu

J.R. Festa, R.M. Lazar (eds.), *Neurovascular Neuropsychology*, DOI 10.1007/978-0-387-70715-0_10,
© Springer Science+Business Media, LLC 2009

Kuilman et al., 1999), 73% at 7 years (Kuilman et al., 1999), and 18% at 10 years (Graves et al., 1997).

Chart reviews (Graves et al., 1997), telephone interviews (Ladwig et al., 1997), and neuropsychological testing (Roine, Kajaste, & Kaste, 1993) on patients who have survived a cardiac arrest have shown that one quarter to two thirds of all survivors have neurological deficits and one half of all survivors have cognitive or motor deficits of a magnitude that requires a major lifestyle change (Bergner, Hallstrom, Bergner, Eisenberg, & Cobb, 1985; Earnest et al., 1980; Graves et al., 1997).

Based on the reported rates for survival and impairment, we would estimate a yearly incidence of approximately 5/100,000 (12,000) survivors of cardiac arrest who will have persistent neurological deficits and a rolling prevalence of 50,000 impaired survivors in the United States. This is roughly equivalent to the number of patients diagnosed with multiple sclerosis in the United States every year (National Multiple Sclerosis Society, 2005) These numbers may increase with the improvement of the "chain of survival" concept (Cummings et al., 1991), implementation of disease modifying therapy (The Hypothermia after Cardiac Arrest Study Group, 2002), and further refinement of the implantable defibrillator (Hlatky, Saynina, McDonald, Garber, & McClellan, 2002).

Neuropathology

During a cardiac arrest, brain tissue can survive for about 4–5 min without oxygen and blood before irreversible damage occurs (Bass, 1985). The severity of brain damage is dependent upon the duration of ischemia, the degree of ischemia, the core temperature, and the blood glucose level (Auer & Benveniste, 1994). Even though cardiac arrest causes global ischemia and hypoxia, neuronal injury is maximal in specific focal regions, a concept known as selective vulnerability. For reasons still not entirely understood, the small and medium-sized

neurons of the striatum, the Purkinjie cells of the cerebellum, the layer III neurons of the cerebral cortex, and thalamic neurons are the first areas to show degenerative changes (Auer & Benveniste, 1994; Kuroiwa & Okeda, 1994). The pyramidal neurons of the hippocampal formation may not show the earliest damage, but undergo delayed neuronal death (Horn & Schlote, 1992; Petito, Feldmann, Pulsinelli, & Plum, 1987). The etiology of this delayed neuronal death is unknown, but factors thought to play a role include the intracellular formation of oxygen free-radicals and excessive neuronal excitability, as the hippocampal pyramidal neurons are at the end of a major excitatory pathway (Auer & Benveniste, 1994; Murayama, Bouldin, & Suzuki, 1990).

There have been several studies on the temporal sequences of cell death after anoxia. Horn and Schlote (1992) examined the brains of 26 cardiac arrest patients and found the earliest damage occurring in cortical layers three, five, and six appearing within the first few days. Purkinjie cell necrosis was observed up to day 6. Rapid hippocampal pyramidal neuronal cell death was seen from day 4 to day 7. Petito (1987) found a similar pattern in their review of 14 cases and concluded that the cortex and basal ganglia suffered early damage (occurring within the first 18 h), while the hippocampus suffered delayed necrosis at greater than 24 h.

The pathology literature is dominated by patients who suffered a severe anoxic injury and early death. Little is known about possibly regionally specific brain pathology in patients suffering less severe anoxia. Although selective vulnerability is the accepted theory to account for the patterns and distribution of neuronal damage and patterns of clinical impairment, the precise relationship between pathology and clinical signs is incompletely understood.

Hypoxic-ischemic damage to specific regions of the brain is, nevertheless, certainly responsible for the diverse, specific neurological deficits. Immediate (hours to days) complications of cardiac arrest include death, coma (Levy et al., 1985; Yarnell, 1976), severe encephalopathy (Sawada et al., 1990), seizures (Madison & Niedermeyer, 1970), myoclonus (Lance & Adams, 1963), and cortical blindness (Sabah, 1969). Long-term complications include persistent vegetative state (Sazbon, Zabreba, Ronen, Solzi, & Costeff, 1993; Yarnell, 1976), diffuse injury (Parkin, Miller, & Vincent, 1987), amnestic syndrome (Volpe & Hirst, 1983), fronto-executive dysfunction (Armengol, 2000; Reich, Regestein, Murawski, DeSilva, & Lown, 1983), visuo-spatial dysfunction (Howard, Trend, & Ross Russell, 1987; Kase, Troncoso, Court, Tapia, & Mohr, 1977), pyramidal tract weakness (Allison, Bedford, & Meyer, 1956), extra-pyramidal disorders (Hawker & Lang, 1990), ataxia (Lance & Adams, 1963), and spinal cord infarct (Silver & Buxton, 1974) and other very rare disorders. The frequency of each of these complications and whether they co-occur in any particular pattern is not known. Whether the course of recovery or specific outcome conditions (other than death) is tightly related to the severity of the hypoxic-ischemic event is unknown. It is also unknown if any pattern of early deficits is systematically linked to long-term sequelae.

For the clinician, there are several levels of importance: (1) predicting acute survival as a basis for judgment about intensive support; (2) among survivors, managing and predicting short and long term recovery; (3) recognizing the range of residual deficits and the implications for specific vulnerability; (4) working knowledge of the utility of proposed treatments.

Acute Prediction of Survival and Quality of Recovery

Examination

There is no measure of injury that has proven uniformly informative about severity. Neither duration of anoxia, time to CPR and defibrillation, nor cause of cardiac arrest accurately predicts outcome (Wijdicks et al., 2006).

Of the cardiac arrest patients that survive to hospitalization, approximately 25% will be awake upon admission (Longstreth, Inui, Cobb, & Copass, 1983). Relying on the level of consciousness to predict outcome, Longstreth et al. (1983) found that of those patients that awakened after 24 h, 73% had cognitive or motor deficits. After 4 days of coma, no patient ever fully recovered. Other studies confirmed that the early awakeners generally have good outcomes with only between 13 and 23% having any motor or cognitive deficits compared to 52–73% of the patients awakening after 12 h having deficits (Earnest, Breckinridge, Yarnell, & Oliva, 1979; Snyder et al., 1980). Sazbon et al. (1993) followed patients with a history of 30 days or more of unconsciousness for at least 5 years and found that not a single patient recovered to a state of moderate disability or better.

The most straightforward and predictively useful applied evaluation is the clinical examination. The critical aspects of the acute clinical examination are description of the depth of coma and the function of the critical vegetative brainstem functions. Assessment of coma may be complicated by intensive care management. The reliance on using the neurological examination to predict neurological outcome was initially based on the work by Levy et al. (1985). They and others (Edgren, Hedstrand, Kelsey, Sutton-Tyrrell, & Safar, 1994; Zandbergen et al., 2006) have shown that the absent pupillary light reflex after 24 h has a 100% positive predictive value (PPV) for a poor outcome. The sensitivity of this test is only around 20%. Absent motor response to painful stimuli at 72 h is a more sensitive test (around 60%) with two class I studies (Edgren et al., 1994; Levy et al., 1985) having a PPV of 100%, but in the most recent class I study (Zandbergen et al., 2006), 5 out of 105 patients with absent motor responses at 72 h were awake after 1 month.

Specific seizures types can also portent a grim prognosis. Several controlled studies have shown that the presence of myoclonic status epilepticus within the first 24 h also portents a grim prognosis (PPV of 100%) (Wijdicks, Parisi, &

Sharbrough, 1994; Zandbergen et al., 2006), although there has been a case report of a survivor of myoclonic status epilepticus (Arnoldus & Lammers, 1995).

Laboratory Studies

Prolonged cardiac arrest results in metabolic cell death with release of intracellular contents, and recent studies have explored the utility of assays of brain enzymes as a potential marker of injury severity and outcome. Studies have focused on serum neuron-specific enolase (NSE) (Karkela, Bock, & Kaukinen, 1993; Schoerkhuber et al., 1999; Zandbergen et al., 2006), serum astroglial S100 (Pfeifer et al., 2005; Zandbergen et al., 2006), brain-type creatine kinase isoenzyme (Karkela, Pasanen, Kaukinen, Morsky, & Harmoinen, 1992; Karkela et al., 1993), and CSF lactaid (Edgren, Hedstrand, Nordin, Rydin, & Ronquist, 1987). These studies indicate that serum NSE levels > 33 ug/L between day 1 and day 3 following cardiac arrest most accurately predicts poor outcome with a PPV of 100% and sensitivity around 50%. These tests currently offer little practical utility as many hospitals cannot provide rapid turnover of these test results.

Electrophysiology

Electroencephalography (EEG) and somatosensory evoked potentials (SSEP) supplement the clinical examination and laboratory tests as predictive measures of poor outcome. Generalized suppression, burst-suppression, or generalized periodic complexes on a flat background EEG patterns within the week of admission almost invariably results in death or vegetative state (Edgren et al., 1987; Rothstein, Thomas, & Sumi, 1991; Scollo-Lavizzari & Bassetti, 1987), although in a single study, two patients with malignant EEG had a good recovery (Chen, Bolton, & Young, 1996). Absent SSEP within

the first week was also predictive of poor recovery. The only class I study (Zandbergen et al., 2006) and six class III studies (Bassetti, Bomio, Mathis, & Hess, 1996; Berek et al., 1995; Chen et al., 1996; Gendo et al., 2001; Logi, Fischer, Murri, & Mauguiere, 2003; Madl et al., 2000) observed that no patients with bilaterally absent N20 response ever recovered. A single class III study (Young, Doig, & Ragazzoni, 2005) had a false positive rate of 6%. A meta-analysis of these eight studies (Wijdicks et al., 2006) demonstrated a PPV of 99.3% with a sensitivity around 50%.

An earlier meta-analysis and recent comparative prospective study by a group in the Netherlands (Zandbergen, de Haan, Stoutenbeek, Koelman, & Hijdra, 1998; Zandbergen et al., 2006) evaluating various early prediction of poor outcome, including clinical exam, brain enzymes, and electrophysiology demonstrated that absence of SSEP at any time within the first week was the most useful predictor of poor outcome. This has been validated by a recent study (Geocadin et al., 2006) showing that this was the clinical parameter most relied upon by neurologists to estimate prognosis.

Neuroimaging

Imaging is frequently obtained in survivors of cardiac arrest but to date, there is no datum on the utility of these modalities to predict outcome in survivors of cardiac arrest. Early CT findings of comatose patients revealed diffuse cerebral edema and occasional low densities in the basal ganglia and thalamus, or watershed distributions (Fujioka, Okuchi, Sakaki, Hiramatsu, & Iwasaki, 1994; Kjos, Brant-Zawadzki, & Young, 1983). MRI imaging in comatose cardiac arrest patients using fluid-attenuated inversion recovery (FLAIR) and diffusion-weighted (DW) imaging demonstrated early signal abnormalities in the cerebral cortex, cerebellum, thalamus, and hippocampus (Wijdicks, Campeau, & Miller, 2001), and in the cerebral white matter (Chalela, Wolf,

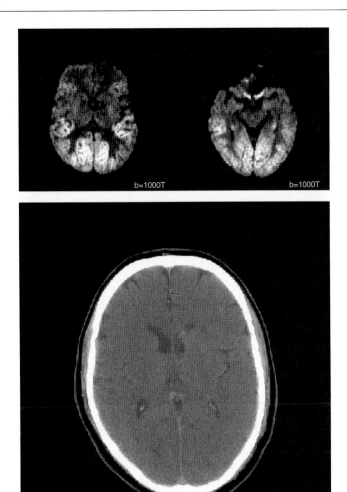

Fig. 1 Diffusion weighted MRI images (A and B) and CT image of a 53-year-old man who suffered a 30-min cardiac arrest. Diffusion images reveal areas of restricted diffusion within the entire cerebral cortex. CT scan shows evidence of gross edema with effacement of sulci and loss of grey/white matter junction

Maldjian, & Kasner, 2001). (See Fig. 1 for representation images of a comatose survivor of a cardiac arrest who died 3 days later.)

Not surprisingly after a direct metabolic injury to neurons, there is a significant reduction in brain metabolic activity in patients with acute cardiac arrest. Mean cerebral glucose utilization in vegetative or comatose subjects is reduced by 38% (Roine et al., 1991) to 50% (DeVolder et al., 1990) compared to a 25% reduction in conscious patients. The reduction is in the watershed distributions of the cerebral cortex, the basal ganglia, and the thalamus. Progressive decline of oxygen metabolism may foretell prolonged coma (Edgren, Enblad, Grenvik, & Langstrom, 2003).

Although non-randomized and non-prospective, these imaging studies do offer some useful markers of a bad outcome (death or severe disability): brain swelling on CT scan on day 3 (Morimoto, Kemmotsu, Kitami, Matsubara, & Tedo, 1993), extensive abnormalities on MRI DWI and FLAIR images (Wijdicks et al., 2001), and >50% perfusion deficits of the supratentorial brain on SPECT scan (Roine et al., 1991). The converse is less useful: structural imaging may be normal in patients who will survive with substantial neurological deficits (Alexander, 1997; Carbonnel, Charnallet, David, & Pellat, 1997; De Renzi & Lucchelli, 1993; Rupright, Woods, & Singh, 1996; Speach, Wong, Cattarin, & Livecchi, 1998).

Summary

The recent study by the Netherlands group (Zandbergen et al., 2006) also examined whether the predictive values of various tests and clinical findings were additive in increasing sensitivity. They found that the combination of the SSEP and NSE raised the sensitivity to 66% and the addition of EEG (burst suppression or worse pattern) increased it to 71% while maintaining 100% PPV.

The current recommendations from the American Academy of Neurology (Wijdicks et al., 2006) involves a decision tree using the following variables: pupillary light reflex, corneal reflex, motor response to pain, myoclonic status epilepticus, NSE, and SSEP to aid in the prediction of outcome in survivors of cardiac arrest. This algorithm involves the prognosis of a poor outcome with the following: (1) the presence of myoclonic status epilepticus on day 1, (2) absent N20 responses on the SSEP after 24 h, (3) Serum NSE > 33 ug/L after 24 h, or (4) Absent pupil or corneal reflexes or absent motor response to pain after 72 h. Even with the adoption of this algorithm, the sensitivity remains poor.

There remains no clinical finding or test result that reliably predicts a good outcome.

Course of Recovery

Caronna and Finklestein (1978) have proposed that patients in coma less than 12 h suffer from a reversible encephalopathy and usually make a rapid and complete recovery, whereas the more severe hypoxic-ischemic patients are in coma for longer than 12 h and suffer structural

damage to specific brain regions. In regards to time to awakening, several studies (Earnest et al., 1979; Longstreth et al., 1983; Snyder et al., 1980) found that 15–27% were awake upon arrival to the hospital and 20–43% of survivors would awaken after 12 h. The most common recovery pattern was of early in-hospital awakening to a confusional state to clearing of cognitive deficits (at least overt ones) during the hospitalization (Levy et al., 1985; Longstreth et al., 1983; Snyder et al., 1980). This has been supported by anecdotal case reports of patients progressing from coma to reportedly normal within 24 h (Sabah, 1969) and of isolated amnestic syndromes recovering over 10 days (Finklestein & Caronna, 1978).

As outlined above, there is a fairly inviolate relationship between duration of coma and the quality of recovery. For coma greater than 2 days, the probability of a good outcome falls dramatically and at 7 days, the probability is essentially zero. The course of recovery is, however, similar for all injuries, albeit for the severe injuries—slower and incomplete. All patients awaken, that is, their eyes open, marking the end of coma in the narrowest sense. More mildly injured patients progress almost immediately into a confusional state. More severely injured patients remain vegetative—eyes open, random eye movements without fixation and without any directed responsiveness—before moving into a confusional state.

Confusional states are conditions of impaired attention with or without impaired arousal. They are characterized by reduced ability to sustain attentional focus, easy distractability, poor registration of new information, and defective recall of experience. Patients are often agitated. Sleep is often disrupted. Over hours to weeks, depending on severity, confusion clears, that is, attention improves. Only when confusion has cleared can the nature and severity of residual deficits be judged.

Determination of the overall distribution of severity of residual deficits will be influenced by the timing and setting of patient accrual and by the measure of severity. One prospective study of patients in coma for at least 12 h

(Caronna & Finklestein, 1978) demonstrated 3-month mortality of 60%, severe disability or vegetative state of 20%, moderate disability of 8%, and good recovery of 12% (30% of all survivors). Differences in "moderate" and "mild" probably reflect differences in measures used. Another prospective study included patients who had already survived at least 3 weeks and were medically stable enough to evaluate for definitive cardiac management. The percentages with good recovery was 28% at initial (3 weeks) evaluation, 43% at about 2 months, and 71% at 6 months (Sauve, Walker, Massa, Winkle, & Scheinman, 1996). This study suggests that there exists a subgroup of patients who will have some late recovery. In a retrospective, population-based chart review, Graves et al. (1997) using the poorly sensitive cerebral performance category[*] (CPC) revealed that after 1 year, 29% of patients in CPC3 and 77% of patients CPC2 improved by at least one performance category. Case reports also mention severely impaired patients who make remarkable recovery within the first 1–3 months of injury (Goh, Heath, Ellis, & Oakley, 2002; Kam, Yoong, & Ganendran, 1978; Kaplan, 1999).

Patients admitted to rehabilitation centers will be the ones with persistent significant deficits once medically stable but not such severe deficits that they cannot participate in therapies. The point of initial assessment will usually be 2–4 weeks after arrest. Fertl (2000) observed that 35% of their patients, all with CPC of 3, improved one performance category and 10% improved two categories during the 3-month rehabilitation. They also noted an improvement of the mean Barthel index of all their patients from 28 to 61. At time of discharge from rehabilitation hospital, 35% had

moderate and 55% had severe deficits. Roine et al. (1993) traced cognitive recovery, albeit with a very coarse instrument for this purpose, the Mini Mental State Exam, and found very little change after 3 months. Others have noted no improvement after 4 months (Groswasser, Cohen, & Cosfeff, 1989), or after 8 months (Drysdale, Grubb, Fox, & O'Carroll, 2000)

Residual Deficits

The focus of this discussion will be on the cognitive deficits as those are almost universally most limiting. The majority of the literature consists of case reports motivated by interest in the cognitive impairment rather than the range of neurological consequences of cardiac arrest. Some investigators were indifferent to the etiology of the hypoxic event. Most group studies followed the same approach, with only a few examining the patterns, frequency, and natural history of the survivors of cardiac arrests. In some reports there was broad latitude in the diagnosis of a hypoxic event, and in others multiple etiologies of hypoxia were considered together without isolating the cardiac arrest patients from other etiologies. We will describe the specific persistent cognitive impairments that have been reported as well as where those impairments fit into the more common characterization of arrest outcomes by severity.

The case reports examining some aspects of cognition after cardiac arrest do offer some insight into the nature of possible impairments. We found 22 case reports with 39 patients who suffered an uncomplicated cardiac arrest (Table 1). There were two cases presenting with virtually unique clinical presentations, one with loss of semantic knowledge (Alexander) and the other with delayed dystonia (Boylan). There were three cases with cognitive deficits in a single domain, with two amnestic (Cummings and Volpe) and one with visual perceptive problems (Rizzo). Based on the clinical description of the cases, we arbitrarily divided the patients into three categories: mild, moderate, or severe.

---

[*] Cerebral Perfomance Category. CPC of 1 indicates good cerebral performance but may have minor psychological or neurological deficits. CPC of 2 indicates moderate cerebral disability typically resulting in impairment of activities of daily living. CPC of 3 is severe cerebral disability with dependence upon others for daily support. CPC of 4 is coma or vegetative state and CPC of 5 is death.

Table 1 Summary of case reports of survivors of isolated cardiac arrest

Study	Case	Age/Sex	Time to Testing	Coma	Category	M	FE	VS	EPS	MO	C	S	L
Alexander		43 M	1 m	5 d	severe	+ +	−	+		+			+
Allison	5	41 M		Yes	severe		+	+					+
	6	19 M			mod			+		+			+
Armengol	2	45 M	13 m	42 h	severe	+ +	+ +	+ +		+			
	5	47 M	15 m	15 d	severe	+ +	+ +	+ +		+			
Barnes		46F	1 y	24 h	mov	+			+ +				
Bengtsson	1	54 M	3 y		n/a	+		+					
	2	78 M	3 y		n/a	+	+	+					
	3	70 M	3 y		n/a	+	+	+					
	6	60 M	2.5 y		n/a	+		+					
	9	54F	2 y		n/a	+	+	+					
	11	73F	1.5 y		n/a	+	+	+					
	12	58 M	1 y		n/a	+	+	+					
	13	74 M	1 y		n/a	+	+	+					+
	15	81F	10 m		n/a	+	+						
	18	63F	7 m		n/a	+							
Boylan		50 M	2 y		n/a				+ +	+			
Bruni		56 M	1 m	4 d	severe		+		+	+	+		
Carbonnel		55 M	1 y	1 w	severe	+		+ +					+
Cummings		53 M	3 m		amn	+ +	+	−		+			−
Dalla Barba		57F	5 m	6 h	mod	+ +	+ +						−
Feve	4	34 M	1 m	1 w	mod		+		+ +	−			
Lance	1	64F	8 y	4 d	n/a			+				+	
	2	62 M	4 y	3 d	mod	+		+				+	
McNeill		49F	6 y		mod	+ +	+	−		+			
Norris	4	49 M	6 m	5 d	mild								
	5	41 M	11 m	Days	severe		+	+	+	+	+		+
Parkin		43F	1 y	16 d	severe	+	+	+	+		+		+
Reich	1	48 M	2 y	hours	mod	+ +	+						
	2	41 M	2 y	15 m	mod	+ +	+						
	3	39 M	2 y	20 h	mod	+ +	+						
	6	56 M	6 m	24 h	mod	+	+						
Rizzo	1	65 M			vis	−			+ +				
Ross		58 M	3 y	Yes	severe	+ +	+ +	+					+
Rupright	1	40 M	2 y		severe	+	+	+					
	4	31F	1 m		severe			+					
Silver	5	54 M	2 m	24 h	severe	+					+		
Szlabowicz		43 M	1 m	8 d	severe								
Volpe	2	42 M	18 m		amn	+ +	−	−		+			−

Abbreviations: M: memory deficit, FE: Frontoexecutive deficit, VS: Visuospatial deficit, EPS: Extrapyramidal deficts, MO: Motor deficits, C: Cerebellar deficits, S: Spinal deficits, L: Language deficits. Mod: Moderate, Diff: Diffuse, Amn: Amnestic syndrome, Vis: Isolated Visuospatial deficit, Mov: Isolated Movement Disorder.
+ neurological deficit by report or mild deficit verified by neuropsychological testing
+ + substantial neurological deficit verified by neuropsychological testing
− no neurological deficit by report or verified by single neuropsychological testing
— no neurological deficit verified by two or more neuropsychological tests

One case had no deficits. Nine cases had multiple deficits of moderate severity. Twelve cases had severe deficits. The remaining 12 cases had insufficient clinical or neuropsychological information to categorize. A large number of case reports did not have an isolated cardiac arrest.

The patients in the moderate injury category presented with a very wide range of signs and symptoms. Coma duration ranged from 15 min to 1 week. Some awoke with no initially reported neurological abnormalities (Reich—case 6) and others were confused and disoriented (McNeill). All patients had deficits in more than one domain.

Of the 12 severe cases, eight reported coma duration, and all were comatose for greater than 24 h. Two other cases were confirmed to have been in coma, but duration was not provided. All four patients whose emergence from coma was described had a severe confusional state. All patients had deficits in every domain tested, with not all domains tested or discussed in each case report.

The group studies, in contrast to the case reports, offer population based information, but often lack the detailed neuropsychological evaluations and frequently involved a mixed population. In 1993, Roine et al. (1993) observed that the most common deficits among 68 consecutive survivors of cardiac arrest at 3 months were disorders of memory (49%), visuoconstructive dyspraxia (43%), and dyspraxia (42%), followed by problems with motivation (37%), depression (35%), programming of activity (34%), and dyscalculia (31%). Language disorders were uncommon (3%). The high frequency of memory disturbances has been confirmed by other with ranges from 80% (Grubb et al., 2000) to 100% of patients examined (Kotila & Kajaste, 1984; Pusswald, Fertl, Faltl, & Auff, 2000). Visuospatial impairments have also been common, occurring in 30–100% of these patients. None of these studies specifically examined executive functions.

Barbara Wilson (1996) performed neuropsychological assessments in 18 survivors of cerebral hypoxia to explore for consistent cognitive profiles. Equipped with an unusually balanced battery of neuropsychological tests for this literature, she identified five distinct patterns: (1) an amnesic syndrome; (2) memory and executive deficits; (3) memory, executive, and visuospatial deficits; (4) isolated visuospatial impairments; and (5) widespread cognitive deficits. With the analysis restricted to survivors of cardiac arrests, there were three profiles: (1) memory and executive deficits; (2) memory, executive, and visuospatial deficits; and (3) widespread cognitive deficits. There were no isolated amnesic or visuospatial syndromes in her pure cardiac arrest patients. These seemed to occur more frequently from other causes of anoxia. Her patient population was small, but if isolated cognitive deficits occur after cardiac arrest, they must be at a very low frequency.

Volpe, Holtzman, and Hirst (1986) have reported the largest series of patients with isolated amnesia after cardiac arrest. These six patients had memory quotients at least 20 points below full scale IQ and normal performance on Ravens Progressive Matrices, the Wisconsin Card Sort task, and the controlled word association test. Neither clinical data nor raw scores nor measures of motor control, mood, or behavior were reported, but these patients appear to represent a pure amnestic syndrome.

It would seem likely that chronically amnestic patients might have hippocampal atrophy and more diffusely impaired patients might have cortical atrophy. This has been explored, although there are limitations because so many of the arrest survivors have implanted defibrillators now and cannot have an MRI. Grubb et al. (2000) compared MRI brain volume in memory impaired and memory intact survivors of cardiac arrest. They did not find selective hippocampal atrophy in their memory impaired patients. Reduction in whole brain volume significantly correlated with memory impairment. Hopkins and colleagues have done MRI volumetric on a number of anoxic patients. In a series of papers comparing anoxic patients to controls, they (Hopkins & Kesner, 1995; Hopkins, Kesner, & Goldstein, 1995) found a reduction in hippocampal areas but not temporal lobe or parahippocampal gyrus volume. Another study (Hopkins, Gale, et al., 1995) did suggest a relationship between morphological abnormalities with performance on cognitive testing, but was limited to three patients. The largest study of 13 patients, of whom only five had had a cardiac arrest, showed a strong correlation between performance on anterograde memory tests with both hippocampal and regional gray matter volume residuals (Allen, Tranel, Bruss, & Damasio, 2006).

We had the opportunity to study eleven cardiac arrest patients under the age of 80 that were referred to a memory disorder clinic for persistent memory deficits (Lim, Alexander, LaFleche, Schnyer, & Verfaellie, 2004). Using standardized neuropsychological tests, we assessed their memory, executive function, perception, language, and motor function (see Table 2). Ten of our patients had moderate to severe memory impairment. Five had severe executive impairments. There was only one patient impaired in lexical-semantic and only one with perceptual difficulties. Nine patients had moderate to severe impairments in motor function. Performing a k-means cluster analysis fixing the results to a 3-cluster solution produced a cluster with no impairments (patient 1), a second cluster with memory and motor impairments and variable executive dysfunction (patients 4, 5, 6), and a third cluster with impairments in all domains (patients 7–11). No patient had an isolated neurological disorder.

Our patient 1 and the small number of case reports with no deficit or only subtle deficits presumably exemplify the largest outcome group of survivors of cardiac arrest. These patients with good recovery usually emerge early from coma. Whether the neural injury was entirely transient and reversible or simply too mild to cause lasting deficits is unknown. As with our patient, there may be relative decrements in performance that are obscured by arbitrary cut-offs on tests, or functional deficits that are not detectable by neuropsychological testing. These patients are likely to be under-represented in the literature.

Patients in our cluster 2, the four patients reported in the Barbara Wilson's study with memory and executive deficits (Wilson, 1996) and several of the case reports reviewed above, all have intermediate outcomes. The relationship between duration of coma and outcome is quite variable. We propose that these patients have not suffered permanent widespread cortical damage and may have damage restricted to the selectively vulnerable brain regions. To our knowledge, this hypothesis has not been directly addressed in any autopsy or adequately sensitive anatomical study. Our patients all had memory and motor impairments. We believe that executive deficits would also consistently have been detected if this group had been evaluated sooner after emergence from coma and confusion.

The patients in our cluster 3 and many of the patients whom we categorized as severe from case reports have similarly poor outcomes. These patients usually have long periods of coma (>24 h). In addition to memory and executive impairments, language and visuospatial functions are disturbed. This suggests that

Table 2 Neuropsychological testing domains of 11 patients who has suffered an isolated cardiac arrest: Mean z-scores or number of tasks on which performance was abnormal

Patient	Memory (z-score)	Executive (z-score)	Boston Naming (z-score)	Perceptual impairment	Motor (z-score)
1	0.4	0.5	0.9	0/3	−1.0
2	−2.6	−0.6	0.1	0/3	−3.3
3	−2.5	−0.5	0.2	1/3	−2.1
4	−3.3	−1.8	−0.1	1/3	−5.0
5	−3.3	−1.2	−1.4	0/3	−2.1
6	−2.0	−1.2	0.8	0/3	−3.8
7	−3.2	−2.8	−1.2	0/3	−2.9
8	−6.5	−2.9	−2.4	0/3	−8.0
9	−3.1	−4.8	−5.1	3/3	−10.0
10	−3.5	−2.6	−9.5	2/3	−1.3
11	−3.6	−3.1	−2.7	1/3	−2.8

the injury likely involves cortex as well as the more vulnerable subcortical and hippocampal regions. Motor deficits might have been prominent if they had been consistently assessed.

Neither the results from our patient group nor a critical review of the literature support the notion that isolated disorders of visual perception or memory occur frequently following cardiac arrest. Thus, the evidence that classic, abrupt CA results in unique damage to the hippocampus and produces long standing isolated amnesia is much weaker than commonly assumed. This is not to conclude that it cannot happen as there exist descriptions of amnesia following cardiac arrest. We propose that the residual deficits in most patients who survive cardiac arrest will fall along a continuum reflecting the severity of injury to those electively vulnerable sites. Impairment will range from no or subtle impairments to a mix of executive, learning, and motor control deficits to such severe executive deficits that all cognitive functions are impaired—a virtual chronic confusional state. Intermixed within these patterns are the rare cases of isolated memory or visuospatial deficits or unusual presentations such as semantic memory loss or delayed dystonia.

Treatment

There are several distinct epochs of management, each with its own treatment imperatives. There are few therapeutic interventions that directly affect the outcome of survivors of out-of-hospital cardiac arrest. Pharmacological interventions that have proven to be ineffective include nimodipine (Roine et al., 1993), thiopental (Group, 1986), magnesium, and/or diazepam (Fatovich, Prentice, & Dobb, 1997; Longstreth et al., 2002), and sodium bicarbonate (Vukmir & Katz, 2006). The single intervention that has significantly improved outcome is hypothermia. Two studies have shown that 24 h of induced hypothermia within the first 4 h of a cardiac arrest will improve overall outcome and survival (Bernard et al., 2002; The Hypothermia after Cardiac Arrest Study Group, 2002).

As described earlier, patients emerge from coma into vegetative states or confusional states. There are no clinical studies of potential treatments for vegetative state after cardiac arrest. Confusional state is usually a transient condition during recovery and in milder injuries it may be rapid enough that no treatment issues emerge. If there is a treatment concern, it is usually agitation. There are no controlled studies of treatment of agitation in this condition. Most adequately controlled studies are in the dementia literature. There are a few basic clinical observations that may assist management of confusion/agitation.

First, confusion and agitation are not synonymous. Treatment of confusion is probably limited to control of the environment around the patient—avoidance of over-stimulation, readily observed orientation material (calendars, clocks, pictures), and vigorous regularization of sleep phases. These should be implemented in every patient. Treatment of agitation should be modulated to the level of distress or inadvertent danger of injury that the patient presents. When possible, use of distractions may be sufficient—visits from family members, opportunities to converse with anyone on staff, recreational activities such as playing cards with a volunteer, watching sports on TV, etc. When the patient is very distressed, possibly becoming in inadvertent danger of injury or disruption of essential medical care, then supervision, passive restraints, and medications are required.

Second, the treatment targets of sleep onset and maintenance and of agitation reduction are not the same. Reduction of agitation should not produce excessive sleep or else sleep phases will become abnormal, probably worsening agitation. Second generation antipsychotics such as quetiapine and olanzapine probably offer the best proportion of tranquilizing without excess sedation. Sleep onset is a separate problem, probably best addressed with standard hypnotics such as trazodone and short half-life benzodiazepines, but these medications will fail at sleep onset in a patient who is agitated, so they may require a preparatory dosage of antipsychotic to achieve a calm enough state that the hypnotic will be effective. Hypnotics should not be repeated too late at night or there will be further disruption of sleep phases due to daytime somnolence. Thus, management may require both treatments, each targeted at a specific factor.

For patients with significant residual deficits, there is at present little direct treatment. We could not identify any controlled studies or even large case reports of late rehabilitation interventions. We are aware of the clinical use of cholinesterase inhibitors, stimulants, and dopaminergic medications but with minimal sense of success and no reported claims of success. To judge by the reports of Grosswasser and Wilson described above—both reports coming from respected cognitive rehabilitation centers—there is little optimism that the fundamental deficits can be treated behaviorally. Whether patients with executive impairments after cardiac arrest might respond to some of the behavioral strategies that have been implemented in patients with trauma or focal frontal lesions is unknown.

There are many obstacles to construction of useful interventions for these patients. We are not entirely clear about the nature of the residual deficits. Are they fundamentally executive function deficits? If so, there is a reasonable possibility of importing useful behavioral and medication treatments from the larger literature on treatment of trauma and focal lesions. When do they stabilize? How malleable are they over the post-acute epoch? Or do the patients who do not recover quickly also always have true memory system (hippocampal) injury as well? If so, behavioral treatments are likely to be insufficient to achieve any functional improvement. Until treatments become more effective or until acute management discovers a biological intervention that prevents acute cell death and apoptosis, there will be a growing population of inadequately treated patients at risk for poor quality of life.

Quality of Life

Impairment does not necessarily lead to disability and handicap, but the reported effects on quality of life have been variable. Bergner observed that cardiac arrest survivors fared significantly worse in all categories of their QOL compared to a random control population (Bergner, Bergner, Hallstrom, Eisenberg, & Cobb, 1984) and when compared to survivors of myocardial infarcts (Bergner et al., 1985). de Vos, de Haes, Koster, and de Haan (1999) showed that the quality of life of their cardiac arrest survivors were worse than an elderly control population, but better than that of patients with strokes. An 8-year follow-up of cardiac arrest patients found that the quality of life in patients was considered good (Kuilman et al., 1999), but the study lacked age-matched controls.

Evaluating the number of patients able to live independently or return to work may be the most sensitive markers of impairment, disability, and handicap. As many as 30–60% of survivors who awaken early are able to return to their previous level of employment (Bergner et al., 1985; Earnest et al., 1980; Graves et al., 1997; Sauve, 1995; Sunnerhagen, Johansson, Herlitz, & Grimby, 1996). On the other hand, of the patients admitted to rehabilitation hospitals, fewer than 10% return to work (Groswasser et al., 1989; Howard et al., 1987). Approximately one half of all survivors achieve full independence in all aspects of daily living (Earnest et al., 1980; Howard et al., 1987; Sunnerhagen et al., 1996), although many require substantial supervision and assistance for instrumental activities, finances, and social activities (Sauve, 1995). There is no datum on return to driving.

References

Alexander, M. P. (1997). Specific semantic memory loss after hypoxic-ischemic injury. *Neurology, 48,* 165–173.

Allen, J. S., Tranel, D., Bruss, J., & Damasio, H. (2006). Correlations between regional brain volumes and memory performance in anoxia. *Journal of Clinical and Experimental Neuropsychology, 28,* 457–476.

Allison, R. S., Bedford, P. D., & Meyer, A. (1956). Discussion on the clinical consequence of cerebral anoxia. *Proceedings of the Royal Society of Medicine, 49,* 609–619.

Armengol, C. G. (2000). Acute oxygen deprivation: Neuropsychological profiles and implications for rehabilitation. *Brain Injury, 14,* 237–250.

Arnoldus, E. P., & Lammers, G. J. (1995). Postanoxic coma: Good recovery despite myoclonus status. *Annals of Neurology, 38,* 697–698.

Auer, R. N., & Benveniste, H. (1994). Hypoxia and related conditions. In S. Greenfield (Ed.), *Neuropathology* (pp. 263–314). London: Arnold.

Bass, E. (1985). Cardiopulmonary arrest. *Annals of Internal Medicine, 103,* 920–927.

Bassetti, C., Bomio, F., Mathis, J., & Hess, C. W. (1996). Early prognosis in coma after cardiac arrest: A prospective clinical, electrophysiological, and biochemical study of 60 patients. *Journal of Neurology, Neurosurgery and Psychiatry, 61,* 610–615.

Becker, L. B., Ostrander, M. P., Barrett, J., & Kondos, G. T. (1991). Outcome of CPR in a large metropolitan area – Where are the survivors. *Annals of Emergency Medicine, 20,* 355–361.

Berek, K., Lechleitner, P., Luef, G., Felber, S., Saltuari, L., Schinnerl, A., et al. (1995). Early determination of neurological outcome after prehospital cardiopulmonary resuscitation. *Stroke, 26,* 543–549.

Bergner, L., Bergner, M., Hallstrom, A. P., Eisenberg, M. S., & Cobb, L. A. (1984). Health status of survivors of out-of-hospital cardiac arrest six months later. *American Journal of Public Health, 74,* 508–510.

Bergner, L., Hallstrom, A. P., Bergner, M., Eisenberg, M. S., & Cobb, L. A. (1985). Health status of survivors of cardiac arrest and of myocardial infarction controls. *American Journal of Public Health, 75,* 1321–1323.

Bernard, S. A., Gray, T. W., Buist, M. D., Jones, B. M., Silvester, W., Gutteridge, G., et al. (2002). Treatment of comatose survivors of out-of-hospital cardiac arrest with induced hypothermia. *New England Journal of Medicine, 346,* 557–563.

Carbonnel, S., Charnallet, A., David, D., & Pellat, J. (1997). One of several semantic systems(s)? Maybe none: Evidence form a case study of modality and category-specific "semantic" impairement. *Cortex, 33,* 391–417.

Caronna, J. J., & Finklestein, S. (1978). Neurologiclal syndromes after cardiac arrest. *Stroke, 9,* 517–520.

Chalela, J. A., Wolf, R. L., Maldjian, J. A., & Kasner, S. E. (2001). MRI identification of early white matter injury in anoxic-ischemic encephalopathy. *Neurology, 56,* 481–485.

Chen, R., Bolton, C. F., & Young, G. B. (1996). Prediction of outcome in patients with anoxic coma: A clinical and electrophysiologic study. *Critical Care Medicine, 24,* 672–678.

Cummings, R. O., Chamberlain, D. A., Abramson, N. S., Allen, M., Baskett, P., Becker, L., et al. (1991). Recommended guidlines for uniform reporting of data from out-of-hospital cardiac arrest: The Utstein style. *Annal of Emergency Medicine, 20,* 861–874.

Cummins, R. O., Ornato, J. P., Thies, W. H., & Pepe, P. E. (1991). Improving survival from sudden cardiac arrest: The "chain of survival" concept. *Circulation, 83,* 1832–1847.

De Renzi, E., & Lucchelli, F. (1993). Dense retrograde amnesia, intact learning capability and abnormal forgetting rate: A consolidation deficit? *Cortex, 29,* 449–466.

de Vos, R., de Haes, H., Koster, R. W., & de Haan, R. J. (1999). Quality of life after cardiopulmonary rescuscitation. *Archives of Internal Medicine, 159,* 249–254.

DeVolder, A. G., Goffinet, A. M., Bol, A., Michel, C., de Barsy, T., & Laterre, C. (1990). Brain glucose metabolism in postanoxic syndrome. *Archives of Neurology, 47,* 197–204.

Drysdale, E. E., Grubb, N. R., Fox, K. A. A., & O'Carroll, R. E. (2000). Chronicity of memory impairment in long-term out-of-hospital cardiac arrest survivors. *Resuscitation, 47,* 27–32.

Earnest, M. P., Breckinridge, J. C., Yarnell, P. Y., & Oliva, P. B. (1979). Quality of survival after out-of-hospital cardiac arrest: Predictive value of early neurologic evaluation. *Neurology, 29,* 56–60.

Earnest, M. P., Yarnell, P. Y., Merrill, S. L., & Knapp, G. L. (1980). Long-term survival and neurologic status after resuscitation from out-of-hospital cardiac arrest. *Neurology, 30,* 1298–1302.

Edgren, E., Enblad, P., Grenvik, A., & Langstrom, B. (2003). Cerebral blood flow and metabolism after cardiopulmonary resuscitation. A pathophysiologic and prognostic positron emission tomography pilot study. *Resuscitation, 57,* 161–170.

Edgren, E., Hedstrand, U., Kelsey, S., Sutton-Tyrrell, K., & Safar, P. (1994). Assessment of neurological prognosis in comatose survivors of cardiac arrest. BRCT I Study Group. *Lancet, 343,* 1055–1059.

Edgren, E., Hedstrand, U., Nordin, M., Rydin, E., & Ronquist, G. (1987). Prediction of outcome after cardiac arrest. *Critical Care Medicine, 15,* 820–825.

Eisenburger, P., List, M., Schorkhuber, W., Walker, R., Sterz, F., & Laggner, A. N. (1998). Long-term cardiac arrest survivors of the Vienna emergency medical service. *Resuscitation, 38,* 137–143.

Fatovich, D. M., Prentice, D. A., & Dobb, G. J. (1997). Magnesium in cardiac arrest (the magic trial). *Resuscitation, 35,* 237–241.

Fertl, E., Vass, K., Sterz, F., Gabriel, H., & Auff, E. (2000) Neurological rehabilitation of severely disabled cardiac arrest survivors. Part I. Course of post-acute treatment. *Resuscitation, 47,* 231–239.

Finklestein, S., & Caronna, J. J. (1978). Amnestic syndrome following cardiac arrest. *Neurology, 28,* 389.

Fischer, M., Fisher, N. J., & Schuttler, J. (1997). One-year survival after out-of-hospital cardiac arrest in

Bonn city: Outcome report according to the 'Utstein style'. *Resuscitation, 33*, 233–243.

Fujioka, M., Okuchi, K., Sakaki, T., Hiramatsu, K. -I., & Iwasaki, S. (1994). Specific changes in human brain following reperfusion after cardiac arrest. *Stroke, 25*, 2091–2095.

Gendo, A., Kramer, L., Hafner, M., Funk, G. C., Zauner, C., Sterz, F., et al. (2001). Time-dependency of sensory evoked potentials in comatose cardiac arrest survivors. *Intensive Care Medicine, 27*, 1305–1311.

Geocadin, R. G., Buitrago, M. M., Torbey, M. T., Chandra-Strobos, N., Williams, M. A., & Kaplan, P. W. (2006). Neurologic prognosis and withdrawal of life support after resuscitation from cardiac arrest. *Neurology, 67*, 105–108.

Goh, W. C., Heath, P. D., Ellis, S. J., & Oakley, P. A. (2002). Neurological outcome prediction in a cardiorespiratory arrest survivor. *British Journal of Anaesthesia, 88*, 719–722.

Graves, J. R., Herlitz, J., Bang, A., Axelsson, A., Ekstrom, L., Holmberg, M., et al. (1997). Survivors of out of hospital cardiac arrest: The prognosis, longevity and functional status. *Resuscitation, 35*, 117–121.

Groswasser, Z., Cohen, M., & Cosfeff, H. (1989). Rehabilitation outcome after anoxic brain damage. *Archives of Physical Medicine and Rehabilitation, 70*, 186–188.

Group, B. R. C. T. I. S. (1986). Randomized clinical study of thiopental loading in comatose survivors of cardiac arrest. Brain Resuscitation Clinical Trial I Study Group. *New England Journal of Medicine, 314*, 397–403.

Grubb, N. R., Fox, K. A. A., Smith, K., Best, J., Blane, A., Ebmeier, K. P., et al. (2000). Memory impairment in out-of-hospital cardiac arrest survivors is associated with global reduction in brain volume, not focal hippocampal injury. *Stroke, 31*, 1509–1513.

Hawker, K., & Lang, A. E. (1990). Hypoxic-ischemic damage of the basal ganglia. *Movement Disorders, 5*, 219–224.

Hlatky, M. A., Saynina, O., McDonald, K. M., Garber, A. M., & McClellan, M. B. (2002). Utilization and outcomes of the implantable cardioverter defibrillator, 1987 to 1995. *American Heart Journal, 144*, 397–403.

Hopkins, R. O., Gale, S. D., Johnson, S. C., Anderson, C. V., Bigler, E. D., Blatter, D. D., et al. (1995). Severe anoxia with and without concomitant brain atrophy and neuropsychological impairments. *Journal of the International Neuropsychological Society, 1*, 501–509.

Hopkins, R. O., & Kesner, R. P. (1995). Item and order recognition memory in subjects with hypoxic brain injury. *Brain and Cognition, 27*, 180–201.

Hopkins, R. O., Kesner, R. P., & Goldstein, M. (1995). Memory for novel and familiar spatial and linguistic temporal distance information in hypoxic subject. *Journal of the International Neuropsychological Society, 1*, 454–468.

Horn, M., & Schlote, W. (1992). Delayed neuronal death and delayed neuronal recovery in the human brain following global ischemia. *Acta Neuropathologica (Berlin), 85*, 79–87.

Howard, R., Trend, P., & Ross Russell, R. W. (1987). Clinicial features of ischemia in cerebral arterial border zones after periods of reduced cerebral blood flow. *Archives of Neurology, 44*, 934–940.

Kam, C. A., Yoong, F. F. Y., & Ganendran, A. (1978). Cortical blindness following hypoxia during cardiac arrest. *Anaesthesia and Intensive Care, 6*, 143–145.

Kaplan, C. P. (1999). Anoxic-hypotensive brain injury: Neuropsychological performance at 1 month as an indicator of recovery. *Brain Injury, 13*, 305–310.

Karkela, J., Bock, E., & Kaukinen, S. (1993). CSF and serum brain-specific creatine kinase isoenzymes (CK-BB), neuron-specific enolase (NSE), and neural cell adhesion molecule (NCAM) as prognostic makers for hypoxic brain injury after cardiac arrest in man. *Journal of Neurological Sciences, 116*, 100–109.

Karkela, J., Pasanen, M., Kaukinen, S., Morsky, P., & Harmoinen, A. (1992). Evaluation of hypoxic brain injury with spinal fluid enzymes, lactate, and pyruvate. *Critical Care Medicine, 20*, 378–386.

Kase, C. S., Troncoso, J. F., Court, J. E., Tapia, J. E., & Mohr, J. P. (1977). Global spatial disorientation. *Journal of the Neurological Sciences, 34*, 267–278.

Kjos, B. O., Brant-Zawadzki, M., & Young, R. G. (1983). Early CT findings of global central nervous system hypoperfusion. *American Journal of Neuroradiology, 4*, 1043–1048.

Kotila, M., & Kajaste, S. (1984). Neurological and neuropsychological symptoms after cardiac arrest. *Acta Neurologica Scandinavica, 69*(Suppl. 98), 337.

Kuilman, M., Bleeker, J. K., Hartman, J. A. M., & Simoons, M. L. (1999). Long-term survival after out-of-hospital cardiac arrest: An 8-year follow-up. *Resuscitation, 41*, 25–31.

Kuisma, M., & Maata, T. (1996). Out-of-hospital cardiac arrest in Helsinki: Utstein style reporting. *Heart, 76*, 18–23.

Kuroiwa, T., & Okeda, R. (1994). Neuropathology of cerebral ischemia and hypoxia: Recent advances in experimental studies on its pathogenesis. *Pathology International, 44*, 171–181.

Ladwig, K. -H., Schoefinius, A., Danner, R., Rolf, G., Herman, R., Koeppel, A., et al. (1997). Effects of early defibrillation by ambulance personnel on short- and long-term outcomes of cardiac arrest survival: The Munich experiment. *Chest, 112*, 1584–1591.

Lance, J. W., & Adams, R. D. (1963). The syndrome of intention or action myoclonus as a sequel to hypoxic encephalopathy. *Brain, 86*, 111–136.

Levy, D. E., Caronna, J. J., Singer, B. H., Lapinski, R. H., Frydman, H., & Plum, F. (1985). Predicting outcome from hypoxic-ischemic coma. *Journal of the American Medical Association, 253*, 1420–1426.

Lim, C., Alexander, M. P., LaFleche, G., Schnyer, D. M., & Verfaellie, M. (2004). The neurological and cognitive sequelae of cardiac arrest. *Neurology*, *63*, 1774–1778.

Logi, F., Fischer, C., Murri, L., & Mauguiere, F. (2003). The prognostic value of evoked responses from primary somatosensory and auditory cortex in comatose patients. *Clinical Neurophysiology*, *114*, 1615–1627.

Lombardi, G., Gallagher, E. J., & Gennis, P. (1994). Outcome of out-of-hospital cardiac arrest in New York City. *Journal of the American Medical Association*, *271*, 678–683.

Longstreth, W. T., Jr., Fahrenbruch, C. E., Olsufka, M., Walsh, T. R., Copass, M. K., & Cobb, L. A. (2002). Randomized clinical trial of magnesium, diazepam, or both after out-of-hospital cardiac arrest. *Neurology*, *59*, 506–514.

Longstreth, W. T., Inui, T. S., Cobb, L. A., & Copass, M. K. (1983). Neurologic recovery after out-of-hospital cardiac arrest. *Annals of Internal Medicine*, *98*, 588–592.

Madison, D., & Niedermeyer, E. (1970). Epileptic seizures resulting from acute cerebral anoxia. *Journal of Neurology, Neurosurgery and Psychiatry*, *33*, 381–386.

Madl, C., Kramer, L., Domanovits, H., Woolard, R. H., Gervais, H., Gendo, A., et al. (2000). Improved outcome prediction in unconscious cardiac arrest survivors with sensory evoked potentials compared with clinical assessment. *Critical Care Medicine*, *28*, 721–726.

Minino, A. M., & Smith, B. L. (2001). Deaths: Preliminary data for 2000. National vital statistics report. *National Vital Statistics Reports*, *49*, 1–40.

Morimoto, Y., Kemmotsu, O., Kitami, K., Matsubara, I., & Tedo, I. (1993). Acute brain swelling after out-of-hsopital cardiac arrest: Pathogenesis and outcome. *Critical Care Medicine*, *21*, 104–110.

Murayama, S., Bouldin, T. W., & Suzuki, K. (1990). Selectve sparing of Betz cells in primary motor area in hypoxia-ischemic encephalopathy. *Acta Neuropathologica (Berlin)*, *80*, 560–562.

National Multiple Sclerosis Society. (2005). Just the Facts 2005–2006, Brochure.

Parkin, A. J., Miller, J., & Vincent, R. (1987). Multiple neuropsychological deficits due to anoxic encephalopathy: A case study. *Cortex*, *1987*, 655–665.

Petito, C. K., Feldmann, E., Pulsinelli, W., & Plum, F. (1987). Delayed hippocampal damage in humans following cardiorespiratory arrest. *Neurology*, *37*, 1281–1286.

Pfeifer, R., Borner, A., Krack, A., Sigusch, H. H., Surber, R., & Figulla, H. R. (2005). Outcome after cardiac arrest: Predictive values and limitations of the neuroproteins neuron-specific enolase and protein S-100 and the Glasgow Coma Scale. *Resuscitation*, *65*, 49–55.

Pusswald, G., Fertl, E., Faltl, M., & Auff, E. (2000). Neurological rehabilitation of severely disabled cardiac arrest survivors. Part II. Life situation of patients and families after treatment. *Resuscitation*, *47*, 241–248.

Reich, P., Regestein, Q. R., Murawski, B. L., DeSilva, R. A., & Lown, B. (1983). Unrecognized organic mental disorders in survivors of cardiac arrest. *American Journal of Psychiatry*, *140*, 1194–1197.

Roine, R. O., Kajaste, S., & Kaste, M. (1993). Neuropsychological sequelae of cardiac arrest. *Journal of the American Medical Association*, *269*, 237–242.

Roine, R. O., Launes, J., Nikkinen, P., Phil, L., Lindroth, L., & Kaste, M. (1991). Regional cerebral blood flow after human cardiac arrest. *Archives of Neurology*, *48*, 625–629.

Rothstein, T. L., Thomas, E. M., & Sumi, S. M. (1991). Predicting outcome in hypoxic-ischemic coma. A prospective clinical and electrophysiological study. *Electroencephalography and Clinical Neurophysiology*, *79*, 101–107.

Rupright, J., Woods, E. A., & Singh, A. (1996). Hypoxic brain injury: Evaluation by single photon emission computed tomography. *Archives of Physical Medicine and Rehabilitation*, *77*, 1205–1208.

Sabah, A. H. (1969). Blindness after cardiac arrest. *Postgraduate Medical Journal*, *44*, 513–516.

Sauve, M. J. (1995). Long-term physical functioning and psychosocial adjustment in survivors of sudden cardiac death. *Heart and Lung*, *24*, 1–20.

Sauve, M. J., Walker, J. A., Massa, S. M., Winkle, R. A., & Scheinman, M. (1996). Patterns of cognitive recovery in sudden cardiac arrest survivors: The pilot study. *Heart and Lung*, *25*, 172–181.

Sawada, H., Udaka, F., Seriu, N., Shindou, K., Kameyama, M., & Tsujimura, M. (1990). MRI demonstration of cortical laminar necrosis and delayed white matter injury in anoxic encephalopathy. *Neuroradiology*, *32*, 319–321.

Sazbon, L., Zabreba, F., Ronen, J., Solzi, P., & Costeff, H. (1993). Course and outcome of patients in vegetative state of nontraumatic aetiology. *Journal of Neurology, Neurosurgery and Psychiatry*, *56*, 407–409.

Schoerkhuber, W., Kittler, H., Sterz, F., Behringer, W., Holzer, M., Frossard, M., et al. (1999). Time course of serum neuron-specific enolase. *Stroke*, *30*, 1598–1603.

Scollo-Lavizzari, G., & Bassetti, C. (1987). Prognostic value of EEG in post-anoxic coma after cardiac arrest. *European Neurology*, *26*, 161–170.

Sedgwick, M. L., Dalzeil, K., Watson, J., Carrington, D. J., & Cobbe, S. M. (1993). Performance of an established system of first responder out-of-hospital defibrillation. The results of the second year of the Heartstart Scotland Project in the 'Utstein style'. *Resuscitation*, *26*, 75–88.

Silver, J. R., & Buxton, P. H. (1974). Spinal stroke. *Brain*, *97*, 539–550.

Snyder, B. D., Loewenson, R. B., Gumnit, R. J., Hauser, W. A., Leppik, I. E., & Ramirez-Lassepas, M. (1980). Neurologic prognosis after cardiopulmonary arrest: II. Level of consciousness. *Neurology*, *30*, 52–58.

Speach, D. P., Wong, T. M., Cattarin, J. A., & Livecchi, M. A. (1998). Hypoxic brain injury with motor apraxia following an anaphylactic reaction to hymenoptera venom. *Brain Injury*, *12*, 239–244.

Sunnerhagen, K. S., Johansson, O., Herlitz, J., & Grimby, G. (1996). Life after cardiac arrest; a retrospective study. *Resuscitation*, *31*, 135–140.

The Hypothermia after Cardiac Arrest Study Group. (2002). Mild therapeutic hypothermia to improve the neurologic outcome after cardiac arrest. *New England Journal of Medicine*, *346*, 549–556.

Volpe, B. T., & Hirst, W. (1983). The characterization of an amnesic syndrome following hypoxic ischemic injury. *Archives of Neurology*, *40*, 436–440.

Volpe, B. T., Holtzman, J. D., & Hirst, W. (1986). Further characterization of patients with amnesia after cardiac arrest: Preserved recognition memory. *Neurology*, *36*, 408–411.

Vukmir, R. B., & Katz, L. (2006). Sodium bicarbonate improves outcome in prolonged prehospital cardiac arrest. *American Journal of Emergency Medicine*, *24*, 156–161.

Waalewijn, R. A., de Vos, R., & Koster, R. W. (1988). Out-of-hospital cardiac arrests in Amsterdam and its surrounding areas: Results from the Amsterdam resuscitation study (ARREST) in Utstein style. *Resuscitation*, *38*, 157–167.

Wijdicks, E. F. M., Campeau, N. G., & Miller, G. M. (2001). MR Imaging in comatose survivors of cardiac arrest. *American Journal of Neuroradiology*, *22*, 1561–1565.

Wijdicks, E. F., Hijdra, A., Young, G. B., Bassetti, C. L., & Wiebe, S. (2006). Practice parameter: Prediction of outcome in comatose survivors after cardiopulmonary resuscitation (an evidence-based review): Report of the Quality Standards Subcommittee of the American Academy of Neurology. *Neurology*, *67*, 203–210.

Wijdicks, E. F., Parisi, J. E., & Sharbrough, F. W. (1994). Prognostic value of myoclonus status in comatose survivors of cardiac arrest. *Annals of Neurology*, *35*, 239–243.

Wilson, B. A. (1996). Cognitive functioning of adult survivors of cerebral hypoxia. *Brain Injury*, *10*, 863–874.

Yarnell, P. Y. (1976). Neurological outcome of prolonged coma survivors of out-of-hospital cardiac arrest. *Stroke*, *1976*, 279–282.

Young, G. B., Doig, G., & Ragazzoni, A. (2005). Anoxic-ischemic encephalopathy: Clinical and electrophysiological associations with outcome. *Neurocritical Care*, *2*, 159–164.

Zandbergen, E. G. J., de Haan, R. J., Stoutenbeek, C. P., Koelman, J. H. T. M., & Hijdra, A. (1998). Systematic review of early prediction of poor outcome in anoxic-ischaemic coma. *Lancet*, *352*, 1808–1812.

Zandbergen, E. G., Hijdra, A., Koelman, J. H., Hart, A. A., Vos, P. E., Verbeek, M. M., et al. (2006). Prediction of poor outcome within the first 3 days of postanoxic coma. *Neurology*, *66*, 62–68.

Zheng, Z. -J., Croft, J. B., Giles, W. H., & Mensah, G. A. (2001). Sudden cardiac death in the United States 1989 to 1998. *Circulation*, *104*, 2158–2163.

Chapter 11
Congestive Heart Failure/Heart Transplant

Giuseppe Zuccalà, Giuseppe Colloca, and Matteo Tosato

Introduction

The term "cardiogenic dementia" was coined in 1977, in an editorial that dealt with the effects of bradycardia on cerebral electrical activity and cognition among older subjects (Editorial, 1977). The author suggested that older subjects might be particularly vulnerable to reduced cerebral perfusion due to several causes, including bradycardia. Subsequently, a study documented multiple cognitive deficits, including memory impairment, in 70% of patients undergoing cardiac rehabilitation (Barclay, Weiss, Mattis, Bond, & Blass, 1988). The authors proposed the term "circulatory dementia" to describe this form of cognitive impairment.

In the late 1990s, the issue of "cardiogenic" or "circulatory" dementia has been revisited by repeated reports on the effect of pace-maker implantation and cardiac transplantation on cognitive function (Koide, Kobayashi, Kitani, Tsunematsu, & Nakazawa, 1994; Bornstein, Starling, Myerowitz, & Haas, 1995; Grimm et al., 1996). In these studies, cognitive impairment was thought to affect only patients with severe cardiac dysfunction. However, subsequent studies demonstrated an excess prevalence of cognitive impairment (ranging from 35% to 58%) in older populations with only mild to moderate heart failure (Cacciatore et al., 1998; Zuccalà et al., 1997, 2003; Almeida & Flicker, 2001). Among such patients, cognitive dysfunction is independently associated with a fivefold increase in the risk of mortality and a sixfold increase in the probability of disability (Zuccalà et al., 2001b, 2003). These figures are important because according to several observations, the spreading of state-of-the-art treatment for heart failure in clinical practice did not affect either mortality or disability rates in older populations with heart failure over the last decades (Barker, Mullooly, & Getchell, 2006). Such observations cast doubts on our knowledge of the determinants of survival in older patients with heart failure, as well as on the efficacy and safety of "acknowledged" drug treatment for heart failure in older populations (Konstam, 2000). This concern was reinforced by the finding of an inverse association between systolic blood pressure levels and cognitive performance among older patients with heart failure who received vasodilating agents (Zuccalà et al., 2001a). This observation, along with several epidemiological reports on increased risk of cognitive impairment in older subjects with lower baseline blood pressure levels, raised the issue of a potential detrimental effect of vasodilating agents on cerebral perfusion (Pullicino & Hart, 2001; Mathias, 2000). However, a subsequent study indicated that, among

G. Zuccalà (✉)
Department of Gerontology, Catholic University of the Sacred Heart, L.go F. Vito, 1 - 00168 Rome, Italy
e-mail: giuseppe_zuccala@rm.unicatt.it

J.R. Festa, R.M. Lazar (eds.), *Neurovascular Neuropsychology*, DOI 10.1007/978-0-387-70715-0_11,
© Springer Science + Business Media, LLC 2009

hospitalized elderly with heart failure, starting treatment with ACE-inhibitors was associated with an increased probability of improving cognitive performance, independent of baseline or discharge blood pressure levels (Zuccalà et al., 2005b).

Such results confirmed the potential reversibility of cognitive impairment associated with heart failure. This issue is crucial from the clinical and economic perspective, since cognitive impairment is a major determinant of the loss of functional ability, and thus of the increased resource consumption associated with heart failure, that currently represents the most costly medical illness in the United States (Zuccalà et al., 2001b; Konstam et al., 1996; Wolinsky, Smith, Stump, Overhage, & Lubitz, 1997; Haldeman, Croft, Giles, & Rashidee 1999; Rich & Nease, 1999). Thus, even moderate gains in cognitive functioning among these patients might yield substantial reductions of mortality rates and resource consumption (Rich & Nease, 1999; Roman, 2004). Reversibility of cognitive impairment following cardiac transplantation has also been reported. Cerebral blood flow (CBF) is reduced approximately by 30% in patients with severe heart failure; however, CBF normalizes following cardiac transplantation (Gruhn, Larsen & Boesgaard, 2001). This improvement in cognitive function might be hindered by treatment with cyclosporine (Grimm et al., 1996).

In the 2003 annual congress of the Heart Failure Society of America, a symposium was dedicated to cognitive impairment in heart failure (Normand, et al., 2005). Subsequently, a position statement of the society highlighted the opportunity of including variations in cognitive functioning among the outcomes of trials on ventricular assist devices (Konstam et al., 2004); this aim is being pursued by researchers (Zimpfer et al., 2006). In addition, assessment and monitoring of cognitive performance has been suggested as a primary endpoint of any pharmacological trials in heart failure (Lang & Mancini, 2006), and is being introduced into clinical guidelines (Arnold

et al., 2006). Research on the determinants and potential treatment of "cardiogenic dementia" has been included among the most relevant studies in the field of heart failure in 2005 (Tang & Francis, 2005).

Currently available epidemiological data indicate that vascular cognitive impairment is the second most common form of dementia after Alzheimer's disease; in fact, this form of cognitive dysfunction might represent 15–20% of all dementias (Roman, 2004). However, this figure is thought to underestimate the true prevalence of this form of cognitive impairment that should probably be considered the most common cause of dementia in western countries, at least among subjects older than 85 (Neuropathology Group of the Medical Research Council Cognitive Function and Ageing Study, 2001). Indeed, some studies performed in eastern populations seem to indicate that this form of dementia is far more common than Alzheimer's disease; such differences in incident rates have not yet been explained, even though genetic factors might play a role (Slooters et al., 1997). Independently of current prevalence rates, it is generally agreed that due to progressive aging of the world population both the incidence and prevalence of vascular dementias will increase in the next decades (Roman, 2004). Also, the prevalence rates of heart failure are increasing, chiefly among the older age strata of populations (McCullough et al., 2002). Accordingly, heart failure represents by far the most common diagnosis in hospitalized elderly patients; a recent study of incident cases has found that patients older than 60 years represent 88% of patients admitted with heart failure as first diagnosis; of these, 49% are older than 80, so that heart failure has been defined a "cardio-geriatric syndrome" (Rich, 2001). In addition, these data and projections are likely to underestimate the true epidemiological reality, as it has been demonstrated that more than 50% of older subjects with left ventricular systolic dysfunction have never been diagnosed with heart failure (Mosterd et al., 1999).

As aforementioned, the reported prevalence of cognitive dysfunction in older populations with heart failure varies across studies according to diagnostic criteria, as well as to the criteria adopted to rule out primary neurodegenerative disorders and cerebrovascular disease. In a large study of ambulatory, unselected older subjects with reported diagnosis of heart failure, cognitive impairment has been detected in nearly 60% of participants (Cacciatore, et al., 1998). In the GIFA (Gruppo Italiano di Farmacoepidemiologia nell' Anziano) database, after the exclusion of patients with any ICD-9 CM codes of Alzheimer's or cerebrovascular disease, cognitive impairment, as diagnosed by a user-friendly screening tool (the Hodkinson Abbreviated Mental Test) was found in 35% (647 of 1,860) of participants with verified diagnosis of heart failure, but only in 28% (4,229 of 15,053) of subjects without such a diagnosis (Zuccalá et al., 2003). In another population of older patients with heart failure, after excluding subjects who met the NINCDS/ADRDA criteria for Alzheimer's disease and those with an Hachinski ischemic score suggestive of possible cerebrovascular disease, use of a thorough mental deterioration battery identified cognitive dysfunction in 53% of cases (Zuccalá et al., 1997).

Even when considering the most conservative estimate (26%) of prevalence rates, it has been calculated that, in the United States alone, over one million individuals might be affected by undiagnosed cognitive dysfunction associated with heart failure (Roman, 2004). Hence, a relevant proportion of "cardiogenic dementia" cases, and thus a relevant source of functional disability and reduced survival, is currently being missed in clinical practice. Notably, a study of comorbid conditions reported in 122,630 Medicare beneficiaries with heart failure found a diagnosis of any form of dementia (thus including Alzheimer's disease and post-stroke cases along with cardiogenic dementia) only in 9% of patients (Braunstein et al., 2003).

Pathophysiology

Cerebral embolism has been initially considered the major culprit for the development of cognitive impairment among patients with heart failure (Pullicino & Hart, 2001). Extracorporeal support during cardiac transplantation might be associated with cerebral embolization. However, an excess prevalence of cognitive dysfunction has also been demonstrated among elderly with heart failure after the exclusion of cases with cerebrovascular disease (Zuccalá et al., 1997, 2003); in addition, either chronic or paroxysmal atrial fibrillation in these patients is not associated with increased probability of cognitive impairment (Zuccalà et al., 2001a). Indeed, the incidence of cerebral embolism among patients with heart failure is too low to account for most cases of cognitive dysfunction in these subjects (Katz et al., 1993). On the other hand, cognitive dysfunction among older patients with heart failure has been associated with left ventricular dysfunction (i.e., left ventricular ejection fraction below 30%), (Zuccalà et al., 1997) and with systolic blood pressure levels lower than 130 mmHg (Zuccalá et al., 2001b). Cohort studies have generally shown that hypertension is a risk factor for development of cognitive impairment or dementia (Kilander, Nyman, Boberg, Hansson, & Lithell, 1998; Whitmer, Sidney, Selby, Johnston, & Yaffe, 2005) and that antihypertensive treatment can prevent cognitive dysfunction (Tzourio et al., 2003). However, in several cohort studies blood pressure has been found to decrease well before the onset of dementia (Launer, Masaki, Petrovich, Foley, & Havlik, 1995; Skoog et al., 1996). Recently, worsening cognitive function has been documented in cohort studies among subjects with baseline systolic blood pressure below 130 mmHg (Glynn et al., 1999; Verghese, Lipton, Hall, Kuslansky, & Katz, 2003). Among older subjects, both heart failure and systolic hypotension have been associated with the presence of white matter lesions; such lesions, in turn, have been associated with increased prevalence of dementia (Tarvonen, et al., 1996). Subcortical alterations have also been associated with conditions of chronic hypoperfusion in neuro-pathologic studies (Cummings, 1994); the pattern of cognitive dysfunction in older subjects with heart failure and reduced left ventricular function further supports the involvement of subcortical areas (Zuccalà et al., 1997) Noticeably, CBF is heavily dependent upon systolic blood pressure in patients with heart failure (Georgiadis et al., 2000), as well as in general older populations (Melamed, Lavy, Bentin, Cooper, & Rinot, 1980), due to impaired auto-regulation of cerebral circulation. The impairment of cognitive functioning in patients with heart failure is thought to be associated with specific damage in the white subcortical matter of selected cerebral areas that seem to be more ensitive to hypoperfusional damage. These areas include the periventricular white matter, the basal ganglia, and the hippocampus. The damage of subcortical white matter causes disruption of intra- and interhemispheric connections; this has relevant consequences due to the ensuing interruption of neuronal circuits that link prefrontal areas to the basal ganglia, thalamocortical junctions, and the limbic lobe. Such pathways are crucial for memory, attention, executive functions, and continence (Breteler et al, 1994). Most recently, the volume of periventricular white matter hyperintensities has been shown to be associated with declining mental processing speed in a prospective study of older subjects without baseline dementia (Van den Heuvel et al., 2006).

The bulk of these observations clearly supports the role of cerebral hypoperfusion as the major determinant of cognitive impairment in patients with heart failure (Pullicino & Hart, 2001; Mathias, 2000; Roman, 2004). This issue does not represent a mere academic matter. In fact, while cerebral embolism would result in permanent damage of cognitive processes, the hypoperfusive mechanism implies potential reversibility of cognitive deficits, at least before the development of structural cerebral alterations (Pullicino & Hart, 2001; Zuccalà 2005b; Roman, 2004). However, other mechanisms might underlie the development of cognitive dysfunction in subjects with heart failure, together with reduced cerebral perfusion. In fact, the rapid changes in cognitive performance produced by both angiotensin-converting enzyme (ACE) inhibitors and angiotensin-I receptor blockers in patients with hypertension or heart failure suggest that activation of the renin-angiotensin system might play a role in the pathogenesis of vascular dementia (Zuccalà, 2005b). Indeed, cerebral AT-1 receptors are thought to be involved in the development of neurologic deficits, as well as neuronal injury, apoptosis, and inflammatory responses (probably via the expression of c-Fos and c-Jun proteins) after cerebral ischemia (Lou et al., 2004; Dai, Funk, Herdegen, Unger, & Culman 1999).

Inflammation is another potential cause, or contributing factor, of cognitive impairment in patients with heart failure. In fact, increased secretion of proinflammatory cytokines is a hallmark of heart failure (Deswal et al., 2001); however, increased serum and cerebral proinflammatory cytokine levels have been associated with both Alzheimer's disease and multi-infarct dementia (Yaffe et al., 2004).

Characteristic Neurobehavioral Syndrome

Neurocognitive dysfunction is common among advanced heart failure patients, worsening with cardiac decompensation (Petrucci et al., 2006; Trojano, et al., 2003). Cognitive deficits are found in 30% to 80% of heart failure patients and range from mild to severe, depending on the measures and methodology used (Bennett & Sauve, 2003). One of the earliest detected abnormalities is in fine motor speed (Petrucci et al., 2006; Putzke et al., 2000). Attention and memory dysfunctions are frequently reported, followed by slowed processing speed and executive dysfunction (Petrucci et al., 2006; Putzke et al., 2000; Deshields, McDonough, Mannen, & Miller,

1996; Schall, Petrucci, Brozena, Cavarocchi, & Jessup, 1989; Bornstein, Starling, Myerowitz, & Haas, 1995). In a database of 760 transplant candidates, 35% of the patients had multiple cognitive impairments on five or more cognitive tests, with impairment defined as ≥ 2 SD below the mean for the normal population (Putzke et al., 1997). One study that examined the effects of age demonstrated greater impairment in patients >50 years old (Schall, Petrucci, Brozena, & Cavarocchi, 1989). Depression and anxiety are also frequent comorbidities in the heart failure population, but studies have not adequately or consistently accounted for the effects of these variables on cognitive functioning.

From the clinical point of view, vascular dementia (that is currently thought to include "cardiogenic dementia") is characterised by early loss of executive function (Buffon et al., 2006). It is generally acknowledged that impairment of executive control functioning in mediates the development of disability (i.e., dependence activities of daily living, such as walking, dressing, bathing, using the toilet, or eating) in subjects with mild cognitive impairment (Royall, Palmer, Chiodo, & Polk, 2005).This might explain the observed development of disability among heart failure elderly with even mild cognitive impairment (Zuccalà et al., 2001b). Impairment in calculation, memory, and language functions seem to occur only later, and the severity of such deficits has no relation, at least initially, with the degree of subcortical damage.

Impairment of executive functions results in psychomotor slowing, postural disturbances, disorganisation of sequential tasks, and difficulty in managing personal effects. Patients may have difficulty initiating activities, have reduced mental flexibility, and are unable to pay attention to relevant aspects of their action. They have a low capacity of discrimination and abstraction. In fact, deterioration of the executive functions causes a dissociation between will and action. For instance, patients do not lose the ability of getting dressed, but are unable to start the action or choose the appropriate

clothes. When considering these features, it is not difficult to explain why cognitive impairment has been associated in older patients with heart failure with a sixfold increase in the probability of dependence for the activities of daily living (Zuccalà et al., 2001b).

As aforementioned, disability is a major determinant of the excess expenditures associated with heart failure (Rich & Nease 1999). However, cognitive dysfunction is also independently associated with a fivefold increase in mortality rates among subjects with diagnosis of heart failure, even 1 year after hospital discharge (Zuccalá, Pedone, Cesari, Onder et al., 2003). We hypothesize that among elderly subjects with heart failure the prognostic role of cognitive impairment might simply reflect the severity of left ventricular dysfunction or, as most recently suggested, of other factors such as anemia, electrolyte imbalance, or renal failure (Zuccalà et al., 2005b). Nevertheless, a study conducted in patients with severe heart failure has proven that reduced perfusion- associated cerebral metabolism, as detected by proton magnetic resonance spectroscopy, is a powerful and independent determinant of decreased survival (Lee et al., 2001). Therefore, cerebral metabolic abnormalities could represent a determinant, rather than a marker, of early mortality among patients with left ventricular dysfunction. It is unclear how brain dysfunction might influence the survival of patients with heart failure; however, impaired autonomic control of cardiac rhythm could represent the link between brain dysfunction and cardiovascular mortality in these subjects. In fact, increased QT dispersion and decreased heart rate variability have been observed in patients with Alzheimer's disease or mild cognitive impairment; in these subjects, the degree of derangement in both electrocardiographic parameters paralleled the severity of cognitive impairment (Zulli et al., 2005). Notably, increased QT dispersion and decreased heart rate variability are associated with decreased survival of patients with heart failure (Adamson, et al., 2004).

At present, there are no individual tests that have both sensitivity and specificity to the known cognitive impairment among patients with heart failure. The extensive neuropsychological battery needed to address the nature and extent of deficits is not readily administered in routine ambulatory cardiac practice. Brief screening instruments, such as the Mini-Mental State Examination and Hodkinson Abbreviated Mental Test have demonstrated impairment in the setting of heart failure, but such tests do not detect dysexecutive syndrome. As yet, there is no consensus in how to assess executive function in outpatient medical practice. The Clock Drawing Test is easily administered and adds some degree of sensitivity over the copying of pentagons in the Mini Mental State Exam (Royall, Cordes, & Polk, 1998). The ecological validity of executive measures such as the Trail Making Test, Wisconsin Card Sorting Test and Controlled Oral Word Association Test remain a matter of debate (Chaytor, Schmitter-Edgecombe, & Bur, 2006). Thus, for the cardiological examiner, a combination of the Mini-Mental State Examination and one of the standard measures of clock drawing will provide a reasonable screening in the outpatient clinic, with a referral for a comprehensive examination indicated when the history or the results of the screening suggest the possibility of cognitive impairment.

Supporting Laboratory Study

The neuroimaging features of cognitive impairment associated with heart failure are those of vascular dementias. Brain imaging, most commonly magnetic resonance imaging or CT, usually demonstrates vascular lesions such as a single strategic lacunar stroke, multiple corticosubcortical strokes, and periventricular white matter ischemia. At present, neuroimaging is thought to play a key role in diagnosing and evaluating vascular dementias, thus including cognitive impairment in the assessment of heart failure. A profile of impairment on tests of executive control and radiological evidence of alterations involving a substantial proportion (about 25%) of the cerebral white matter is considered sufficient for a diagnosis of subcortical vascular dementia (Price, Jefferson, Merino, Heilman, & Libon, 2005). Hippocampal atrophy, cortical gray matter lesions, and white matter lesions are considered strong predictors of cognitive impairment due to vascular disease (Mungas et al., 2001).

Treatment

As described above, neuroanatomical and neuropathological studies indicate that patients with heart failure eventually develop structural cerebral alterations that lead to permanent cognitive dysfunction (Tarvonen et al., 1996; Cummings, 1994) It must be emphasized that, even though some descriptive studies have shown that cognitive impairment associated with heart failure might be improved by cardiac transplantation, pacemaker implantation, or pharmacological treatment (Koide, Kobayashi, Kitani, Tsunematsu, & Nakazawa, 1994; Bornstein et al., 1995; Grimm et al., 1996; Zuccalà et al., 2005b), no intervention has so far been proven to reverse this form of vascular dementia in a randomized trial. Therefore, prevention of cerebral vascular damage based upon the most accurate and early control of vascular risk factors currently represents the key intervention (Roman, 2004).

Older patients, and even physicians, are often uncertain about the benefits of preventive interventions in older age. Nevertheless, even though the relative risk associated with single cardiovascular risk factors decreases with advancing age, the absolute risk increases steeply. Thus, the "number needed to treat" for preventive interventions is markedly reduced in older subjects, so rendering the cost-effectiveness ratio of both primary and secondary prevention more favourable among older subjects (Carbonin, Zuccalà, Marzetti, & Manaco, 2003).

The relevance of healthy lifestyle habits, including smoking cessation, moderate alcohol consumption, and regular physical activity should be stressed to any patient with heart failure. Also, strict control of diabetes and dyslipidemia is essential for preventing structural and functional cerebral damage. Notably, it has been suggested that statins might improve cognition in general, as well as in demented older populations (Sparks et al., 2005; Zamrini, McGwin, & Roseman, 2004). Most recently, analyses performed in 1,511 hospitalized elderly with diagnosis of heart failure enrolled in the GIFA study demonstrated that among the elderly the presence of hyperglycemia was associated with a 33% increased probability of cognitive impairment, after adjusting for potential confounders (Zuccalà, 2005a). On the other hand, restoration of normal serum glucose levels was associated with improved cognitive performance at discharge. The same study found that abnormal sodium and potassium serum levels were independently associated with detection of cognitive dysfunction and that normalization of serum potassium was associated with improving cognition through hospital stay.

Increased serum creatinine, and reduced albumin and hemoglobin levels were other potentially reversible predictors of cognitive impairment among patients with heart failure in the GIFA database; again, normalization of hemoglobin levels was independently associated with improving cognitive performance at discharge (Zuccalà, 2005a). Renal dysfunction is increasingly being found a relevant marker of decreased survival and functional status among patients with heart failure. The issue of anemia deserves particular attention. In fact, neurological symptoms are commonly reported in elderly patients with anemia (Lipschitz, 2003). Although data on specific neurological effects of anemia are limited, the presence of anemia (and consequent hypoxia) appears to contribute to impaired cognitive function in patients with chronic renal failure, who frequently suffer from confusion, inability to concentrate, decreased mental alertness, and impaired memory (Lipschitz, 2003, Nissenson, 1999) Correction of anemia with erythropoietin treatment may reverse brain dysfunction not directly attributable to uremia. In fact, it improves both cognitive function and brain electrophysiology by raising levels of sustained attention, thereby increasing the speed and efficiency of scanning and perceptual motor function, and enhancing learning and memory (Nissenson, 1999). The association between anemia and cognitive function is also suggested by the increasing evidence indicating a relationship between erythropoietin and nervous system function (Lipton, 2004).

Treatment of anemia also yields relevant hemodynamic and metabolic effects. In fact, treatment of anemia by erythropoietin in patients with heart failure has been proven to increase peripheral oxygen delivery and, in older patients undergoing hemodialysis, to increase CBF, oxygen extraction, and metabolic rate for oxygen (Silveberg et al., 2001; Metry et al., 1999) In addition, normalisation of hemoglobin levels in anemic patients with heart failure has been found to improve left ventricular ejection fraction, stroke volume, and cardiac output, which, in turn, might improve cerebral perfusion (Nissenson, Goodnough, & Dubois, 2003). This issue is of particular interest in the view of a potential negative effect of ACE-inhibitors on hemoglobin levels (Ishani et al., 2005). Therefore, treatment of anemia might become a mainstay in the prevention, and possibly treatment, of cognitive dysfunction associated with heart failure.

The issue of the effects of blood pressure control on cognitive functioning of patients with heart failure is more complex. In fact, systolic blood pressure levels below 130 mmHg have been associated with increased probability of cognitive impairment among hospitalized patients with heart failure, including those who received vasodilating agents (Zuccalà, 2001b). Indeed, systolic blood pressure levels below 130 mmHg have also been associated with increased risk of cognitive decline in the general older populations (Glynn et al., 1999; Verghese et al., 2003).These findings, along with other reports on reduced cerebrovascular reactivity in heart failure patients, raised concern about the potential detrimental effects of agents yielding vasodilating effects on cerebral perfusion of subjects with left ventricular dysfunction (Pullicino & Hart, 2001; Mathias, 2000). Nevertheless, a study of 1,220 older inpatients with diagnosis of heart failure indicated that starting treatment with ACE inhibitors was independently associated with increased probability of improving cognitive performance during hospital stay (Zuccalà, 2005b). In this study, the probability of improving cognitive performance was higher for dosages above the median values, as compared with lower doses, and was increased with longer duration of treatment. Most importantly, such effects of ACE inhibitors on cognitive functioning were independent of baseline, as well as of achieved blood pressure levels. Noticeably, ACE inhibitors and angiotensin II receptor blockers have been proven to prevent cognitive decline, or even to reverse cognitive deficits, in hypertensive populations (Tzourio et al., 2003; Fogari et al., 2003). In addition, enalapril has been found to increase CBF in patients with HF (Kamishirado et al., 1997). As a whole, these data indicate that either ACE inhibitors or sartans should be administered to subjects with heart failure also with the aim of improving cognitive performance, independently of blood pressure levels. Also, adequate up-titration of these agents might be required to yield the greatest benefit (Zuccalà, 2005b). Notably, ACE inhibitors are characterized by poor diffusibility through the blood-brain barrier; angiotensin-1 receptor blockers, on the contrary, yield high intracerebral concentrations (Fabris, Chen, Pupic, Perich, & Johnston, 1990; Hu et al., 2001). In addition, selective blockade of cerebral angiotensin-1 receptors by sartans has been shown to blunt neurologic deficits and to reduce neuronal apoptosis following experimental ischemia (Lou et al., 2004; Dai et al., 1999) Also, treatment with angiotensin-1 receptor blockers should allow angiotensin II to interact with AT-2 receptors, yielding non-hemodynamic neuroprotective effects and modulating glutamatergic and GABAergic synaptic transmission (Li et al., 2005; Pan, 2004). Accordingly, several clinical studies found that angiotensin-1 receptor blockers, but not ACE inhibitors, yielded neuroprotective effects in subjects with cerebral ischemia (Pan, 2004; Fournier, Messerli, Achard, & Fernandez, 2004). However, whether sartans might be superior to ACE inhibitors in improving cognitive performance of patients with heart failure has to be ascertained by randomized trials.

A host of data currently indicates that "cardiogenic dementia" is a major, potentially reversible cause of functional disability and reduced survival in patients with heart failure. However, research on the determinants and potential treatment of "cardiogenic dementia" is only the beginning. In fact, there is still a need to achieve consensus on the methods to adopt for the routine assessment of cognitive functioning in patients with heart failure. Moreover, the effects of treatment for heart failure on cognitive performance have yet to be ascertained in randomized trials. The available evidence on cognitive impairment associated with heart failure indicate that mortality and hospitalization rates cannot be considered any longer the only outcomes in the management of older patients with HF. As stated by several authors, research in the field of heart failure should broaden to a comprehensive view of health outcomes, thereby yielding evidence that might support clinical decision making, improve clinical practice, and guide health policy. Focusing on health status outcomes would also be in keeping with the Institute of Medicine's promotion of patient-centered care, among the six strategies designated to improve the quality of care in the US. The course of research on multidimensional assessment of older patients with heart failure is still far from its end.

References

Adamson, P. B., Smith, A. L., Abraham, W. T., Kleckner, K. J., Stadler, R. W., Shih, A. et al. (2004). Continuous autonomic assessment in patients with symptomatic heart failure: prognostic value of heart rate variability measured by an implanted cardiac resynchronization device. *Circulation, 110*:2389–2394.

Almeida, OP, and Flicker, L. (2001). The mind of a failing heart: A systematic review of the association between congestive heart failure and cognitive functioning. *Internal Medicine Journal, 31*:290–295.

Arnold, J. M., Liu, P., Demers, C., Dorian, P., Giannetti, N., Haddad, H., et al. (2006). Canadian cardiovascular society consensus conference recommendations on heart failure 2006: diagnosis and management. *Canadian Journal of Cardiology, 22*(1):23–45.

Barclay, L. L., Weiss, E. M., Mattis, S., Bond, O., and Blass, J. P. (1988). Unrecognized cognitive impairment in cardiac rehabilitation patients. *Journal of the American Geriatrics Society, 36*:22–28.

Barker, W. H., Mullooly, J. P., and Getchell, W. (2006). Changing incidence and survival for heart failure in a well-defined older population, 1970–1974 and 1990–1994. *Circulation, 113*:799–805.

Bennett, S. J. and Sauve, M. J. (2003). Cognitive deficits in patients with heart failure: a review of the literature. *Journal of Cardiovascular Nursing, 18*(3):219–242.

Bornstein, R. A., Starling, R. C., Myerowitz, P., and Haas, G. J. (1995). Neuropsychological function in patients with end-stage heart failure before and after cardiac transplantation. *Acta Neurologica Scandinavica, 91*:260–265.

Braunstein, J. B., Anderson, G. F., Gerstenblith, G. Weller,W., Niefeld, M., Herbert, R., et al. (2003). Noncardiac comorbidity increases preventable hospitalizations and mortality among Medicare beneficiaries with chronic heart failure. *Journal of the American College of Cardiology, 42*:1226–1233.

Breteler, M. M., Van Swieten, J. C., Bots, M. L., Grobbee, D. E., Claus, J. J., van den Hout, J. H. et al. (1994). Cerebral white matter lesions, vascular risk factors, and cognitive function in a population-based study: the Rotterdam study. *Neurology, 44*:1246–1252.

Buffon, F., Porcher, R., Hernandez, K., Kurtz, A., Pointeau, S., Vahedi, K., et al. (2006). Cognitive profile in CADASIL. *Journal of Neurology, Neurosurgery, and Psychiatry, 77*:175–180.

Cacciatore, F., Abete, P., Ferrara, N., Calabrese, C., Napoli, C., Maggi, S., et al. (1998). Congestive heart failure and cognitive impairment in an older population. Osservatorio Geriatrico Campano Study Group. *Journal of the American Geriatrics Society, 46*(11):1343–1348.

Carbonin, P., Zuccala, G.,Marzetti, E., and Monaco, M. (2003). Coronary risk factors in the elderly: Their interactions and treatment. *Current Pharmaceutical Design, 9*(29): 2465–2478.

Chaytor, N., Schmitter-Edgecombe, M., and Burr, R. (2006). Improving the ecological validity of executive functioning assessment. *Archives of Clinical Neuropsychology, 21*:217–227.

Cummings, J. L. (1994). Vascular subcortical dementias: clinical aspects. *Dementia;5*:177–80.

Dai, W. J., Funk, A., Herdegen, T., Unger, T. and Culman, J. (1999). Blockade of central angiotensin AT1 receptors improves neurological outcome and reduces expression of AP-1 transcription factors after focal brain ischemia in rats. *Stroke 30*:2391–2299.

Deshields, T. L., McDonough, E. M., Mannen, R. K., and Miller, L. W. (1996). Psychological and cognitive status before and after heart transplantation. *General Hospital Psychiatry, 18*(6 Suppl):62S–69S.

Deswal, A., Petersen, N. J., Feldman, A. M., Young, J. B., White, B. G., and Mann, D. L. (2001). Cytokines and cytokine receptors in advanced heart failure: an analysis of the cytokine database from the VESnarinone Trial (VEST). *Circulation, 103*:2055–2059.

Editorial. (1977). Cardiogenic dementia. *Lancet, 1*:27–28.

Fabris, B., Chen, B. Z., Pupic, V., Perich, R., and Johnston, C. I. (1990). Inhibition of angiotensin-converting enzyme (ACE) in plasma and tissue. *Journal of Cardiovascular Pharmacology, 15*(S2): S6–S13.

Fogari, R., Mugellini, A., Zoppi, A., Derosa, G., Pasotti, C., Fogari, E., et al. (2003). Influence of losartan and atenolol on memory function in very elderly hypertensive patients. *Journal of Human Hypertension 17*:781–785.

Fournier, A., Messerli, F. H., Achard, J. M., and Fernandez, L. (2004). Cerebroprotection mediated by angiotensin II – a hypothesis supported by recent randomized clinical trials. *Journal of the American College of Cardiology, 43*:1343–1347.

Georgiadis, D., Sievert, M., Cencetti, S., Uhlmann, F., Krivokuca, M., Zierz, S., et al. (2000). Cerebrovascular reactivity is impaired in patients with cardiac failure. *European Heart Journal, 21*:407–413.

Glynn, R. J., Beckett, L. A., Herbert, L. E. , Morris, M. C., Scherr, P. A., and Evans, D. A. (1999). Current and remote blood pressure and cognitive decline. *JAMA 281*:438–445.

Grimm, M., Yeganehfar, W., Laufer, G., Madl, C., Kramer, L. Eisenhuber, E., et al. (1996). Cyclosporine may affect improvement of cognitive brain function after successful cardiac transplantation. *Circulation, 94*:1339–1345.

Gruhn, N., Larsen, F., and Boesgaard, S. (2001). Cerebral blood flow in patients with chronic heart failure before and after heart transplantation. *Stroke, 32*:2530–2533.

Haldeman, G. A., Croft, J. B., Giles, W. H., and Rashidee, A. (1999). Hospitalization of patients with heart failure: National Hospital Discharge Survey, 1985 to 1995. *American Heart Journal, 137*:352–360.

Hu, K., Bahner, U., Gaudron, P., Palkovits, M., Ring, M., Fehle, A., et al. (2001). Chronic effects of ACE-inhibiiton (quinapril) and angiotensin-II type-1 receptor blockade (losartan) on atrial natriuretic peptide in brain nuclei of rats with experimental myocardial infarction. *Basic Research in Cardiology 96*:258–266.

Ishani, A., Weinhandl, E., Zhao, Z., Gilbertson, D. T., Collins, A. J., Yusuf, S., et al. (2005). Angiotensin-converting enzyme inhibitor as a risk factor for the development of anemia, and the impact of incident anemia on mortality in patients with left ventricular dysfunction. *Journal of the American College of Cardiology, 45*:391–399.

Kamishirado, H., Inoue, T., Fujito, T., Kase, M., Shimizu, M., Sakai, Y. et al., (1997). Effect of enalapril maleate on cerebral blood flow in patients with chronic heart failure. *Angiology, 48*:707–713.

Katz, S. D., Marantz, P. R., Biasucci, L., Jondeau, G., Lee, K., Brennan, C., et al. (1993). Low incidence of stroke in ambulatory patients with heart failure: a prospective study. *American Heart Journal, 126*:141–146.

Kilander, L., Nyman, H., Boberg, M., Hansson, L., and Lithell, H. (1998). Hypertension is related to cognitive impairment. *Hypertension 31*:780–786.

Koide, H., Kobayashi, S., Kitani, M., Tsunematsu, T., and Nakazawa, Y. (1994). Improvement of cerebral blood flow and cognitive function following pacemaker implantation in patients with bradycardia. *Gerontology 40*:79–85.

Konstam, M. A. (2000). Progress in heart failure management? Lessons from the real world. *Circulation 102*:1076–1078.

Konstam, M. A., Lindenfeld, J., Pina, I. L., Packer, M., Lazar, R. M., and Warner Stevenson, L. (2004). Key issues in trial design for ventricular assist devices: a position statement of the Heart Failure Society of America. *Journal of Cardiac Failure 10*:91–100.

Konstam, V., Salem, D., Pouleur, H., Kostis, J., Gorkin, L., Shumaker, S., et al. (1996). Baseline quality of life as a predictor of mortality and hospitalization in 5,025 patients with congestive heart failure. SOLVD Investigations. Studies of Left Ventricular Dysfunction Investigators. *The American Journal of Cardiology 78*:890–895.

Lang, C. C., and Mancini, D. M. (2006). Noncardiac comorbidities in heart failure. *Heart, 93*: 665–71.

Launer, L. J., Masaki, K., Petrovich, H., Foley, D., and Havlik, R. J. (1995). Association between midlife blood pressure levels and late-life cognitive function. *JAMA 274*:1846–1851.

Lee, C. W., Lee, J., Lim, T. H., Yang, H. S., Hong, M.-K., Song, J.-K. et al. (2001). Prognostic significance of cerebral metabolic abnormalities in patients with congestive heart failure. *Circulation 103*:2784–2787.

Li, J., Culman, J., Hörtnagl, H., Zhao, Y., Gerova, N., Timm, M., et al. (2005). Angiotensin AT2 receptor protects against cerebral ischemia-induced neuronal injury. *FASEB Journal 19*:617–619.

Lipschitz, D. (2003). Medical and functional consequences of anemia in the elderly. *Journal of the American Geriatrics Society 51*:S10–S13.

Lipton, S. A. (2004). Erythropoietin for neurologic protection and diabetic neuropathy. *The New England Journal of Medicine, 350*:2516–2517.

Lou, M., Blume, A., Zhao, Y., Gohlke, P., Deuschl, G., Herdegen, T., et al. (2004). Sustained blockade of brain AT1 receptors before and after focal cerebral ischemia alleviates neurological deficits and reduces neuronal injury, apoptosis, and inflammatory responses in the rat. *Journal of Cerebral Blood Flow and Metabolism, 24*:536–547.

Mathias, C. J. (2000). Cerebral hypoperfusion and impaired cerebral function in cardiac failure. *European Heart Journal, 21*:346.

McCullough, P. A., Philbin, E. F., Spertus, J. A., Kaatz, S., Sandberg, K. R., and Weaver, W. D. (2002). Confirmation of a heart failure epidemic: findings from the Resource Utilization Among Congestive Heart Failure (REACH) study. *Journal of the American College of Cardiology. 39*:60–69.

Melamed, E., Lavy, S., Bentin, S., Cooper, G., and Rinot, Y. (1980). Reduction in regional cerebral blood flow during normal aging in man. *Stroke 11*:31–35.

Metry, G., Wickstrom, B., Valind, S., Sandhagen, B., Linde, T., Beshara, S., et al. (1999). Effect of normalization of hematocrit on brain circulation and metabolism in hemodialysis patients. *Journal of the American Society of Nephrology, 10*:854–863.

Mosterd, A., Hoes, A. W., de Bruyne, M. C., Deckers, J. W., Linker, D. T., Hofman, A., et al. (1999). Prevalence of heart failure and left ventricular dysfunction in the general population: the Rotterdam Study. *European Heart Journal 20*:447–455.

Mungas, D., Jagust, W. J., Reed, B. R., Jagust, W. J., DeCarli, C., Beckett, L. et al. (2001). MRI predictors of cognition in subcortical ischemic vascular disease and Alzheimer's disease. *Neurology 57*:2229–2235.

Neuropathology Group of the Medical Research Council Cognitive Function and Ageing Study. (2001). Pathological correlates of late-onset dementia in a multicentre, community-based populationin England and Wales. *Lancet 357*:169–175.

Nissenson AR. (1999). Epoetin and cognitive function. *American Journal of Kidney Diseases*. *20*:21–24.

Nissenson, A. R., Goodnough, L. T., Dubois, R. W. (2003). Anemia—not just an innocent bystander? *Archives of Internal Medicine*. *163*:1400–1404.

Normand, S. L., Rector, T. S., Neaton, D. J. Pina, I. L., Lazar, R. M., Proestel, S. E., et al. (2005). Clinical considerations in the study of health status in device trials for heart failure. *Journal of Cardiac Failure*, *11*:396–403.

Pan HL. (2004). Brain angiotensin II and synaptic transmission. *Neuroscientist 10*:422–431.

Petrucci, R. J., Truesdell, K. C., Carter, A., Goldstein, N. E., Russell, M. M., Dilkes, D., et al. (2006). Cognitive dysfunction in advanced heart failure and prospective cardiac assist device patients. *Annals of Thoracic Surgery*, *81*(5):1738–1744.

Price, C. G., Jefferson, A. L., Merino, J. G., Heilman, K. M. and Libon, D. J. (2005). Subcortical vascular dementia. Integrating neuropsychological and neuroradiologic data. *Neurology 65*: 376–382.

Pullicino, P. M., Hart, J. (2001). Cognitive impairment in congestive heart failure? Embolism vs hypoperfusion. *Neurology 57*:1945–1946.

Putzke, J. D., Williams, M. A., Millsaps, C. L., Azrin, R. L., LaMarche, J. A., Bourge, R. C., et al. (1997). Heart transplant candidates: A neuropsychological descriptive database. *Journal of Clinical Psychology in Medical Settings*, *4*(3):343–355.

Putzke, J. D., Williams, M. A., Daniel, F., Foley, B. A., Kirklin, J. K., and Boll, T. J. (2000). Neuropsychological functioning among heart transplant candidates: A case control study. *Journal of Clinical and Experimental Neuropsychology*, *22*(1):95–103.

Rich, M. W. (2001). Heart failure in the 21st century: a cardiogeriatric syndrome. *The Journals of Gerontology. Series A, Biological Sciences and Medical Sciences*. *56*:M88–M96.

Rich, M. W., and Nease, R. F. (1999). Cost-effectiveness analysis in clinical practice. The case of heart failure. *Archives of Internal Medicine 159*: 1690–1700.

Roman, G. C. (2004). Brain hypoperfusion: a critical factor in vascular dementia. *Neurology Research*. *26*:454–58.

Royall, D. R., Cordes, J. A., and Polk, M. (1998). CLOX: an executive clock drawing task. *Journal of Neurology, Neurosurgery, and Psychiatry 64*:588–594.

Royall, D. R., Palmer, R., Chiodo, L. K., and Polk, M. J. (2005). Executive control mediates memory's association with change in instrumental activities of daily living: the Freedom House Study. *Journal of the American Geriatrics Society 53*:11–17.

Schall, R. R.. Petrucci, R. J., Brozena, S. C., Cavarocchi, N. C., and Jessup, M. (1989). Cognitive function in patients with symptomatic dilated cardiomyopathy before and after cardiac transplantation. *Journal of the American College of Cardiology*, *14*(7):1666–1672.

Silverberg, D. S., Wexler, D., Sheps, D., Blum, M., Keren, G., Baruch, R., et al. (2001). The effect of correction of mild anemia in severe, resistant congestive heart failure using subcutaneous erythropoietin and intravenous iron: a randomized controlled study. *Journal of the American College of Cardiology*. *37*:1775–1780.

Skoog I, Lernfelt B, Landahal S Palmertz, B., Andreasson, L.-A., Nilsson, L., et al. (1996). A 15 year longitudinal study on blood pressure and dementia. *Lancet 347*:1141–1145.

Slooter, A. J., Tang, M. X., van Duijn, C. M., Stern, Y., Ott, A., Bell, K., et al. (1997). Apolipoprotein E epsilon 4 and the risk of dementia with stroke. A population-based investigation. *JAMA 277*:818–821.

Sparks, D. L., Sabbagh, M. N., Connor, D. J., Lopez, J., Launer, L. J., Browne, P., et al. (2005). Atorvastatin for the treatment of mild to moderate Alzheimer disease: preliminary results. *Archives of Neurology 62*:753–757.

Tang, W. H. W., and Francis, G. S. (2005). The year in heart failure. Journal of the *American College of Cardiology 46*:2125–2133.

Tarvonen, S., Roytta, M., Raiha, I., Kurki, T., Rajala, T., and Sourander, L. (1996). Clinical features of leukoaraiosis. *Journal of Neurology, Neurosurgery, and Psychiatry*, *60*:431–436.

Trojano, L., Antonelli Incalzi, R., Acanfora, D., Picone, C., Mecocci, P., Rengo, F., et al. (2003). Cognitive impairment: a key feature of congestive heart failure in the elderly. *Journal of Neurology*, *250*(12):1456–1463.

Tzourio, C., Anderson, C., Chapman, N., Woodward, M., Neal, B., MacMahon S., et al. (2003). Effects of blood pressure lowering with perindopril and indapamide therapy on dementia and cognitive decline in patients with cerebrovascular disease. *Archives of Internal Medicine 163*:1069–1075.

van den Heuvel, D. M., ten Dam, V. H., de Craen, A. J., Admiraal-Behloul, F., Olofsen, H., Bollen, E. L., et al. (2006). Increase in periventricular white matter hyperintensities parallels decline in mental processing speed in a non-demented elderly population. *Journal of Neurology, Neurosurgery, and Psychiatry 77*:149–153.

Verghese, J., Lipton, R. B., Hall, C. B., Kuslansky, G., and Katz, M. J. (2003). Low blood pressure and the risk of dementia in very old individuals. *Neurology 61*:1667–1672.

Whitmer, R. A., Sidney, S., Selby, J., Johnston, S. C., and Yaffe, K. (2005). Midlife cardiovascular risk factors and risk of dementia in late life. *Neurology 64*:277–281.

Wolinsky, F. D., Smith, D. M., Stump, T. E., Overhage, J. M., and Lubitz, R. M. (1997). The sequelae of hospitalization for congestive heart failure among older adults. *Journal of the American Geriatrics Society*. *45*:558–563.

Yaffe, K., Kanaya, A., Lindquist, K., Simonsick, E. M., Harris, T., Shorr, R. I., et al. (2004). The metabolic syndrome, inflammation, and risk of cognitive decline. *JAMA 292*:2237–2242.

Zamrini, E., McGwin, G., and Roseman, J. M. (2004). Association between statin use and Alzheimer's disease. *Neuroepidemiology 23*:94–98.

Zimpfer, D., Wieselthaler, G., Czerny, M., Fakin, R., Haider, D., Zrunek, P., et al. (2006). Neurocognitive function in patients with ventricular assist devices. A comparison of pulsatile and continuous blood flow devices. *ASAIO Journal 52*:24–27.

Zuccalá, G., Cattel, C., Gravina-Manes, E., Di Niro, M. G., Cocchi, A., and Bernabei, R., (1997). Left ventricular dysfunction: a clue to cognitive impairment in older patients with heart failure. *Journal of Neurology, Neurosurgery, and Psychiatry, 63*:509–512.

Zuccalà, G., Onder, G., Pedone, C., Carosella, L., Pahor, M., Bernabei, R., et al. (2001a). Hypotension and cognitive impairment: selective association in patients with heart failure. *Neurology 59*:1986–1992.

Zuccalà, G., Onder, G., Pedone, C., Cocchi, A., Cattel, C., Carbonin, P. U. et al. (2001b). Cognitive dysfunction as a major determinant of disability in patients with heart failure: results from a multicentre survey. *Journal of Neurology, Neurosurgery, and Psychiatry 70*:109–112.

Zuccalá, G., Pedone, C., Cesari, M., Onder, G., Pahor, M., Marzetti, E., et al. (2003). The effects of cognitive impairment on mortality among hospitalized patients with heart failure. *The American Journal of Medicine 115*:97–103.

Zuccalà, G., Marzetti, E., Cesari, M., Lo Monaco, MR., Antonica, L., Cocchi, A.,, et al. (2005a). Correlates of cognitive impairment among patients with heart failure: Results of a multicenter survey. *The American Journal of Medicine 118*:496–502.

Zuccalà, G., Onder, G., Marzetti, E., Monaco, M. R., Cesari, M., Cocchi, A., et al. (2005b). Use of angiotensin-converting enzyme inhibitors and variations in cognitive performance among patients with heart failure. *European Heart Journal 26*: 226–233.

Zulli, R., Nicosia, F., Borroni, B., Agostil, C.,. Prometti, P., Donati, P., et al. (2005). QT dispersion and heart rate variability abnormalities in Alzheimer's disease and in mild cognitive impairment. *Journal of the American Geriatrics Society, 53*:2135–2139.

Chapter 12
Cognition After Cardiac Surgery

Ola A. Selnes and Rebecca F. Gottesman

Introduction

Cardiopulmonary bypass (CPB) was introduced more than five decades ago, and although there has been a dramatic reduction in both morbidity and mortality associated with this procedure, both short- and long-term cognitive impairment after coronary artery bypass grafting (CABG) continue to be significant concerns. The search for the etiology of these adverse neurocognitive outcomes has focused mainly on procedure-related factors such as embolic injury and hypoperfusion, but more recent studies have also considered patient-related factors, in particular the overall vascular burden of the patient's brain before surgery.

Progress in our understanding of the cognitive consequences of the use of CPB has been slow for several reasons. First, the technology of CPB has been continuously evolving since its introduction, and results of studies published more than 10 years ago are therefore less applicable to the way in which CABG is being performed today. Second, the patient population has also changed during the past several decades, from younger and relatively healthy individuals to older patients with a

greater overall burden of vascular disease. Third, and perhaps most important, the design of many cognitive outcome studies has been limited by serious methodological shortcomings, including lack of appropriate controls and the use of arbitrary statistical criteria for defining incidence of decline. Several of these methodological issues were addressed in a consensus statement regarding the assessment of cognitive and neurological outcomes after cardiac surgery published in 1995 (Murkin, Newman, Stump, & Blumenthal, 1995).

Methodological Issues

One of the factors that significantly influences the reported incidence of postoperative cognitive impairment is the choice of follow-up interval. Some studies have tested patients at the time of hospital discharge after CABG, but such brief follow-up intervals may be associated with confounding effects of anesthetic drugs, pain medications, or other clinical issues (Johnson, 2000). Therefore, other investigators have chosen to defer follow-up testing until several weeks after surgery. Although this strategy may yield follow-up data that are less contaminated by nonspecific surgical factors, extending the follow-up time may also mask transient changes in cognition.

A second factor of critical importance for determining the incidence of cognitive decline

O.A. Selnes (✉)
Neurology, Division of Cognitive Neuroscience,
Reed Hall East – 2, 1620 McElderry St., Baltimore,
MD 21287, USA
e-mail: oselnes@jhmi.edu

J.R. Festa, R.M. Lazar (eds.), *Neurovascular Neuropsychology*, DOI 10.1007/978-0-387-70715-0_12,
© Springer Science + Business Media, LLC 2009

after CABG is the choice of statistical criteria for defining decline. Mahanna and colleagues compared five different criteria for decline using the same data set and found that the incidence of cognitive decline at 6 weeks after surgery ranged from a low of 1% to a high of 34% depending on which criterion was used (Mahanna et al., 1996). They concluded that the "large variation in the reported incidence of cognitive decline after CABG can be attributed to the different criteria used to define impairment." Despite the arbitrary nature of statistical criteria such as "20% decline on 20% of tests," they are nonetheless still being used in some studies.

A third, and closely related methodological issue, is the inclusion of a control group. Some studies have controlled for the effect of age on cognitive performance (Keith et al., 2002), while others have chosen control patients with diagnosed coronary artery disease (Selnes et al., 2003) or hospitalized inpatients having noncardiac procedures (Mullges, Babin-Ebell, Reents, & Toyka, 2002). The choice of controls should be guided by the specific research questions being asked, and sometimes more than one control group may be required. Because candidates for CABG typically have a long-standing history of hypertension, hypercholesterolemia, and other risk factors for cerebrovascular disease, the use of published normative data from healthy controls will overestimate the degree of cognitive decline attributable to the surgery.

A recent example of the importance of including a control group is the reanalysis of data from the Octopus Study group, which originally used the 20% decline on 20% of tests criterion in the analysis of cognitive change after conventional and off-pump CABG (van Dijk et al., 2002). In their original analysis, 31% of the CABG patients were classified as having decline at 3 months. In a follow-up to this study, they recruited healthy controls, not undergoing surgery, and found that only 8% of the CABG and 5% of the controls met criteria for postoperative decline at 3 months (Keizer, Hijman, Kalkman, Kahn, &

Van, 2005). The authors concluded that their previous use of the 20% decline of 20% of test criterion had greatly overestimated the incidence of cognitive decline after CABG.

The Syndrome of Post-Cabg Cognitive Impairment

The focus of most studies examining cognitive outcomes after CABG has been on the incidence of clinically significant cognitive impairment at different follow-up points after surgery, and there is little consensus with respect to which specific cognitive functions are most vulnerable during the immediate postoperative period. Some studies have reported early decline in several cognitive domains, including memory, psychomotor speed, executive functions, and visuoconstructional abilities, suggesting that multiple brain regions may be involved (Selnes et al., 1999). From the perspective of the patient and family members, the most frequent complaint involves changes in concentration and memory (Bergh, Backstrom, Jonsson, Havinder, & Johnsson, 2002). Because subjective cognitive complaints do not always correlate well with objective neuropsychological test performance, some investigators have dismissed such subjective complaints as being secondary to depression.

One of the few studies that have attempted to define the nature of the postoperative cognitive impairment is by Kneebone and colleagues (Kneebone, Luszcz, Baker, & Knight, 2005). They investigated cognitive outcomes in 85 patients before and 6 months after CABG, and attempted to determine if the profile of cognitive outcomes could be classified as principally cortical or subcortical. Their cognitive test battery covered most cognitive domains, with the notable exception that a measure of constructional praxis was not included. They identified three subtypes of memory outcomes: (1) memory within normal limits (48%); (2) retrieval deficit (38%); and

(3) encoding/storage deficit (17%). These findings suggest that of those patients who do have memory changes after CABG, the majority have a subcortical pattern, characterized by relative preservation of recognition memory. Only a small subset of their patients had storage/encoding deficits consistent with cortical or medial temporal lobe involvement. The authors did not examine their preoperative (baseline) data for similar patterns of cortical or subcortical deficits, and it is therefore unclear to what extent the 6-month findings in part represented pre-existing deficits. There is now increasing evidence that a substantial number of patients undergoing CABG have impaired neuropsychological test performance even before the surgery (Browndyke et al., 2002; Millar, Asbury, & Murray, 2001; Rosengart et al., 2005).

performance (Aleman, Muller, De Haan, & van der Schouw, 2005; Vingerhoets, Van Nooten, & Jannes, 1997). The pattern of the preoperative cognitive deficits, with psychomotor slowing and impaired performance on measures of verbal memory and executive functioning, is also generally consistent with predominantly subcortical disease (Rankin, Kochamba, Boone, Petitti, & Buckwalter, 2003; Vingerhoets et al., 1997). The high prevalence of preoperative cognitive deficits is also in agreement with findings from neuroimaging studies, which have demonstrated that nearly half the candidates for CABG have white matter abnormalities on magnetic resonance imaging (MRI) (Goto et al., 2001b). In addition, given the age range of candidates for CABG, a small percentage might be expected to have mild-to-moderate Alzheimer-type pathology preoperatively (Emmrich et al., 2003).

Baseline Cognitive Abnormalities

When compared with normal controls free of coronary artery disease, the pre-operative cognitive performance of candidates for CABG has been found to be lower than expected in several cognitive domains (Rosengart et al., 2005). Moreover, patients with preoperative cognitive impairment are also more likely to have impaired cognitive performance at 6 days and 6 months after surgery (Millar et al., 2001).

Because some patients have their preoperative baseline evaluation in the hospital room shortly before surgery, some have speculated that the lower than expected preoperative cognitive performance may be related to situational factors, such as anxiety and suboptimal testing conditions (Keith et al., 2002). However, Studies that have examined the effects of preoperative anxiety on cognitive test performance have not confirmed this. There is considerable evidence, on the other hand, that poor cardiac functioning and risk factors for subcortical small vessel cerebrovascular disease are associated with lower cognitive

Incidence of Early Cognitive Decline

As discussed above, estimates of cognitive decline after CABG have been highly variable because of differences in patient inclusion criteria, choice of time points for measuring follow-up, and differences in the statistical criteria for defining decline. Only a handful of contemporary studies have included either healthy or cardiovascular disease controls. In a study of acute postoperative cognitive outcomes from Germany, a group of 67 CABG patients were examined before surgery and at days 3, 6, and 9 after surgery (Mullges, Berg, Schmidtke, Weinacker, & Toyka, 2000). Patients with a history of previous stroke, carotid stenosis, or general medical disorders and those with low baseline cognitive test scores were excluded, thus resulting in a relatively healthy study group. Hospitalized patients with peripheral neuropathy served as controls. The CABG patients had a significant decline in neuropsychological test performance at days 3 and 6, but had return to baseline levels of performance or above by day 9.

Thus, in a relatively "low-risk" group of CABG patients, postoperative cognitive decline appears to be mild and reversible within a period of less than 2 weeks.

Keith and colleagues compared the neurocognitive performance of 57 CABG patients with 55 controls from a senior citizen wellness program. Patients with previous CABG and those with a history of visual impairments were excluded. The CABG patients had significantly lower performance than the controls at baseline for some tests of motor speed and verbal memory. The follow-up evaluation was performed 3–4 weeks after surgery, with 65% of the CABG patients being available for testing. Although the cognitive performance of the CABG group did not decline for any of the tests at follow-up, they had less improvement from practice effects in comparison with the control subjects. Thus, in this relatively unselected group of CABG patients, lower than expected cognitive performance was observed preoperatively, but no significant decline in the CABG group when compared to healthy controls at 3–4 weeks after surgery (Keith et al., 2002).

Selnes and colleagues prospectively evaluated a group of 140 CABG patients and 92 demographically similar nonsurgical controls with diagnosed coronary artery disease (Selnes et al., 2003). Both groups improved from baseline to 12 weeks, and apart from somewhat greater improvement in verbal memory among the CABG patients, there were no statistically significant differences between the two groups. In the context of findings from other studies of earlier postoperative outcomes, this study thus demonstrates that cognitive decline after CABG is transient and reversible and that the majority of patients return to their baseline cognitive performance between 3 and 12 weeks after surgery.

Because every longitudinal study has some attrition, one cannot rule out that patients who are not seen for follow-up may have more significant or persistent cognitive decline. Patients who are lost to follow-up typically have worse baseline cognitive performance,

and it is probable that some of the more severe adverse cognitive outcomes after CABG may represent exacerbation of pre-existing deficits.

Pathophysiology of Early Cognitive Changes

No single intraoperative factor that can account for the early postoperative cognitive changes has been identified. Several previous investigations have focused on neural injury secondary to procedure-related factors, including microemboli, hypoperfusion, and the systemic inflammatory response. It has proven surprisingly difficult, however, to find evidence that these variables, either individually or in combination with other risk factors, can predict short-term cognitive changes. More recent studies, therefore, have also considered patient-related factors, such as the number and type of risk factors for cerebrovascular disease.

Microemboli

Several studies that used transcranial Doppler have demonstrated that showers of emboli commonly occur during cardiac surgery (Mullges, Franke, Reents, & Babin-Ebell, 2001), particularly during manipulation of the aorta. These emboli vary in size and composition. Some studies have found that the majority of emboli are gaseous rather than solid (Abu-Omar, Balacumaraswami, Pigott, Matthews, & Taggart, 2004). The number of emboli that are required to produce detectable cognitive or neurological symptoms remains to be determined, however, and is likely to differ from one patient to another. Some earlier studies demonstrated a modest association between total numbers of emboli and short-term cognitive outcomes (Clark et al., 1995; Fearn et al., 2001), but others have not reported any statistically significant associations (Braekken, Reinvang, Russell, Brucher, &

Svennevig, 1998; Browndyke et al., 2002; Neville, Butterworth, James, Hammon, & Stump, 2001). It is unclear whether these discrepant findings are due to technical aspects, such as problems distinguishing between solid versus gaseous emboli, or other aspects of quantification of the embolic load.

It has been suggested that the cognitive manifestations of microemboli may depend as much on patient-related risk factors, such as the degree of pre-existing cerebrovascular disease, as on the number and size of the emboli reaching the brain (Andrell et al., 2005). Patients with significant pre-existing cerebrovascular disease may have a lower tolerance for showers of emboli than do those without such disease. Consistent with this, the strongest predictors of cognitive decline in a large multicenter Veterans Administration study included cerebrovascular disease, peripheral vascular disease, and a history of chronic disabling neurological illness (Ho et al., 2004).

The cognitive consequences of embolic injury may also depend on which regions of the brain circulation are most heavily exposed. Special staining techniques have demonstrated numerous capillary and arteriolar dilatations in the brains of patients who die shortly after their surgery, but the regional brain distribution of these emboli has not been described. Most of these presumed embolic changes disappear over time, and are not typically seen in brains that come to autopsy a week or longer after the surgery (Brown, Moody, & Challa, 1999). Autopsy studies have reported relatively low numbers of embolic injuries in the brains of patients who die shortly after CABG, but cerebral microbleeds are relatively common (Emmrich et al., 2003).

Hypoperfusion

Longstanding hypertension and aging are associated with morphological alterations of the brain vasculature that may make elderly patients less tolerant of episodes of transient hypoperfusion. Certain regions of the brain, including the hippocampus, periventricular white matter areas, and watershed areas may be more vulnerable to periods of hypoperfusion. Abildstrom and colleagues reported that preoperatively, candidates for CABG had lower global cerebral blood flow than controls, but found no correlation between neuropsychological test performance and postoperative global or regional blood flow (Abildstrom et al., 2002). Caplan and colleagues have suggested that emboli and hypoperfusion may play a synergistic role: decreased blood flow during the surgery may result in reduced washout of embolic materials from the brain, particularly in the watershed areas of the brain (Caplan & Hennerici, 1998).

Atrial Fibrillation

Atrial fibrillation is a common complication after coronary artery bypass graft surgery and may be associated with increased risk for adverse neurological outcomes and prolonged hospitalization. Approximately one third of patients undergoing cardiac surgery with CPB have new onset postoperative atrial fibrillation (Crystal & Connolly, 2004; Mathew et al., 2004). Older age is the only variable that has been consistently associated with the development of postoperative atrial fibrillation (Zangrillo et al., 2004). Patients who have recurrent episodes of atrial fibrillation are at increased risk of stroke (Lahtinen et al., 2004) as well as cognitive impairment (Stanley et al., 2002).

Anesthesia

A subset of elderly patients undergoing major noncardiac surgery with general anesthesia also suffer short- or long-term cognitive dysfunction. Although increasing age appears to be the principal risk factor, postoperative cognitive decline has been reported in younger patients as well (Johnson et al., 2002). A study comparing regional versus general anesthesia did not find any difference in the incidence of cognitive decline 3 months after surgery, thus questioning a direct causal relationship between general anesthesia and postoperative cognitive impairment (Rasmussen et al., 2003). Regardless of the specific etiology of postoperative cognitive impairment after general anesthesia, there is evidence of short-term cognitive decline in some patients even after major *noncardiac surgery* with general anesthesia.

Depression

Mild to moderate depression is common after CABG, but one of the best predictors of post-operative depression is being depressed preoperatively, thus suggesting that postoperative depression is not caused by CABG. Anecdotally, short-term cognitive decline after CABG was often attributed to depression, and some cross-sectional investigations in noncardiac populations have reported an association between depression and performance on neuropsychological tests (Vinkers, Gussekloo, Stek, Westendorp, & van der Mast, 2004). In prospective studies, however, there is no evidence that new onset of depression after CABG correlates with either short- or long-term changes in cognitive performance (Andrew, Baker, Kneebone, & Knight, 2000).

The etiology of short-term cognitive changes after CABG is thus likely to be multi-factorial (Selnes et al., 1999). There is increasing evidence that procedure-related variables, such as number of emboli and degree of hypoperfusion, interact with patient-related variables. In an otherwise healthy brain, showers of emboli and transient hypoperfusion may not result in significant neurocognitive sequelae, but in the brain of a patient with long-standing, pre-existing cerebrovascular disease, the consequences may entail significant neurocognitive decline (Goto et al., 2001a; Ho et al., 2004). Further evidence that the use of CPB by itself is not the sole cause of postoperative

cognitive impairment comes from randomized trials comparing cognitive outcomes after conventional on-pump surgery with off-pump surgery without the use of CPB. With the exception of one smaller study (Zamvar et al., 2002), these trials have not found evidence of reduced incidence of cognitive impairment with off-pump surgery (Jensen, Hughes, Rasmussen, Pedersen, & Steinbruchel, 2006; van Dijk et al., 2002).

Late Cognitive Decline

A recent study from Duke University raised the possibility of late or delayed cognitive decline after CABG. Newman and colleagues studied a group of 261 patients before surgery and followed them prospectively before discharge, and at 6 weeks, 6 months, and 5 years after CABG surgery (Newman et al., 2001). The incidence of decline at the time of discharge was 53%, dropping to 24% at 6 months. At 5 years, an unexpected 42% of the patients available for follow-up performed below their baseline performance on a global measure of cognition. Similar rates of late decline have been reported by subsequent studies (Selnes et al., 2001; Stygall et al., 2003), but none of these studies have included a control group.

Only two long-term follow-up studies published to date have included a control group. Hlatky and colleagues obtained cross-sectional neuropsychological test performance on a group of patients who had been randomized to either standard CABG ($n = 125$) or angioplasty ($n = 64$) 5 years earlier (Hlatky et al., 1999). In an intention-to-treat analysis, there were no significant differences in the 5-year cognitive test scores for these two groups. Although this study did not evaluate cognitive changes prospectively, the findings nonetheless confirm that 5 years after the procedure, the cognitive performance of patients treated with coronary artery bypass surgery did not differ from that of patients treated with angioplasty.

In a study of twins, the postoperative cognitive performance of 232 CABG patients, stratified across three age categories, was compared to that of their twins who had not had CABG. Surprisingly, CABG patients who had their surgery at a relatively young age (between ages 63 and 70 years) had better cognitive performance 1–2 years postoperatively than did their co-twins without the surgery. No significant differences in cognitive performance was found for the twin pairs in the older age groups (Potter, Plassman, Helms, Steffens, & Welsh-Bohmer, 2004).

There is thus evidence from some studies that late cognitive decline does occur between baseline and 5 years. The degree of decline relative to baseline performance appears to be relatively minor, and is observed mainly in the domains of motor or psychomotor speed, with no significant decline in memory performance. The pattern of these late cognitive changes is thus similar to that is seen in patients with mild subcortical vascular disease.

Pathophysiology of Late Cognitive Decline

Normal Aging

Although the occurrence of late cognitive decline after CABG is by now well-established, it remains unclear whether the mild cognitive changes observed 5 years after surgery are causally related to the use of CPB, normal aging, development of Alzheimer's disease during the follow-up period, or other causes. The cognitive domain with the most pronounced late decline in the studies to date has been psychomotor speed (Trail Making test), with little or no decline in areas of verbal learning and memory. Progressive decline in psychomotor speed has also been reported in longitudinal community-based studies of normal elderly subjects (Ratcliff, Dodge, Birzescu, & Ganguli, 2003), raising the possibility that the late cognitive changes after CABG may at least in part be related to normal aging rather than the use of CPB. Future studies with appropriate control groups are needed to answer this question.

Alzheimer's Disease

In a recent study comparing the incidence of Alzheimer's disease in patients having either CABG or percutaneous transluminal angioplasty (PTCA) 5 years earlier, the authors concluded that the risk of developing AD was significantly greater among the CABG patients (Lee, Wolozin, Weiss, & Bednar, 2005). Given that both groups would be expected to have high rates of coexisting cerebrovascular disease, the rates of dementia were surprisingly low, with only 1.5% of the CABG and 1.0% of the PTCA patients being classified as having Alzheimer's disease. In the absence of MRI to rule out cerebrovascular disease, it is likely that a substantial number of these cases may have met criteria for vascular dementia. In a recent community based study of dementia diagnosis, 44% of incident dementia cases were classified as having possible or probable vascular dementia when MRI information was taken into account (Kuller et al., 2005). Using a case-control approach, Knopman and colleagues did not find any evidence of an association of CABG and dementia in a sample from the Mayo clinic (Knopman, Petersen, Cha, Edland, & Rocca, 2005).

Progression of Cerebrovascular Disease

There is considerable evidence from epidemiological studies that the presence of one or more risk factors for cerebrovascular disease is associated with cognitive decline over time even without cardiac surgery (Bennett et al., 2003; Elwood, Pickering, Bayer, & Gallacher, 2002; Piguet et al., 2003; Saxton et al., 2000). In a community-based study, Knopman and colleagues found that participants with a history of diabetes or hypertension at baseline had greater cognitive decline over a 4- to 6-year follow-up period than did those without such risk factors (Knopman et al., 2001). Others have reported that diabetes alone may be associated with cognitive decline over time (Fontbonne, Berr, Ducimetiere, & Alperovitch, 2001). Longer duration of diabetes appears to be associated with worse cognitive performance (Logroscino, Kang, & Grodstein, 2004) and individuals with multiple risk factor have greater cognitive decline in late life (Hassing et al., 2004). Finally, there are data to suggest that treatment of these risk factor for vascular disease may prevent late cognitive consequences (Hebert et al., 2004; Logroscino et al., 2004). These findings are thus consistent with the findings from a 5-year CABG follow-up study by Mullges and colleagues, who hypothesized that better control of risk factors for vascular disease during the 5 years after surgery may have accounted for the lack of late decline in their study (Mullges et al., 2002). Accumulating evidence from epidemiological studies, therefore, demonstrates an association between the duration and degree of vascular disease and risk of cognitive decline during the later years of life even in community-dwelling elderly individuals who have not undergone CABG.

In summary, there is thus evidence from several studies that mild cognitive decline occurs 5 years after CABG. The etiology may include normal aging, progression of underlying cerebrovascular disease, and progression of pre-existing neurodegenerative disorders. Controlled studies demonstrating an etiological link of the late cognitive changes to the use of CPB 5 years earlier have not yet been reported.

Neuropathological Studies

Contemporary bypass surgery is associated with a low mortality rate and there are therefore relatively few neuropathological studies. In a recent study from Germany, the authors examined the brains of 262 patients who died after heart surgery (Emmrich et al., 2003). Of these patients, 125 had isolated CABG, while the remainder had combined CABG/valve surgery, valve surgery only, or heart transplantation. The most common neuropathological findings included large infarcts and bleeds. Microinfarcts were less common. Old infarcts were present in about one third of the patients with isolated CABG. As an incidental finding, 37 of the 239 patients with heart surgery had Alzheimer-type pathological changes. The majority of these cases (28/37) had very mild findings (stage I or II), while the remaining nine cases had more advanced pathology (stage III; $n = 8$ and IV; $n = 1$). These data were not stratified by type of surgery, and it cannot be determined if the rate of AD changes differed between isolated CABG and valve surgery. Previous studies have reported higher than expected Alzheimer-type pathology (senile plaque formation) in patients dying with or as a result of coronary artery disease (Sparks et al., 1990; Soneira & Scott, 1996), suggesting that these findings pre-dated the cardiac surgery. In addition, since the majority of the patients with isolated CABG survived for only a relatively short time (1–30 days) after surgery, it would be unlikely that the CABG could be construed as the "cause" of these neuropathological changes.

The clinical significance of Alzheimer type pathology by itself cannot be readily determined because mild to moderate Alzheimer pathology is also found in otherwise cognitively normal individuals. One recent study reported such findings in more than one third of their cognitively normal subjects (Bennett et al., 2006). Stronger evidence that some candidates for CABG have cognitive abnormalities consistent with possible Alzheimer disease even before surgery comes from studies that have reported baseline Mini Mental State Exam (MMSE) scores. One such study found that 20% of their otherwise eligible study patients had MMSE scores in a range consistent with possible Alzheimer disease (Jensen et al., 2006).

Neuroimaging

Magnetic Resonance Imaging

Community-based studies have shown that clinically silent abnormalities on MRI are surprisingly common, with nearly one third of neurologically asymptomatic individuals having such findings. Candidates for CABG often have multiple risk factors for cerebrovascular disease, and therefore, such abnormalities would be expected to be even more common in this population. Because of the relatively short time between admission and surgery, however, preoperative brain imaging has been difficult to obtain. In a study from Japan, preoperative MRIs were performed in a group of 421 candidates for CABG (Goto et al., 2001b). Of these patients, 30% were found to have single, small brain infarctions and an additional 20% had multiple infarctions. Thus, nearly half of this group had evidence of chronic silent brain abnormalities before surgery. Patients with single or multiple infarctions had lower baseline cognitive performance and were more likely to have decline in cognitive test performance postoperatively.

A more recent study has confirmed a high frequency of chronic cerebrovascular disease in candidates for CABG. Nakamura and colleagues obtained preoperative MRI in 91 patients and found that 33 patients had small infarctions, 38 had multiple small infarctions, and 8 had infarctions greater than 15 mm (Nakamura et al., 2004). Thus, clinically silent ischemic cerebral disease is commonly seen preoperatively in patients undergoing CABG, and it is predictive of an increased risk of postoperative cognitive decline in the short term. The association of pre-existing silent MRI abnormalities with late cognitive changes has not yet been examined.

Diffusion Weighted Imaging Studies

The advent of magnetic resonance diffusion-weighted imaging (DWI) has allowed improved detection of acute ischemic lesions, and has become a valuable tool in the study of postoperative ischemic complications (Fig. 1). The first study of DWI after CABG reported new ischemic lesions in 9/35 patients when they were imaged during the first week

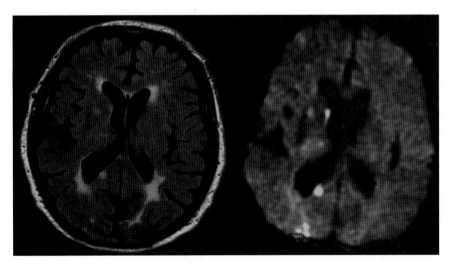

Fig. 1 MRI Fluid-attenuated inversion recovery (FLAIR) and diffusion-weighted imaging (DWI) of a patient with chronic cerebrovascular disease and superimposed acute infarction 3 days after CABG. The FLAIR image (left) demonstrates an old left occipital stroke and moderate chronic white matter ischemic disease. The DWI image on the right shows acute infarction in the right occipital lobe as well as multiple other locations

after surgery (Bendszus et al., 2002). None of these patients had focal neurological findings postoperatively. More recent studies have confirmed new postoperative ischemic lesions in 31–45% of patients undergoing CABG, depending on presence of vascular risk factors. Postoperative DWI lesions have also been reported in patients having off-pump surgery (Friday et al., 2005), suggesting that CPB may not be the only cause of these ischemic lesions. It is unclear whether the rate of new DWI lesions is different in patients having surgery for cardiac valve replacement (Floyd et al., 2006; Knipp et al., 2005). DWI allows for better differentiation between acute postoperative infarction and older cerebrovascular disease, as well as the potential interplay between these two. Figure 1 demonstrates the MRI fluid-attenuated inversion recovery (FLAIR) image of a CABG patient, showing extensive chronic vascular disease, including an old left occipital stroke. The corresponding DWI image on the right shows acute infarction (bright white) involving the right occipital as well as other locations.

None of the DWI studies published to date have found an association between new ischemic lesions and postoperative decline in neuropsychological test performance. Although the lack of such an association may seem somewhat paradoxical, it might be explained by the fact that many of the DWI lesions are quite small, and some are in areas of the brain with no known cognitive functions.

Cognitive Change After Cardiac Procedures Other Than CABG

The incidence and time course of cognitive changes after other cardiac surgeries, such as cardiac valve replacement, has been less well documented. Most studies have been based on relatively small numbers of patients, and

controls have not typically been included (Knipp et al., 2005). Some studies have relied on noncognitive endpoints, such as auditory evoked potentials (Zimpfer et al., 2003, 2006) or new lesions on diffusion-weighted magnetic resonance imaging (DWI) (Floyd et al., 2006; Stolz et al., 2004). As with studies of CABG patients, the appearance of new DWI lesions after valve surgery does not appear to correlate with neuropsychological outcomes (Knipp et al., 2005). Most of the studies of neurocognitive outcomes after valve surgery have concluded that while there are some short term cognitive changes, the majority of patients return to their baseline level of functioning with no long-term adverse cognitive changes (Zimpfer et al., 2006).

Conclusions

Cardiac surgery with CPB, as currently practiced, may be associated with transient changes in memory, executive functions, and motor speed in a subset of patients during the first few days to weeks after CABG. The etiology is most likely multifactorial and is believed to include a synergistic effect of procedure-related variables such as microemboli and hypoperfusion and patient-related variables such as age and degree of pre-existing cerebrovascular disease. For the great majority of patients, the short term cognitive changes appear to be reversible by 3 months after surgery. Cases of more severe or progressive postoperative cognitive decline may reflect emergence of pre-existing but clinically silent vascular or neurodegenerative disease. Mild late cognitive decline after CABG, occurring between 1 and 5 years after the surgery, has been well-documented in several prospective studies. Whether this decline is specifically related to the use of CPB itself, rather than to progression of underlying cerebrovascular disease or other age-related changes, awaits clarification by prospective controlled studies.

Acknowledgements This research was supported by grant 35610 from the National Institute of Neurological Disorders and Stroke, NIH, Bethesda, MD and by the Dana Foundation, New York, NY, and the Johns Hopkins Medical Institutions GCRC grant RR 00052.

We also thank the staff and participants in our study and Dr. Talalay for her editorial assistance. We are also grateful for the ongoing collaboration with Dr. W. Baumgartner as well as other participating cardiac surgeons and cardiologists.

References

Abildstrom, H., Hogh, P., Sperling, B., Moller, J. T., Yndgaard, S., & Rasmussen, L. S. (2002). Cerebral blood flow and cognitive dysfunction after coronary surgery. *Annals of Thoracic Surgery, 73,* 1174–1178.

Abu-Omar, Y., Balacumaraswami, L., Pigott, D. W., Matthews, P. M., & Taggart, D. P. (2004). Solid and gaseous cerebral microembolization during off-pump, on-pump, and open cardiac surgery procedures. *Journal of Thoracic and Cardiovascular Surgery, 127,* 1759–1765.

Aleman, A., Muller, M., De Haan, E. H., & van der Schouw, Y. T. (2005). Vascular risk factors and cognitive function in a sample of independently living men. *Neurobiology of Aging, 26,* 485–490.

Andrell, P., Jensen, C., Norrsell, H., Ekre, O., Ekholm, S., Norrsell, U., et al. (2005). White matter disease in magnetic resonance imaging predicts cerebral complications after coronary artery bypass grafting. *Annals of Thoracic Surgery, 79,* 74–79.

Andrew, M. J., Baker, R. A., Kneebone, A. C., & Knight, J. L. (2000). Mood state as a predictor of neuropsychological deficits following cardiac surgery. *Journal of Psychosomatic Research, 48,* 537–546.

Bendszus, M., Reents, W., Franke, D., Mullges, W., Babin-Ebell, J., Koltzenburg, M., et al. (2002). Brain damage after coronary artery bypass grafting. *Archives of Neurology, 59,* 1090–1095.

Bennett, H. P., Piguet, O., Grayson, D. A., Creasey, H., Waite, L. M., Broe, G. A., et al. (2003). A 6-year study of cognition and spatial function in the demented and non-demented elderly: The Sydney Older Persons Study. *Dementia and Geriatric Cognitive Disorders, 16,* 181–186.

Bennett, D. A., Schneider, J. A., Arvanitakis, Z., Kelly, J. F., Aggarwal, N. T., Shah, R. C., et al. (2006). Neuropathology of older persons without cognitive impairment from two community-based studies. *Neurology, 66,* 1837–1844.

Bergh, C., Backstrom, M., Jonsson, H., Havinder, L., & Johnsson, P. (2002). In the eye of both patient and spouse: memory is poor 1 to 2 years after coronary

bypass and angioplasty. *Annals of Thoracic Surgery, 74,* 689–693.

Braekken, S. K., Reinvang, I., Russell, D., Brucher, R., & Svennevig, J. L. (1998). Association between intraoperative cerebral microembolic signals and postoperative neuropsychological deficit: Comparison between patients with cardiac valve replacement and patients with coronary artery bypass grafting. *Journal of Neurology, Neurosurgery, and Psychiatry, 65,* 573–576.

Brown, W. R., Moody, D. M., & Challa, V. R. (1999). Cerebral fat embolism from cardiopulmonary bypass. *Journal of Neuropathology and Experimental Neurology, 58,* 109–119.

Browndyke, J. N., Moser, D. J., Cohen, R. A., O'Brien, D. J., Algina, J. J., Haynes, W. G., et al. (2002). Acute neuropsychological functioning following cardiosurgical interventions associated with the production of intraoperative cerebral microemboli. *Clinical Neuropsychologist, 16,* 463–471.

Caplan, L. R., & Hennerici, M. (1998). Impaired clearance of emboli (washout) is an important link between hypoperfusion, embolism, and ischemic stroke. *Archives of Neurology, 55,* 1475–1482.

Clark, R. E., Brillman, J., Davis, D. A., Lovell, M. R., Price, T. R., & Magovern, G. J. (1995). Microemboli during coronary artery bypass grafting. Genesis and effect on outcome. *Journal of Thoracic and Cardiovascular Surgery, 109,* 249–257; discussion 257–258.

Crystal, E., & Connolly, S. J. (2004). Atrial fibrillation: Guiding lessons from epidemiology. *Cardiology Clinics, 22,* 1–8.

Elwood, P. C., Pickering, J., Bayer, A., & Gallacher, J. E. (2002). Vascular disease and cognitive function in older men in the Caerphilly cohort. *Age Ageing, 31,* 43–48.

Emmrich, P., Hahn, J., Ogunlade, V., Geiger, K., Schober, R., & Mohr, F. W. (2003). Neuropathological findings after cardiac surgery-retrospective study over 6 years. *Zeitschrift für Kardiologie, 92,* 925–937.

Fearn, S. J., Pole, R., Wesnes, K., Faragher, E. B., Hooper, T. L., & McCollum, C. N. (2001). Cerebral injury during cardiopulmonary bypass: Emboli impair memory. *Journal of Thoracic and Cardiovascular Surgery, 121,* 1150–1160.

Floyd, T. F., Shah, P. N., Price, C. C., Harris, F., Ratcliffe, S. J., Acker, M. A., et al. (2006). Clinically silent cerebral ischemic events after cardiac surgery: Their incidence, regional vascular occurrence, and procedural dependence. *Annals of Thoracic Surgery, 81,* 2160–2166.

Fontbonne, A., Berr, C., Ducimetiere, P., & Alperovitch, A. (2001). Changes in cognitive abilities over a 4-year period are unfavorably affected in elderly diabetic subjects: Results of the Epidemiology of Vascular Aging Study. *Diabetes Care, 24,* 366–370.

Friday, G., Sutter, F., Curtin, A., Kenton, E., Caplan, B., Nocera, R., et al. (2005). Brain magnetic resonance imaging abnormalities following off-pump cardiac surgery. *Heart Surgery Forum*, *8*, E105–E109.

Goto, T., Baba, T., Honma, K., Shibata, Y., Arai, Y., Uozumi, H., et al. (2001a). Magnetic resonance imaging findings and postoperative neurologic dysfunction in elderly patients undergoing coronary artery bypass grafting. *Annals of Thoracic Surgery*, *72*, 137–142.

Goto, T., Baba, T., Honma, K., Shibata, Y., Arai, Y., Uozumi, H., et al. (2001b). Magnetic resonance imaging findings and postoperative neurologic dysfunction in elderly patients undergoing coronary artery bypass grafting. *Annals of Thoracic Surgery*, *72*, 137–142.

Hassing, L. B., Hofer, S. M., Nilsson, S. E., Berg, S., Pedersen, N. L., McClearn, G., et al. (2004). Comorbid type 2 diabetes mellitus and hypertension exacerbates cognitive decline: Evidence from a longitudinal study. *Age Ageing*, *33*, 355–361.

Hebert, L. E., Scherr, P. A., Bennett, D. A., Bienias, J. L., Wilson, R. S., Morris, M. C., et al. (2004). Blood pressure and late-life cognitive function change: A biracial longitudinal population study. *Neurology*, *62*, 2021–2024.

Hlatky, M. A., Bacon, C., Boothroyd, D., Mahanna, E., Reves, J. G., Newman, M. F., et al. (1999). Cognitive function 5 years after randomization to coronary angioplasty or coronary artery bypass graft surgery. *Circulation*, *96*(Suppl. II), 11–15.

Ho, P. M., Arciniegas, D. B., Grigsby, J., McCarthy, M., Jr., McDonald, G. O., Moritz, T. E., et al. (2004). Predictors of cognitive decline following coronary artery bypass graft surgery. *Annals of Thoracic Surgery*, *77*, 597–603.

Jensen, B. O., Hughes, P., Rasmussen, L. S., Pedersen, P. U., & Steinbruchel, D. A. (2006). Cognitive outcomes in elderly high-risk patients after off-pump versus conventional coronary artery bypass grafting: A randomized trial. *Circulation*, *113*, 2790–2795.

Johnson, R. G. (2000). Abnormal neuropsychometrics early after coronary artery bypass grafting. *Critical Care Medicine*, *28*, 2142–2143.

Johnson, T., Monk, T., Rasmussen, L. S., Abildstrom, H., Houx, P., Korttila, K., et al. (2002). Postoperative cognitive dysfunction in middle-aged patients. *Anesthesiology*, *96*, 1351–1357.

Keith, J. R., Puente, A. E., Malcolmson, K. L., Tartt, S., Coleman, A. E., & Marks, H. F., Jr. (2002). Assessing postoperative cognitive change after cardiopulmonary bypass surgery. *Neuropsychology*, *16*, 411–421.

Keizer, A. M., Hijman, R., Kalkman, C. J., Kahn, R. S., & Van, D. D. (2005). The incidence of cognitive decline after (not) undergoing coronary artery bypass grafting: The impact of a controlled definition. *Acta Anaesthesiologica Scandinavica*, *49*, 1232–1235.

Kneebone, A. C., Luszcz, M. A., Baker, R. A., & Knight, J. L. (2005). A syndromal analysis of

neuropsychological outcome following coronary artery bypass graft surgery. *Journal of Neurology, Neurosurgery, and Psychiatry*, *76*, 1121–1127.

Knipp, S. C., Matatko, N., Schlamann, M., Wilhelm, H., Thielmann, M., Forsting, M., et al. (2005). Small ischemic brain lesions after cardiac valve replacement detected by diffusion-weighted magnetic resonance imaging: Relation to neurocognitive function. *European Journal of Cardio-Thoracic Surgery*, *28*, 88–96.

Knopman, D., Boland, L. L., Mosley, T., Howard, G., Liao, D., Szklo, M., et al. (2001). Cardiovascular risk factors and cognitive decline in middle-aged adults. *Neurology*, *56*, 42–48.

Knopman, D. S., Petersen, R. C., Cha, R. H., Edland, S. D., & Rocca, W. A. (2005). Coronary artery bypass grafting is not a risk factor for dementia or Alzheimer disease. *Neurology*, *65*(7), 986–990.

Kuller, L. H., Lopez, O. L., Jagust, W. J., Becker, J. T., Dekosky, S. T., Lyketsos, C., et al. (2005). Determinants of vascular dementia in the Cardiovascular Health Cognition Study. *Neurology*, *64*, 1548–1552.

Lahtinen, J., Biancari, F., Salmela, E., Mosorin, M., Satta, J., Rainio, P., et al. (2004). Postoperative atrial fibrillation is a major cause of stroke after on-pump coronary artery bypass surgery. *Annals of Thoracic Surgery*, *77*, 1241–1244.

Lee, T. A., Wolozin, B., Weiss, K. B., & Bednar, M. M. (2005). Assessment of the emergence of Alzheimer's disease following coronary artery bypass graft surgery or percutaneous transluminal coronary angioplasty. *Journal of Alzheimer's Disease*, *7*, 319–324.

Logroscino, G., Kang, J. H., & Grodstein, F. (2004). Prospective study of type 2 diabetes and cognitive decline in women aged 70–81 years. *British Medical Journal*, *328*, 548.

Mahanna, E. P., Blumenthal, J. A., White, W. D., Croughwell, N. D., Clancy, C. P., Smith, L. R., et al. (1996). Defining neuropsychological dysfunction after coronary artery bypass grafting. *Annals of Thoracic Surgery*, *61*, 1342–1347.

Mathew, J. P., Fontes, M. L., Tudor, I. C., Ramsay, J., Duke, P., Mazer, C. D., et al. (2004). A multicenter risk index for atrial fibrillation after cardiac surgery. *Journal of the American Medical Association*, *291*, 1720–1729.

Millar, K., Asbury, A. J., & Murray, G. D. (2001). Preexisting cognitive impairment as a factor influencing outcome after cardiac surgery. *British Journal of Anaesthesia*, *86*, 63–67.

Mullges, W., Babin-Ebell, J., Reents, W., & Toyka, K. V. (2002). Cognitive performance after coronary artery bypass grafting: A follow-up study. *Neurology*, *59*, 741–743.

Mullges, W., Berg, D., Schmidtke, A., Weinacker, B., & Toyka, K. V. (2000). Early natural course of transient encephalopathy after coronary artery bypass grafting. *Critical Care Medicine, 28,* 1808–1811.

Mullges, W., Franke, D., Reents, W., & Babin-Ebell, J. (2001). Brain microembolic counts during extracorporeal circulation depend on aortic cannula position. *Ultrasound in Medicine and Biology, 27,* 933–936.

Murkin, J. M., Newman, S. P., Stump, D. A., & Blumenthal, J. A. (1995). Statement of consensus on assessment of neurobehavioral outcomes after cardiac surgery. *Annals of Thoracic Surgery, 59,* 1289–1295.

Nakamura, Y., Kawachi, K., Imagawa, H., Hamada, Y., Takano, S., Tsunooka, N., et al. (2004). The prevalence and severity of cerebrovascular disease in patients undergoing cardiovascular surgery. *Annals of Thoracic and Cardiovascular Surgery, 10,* 81–84.

Neville, M. J., Butterworth, J., James, R. L., Hammon, J. W., & Stump, D. A. (2001). Similar neurobehavioral outcome after valve or coronary artery operations despite differing carotid embolic counts. *Journal of Thoracic and Cardiovascular Surgery, 121,* 125–136.

Newman, M. F., Kirchner, J. L., Phillips-Bute, B., Gaver, V., Grocott, H., Jones, R. H., et al. (2001). Longitudinal assessment of neurocognitive function after coronary artery bypass surgery. *New England Journal of Medicine, 344,* 395–402.

Piguet, O., Grayson, D. A., Creasey, H., Bennett, H. P., Brooks, W. S., Waite, L. M., et al. (2003). Vascular risk factors, cognition and dementia incidence over 6 years in the Sydney Older Persons Study. *Neuroepidemiology, 22,* 165–171.

Potter, G. G., Plassman, B. L., Helms, M. J., Steffens, D. C., & Welsh-Bohmer, K. A. (2004). Age effects of coronary artery bypass graft on cognitive status change among elderly male twins. *Neurology, 63,* 2245–2249.

Rankin, K. P., Kochamba, G. S., Boone, K. B., Petitti, D. B., & Buckwalter, J. G. (2003). Presurgical cognitive deficits in patients receiving coronary artery bypass graft surgery. *Journal of the International Neuropsychological Society, 9,* 913–924.

Rasmussen, L. S., Johnson, T., Kuipers, H. M., Kristensen, D., Siersma, V. D., Vila, P., et al. (2003). Does anaesthesia cause postoperative cognitive dysfunction? A randomised study of regional versus general anaesthesia in 438 elderly patients. *Acta Anaesthesiologica Scandinavica, 47,* 260–266.

Ratcliff, G., Dodge, H., Birzescu, M., & Ganguli, M. (2003). Tracking cognitive functioning over time: Ten-year longitudinal data from a community-based study. *Applied Neuropsychology, 10,* 76–88.

Rosengart, T. K., Sweet, J., Finnin, E. B., Wolfe, P., Cashy, J., Hahn, E., et al. (2005). Neurocognitive functioning in patients undergoing coronary artery bypass graft surgery or percutaneous coronary intervention: Evidence of impairment before intervention compared with normal controls. *Annals of Thoracic Surgery, 80,* 1327–1334.

Saxton, J., Ratcliff, G., Newman, A., Belle, S., Fried, L., Yee, J., et al. (2000). Cognitive test performance and presence of subclinical cardiovascular disease in the cardiovascular health study. *Neuroepidemiology, 19,* 312–319.

Selnes, O. A., Goldsborough, M. A., Borowicz, L. M., Enger, C., Quaskey, S. A., & McKhann, G. M. (1999). Determinants of cognitive change after coronary artery bypass surgery: A multifactorial problem. *Annals of Thoracic Surgery, 67,* 1669–1676.

Selnes, O. A., Grega, M. A., Borowicz, L. M., Jr., Royall, R. M., McKhann, G. M., & Baumgartner, W. A. (2003). Cognitive changes with coronary artery disease: A prospective study of coronary artery bypass graft patients and nonsurgical controls. *Annals of Thoracic Surgery, 75,* 1377–1384.

Selnes, O. A., Royall, R. M., Grega, M. A., Borowicz, L. M., Jr., Quaskey, S., & McKhann, G. M. (2001). Cognitive changes 5 years after coronary artery bypass grafting: Is there evidence of late decline? *Archives of Neurology, 58,* 598–604.

Soneira, C. F., & Scott, T. M. (1996). Severe cardiovascular disease and Alzheimer's disease: senile plaque formation in cortical areas. *Clinical Anatomy, 9,* 118–127.

Sparks, D. L., Hunsaker, J. C., Scheff, S. W., Kryscio, R. J., Henson, J. L., & Markesberry, W. R. (1990). Cortical senile plaques in coronary artery disease, aging and Alzheimer's disease. *Neurobiology of Aging, 11,* 601–607.

Stanley, T. O., Mackensen, G. B., Grocott, H. P., White, W. D., Blumenthal, J. A., Laskowitz, D. T., et al. (2002). The impact of postoperative atrial fibrillation on neurocognitive outcome after coronary artery bypass graft surgery. *Anesthesia and Analgesia, 94,* 290–295.

Stolz, E., Gerriets, T., Kluge, A., Klovekorn, W. P., Kaps, M., & Bachmann, G. (2004). Diffusion-weighted magnetic resonance imaging and neurobiochemical markers after aortic valve replacement: Implications for future neuroprotective trials? *Stroke, 35,* 888–892.

Stygall, J., Newman, S. P., Fitzgerald, G., Steed, L., Mulligan, K., Arrowsmith, J. E., et al. (2003). Cognitive change 5 years after coronary artery bypass surgery. *Health Psychology, 22,* 579–586.

van Dijk, D., Jansen, E. W., Hijman, R., Nierich, A. P., Diephuis, J. C., Moons, K. G., et al. (2002). Cognitive outcome after off-pump and on-pump coronary artery bypass graft surgery: A randomized trial. *Journal of the American Medical Association, 287,* 1405–1412.

Vingerhoets, G., Van Nooten, G., & Jannes, C. (1997). Neuropsychological impairment in candidates for cardiac surgery. *Journal of the International Neuropsychological Society, 3,* 480–484.

Vinkers, D. J., Gussekloo, J., Stek, M. L., Westendorp, R. G., & van der Mast, R. C. (2004). Temporal relation between depression and cognitive impairment in old age: Prospective population based study. *British Medical Journal, 329*, 881.

Zamvar, V., Williams, D., Hall, J., Payne, N., Cann, C., Young, K., et al. (2002). Assessment of neurocognitive impairment after off-pump and on-pump techniques for coronary artery bypass graft surgery: Prospective randomised controlled trial. *British Medical Journal, 325*, 1268–1271.

Zangrillo, A., Landoni, G., Sparicio, D., Benussi, S., Aletti, G., Pappalardo, F., et al. (2004). Predictors of atrial fibrillation after off-pump coronary artery bypass graft surgery. *Journal of Cardiothoracic and Vascular Anesthesia, 18*, 704–708.

Zimpfer, D., Czerny, M., Schuch, P., Fakin, R., Madl, C., Wolner, E., et al. (2006). Long-term neurocognitive function after mechanical aortic valve replacement. *Annals of Thoracic Surgery, 81*, 29–33.

Zimpfer, D., Kilo, J., Czerny, M., Kasimir, M. T., Madl, C., Bauer, E., et al. (2003). Neurocognitive deficit following aortic valve replacement with biological/mechanical prosthesis. *European Journal of Cardio-Thoracic Surgery, 23*, 544–551.

Chapter 13
Pulmonary Disease and Lung Transplantation

Donna K. Broshek, George W. Shaver, and Mark D. Robbins

Patients and physicians alike are often surprised to learn that neuropsychologists play a role in the evaluation of patients with pulmonary disease. Given that the brain requires 20% of the body's oxygen supply despite weighing only 2% of total body mass and that the primary function of the lungs is to provide a place for oxygen from the air to enter the bloodstream, it seems quite logical that pulmonary and cerebral functioning are closely linked (Brigham and Women's Hospital Neurosurgery Group, 2006). In addition, since neurons have no oxygen storage, they are exquisitely sensitive to hypoxic states that can arise due to pulmonary disease. As a result, neuropsychology can provide valuable information in the clinical and empirical understanding of patients with compromised pulmonary functioning. This chapter will describe various types of chronic and end-stage pulmonary disease, associated neurocognitive deficits, and lung transplant evaluations.

Overview of Pulmonary Disease

Types of Pulmonary Disease

Obstructive Pulmonary Disease

Obstructive airway diseases include chronic obstructive pulmonary disease (COPD), asthma, bronchiectasis, and cystic fibrosis. Chronic obstructive pulmonary disease is common with an estimated prevalence rate of 6–14% in adults (Ries, 2005b). The primary risk factor is tobacco smoking, accounting for approximately 90% of cases. Other etiologies include toxic exposure and genetic factors. Due to the large reserve of lung function and an insidious onset, there is typically a lengthy preclinical period of increasing shortness of breath upon exertion (Ries, 2005a). Patients may attribute their breathlessness to aging or reduced fitness and may not seek medical attention until they experience a more acute situation, such as significant difficulty recovering from a winter cold. Typical symptoms include a productive cough with sputum (often called a "smokers cough") and frequent respiratory infections from which recovery becomes increasingly difficult.

Although the two primary types of COPD, emphysema and chronic bronchitis, are marked by obstruction of expiratory flow and dyspnea upon exertion, the disease process is different. While the clinical distinction may be difficult to discern, the pathological process occurs in

D.K. Broshek (✉)
Neurocognitive Assessment Laboratory, Box 800203, University of Virginia Health System, Charlottesville, VA 22908-0203, USA
e-mail: broshek@virginia.edu

J.R. Festa, R.M. Lazar (eds.), *Neurovascular Neuropsychology*, DOI 10.1007/978-0-387-70715-0_13,
© Springer Science+Business Media, LLC 2009

the airways for chronic bronchitis and in the pulmonary parenchyma for emphysema (Ries, 2005b). Emphysema involves overall lung destruction resulting in abnormal enlargement of the airspaces and overinflation of the lung and chest from airway destruction. Despite the large barrel shaped appearance of their chest, these patients actually have less lung tissue and often have low oxygen levels. The lung overinflation results in significant dyspnea and air hunger (perception of the need to breathe). Notably, inhalation/inspiration of oxygen is normal, but there is a significant obstruction of expiratory flow (Ries, 2005b).

Chronic bronchitis is marked by a chronic productive cough with excessive sputum production. Patients with pure chronic bronchitis typically have generally normal total lung capacity and some obstruction of both expiration and inspiration (Ries, 2005b). In clinical practice, however, there is typically significant overlap between chronic bronchitis and emphysema. A subtype of emphysema, alpha-1, is a genetically transmitted autosomally recessive disease and is caused by a deficiency in a key protective protein called alpha-1 antitrypsin. The incidence rate of alpha-1 antitrypsin deficiency is less than 1 in 2,000 (Ries, 2005b). These patients are highly sensitive to tobacco smoke and they often develop emphysema at a young age with minimal smoking history.

Infected Obstructive Lung Diseases

Bronchiestasis. Infected obstructive lung diseases include bronchiectasis and cystic fibrosis. Bronchiectasis is an acquired disease process that may develop in early childhood or later and is marked by distortion and chronic irreversible dilation and thickening of bronchi walls (Lichter, 2005). Bronchiectasis may be caused by any number of infectious pulmonary insults and causes impaired drainage, obstruction of airflow, and impaired host defense. Treatment often consists of prolonged antibiotic therapy.

Cystic Fibrosis. Cystic fibrosis is the most common lethal genetic disease in Caucasians and is characterized by progressive bronchiectasis, malabsorption of nutrients from the pancreas, and acute and chronic sinusitis (Conrad, 2005). A protein defect in the CFTR membrane protein leads to lung, pancreas, sweat, and male reproductive disorders. The lung defect leads to chronic infected sputum resulting in lung destruction and chronic pulmonary infection. Once considered to be a fatal disease of childhood, the median survival is now 36.8 years according to the Cystic Fibrosis Foundation, (www.cff.org, 2006). As a result of the many different medical therapies that patients undergo to improve or maintain lung function, patients can now maintain pulmonary lung function well into their adult years. The cornerstone of therapy is antibiotics, nutritional enzymes, and secretion clearance.

Occupational/Environmental Pulmonary Disease

Select professions and job occupations may result in chronic lung disease. Coal mining and hard rock industries can result in a type of lung disease referred to as coal workers' pneumoconiosis or black lung disease. The inhaled coal dust can lead to chronic scarring and nodules and the disease progression may continue even after the exposure is stopped. Unfortunately, the disease is unresponsive to medical therapy. Cigarette smoking is a major contributor to pulmonary disease in coal miners, but does not increase the incidence of simple coal worker's pneumoconiosis or the progression of the disease to progressive massive fibrosis (Hughson, 2005b). Asbestosis is a lung condition seen in ship builders, plumbers, and mechanics and is characterized by parenchymal fibrosis due to asbestos exposure (Hughson, 2005a). These patients also have an increased risk of lung cancer.

Interstitial/Inflammatory Pulmonary Disease

Sarcoidosis. Sarcoidosis is an inflammatory multi-systemic disease of unknown etiology. Many organs can be affected including the lung, heart, liver, kidney, skin, and lymph nodes. Pulmonary disease may be severe, leading to death. Although the disease affects all races, in the United States it occurs more frequently in African American women (Stenbit, 2005). While most patients with sarcoidosis may have restrictive lung disease, a subgroup may have airway obstruction. Hypoxemia may be present during exertion and at rest. While the large majority of patients may not require treatment and may even experience spontaneous remission, patients with more severe pulmonary disease are treated with corticosteroids and some will eventually need a lung transplant.

Idiopathic Pulmonary Fibrosis. Idiopathic pulmonary fibrosis (IPF), a form of interstitial pneumonia with chronic fibrosis, is the most common restrictive lung disease leading to death. It tends to occur more frequently in males and the average age at diagnosis is 66 years (Han, Parrish, & Smith, 2005). The course is progressive and insidious and the average length of survival after diagnosis is 2.8 years. For those who are generally unresponsive to medical treatment, including immunosuppressant therapy, additional medications for IPF are currently being investigated in several ongoing multi-center drug studies.

Lymphangioleiomyomatosis. Lymphangioleiomyomatosis (LAM) is a rare, infiltrative lung disease characterized by proliferation of smooth muscle in the lungs. Other organs may also be involved. The disease occurs exclusively in women, typically during childbearing years, and progresses to respiratory failure and death (Parrish, Han, & Smith, 2005). Hormonal factors are presumed to be important in the development of LAM and the disease may worsen during pregnancy and estrogen therapy and some women experience a remission during menopause. Progesterone therapy and surgical removal of the ovaries appear to be the most effective treatment for slowing or even reversing the disease if treatment is initiated before destructive changes occur. For those with end-stage disease, lung transplant is an option.

Pulmonary Circulation Disorder

Pulmonary hypertension. Pulmonary hypertension is a rare disease causing high pressure in the pulmonary arteries leading to hypertrophy of the right ventricle followed by heart failure and death. Pulmonary hypertension may occur independently or in association with other lung disorders, such as COPD or interstitial lung disease (Chin, Channick, & Rubin, 2005). Pulmonary arterial hypertension (PAH) is one of the primary categories of pulmonary hypertension and occurs more frequently in women, typically during their thirties and fourties. There are now multiple approved drug therapies for PAH and these patients seldom require a transplant. These therapies include intravenous Flolan, IV Remodulin, inhaled iloprost, and oral medications, including Bosentan and sildenafil.

Measuring Pulmonary Function

A spirometer is a recording device that measures how quickly the lungs can move air in and out and the quantity of air moved. The patient places his or her mouth on the mouthpiece at the end of a flexible tube attached to the spirometer and is instructed to inhale as deeply as possible. The patient is then asked to exhale as forcefully and rapidly as possible. The volume of air expelled in the first second is the FEV_1, which is an indicator of lung elasticity and airway obstruction. In obstructive pulmonary disease, the time to exhale a particular volume of air is increased. See Table 1 for

Table 1 Terms related to Pulmonary function

Measures of Pulmonary function	Definition
Arterial Blood Gas Sampling (ABG)	Provides measure of partial pressure of oxygen via arterial puncture.
Forced Expiratory Volume (FEV$_1$)	Volume of air expelled in the first second of maximum forced exhalation following full lung inhalation.One of the most frequently used measures of pulmonary functioning.
Forced Vital Capacity (FVC)	Total volume of air expelled during the FEV test.
Peak Expiratory Flow Rate	How quickly air is expelled during the FEV test.
Partial Pressure of Oxygen (PaO$_2$/PO$_2$)	Measures arterial oxygen through blood gas analysis.
Pulmonary Artery Pressure (PAP)	Blood pressure in the pulmonary artery, which reflects the pressure generated by the heart to pump blood through the lungs.
Pulmonary Capillary Wedge Pressure	Pressure that must be overcome by blood returning to the heart from the lungs.
Pulse Oximetry ("pulse ox")	Non-invasive measure of blood oxygen saturation. Normal level is 95% or higher.

a description of other terms used to assess pulmonary function.

Neurocognitive Deficits Associated With Pulmonary Disease

During the past 20 years, there have been few studies examining the neuropsychological profiles of patients with chronic pulmonary disease. This is somewhat surprising given the risk of neuropsychological compromise due to chronic hypoxia (see Table 2) and chronic physical and/or emotional decline in general. Most of the work that has been done focused on patients with COPD, which is the fourth leading cause of death as of 1990 and is also a major cause of disability (Ries, 2005b).

Interest in the neuropsychological correlates of COPD was raised as early as 1973 when Krop, Block, and Cohen (1973) reported the effects of oxygen treatment on neuropsychological and personality variables in a small group of patients. They found that hypoxemic patients

Table 2 Hypoxia, hypoxemia, and hypercapnea

Pulmonary terms	
Hypoxia	Low oxygen levels in body tissue despite adequate blood perfusion.
Hypoxemia	Decreased arterial oxygen partial pressure (Pao$_2$); refers to low oxygen levels in arterial blood.
Hypercapnea	Increased blood carbon dioxide levels.

with COPD exhibited impairments on measures of visual-spatial function and simple motor speed, within the context of generally preserved intellectual and memory functioning. With regard to personality functioning, these patients obtained significant elevations on scales 1, 2, and 3 of the Minnesota Multiphasic Personality Inventory (MMPI) prior to oxygen treatment. The first large-scale studies of the neuropsychological functioning of patients with COPD, the Nocturnal Oxygen Therapy Trial (NOTT), and the Intermittent Positive Pressure Breathing study (IPPB) were not published until nearly a decade later.

The NOTT study (Grant, Heaton, McSweeny, Adams, & Timms, 1982) was the first study with the COPD patient population to include adequate control groups. The study was aimed at assessing the effectiveness of continuous versus only nighttime oxygen therapy in patients with advanced COPD. The 203 hypoxemic patients (mean paO$_2$ = 51.2) in this study had a mean age of 65.5 years (SD = 8.4) and were compared to 74 matched controls on a variety of neuropsychological measures, including the Halstead-Reitan Battery. Although the group with COPD performed worse than controls on nearly every measure in the battery, the most prominent and reliable deficits were noted on tests of abstraction/conceptual skill, flexible thinking, perceptual-motor integration, and simple motor speed and strength. Relative to controls, hypoxemic patients with COPD also exhibited milder deficits in verbal ability and immediate verbal memory, though these skills were, on average, in the borderline to normal range. Overall, 77% of the patient group exhibited significant neuropsychological impairment, with 42% showing moderate to severe impairment.

In a follow-up study by the same authors (Heaton, Grant, McSweeny, Adams, & Petty, 1983), 42% of the hypoxemic patient group showed modest improvement (compared to 6% of the control group) in neuropsychological functioning at 6 and 12 months following the initial evaluation and initiation of oxygen therapy. Despite the modest improvement noted, the nature and rate of impairment remained comparable to the initial evaluations, providing support for the reliability of observed neuropsychological impairment in hypoxemic patients with COPD.

The IPPB study (Prigatano, Parsons, Wright, Levin, & Hawryluk, 1983) compared the neuropsychological performance of 100 mildly hypoxemic patients to that of 25 matched controls. The patients in this study were slightly younger (mean age = 61.5 years) and less hypoxemic (mean paO$_2$ = 66.3) than those in the NOTT study. Overall, individuals with COPD in the IPPB study demonstrated deficits in abstract reasoning, memory, and performance speed. While the severity of some neuropsychological deficits in this sample of mildly hypoxemic patients was comparable to those found in the NOTT patient group with greater hypoexemia (e.g., abstract reasoning), the severity of other deficits was less in the IPPB study (e.g., memory and simple motor speed). Thus, the authors of the IPPB and NOTT studies combined the data in order to examine the effects of hypoxemia severity on neuropsychological functioning.

Analyses of the merged data sets (Grant et al., 1987) found a significant relationship between degree of hypoxemia and neuropsychological impairment. In general, patients with more severe hypoxemia tended to perform worse on most neuropsychological measures, and even the mildly hypoxemic patients performed worse than controls on some measures. The rate of neuropsychological impairment was found to

increase from 27% in the mildly hypoxemic group to 61% in the severely hypoxemic group. Furthermore, as the degree of hypoxemia increased, the patients with COPD tended to perform worse on neuropsychological tests related to three specific factors that had been defined by a factor analysis: (1) perceptual learning—problem solving; (2) alertness—psychomotor speed; and (3) simple motor functions. Notably, patients with COPD generally exhibited relatively preserved abilities on a factor measuring language and intellectual skills (i.e., verbal-intelligence factor). The authors of these studies suggested that their findings implicate both generalized (e.g., reduced abstract reasoning skill) and specific (e.g., motor and psychomotor speed) effects related to the neuropsychological sequelae of COPD.

More recent studies have also demonstrated a significant relationship between chronic hypoxemia and neuropsychological dysfunction in patients with COPD. Stuss, Peterkin, Guzman, Guzman, and Troyer (1997) found evidence of increasing neuropsychological deficits with increased hypoxemia in 18 patients with COPD. These researchers found that chronic hypoxemia and hypercapnea were related to progressive deficits in verbal memory and sustained attention on tasks requiring significant allocation of attentional resources, such as the PASAT and Trailmaking Test, Part B. Furthermore, even mildly hypoxic patients demonstrated significantly impaired neuropsychological performance. Interestingly, the degree of hypercapnea was more strongly related to neurocognitive impairment than the degree of hypoxemia. Similar to the NOTT and IPPB studies, language skills were generally preserved. In contrast to the previous research, however, Stuss and his co-authors did not find a significant relationship between simple motor speed and measures of pulmonary functioning. These researchers attributed the observed memory dysfunction to disruptions in limbic system functioning, while deficits in attention were attributed to more diffuse brain involvement.

The impact of hypoxemia was also examined by Incalzi and colleagues (2003) using perfusion single photon emission computed tomography (SPECT). They compared the cognitive performances and SPECT scans of 15 hypoxemic and 18 non-hypoxemic COPD patients to 15 patients with mild Alzheimer's dementia (AD) and 10 healthy controls. In almost half of their patients with COPD, these researchers found a pattern of test results characterized by impaired verbal fluency and memory within the context of preserved visual attention and diffuse worsening of other cognitive functions. This pattern of test results distinguished patients with COPD from the control group and from the AD group. Although no significant group differences were found between the hypoxemic and non-hypoxemic groups with respect to their performances on the cognitive tests included in the study, when compared with standardized reference norms, there was a steady decline in cognitive functioning from non-hypoxemic to hypoxemic patients. Furthermore, the SPECT scans of the non-hypoxemic group were similar to the normal controls, while the hypoxemic group showed hypoperfusion intermediate to these groups and the mild AD group. In contrast to both COPD groups, the AD group was uniquely characterized by hypoperfusion of the brain's associative areas. The hypoxemic group, however, was similar to the AD group in its demonstration of reduced perfusion in frontal, anterior temporal, and ventral thalamic regions. These authors suggested that advanced COPD, marked by increased hypoxemia, is likely characterized by deficient frontal and/or subcortical metabolism, and such findings may signal a frontal-type cognitive decline. It is important to note, however, that the neurocognitive deficits in the COPD group were attributed to other factors in addition to chronic hypoxemia, including hypercapnea, acidosis, and hypocapnea. In another SPECT study conducted by a different group of researchers, patients with hypoxemic COPD demonstrated significant deficits relative to healthy controls on the attention, delayed recall, and verbal memory indices from the Wechsler Memory Scale-Revised (Ortapamuk & Naldoken, 2006). In contrast, patients with non-hypoxemic COPD

only had deficits in verbal memory relative to controls.

Chronic hypoxemia is likely not the only contributor to significant neurocognitive dysfunction in patients with COPD. Liesker and fellow researchers (2004) compared the neurocognitive profiles of 30 non-hypoxemic patients with COPD ($paO_2 > 60$ mmHg) to those of 20 healthy matched controls and found that the COPD group generally demonstrated worse performance on tasks related to speed of information processing (i.e., Digit Symbol Test, Trailmaking Test B, and Addition subtest of the Groningen Intelligence Test). No significant group differences were observed on tasks of memory or mental flexibility, and cognitive performance in the COPD group was generally unrelated to measures of overall health (i.e., FEV_1, quality of life as measured by the Chronic Respiratory Questionnaire, and pack-years of smoking). While the researchers concede that it is possible that less than optimal arterial blood oxygen levels due to either nocturnal desaturation or marginally below normal daytime levels contributed to poorer cognitive performance in the non-hypoxemic group, PaO_2 was not correlated with cognitive performance on any of the cognitive tests included in the study.

Although much less prevalent in the literature, there have been studies examining the relationship between cognitive function and pulmonary function in general (i.e., apart from the presence of COPD). Anstey, Windsor, Jorm, Christensen, and Rodgers (2004) examined the relationship between cognitive performance and pulmonary function measured by FEV_1 in a large sample distributed across three age cohorts: 20–24 ($n = 2,404$), 40–44 ($n = 2,530$), and 60–64 ($n = 2,551$). After controlling for demographic variables, smoking, physical activity, and respiratory disease, these researchers found significant associations in all age groups between FEV_1 and most of the cognitive measures, which included measures of vocabulary knowledge, attention/concentration, processing speed, immediate verbal memory, and reaction time. Although the relationship between FEV_1 and processing speed was found to increase with age, the fact that pulmonary function was independently associated with cognitive function even in the younger cohort suggests that "FEV_1 does not become important in old age, but is a correlate of neurological function throughout adulthood" (p. 233).

Using a subgroup of participants aged 60–64 years old ($n = 469$) who are participating in an Australian longitudinal study of personality and health in randomly recruited citizens, researchers found that impaired pulmonary function was significantly associated with subcortical atrophy on magnetic resonance imaging (MRI) (Sachdev et al., 2006). Decreased pulmonary functioning was also associated with deficits on neuropsychological measures of information processing speed and fine motor speed. Regression models that controlled for sex, age, height, level of activity, smoking, chronic respiratory disease, and education revealed a significant relationship between measures of pulmonary function (FEV1 and FVC) and MRI measures of subcortical atrophy. Furthermore, in a subgroup with chronic respiratory disease ($n = 45$), the males had more deep white matter hyperintensities compared to controls, but this result did not persist after controlling for diabetes and hypertension. The studies by Sachdev, Anstey, and their colleagues are important because they demonstrate an association between pulmonary function and cognitive performance that may be independent of pulmonary disease.

greater periventricular white matter disease (van Dijk et al., 2004). Notably, lower arterial oxygen saturation was not associated with lacunar infarcts or subcortical white matter lesions. Since the majority of the participants had arterial oxygen saturation values within normal limits, it is unclear whether the latter findings would hold up in a clinical sample with more severe COPD. The results of a SPECT scan study revealed decreased cerebral perfusion in the frontal and parietal regions of patients with stable hypoxemic COPD ($n = 8$) compared to age-matched healthy controls ($n = 10$) (Ortapamuk & Naldoken, 2006). Patients with stable non-hypoxemic COPD in the same study ($n = 10$) demonstrated significantly less perfusion in left frontal regions relative to controls. The authors speculated that chronic deficits in arterial blood gases resulted in reduced cerebral blood flow in patients with COPD.

A small study using transcranial magnetic stimulation examined motor cortex excitability in patients experiencing an acute exacerbation of COPD ($n = 4$) relative to age-matched healthy controls ($n = 8$) (Oliviero et al., 2002). The results revealed reduced intracortical inhibition and duration of cortical silent period in the COPD patients. Follow-up evaluations conducted 3–4 months after oxygen therapy indicated that treatment with oxygen therapy improved these two parameters toward the normal range. Oliviero and colleagues interpret their findings as preliminary evidence of impaired GABAergic cortical circuits associated with acute episodes of COPD-related hypoxia.

Cerebral Compromise Associated With Pulmonary Disease

Studies have also been completed which examined cerebral compromise due to pulmonary disease, but without neuropsychological data on functional deficits. A large population based study ($n = 1077$) of elderly individuals without dementia revealed that COPD and lower arterial oxygen saturation were associated with

End-Stage Pulmonary Disease

Until recently, no studies examining neurocognitive profiles in end stage pulmonary disease existed. Beginning in 2000, our research group began conducting clinical studies of patients with end-stage pulmonary disease who were presenting for potential lung transplant. These studies resulted in the reporting of neuropsychological prevalence data for patients with end-stage cystic fibrosis ($n = 18$; Crews, Jefferson, Broshek, Barth, & Robbins, 2000), alpha-1 antitrypsin deficiency ($n = 4$; Jefferson, Crews, Broshek, Barth, & Robbins, 2003), and COPD ($n = 47$; Crews et al., 2001). These end-stage studies were ultimately combined with additional patients, yielding a total sample of 134 patients diagnosed with a variety of end-stage pulmonary diseases in order to provide consolidated prevalence data on neuropsychological profiles associated with end-stage pulmonary disease (Crews et al., 2003).

The patients included in this series of investigations were classified as end-stage and in need of a lung transplant if they met either of the following criteria: a forced expiratory volume (FEV_1) < 25% predicted or a Pao_2 < 60 mmHg on room air. Patients who had a Pao_2 < 55 mmHg were given supplemental oxygen therapy in an effort to reverse any hypoxia, but Pao_2 was not measured at the time of testing. The patient population was relatively young compared to that of studies examining neurocognitive profiles of COPD patients who were not end-stage (mean age = 48.27, SD = 13.96). The neuropsychological test battery used in these studies was necessarily brief because patients were unable to tolerate more extensive batteries due to their fragile medical condition, but included measures of intelligence, executive functioning, processing speed, verbal and visual memory, and personality functioning. Neuropsychological test scores that fell more than one standard deviation below their respective normative means were judged to be impaired. These studies did not include healthy control groups, but instead, they compared the frequency of impairment on the various neuropsychological measures with the expected frequency of impairment derived from normalized distributions of published normative data (i.e., 16th percentile).

The findings of the combined study were generally consistent with those of the previous component investigations. Overall, these investigations revealed a variety of neurocognitive impairments in patients with end-stage pulmonary disease. In the combined study, notable rates of impairment were found on measures of contextual verbal and non-verbal memory and aspects of executive functioning (i.e., cognitive processing speed, visuomotor scanning abilities, cognitive flexibility/sequencing skills, maintaining response strategies, and concept formation/reasoning skills). However, impairment rates in these domains did not occur more frequently than expected when compared to normalized distributions of the published normative data for each respective measure. The most prevalent deficits across studies were noted on tasks involving immediate free recall and long term retrieval of non-contextual verbal information as measured by the Selective Reminding Test (SRT) with impairment rates ranging from 41.67% to 51.19%. The rates of impairment on the SRT were significantly greater than those observed in the frequency distributions of the published normative data. Of note, deficits in non-contextual verbal memory were not found for those patients who were given the Rey Auditory Verbal Learning Test (RAVLT) instead of the SRT, suggesting that "the SRT, as compared to the RAVLT, may be a more sensitive index of impaired immediate and delayed free recall of non-contextual verbal material in patients with end-stage pulmonary disease" (Crews et al., 2003, p. 359).

This series of studies also examined personality functioning in patients with end-stage pulmonary disease via the Minnesota Multiphasic Personality Inventory—Second Edition (Hathaway & McKinley, 1989) and the Minnesota Multiphasic Personality Inventory—Adolescent (Butcher, Graham, Williams, & Kaemmer, 1992; MMPI-2/A). In the combined study, mean MMPI-2/A profiles revealed significant elevations on Scales 1 (Hypochondriasis) and 3 (Conversion Hysteria), with a subclinical elevation on Scale 2 (Depression). The mean profile was interpreted as suggesting that this patient population tends to experience a diversity of somatic symptoms that fluctuate with degree of stress, as well as significant lethargy/fatigue and a reduction in the efficiency of their overall functioning (Crews et al., 2003). Many of these patients also experienced symptoms of depression. The 1–3 code-type exhibited in this patient population is not unexpected, as these patients typically are medically fragile, with multiple physical symptoms and complications. Another study of patients with end-stage lung disease revealed five cluster profiles consisting of mild somatic concern, mild depression, no psychological distress, significant psychological distress, and a small group of patients with antisocial characteristics (Singer, Ruchinskas, Riley, Broshek, & Barth, 2001). The psychological findings of the end-stage studies are generally consistent with those of previous investigations of patients with less severe COPD, which reported reactive depression, generalized dissatisfaction with life, and preoccupation with somatic complaints, and found similar clinical elevations on Scales 1, 2, and 3 of the MMPI (McSweeny, Grant, Heaton, Adams, & Timms, 1982; Prigatano, Wright, & Levin, 1984).

This series of end-stage studies demonstrated the neuropsychological impact of progressive declines in pulmonary functioning and resulting chronic hypoxia. Some memory disruption is likely due to localized dysfunction in hippocampal formation and basal ganglia, both of which are especially vulnerable to hypoxia/anoxia (Lezak, Howieson, & Loring, 2004). However, Liesker and colleagues (2004) demonstrated that even non-hypoxemic patients with COPD show significant impairments in cognitive performance, suggesting that other factors may play a role in the neuropsychological dysfunction demonstrated by patients with pulmonary disease. With regard to patients with end-stage pulmonary disease, possible contributing factors include hypercapnea (Stuss et al., 1997), other disease processes (Grant et al., 1982), accelerated aging due to enhanced preexisting vascular disease (Prigatano et al., 1983), and exacerbations of neuropsychological deficits by psychological distress (Lezak et al., 2004).

Lung Transplantation

Dr. James Hardy at the University of Mississippi performed the first single lung transplant in 1963 (Grover et al., 1997). Unfortunately, the recipient died of renal failure 18 days later. From 1963 to 1983, 40 other lung transplants were performed, but there were no long-term survivors with the exception of one patient who survived 10 months. The patient spent the majority of his post-transplant life in the hospital and eventually succumbed to pneumonia with chronic rejection. In 1983, Dr. Joel Cooper at the University of Toronto investigated immunosuppressant medications and performed what is considered the "landmark" single lung transplant as it resulted in long-term survival for the patient. In the early years of lung transplantation, most patients who underwent the procedure had pulmonary fibrosis, whereas COPD, cystic fibrosis, and pulmonary hypertension were considered contraindications to transplant.

Since 1988, over 14,000 lung transplants have been performed in the United States (Organ Procurement and Transplantation Network, 2006). In contrast to the early years in which COPD was a contraindication to transplant, the majority of single lung transplants now performed internationally are in patients with COPD/alpha-1 antitrypsin deficiency (61.2%), followed by IPF (24%) (Estenne & Kotloff, 2006). The majority of double lung transplants performed internationally are for COPD (32%) and cystic fibrosis (32%). According to data provided by the Organ Procurement and Transplantation Network (2006), the 1-year survival rate for transplants performed between 1995 and 2002 is 77.7% for single lung transplants and 78.6% for double lung transplants. At 5 years, the survival rate drops to 40.8% for the unilateral procedure and 46.2% for the bilateral lung transplant.

Change in Allocation Policy

Prior to the spring of 2005, lungs were allocated by patients' accrued time on the waiting list. A large number of patients died while awaiting available cadaveric lungs for transplantation. Determining how to allocate such a scarce resource became a matter of debate (Egan & Kotloff, 2005). According to Egan, people generally comprehend the concept of "waiting in line," but also understand that triage is an accepted medical practice in which the most critically ill patients receive higher priority for health care. Egan notes that the system of time accrued on the wait list did not take into account the severity of illness or the rapidity of disease progression. As such, there was no mechanism for hastening transplant for patients with an acutely increased mortality risk. Due to the ethical and moral belief that inaction is not acceptable when an individual's life is in jeopardy and potential lifesaving measures are available, a new national lung allocation system (LAS) was developed. The LAS is an algorithm based on numerous physiological measures (e.g., forced vital capacity), health status (e.g., co-morbid insulin dependent diabetes), diagnosis, and age. The LAS reflects the ratio of estimated length of survival without transplant to likelihood of post-transplant survival and is normalized on a scale from 0 to 100 with higher scores indicating greater urgency.

The LAS has been criticized on the grounds that this new system "is potentially flawed in its attempt to make an exact science out of the imperfect art of predicting the natural history of lung disease" (p.412; Egan & Kotloff, 2005). Although the LAS was based on multivariate analysis, there is no information on the confidence intervals for the factors identified as critical in predicting death on the wait list or after transplant and the validity of the new system has been questioned.

Living Lobar Transplants

Due to the shortage of available organs, Dr. Starnes and his colleagues at the University of Southern California and the Children's Hospital of Los Angeles pioneered living lobar transplantation in 1993 (Barr, Schenkel, Bowdish, & Starnes, 2005; Barr et al., 2001). This procedure involves two donors, each of whom donates a lower lobe, and three operating rooms. As such, it is a complex and expensive procedure and two healthy donors are exposed to potential medical risks. While there have been no fatalities for donors to date and the perioperative risks are similar to standard lung resection, this procedure raises complex ethical issues, particularly when the recipient is critically ill. Neuropsychologists or medical psychologists can play an important role in such evaluations by assessing the motives of the donors, their competency and capacity to make the decision to donate, their psychological status, and identifying potential implicit or explicit coercion that may be unduly influencing the potential donor to expose themselves to medical risk.

Criteria for Referral for Lung Transplant Evaluation

In general, patients are referred for a lung transplant evaluation when they have end-stage pulmonary disease with an 18- to 24-month life expectancy, are severely disabled, have an unacceptable quality of life, and have failed maximal medical therapy. Optimally, referred patients should be medically adherent and have a strong personal and family commitment to transplant.

Components of Transplant Evaluation and Contraindications to Transplant

Patients undergo extensive medical testing to determine their suitability for transplant. Basic studies that should be completed prior to or as part of the initial evaluation include pulmonary function tests, exercise tolerance (e.g., 6-min walk), electrocardiogram, echocardiogram, creatinine clearance, and assessment of liver function (Maurer, Frost, Estenne, Higenbottam, & Glanville, 1998). In select patients, a stress echocardiogram and/or high resolution CT of the thorax may also be required. As part of the evaluation process, patients may also undergo cardiac catheterization, bone density testing, abdominal ultrasound, and other procedures required by their specific medical history and health status. Patients also typically undergo psychosocial evaluation, which may be conducted by a spectrum of mental health professionals, including social workers, psychologists, neuropsychologists, or psychiatrists. Part of the evaluation process involves identifying absolute and relative contraindications to transplant due to the relationship between those variables and long-term outcome (see Table 3).

Table 3 International guidelines for the selection of lung transplant candidates

Absolute Contraindications to Lung Transplantation

- Creatinine clearance of < 50 mg/ml/min, indicating renal dysfunction
- HIV infection
- Active malignancy within 2 years (except for basal cell and squamous cell skin cancer)
- Active malignancy within 5 years of the following: extracapsular renal cell cancer, stage 2 or higher breast cancer, higher than Dukes A colon cancer, and level III or higher melanoma
- Positive hepatitis B antigen
- Hepatitis C with liver disease indicated by biopsy
- Progressive neuromuscular disease

Relative Contraindications to Lung Transplantation

- Severe osteoporosis
- Severe musculoskeletal disease involving the thorax
- Corticosteroid use of > 20 mg daily
- Severe malnutrition or obesity (less than 70% or greater than 130% of ideal body weight)
- Substance addiction within the past six months (e.g., narcotics, alcohol, tobacco)
- Unresolved psychosocial issues that are likely to have a negative impact on medical outcome
- Documented history of medical non-adherence regardless of psychiatric history
- Invasive ventilation
- Pan-resistant organisms in sputum

Source: Maurer et al. (1998)

Role of Neuropsychology in Lung Transplant Evaluations

Given the increasing number of patients referred for evaluation and the scarcity of organs available, neurocognitive, behavioral, and psychosocial factors have played an increasingly important role in the selection of lung transplant candidates (Dobbels, Verleden, Dupont, Vanhaecke, & De Geest, 2006). These factors are important because they may be correlated with poor outcome after transplant and increase the risk of medical non-adherence. Compared to other organ transplant patients (e.g., heart, liver, and kidney), patients who have undergone lung transplantation require more intensive immunosuppressant treatment (Dobbels et al., 2006). Identification of factors that affect patients' ability to comprehend, remember, and carry out complex medical instructions is critical. A neuropsychological evaluation that targets verbal memory, problem solving skills, and processing speed is very helpful in identifying those patients who will require modification of standard verbal medical instructions. Since patients are often given transplant manuals that contain complex and detailed information about the transplant and medication regimens, assessment of reading ability is particularly important for those candidates who did not complete high school. Health care professionals may negatively judge patients' motivation for transplant because they have not read the transplant manual without realizing that the patient is functionally illiterate. The neuropsychologist's role in these situations is particularly critical in identifying cognitive and academic weaknesses, as well as noting strategies that will enable the patient to compensate in order to increase the likelihood of positive medical outcome. Common recommendations for those patients with memory impairment include providing important medical instructions in writing, use of pill boxes and/or alarm wrist watches for maximizing medication adherence, posting the medical regimen in an easily seen location such as the refrigerator, and family assistance oversight and monitoring. When patients have limited intellectual ability or difficulty with problem solving, compensatory strategies include avoiding the use of medical jargon, requiring the patient to contact the nurse coordinator regarding any unusual symptoms rather than trying to cope with them on their own, and providing medical follow-up when the medical regimen has been changed.

The clinical interview conducted as part of a neuropsychological evaluation also provides critical information related to the patient's quality of life and medical outcome. Many patients facing their own mortality and the prospect of organ transplant in order to save their lives, as well as reduced quality of life and limitations in ability to perform physical activities, experience some degree of depression and/or anxiety. In addition, many patients with pulmonary disease develop anxiety and panic attacks as a result of air hunger. Evaluation of more severe depression and anxiety is invaluable in identifying those patients who would benefit from psychotropic medication, psychotherapy, or behavioral interventions such as relaxation training, biofeedback, or attending a support group. The interview can also provide important information about support systems and identification of family members or friends who will provide assistance to the patient during convalescence and aid the patient in adhering to medical instructions and communicating with medical professionals.

Summary

Pulmonary disease is a common disorder in the United States and causes significant morbidity and mortality. Research has revealed that pulmonary compromise is associated with functional neurocognitive deficits and cerebral compromise as indicated by neuroimaging. Neuropsychology has an important role to play in the clinical evaluation and management of these patients, as well as in future research on the neurocognitive sequelae of pulmonary disease. Follow-up data is still lacking on how patients' neurocognitive functioning might be affected by lung transplant and this is an important area of future study. Given the scarcity of available organs for transplant, identifying potential indicators of a poor outcome via a neuropsychological evaluation and strategies for remediating those factors is critical for maximizing the likelihood of positive medical outcomes.

References

Anstey, K. J., Windsor, T. D., Jorm, A. F., Christensen, H., & Rodgers, B. (2004).

Association of pulmonary function with cognitive performance in early, middle and late adulthood. *Gerontology, 50,* 230–234.

Barr, M. L., Baker, C. J., Schenkel, F. A., Bowdish, M. E., Bremner, R. M., Cohen, R. G., et al. (2001). Living donor lung transplantation: Selection, technique, and outcome. *Transplantation Proceedings, 33,* 3527–3532.

Barr, M. L., Schenkel, F. A., Bowdish, M. E., & Starnes, V. A. (2005). Living donor lobar lung transplantation: Current status and future directions. *Transplantation Proceedings, 37,* 3983–3986.

Brigham and Women's Hospital Neurosurgery Group. (2006). Principles of cerebral oxygenation and blood flow in the neurological critical care unit. *Neurocritical Care, 4,* 77–82.

Butcher, J. N., Graham, J. R., Williams, C. L., & Kaemmer, B. (1992). *Minnesota multiphasic personality inventory – adolescent.* Minneapolis, MN: University of Minnesota Press.

Chin, K. M., Channick, R. N., & Rubin, L. J. (2005). Pulmonary hypertension: Pathogenesis and etiology. In R. A. Bordow, A. L. Ries, & T. A. Morris (Eds.), *Manual of clinical problems in pulmonary medicine* (6th ed., pp. 392–397). Philadelphia, PA: Lippincott, Willams & Wilkins.

Conrad, D. J. (2005). Cystic fibrosis. In R. A. Bordow, A. L. Ries, & T. A. Morris (Eds.), *Manual of clinical problems in pulmonary medicine* (6th ed., pp. 417–423). Philadelphia, PA: Lippincott, Willams & Wilkins.

Crews, W. D., Jefferson, A. L., Broshek, D. K., Barth, J. T., & Robbins, M. K. (2000). Neuropsychological sequelae in a series of patients with end-stage cystic fibrosis: Lung transplant evaluation. *Archives of Clinical Neuropsychology, 15,* 59–70.

Crews, W. D., Jefferson, A. L., Broshek, D. K., Rhodes, R. D., Williamson, J., Brazil, A. M., et al. (2003). Neuropsychological dysfunction in patients with end-stage pulmonary disease: Lung transplant evaluation. *Archives of Clinical Neuropsychology, 18,* 353–362.

Crews, W. D., Jefferson, A. L., Bolduc, T., Elliot, J. B., Ferro, N. M., Broshek, D. K., et al. (2001). Neuropsychological dysfunction in patients suffering from end-stage chronic obstructive pulmonary disease. *Archives of Clinical Neuropsychology, 16,* 643–652.

Dobbels, F., Verleden, G., Dupont, L., Vanhaecke, J., & De Geest, S. (2006). To transplant or not? The importance of psychosocial and behavioral factors before lung transplantation. *Chronic Respiratory Disease, 3,* 39–47.

Egan, T. M., & Kotloff, R. M. (2005). Pro/con debate: Lung allocation should be based on medical urgency and transplant survival and not on waiting time. *Chest, 128,* 407–415.

Estenne, M., & Kotloff, R. M. (2006). Update in transplantation 2005. *American Journal of Respiratory and Critical Care Medicine, 173,* 593–598.

Grant, I., Heaton, R. K., McSweeny, A. J., Adams, K. M., & Timms, R. M. (1982). Neuropsychologic findings in hypoxemic chronic obstructive pulmonary disease. *Archives of Internal Medicine, 142,* 1470–1476.

Grant, I., Prigatano, G. P., Heaton, R. K., McSweeny, A. J., Wright, E. C., & Adams, K. M. (1987). Progressive neuropsychological impairment in relation to hypoxemia in chronic obstructive pulmonary disease. *Archives of General Psychiatry, 44,* 999–1006.

Grover, F. L., Fullerton, D. A., Zamora, M. R., Mills, C., Ackerman, B., Badesch, D. et al. (1997). The past, present, and future of lung transplantation. *American Journal of Surgery, 173,* 523–533.

Han T., Parrish, J. S., & Smith, C. M. (2005). Idiopathic interstitial pneumonia. In R. A. Bordow, A. L. Ries, & T. A. Morris (Eds.), *Manual of clinical problems in pulmonary medicine* (6th ed., pp. 529–535). Philadelphia, PA: Lippincott, Willams & Wilkins.

Hathaway, S. R., & McKinley, J. C. (1989). *Minnesota multiphasic personality inventory* (2nd ed.). Minneapolis, MN: University of Minnesota Press.

Heaton, R. K., Grant, I., McSweeny, A. J., Adams, K. M., & Petty, T. L. (1983). Psychologic effects of continuous and nocturnal oxygen therapy in hypoxemic chronic obstructive pulmonary disease. *Archives of Internal Medicine, 143,* 1941–1947.

Hughson, W. G. (2005a). Asbestos-related disease. In R. A. Bordow, A. L. Ries, & T. A. Morris (Eds.), *Manual of clinical problems in pulmonary medicine* (6th ed., pp. 461–464). Philadelphia, PA: Lippincott, Willams & Wilkins.

Hughson, W. G. (2005b). Coal workers' pneumoconiosis. In R. A. Bordow, A. L. Ries, & T. A. Morris (Eds.), *Manual of clinical problems in pulmonary medicine* (6th ed., pp. 457–460). Philadelphia, PA: Lippincott, Willams & Wilkins.

Incalzi, R. A., Marra, C., Giordano, A., Calcagni, M. L., Cappa, A., Basso, S., et al. (2003). Cognitive impairment in chronic obstructive pulmonary disease: A neuropsychological and spect study. *Journal of Neurology, 250,* 325–332.

Jefferson, A. L., Crews, W. D., Broshek, D. K., Barth, J. T., & Robbins, M. K. (2003). An examination of the neuropsychological sequelae associated with end-stage pulmonary disease secondary to alpha-1 antitrypsin deficiency. *Advances in Medical Psychotherapy and Psychodiagnosis, 11,* 35–44.

Krop, H., Block, A. J., & Cohen, E. (1973). Neuropsychological effects of continuous oxygen therapy in chronic obstructive pulmonary disease. *Chest, 64,* 317–322.

Lezak, M. D., Howieson, D. B., & Loring, D. W. (2004). *Neuropsychological Assessment* (4th ed.). New York: Oxford University Press.

Lichter, J. P. (2005). Bronchiectasis. In R. A. Bordow, A. L. Ries, & T. A. Morris (Eds.), *Manual of clinical problems in pulmonary medicine* (6th ed., pp. 306–313). Philadelphia, PA: Lippincott, Willams & Wilkins.

Liesker, J. J. W., Postma, D. S., Beukema, R. J., ten Hacken, N. H. T., van der Molen, T., Riemersma, R. A., et al. (2004). Cognitive performance in patients with COPD. *Respiratory Medicine, 98,* 351–356.

Maurer, J. R., Frost, A. E., Estenne, M., Higenbottam, T., & Glanville, A. R. (1998). International guidelines for the selection of lung transplant candidates. *Transplantation, 66,* 951–956.

McSweeny, A. J., Grant, I., Heaton, R. K., Adams, K. M., & Timms, R. M. (1982). Life quality of patients with chronic obstructive pulmonary disease. *Archives of Internal Medicine, 142,* 473–478.

Oliviero, A., Corbo, G., Tonali, P. A., Pilato, F., Saturno, E., Dileone, M., et al. (2002). Functional involvement of central nervous system in acute exacerbation of chronic obstructive pulmonary disease: A preliminary transcranial magnetic stimulation study. *Journal of Neurology, 249,* 1232–1236.

Organ Procurement and Transplantation Network. (2006). Retrieved August 10, 2006, from http://www.unos.org/data/about/viewDataReports.asp

Ortapamuk, H., & Naldoken, S. (2006). Brain perfusion abnormalities in chronic obstructive pulmonary disease: comparison with cognitive impairment. *Annals of Nuclear Medicine, 20,* 99–106.

Parrish, J. S., Han, T. S., & Smith, C. M. (2005). Neurofibromatosis, lymphangiomyomatosis, and tuberous sclerosis. In R. A. Bordow, A. L. Ries, & T. A. Morris (Eds.), *Manual of clinical problems in pulmonary medicine* (6th ed., pp. 556–562). Philadelphia, PA: Lippincott, Willams & Wilkins.

Prigatano, G. P., Parsons, O. A., Wright, E. C., Levin, D. C., & Hawryluk, G. (1983). Neuropsychological test performance in mildly hypoxemic patients with chronic obstructive pulmonary disease.

Journal of Consulting and Clinical Psychology,
51, 108–116.

Prigatano, G. P., Wright, E. C., & Levin, D. (1984). Quality of life and its predictors in patients with mild hypoxemia and chronic obstructive pulmonary disease. *Archives of Internal Medicine, 144,* 1613–1619.

Ries, A. L. (2005a). Chronic obstructive pulmonary disease: Clinical and laboratory manifestations, pathophysiology, and prognosis. In R. A. Bordow, A. L. Ries, & T. A. Morris (Eds.), *Manual of clinical problems in pulmonary medicine* (6th ed., pp. 293–296). Philadelphia, PA: Lippincott, Willams & Wilkins.

Ries, A. L. (2005b). Chronic obstructive pulmonary disease: Definition and epidemiology. In R. A. Bordow, A. L. Ries, & T. A. Morris (Eds.), *Manual of clinical problems in pulmonary medicine* (6th ed., pp. 287–292). Philadelphia, PA: Lippincott, Willams & Wilkins.

Sachdev, P. S., Anstey, K. J., Parslow, R. A., Wen, W., Maller, J., Kumar, R., et al. (2006). Pulmonary function, cognitive impairment and brain atrophy in a middle-aged community sample. *Dementia and Geriatric Cognitive Disorders, 21,* 300–308.

Singer, H. K, Ruchinskas, R. A, Riley, K. C., Broshek, D. K., & Barth, J. T. (2001). The psychological impact of end-stage lung disease. *Chest, 120,* 1246–1252.

Stenbit, A. E. (2005). Sarcoidosis. In R. A. Bordow, A. L. Ries, & T. A. Morris (Eds.), *Manual of clinical problems in pulmonary medicine* (6th ed., pp. 511–515). Philadelphia, PA: Lippincott, Willams & Wilkins.

Stuss, D. T., Peterkin, I., Guzman, D. A., Guzman, C., & Troyer, A. K. (1997). Chronic obstructive pulmonary disease: Effects of hypoxia on neurological and neuropsychological measures. *Journal of Clinical and Experimental Neuropsychology, 19,* 515–524.

Van Dijk, E. J., Vermeer, S. E., de Groot, J. C., van de Minkelis, J., Prins, N. D., Oudkerk, M., et al. (2004). Arterial oxygen saturation, COPD, and cerebral small vessel disease. *Journal of Neurology, Neurosurgery, and Psychiatry, 75,* 733–736.

Chapter 14
Diabetes and Hypertension

Lenore J. Launer and Clinton Wright

Introduction

Cognitive impairment and dementia are very prevalent conditions in persons 60 years and older. Estimates of persons with a mild level of cognitive impairment (MCI) vary widely depending on the definition of MCI and the sample (Panza et al., 2005), but in community based studies, it is estimated to be at least twice the overall prevalence of dementia. Many persons with cognitive impairment go on to develop dementia, which doubles in prevalence and incidence every additional 5 years of age (Lobo et al., 2000). Between 65 years and 85 years and older, the prevalence of dementia increases from <1% to approximately 30% of the population, and number of new cases that develop increases from <1 to 80 per 1,000 person years of observation (Launer et al. 1999).

Vascular disease is also highly prevalent in older individuals. Hypertension represents a very large public health problem with a prevalence in 2000 estimated at 65 million in the US and almost a billion worldwide (Fields et al. 2004; Kearney et al. 2005). In the elderly at greatest risk of dementia, the prevalence of hypertension can be as high as 73% (Sacco et al. 2004). Type 2 diabetes (T2D) is also

rapidly emerging as a global epidemic and challenge to the public health system (Amos et al. 1997; Resnick et al. 2000; Philippe 2002). Currently approximately 18–20% of older persons suffer from T2D, and with the aging of the population, this number is projected to increase (Harris et al. 1998).

An increase in the prevalence of both hypertension and T2D has implications for vascular cognitive disorders due to the different mechanisms through which they may affect cognition. In general, the main cerebral consequence of both hypertension and T2D has been macrovascular clinical stroke. However, studies suggest patients with each of these disorders can have impaired neuropsychologic functioning in the absence of major clinical stroke (Strachan et al. 1997; Coker et al. 2003). Importantly, recent improvements in neuroimaging, and the administration of neuropsychologic tests in large samples with varied clinical and cultural backgrounds, have shed new light on the potential subclinical, or "silent", as well as clinical, damage hypertension and T2D can do to the brain.

In epidemiologic samples of older persons, where Type 2 is the main type of diabetes, T2D has been associated with a higher prevalence of global cognitive impairment (Kalmijn et al. 1995) and a higher incidence of cognitive decline (Gregg et al. 2000). In the Cardiovascular Health Study (CHS) of persons over 65 years of age, T2D and high levels of glucose were significantly associated

L.J. Launer (✉)
Neuroepidemiology Section, Laboratory of Epidemiology, Demography and Biometry, National Institute on Aging, Bethesda, MD, USA
e-mail: launerl@nia.nih.gov

J.R. Festa, R.M. Lazar (eds.), *Neurovascular Neuropsychology*, DOI 10.1007/978-0-387-70715-0_14,
© Springer Science+Business Media, LLC 2009

with a 7-year decline in cognitive function (Haan et al. 1999). Data from population-based studies also suggest that T2D is not only a risk factor for vascular dementia (Curb et al. 1999), but also for Alzheimer's disease (AD) (Leibson et al. 1997; Ott et al. 1999), the most common form of dementia. Together, prospective cohort studies suggest diabetics have approximately two times increased risk for AD, in particular, AD combined with cerebrovascular disease. This is a fairly robust finding, as studies are based on different ethnic/race/lifestyle groups, including Japanese-American men (Peila et al. 2002), a mixed ethnic/race cohort (Luchsinger et al. 2001), European Caucasian (Leibson et al. 1997; Ott et al. 1999), and religious order members (Arvanitakis et al. 2004).

Hypertension has also been associated with a greater risk of cognitive impairment (Kilander et al. 1998) and dementia (Skoog et al. 1996), including the subtype of vascular dementia (Hofman et al. 1997). A relationship between blood pressure and AD has been found when BP was measured in mid-life (Kivipelto, 2001; Launer, 2000), but the relationship between Alzheimer's and blood pressure is inconsistent when measured close to the time of dementia onset (Morris et al. 2001; Posner et al. 2002). Other population based studies have shown that systolic blood pressure, if untreated, was related to cognitive impairment (Elias M. F. et al. 1993; Guo et al. 1997; Launer et al. 2000) and that treatment was associated with a lower risk of cognitive impairment (Murray et al. 2002).

Randomized double blind clinical trials have been less consistent and the authors of a recent meta-analysis that included three such trials showed no convincing evidence that treatment of hypertension prevents the development of cognitive impairment or dementia (Cochrane_Review 2007). The Syst Eur trial did show a reduced risk of dementia in the group treated for hypertension, but 50% of the placebo group received active treatment,

raising questions about the conclusions. In this chapter, the pathophysiologic mechanisms that are hypothesized to contribute to the changes in brain function caused by hypertension and diabetes as well as characteristic neurobehavioral changes will be reviewed.

Neuropathology and Pathophysiology

Both hypertension and T2D are strong risk factors for arterial damage of large (>2 mm diameter) and small-sized (usually <0.8 mm diameter) vessels of the heart, systemic circulation, and other organs including the brain. As a result, the effects on cognition vary by the type of injury.

Large Vessel Disease

Hypertension and T2D can lead to ischemic heart disease (IHD) and atrial and ventricular chamber abnormalities that increase the likelihood of clot formation, embolization to the brain, and resulting ischemic stroke. Ruptured atherosclerotic plaque of the large vessels with distal embolization may have the same result. Both of these pathologic mechanisms most commonly result in damage to the brain territory of one of the major intracranial vessels such as the middle, anterior, and posterior cerebral arteries and can result in cognitive deficits or frank dementia depending on the size, location, and number of lesions (see Chapter 3 for cognitive effects of stroke).

Aside from embolism to the brain, IHD can lead to heart failure (Chapter 11) and large vessel atherosclerosis with stenosis or occlusion of one or more vessels supplying the brain (e.g., the carotid artery, Chapter 9), resulting in severe reductions in blood flow that can cause cognitive dysfunction.

Small Vessel Disease

Small vessel damage, or microangiopathy, is an important mediator of the effects of both hypertension and diabetes on cognition. Small vessel disease has been of great interest since Maxime Durand-Fardel described three common brain lesions associated with such damage, in the 1850s. The first of these, called "Atrophie interstitielle du cerveau" by Durand-Fardel, corresponds to modern day imaging findings of periventricular and deep white matter lucencies (on computed tomography (CT) scans) or hyperintensities (on magnetic resonance (MR) scans). Vladimir Hachinski coined the term "leukoaraiosis" for these changes to avoid *presuming* an etiology (Hachinski et al. 1987). However, pathological studies have found that leukoaraiosis often corresponds to ischemic damage of varying degrees that has been caused by injury to the small penetrating vessels that supply the basal ganglia and subcortical white matter.

Small penetrating arterioles of the deep gray nuclei and white matter tracts are end-arteries without significant overlap with other vascular beds. As such, a key contributor to damage is the reduction in cerebral perfusion that accompanies chronic hypertension and diabetes. Normally the brain is able to modulate the diameter of small "resistance" vessels in the brain parenchyma, dilating them to increase, and constricting them to decrease, the amount of cerebral perfusion to keep it within an acceptable range. However, chronic exposure to raised blood pressure reduces this "vasodilatory capacity." Resistance vessels are no longer able to constrict in the face of daily fluctuations in blood pressure, such as nocturnal dips, and adequate perfusion may not be maintained resulting in ischemic damage (Isaka et al. 1994).

Based on autopsy studies, lacunae and leukoaraiosis are thought to result from four lesions—small vessel atherosclerosis, lipohyalinosis (complex small vessel disease), arteriolosclerosis (simple small vessel disease), and enlarged perivascular spaces—but their relationship to each other is not completely understood (Donnan 2002). For example, to what extent is arteriolosclerosis a stage that precedes lipohyalinosis? In addition, some lacunae are due to infarcts caused by thrombosis of a small vessel. In other cases, ischemic damage can also result from increased vascular permeability of damaged vessels causing chronic edema resulting in local hypoxia, or impaired nutrient supply to peri-vascular regions (Donnan 2002).

Three subtypes of lacunae have been described pathologically and include the following: (1) incomplete infarctions in which not all cellular elements are damaged as well as complete infarctions that are gliotic cavitated lesions (Type I); (2) lacunae with a significant number of macrophages (Type II); and (3) enlarged peri-vascular spaces (Type III)(Poirier et al. 1984). Types I and II are very similar and probably represent different extremes rather than distinct entities. Type III lacunae may be due to disruption of the blood brain barrier with damage to peri-arteriolar tissue or trauma to the brain tissue that surrounds small vessels due to high blood pressure. Thus, small vessel damage may first lead to ischemic demyelination in the deep white matter and, later, lacunar infarction (Fazekas et al. 1993).

Brain Atrophy

High blood pressure and T2D have also been associated with brain atrophy in addition to subcortical vascular lesions. Such reductions in brain volume may represent damage to the cortex that could have a detrimental effect on cognition. However, the importance of brain atrophy as a mechanism separate from microangiopathy is difficult to sort out because ischemic damage can cause reductions in brain volume as well (Schmidt et al. 2004; Wiseman et al. 2004; Goldstein et al. 2005). In addition, cortical volume loss can also be caused by AD, with hypertension or diabetes as important mediators. For example, midlife hypertension has been associated with greater brain atrophy and an increased burden of Alzheimer pathology in autopsied cases (Petrovitch et al. 2000). In the ARIC study of middle-aged and young-elderly men and women, T2D was associated with greater ventricular size, an indicator of general atrophy (Knopman et al. 2005). Using a similar methodology, similar findings were reported for older men and women in the CHS (Longstreth et al. 2000). Other research (den Heijer et al. 2003) has also found smaller hippocampal and amygdalar volumes, regardless of vascular pathology, were associated with T2D. Similarly, compared to non-diabetics, diabetics had smaller hippocampal volumes and more lacunas in a study of very old Japanese Americans followed as a part of the HAAS study (Korf et al. 2006). In the HAAS study, there was evidence that insulin users had smaller hippocampi than non-insulin using diabetics. In addition, results showed proportionately more brain pathology in those who have been diabetic for at least 20 years. In a multi-center MRI study of 65- to 75-year olds, an interaction between T2D and hypertension was noted: those with both conditions had an increased risk for brain atrophy that was greater than those having only one or none of the conditions (Schmidt et al. 2004). These findings suggest that the amount of brain pathology may increase with disease severity, co-morbidity, or duration, but further investigation is needed in a larger sample that is prospectively followed.

Intermediary Metabolic, Inflammatory and Oxidative Mechanism: Hypertension

Studies suggest various pathways through which elevated BP or diabetes could alter the structure of the brain and cause cognitive impairment. Direct effects of high blood pressure on Alzheimer's disease pathology can be hypothesized. Endothelial damage caused by hypertension itself may lead to pro-inflammatory, pro-coagulant, and oxidative responses similar to those hypothesized to trigger the formation of neuritic plaques in Alzheimer's disease (Tanzi et al. 2004).

Intermediary Physiologic Changes in Type II Diabetes

T2D is associated with oxidative stress, inflammation, (Klein et al. 2003) an increase in O-linked glycoprotein, and increased formation of advanced glycosylation end products (AGES) (Singh R. et al. 2001), which may have a detrimental effect on cognition.

In addition to vascular damage, there has been considerable debate in the literature about whether those with T2D are at increased risk for degenerative changes in the brain that lead to cognitive problems (Halter 1996; Hoyer 1998; Grossman 2003; Forrester 2004). Several of the above mechanisms also contribute to neurodegeneration (Hardy, 2002). Other diabetes-related pathology, such as AGES, can contribute directly to neurodegeneration and the formation of neuritic plaques (NP) and neurofibrillary tangles (NFT). Consistent with these mechanisms, autopsy data based on the Honolulu Asia Aging Study (HAAS) cohort, shows a significant association of T2D to infarcts as well as hippocampal NFT and NP (Peila et al. 2002); another study, however, did not confirm this association (Arvanitakis et al. 2006). It is also likely that a vicious cycle develops with T2D and neurodegenerative processes. A hyperglycemic environment can lead to neuronal degeneration, and neuronal degeneration can lead to impaired glucose regulation. For example, there may be a direct effect of hyperglycemia on the calcium balance in hippocampal neurons that could lead to degeneration (McEwen et al. 2002). Such neuronal damage could interfere with the hippocampus role in regulating peripheral glucose (Gispen et al. 2000; Magarinos et al. 2000), as well as the synaptic plasticity in hippocampal neurons as demonstrated in animal studies (Klein et al. 2003). It has also been suggested that hyperglycemia leads to increased vasopressin, which is part of a cascade that eventually results in degeneration of hypothalamic neurons (Magarinos et al. 2000) and impaired hypothalamic function. Since the hypothalamus is central to the regulation of many physiologic mediators, including vasopressin, leptin, ghrelin, insulin, and glucose (Elmquist et al. 2003), changes in the neurons in this structure could lead to dysregulation of the pathways that depend on these metabolic products.

Diabetics are also at increased risk for hypoglycemic events, which disturb delivery of nutrients to the brain, may down regulate different markers of neuronal plasticity (Singh P. et al. 2003), and increase the amount of neurotoxic glutamate. Further, the brains of people with T2D are at risk for adverse sequela following repeated hypoglycemic events (Langan et al. 1991; Perros et al. 1997).

Hyperinsulinemia

In the brain, insulin modulates glucose availability as well as the activity of neurotransmitters and neuronal health (Craft et al. 2004). Central nervous system (CNS) insulin is derived mainly from the peripheral circulation (Schwartz et al. 1991) and is proportionally related to plasma insulin levels (Schwartz et al. 1992). Under physiological conditions, a higher serum insulin level may reflect a higher level of brain insulin, and a low level could reflect an insufficient insulinization of the brain. In hyperinsulinemic conditions the transport of insulin into the CNS is altered and insulin resistance can ensue (Bonora et al. 1998).

Insufficient insulinization in the brain could lead to multiple cerebral changes. Studies of the relatively acute effects of insulin in the brain have shown that insulin potentiates memory. It does this through several hypothesized pathways such as modulation of cellular glucose uptake, neurotransmitter levels, and long term potentiation critical in the communication of memory-related impulses from neuron to neuron (Craft et al. 2004). Both peripheral and central levels of inflammatory markers and oxidative stress are also increased in hyperinsulinemic conditions. Metabolic dysregulation of insulin can cause endothelial damage and impair the health of the vasculature; it can also lead to phosphorylation of tau, disrupture of microtubles in the neuron, and neurofibrillary tangles, a hallmark of AD pathology (Hong et al. 1997).

Dysfunction of the insulin degrading enzyme (IDE) may also provide a pathological link between neurodegeneration and T2D. This enzyme degrades insulin as well as β-amyloid, a major component of the extracellular plaques that characterize AD. In T2D, dysfunction of IDE leads to high levels of insulin and β-amyloid, (Qiu et al. 1998; Edbauer et al. 2002). In AD, hyperinsulinemia is more prevalent compared to controls, and the activity and amount of IDE is diminished (Perez et al. 2000; Cook et al. 2003). Interestingly, IDE is located on chromosome 10; there is some evidence for genetic linkage of Alzheimer's disease on this chromosome (Bertram et al. 2000).

Diabetes and Genetic Susceptibility

Interactions between genetic susceptibility and T2D have been reported. Data from the Zutphen Study (Kalmijn et al. 1996), suggests that men who carry an Apolipoprotein E ε4 allele *and* have T2D had a higher risk for cognitive decline compared to those with no T2D or no Apo E ε4 genotype. Similarly, the HAAS study found that diabetics with an Apo E ε4 allele had a significantly higher risk for AD compared to those with none or one condition (Peila et al. 2002). An interaction of T2D and Apo E ε4 allele on the risk for dementia was also reported in the CHS (Irie et al. 2008).

Characteristic Neurobehavioral Syndromes

The cognitive consequences of hypertension and diabetes depend on the mechanisms of damage noted in the preceding section. To review the cognitive deficits associated with specific lesion locations, such as with lacunar infarcts, is beyond the scope of this chapter (see Chapter 2). Infarcts in specific locations can result in cognitive deficits depending on the cognitive functions subserved by the area involved. For example, thalamic infarcts have been shown to impair memory function, while infarcts in the frontal lobe are more likely to affect speed of processing and executive function (Vermeer et al. 2003). Multiple infarcts can likewise cause deficits in several domains.

Nineteenth-century authors, including Durand-Fardel and most famously Otto Binswanger, were the first to posit an effect of leukoaraiosis on cognition but it was not until modern brain imaging with CT and MR that the issue has been addressed in large samples. The question is far from simple because leukoaraiosis is often seen incidentally on the brain scans of elderly individuals without dementia and the amount required to cause cognitive problems is not known. In addition, elderly individuals with cognitive problems often have Alzheimer's disease in addition to hypertension and/or T2D, making the contribution of leukoaraiosis to the cognitive profile difficult to sort out. The above notwithstanding, leukoaraiosis has been associated with cognitive decline and dementia (Barber et al. 1999; Vermeer et al. 2003).

The cognitive deficits associated with leukoaraiosis include psychomotor slowing and executive dysfunction and represent a typical subcortical pattern of injury (Prins et al. 2005; Sachdev et al. 2005). Executive functions involving planning, decision making, and cognitive flexibility managed by the frontal cortex.

In order to explain how executive dysfunction might be caused by leukoaraiosis, microvascular damage has been posited to disrupt projections from cortical areas to subcortical structures (Cummings 1993). Imaging studies of the topography of white matter hyperintensities in the coronal plane have shown that as the volume of damage increases, white matter damage extends further and further away from the ventricular wall in a uniform manner (DeCarli et al. 2005). In this way, frontal subcortical circuits most adjacent to the ventricular wall might be progressively disrupted. This concept is supported by data showing that leukoaraiosis affects frontal lobe function regardless of their location (Tullberg et al. 2004). Another way leukoaraiosis may affect cognition is by slowing neural transmission since somatosenory and visual evoked potentials are delayed in the presence of leukoaraiosis (Kato et al. 1990; Shibata et al. 2000).

The cognitive profile of chronic exposure to hypertension or diabetes independent of leukoaraiosis and lacunar infarction is difficult to sort out for the reasons mentioned earlier. Brain atrophy resulting from such exposure and not due to other causes such as Alzheimer's disease might have an effect on frontal lobe function as well. This is supported by data showing that men with higher systolic blood pressures had lower regional frontal lobe volumes (atrophy) and these lower volumes correlated with worse performance on tests of cognitive flexibility (executive function) and working memory (Gianaros et al. 2006). Experimental models of hypertension can also be helpful. Recent studies in Rhesus monkeys where blood pressure was increased to varying degrees experimentally have shown negative effects on abstraction and shifting set. Loss of neurons in the cortex and of myelin fibers in the white matter predominated in the forebrain, internal capsule, corona radiata, and cortex (Moore et al. 2002).

Diabetes: Special Considerations

Type 1 Diabetes

Observational studies on small samples of persons older than 18 years have had inconsistent findings about whether, and in what domains, Type 1 diabetes is associated with cognitive impairment. However, a recent meta-analysis of the studies on Type 1 diabetes demonstrated relatively small, but significant differences between cases and controls in mental speed and flexibility (Brands et al. 2005). The Diabetes Control and Complications Trial (DCCT) results on Type 1 diabetic cases, however, did not demonstrate any differences in cognitive function between those in the intensive treatment arm and the conventional treatment arm (DCCT 1996). The average age of Type 1 patients in these studies is around 35 years old. A recent study on a sample of relatively older Type 1 diabetics (average age 60 years) and controls found only mild cognitive impairments in the diabetics compared to age-matched controls (Brands et al. 2006).

Type 2 Diabetes

Data in older individuals have been inconclusive regarding the question whether diabetes is associated with global cognitive impairment, or impairment in specific domains. Part of the reason is the great variability in study design and test results that characterize this area of research. Small sample size, relatively young mean age, lack of control for confounders such as depression, or other cardiovascular risk factors characterize much of the literature. (Stewart et al. 1999; Coker et al. 2003); Musselman et al. 2003; Cukierman et al. 2005). However, findings in several large scale studies of persons aged 60 years and older do suggest diabetics are cognitively impaired relative to those with no diabetes. Four studies (Kalmijn et al. 1995; Sinclair et al. 2000; Fontbonne et al. 2001; Grodstein et al. 2001) showed that, compared to non-diabetics, diabetics performed significantly poorer on tests of global cognitive function, such as the Mini-Mental State Exam (MMSE), or equivalent (Folstein et al. 1975; Teng et al. 1987). Very few large studies have included more than one test of cognitive function. A study of religious order members followed for a mean 5.5 years reported that diabetics declined significantly more than non-diabetics in tests of perceptual speed and semantic memory, marginally more in visuospatial ability, and did not differ in measures of working and episodic memory (Arvanitakis et al. 2004). In a study of three cognitive tests administered to participants in the Study of Osteoporotic Fractures, diabetic women 65 years and older demonstrated lower performance than those without diabetes on the Digit Symbol Substitution Test (a measure of psychomotor speed), the Trail Making Test Part B, a measure of executive function, and a modified version of the MMSE (Gregg et al. 2000).

Type 2 diabetes may interact with hypertension to increase the risk for cognitive impairment. A study based on the Framingham cohort suggests that persons with both T2D and hypertension are at a higher risk for impairment in verbal and visual memory, compared to those without these two conditions (Elias P. K. et al. 1997). Inconsistent findings in these studies may reflect the age of the subjects, and therefore the balance and degree of neurodegeneration and vascular damage, non-comparable tests or the sensitivity of the cognitive tests in the specific populations, as well as the length of follow-up. Additional well-designed prospective studies on larger samples are needed to better identify cognitive domains that might specifically be impaired in diabetes, and to identify other factors that interact with diabetes and lead to more impairment.

Plasma Glucose Dose Effects

Current studies provide a mixed picture as to whether the risk for cognitive disorders reflects an underlying linear increase with increasing glucose levels, similar to the linear increase in risk for stroke associated with increasing levels of blood pressure (MacMahon et al. 1990). Specifically, several investigators report no association between impaired glucose tolerance and performance on multiple cognitive tests (Fontbonne et al. 2001; Kanaya et al. 2004). On the other hand, another study found a significant trend of normoglycemia, impaired glucose tolerance and diabetes for greater cognitive decline on a composite score of memory and executive functions(Yaffe et al. 2004). In a Finnish study, men and women with impaired glucose tolerance, compared to normoglycemic subjects, performed more poorly on the MMSE but not other tests of memory and frontal lobe function (Vanhanen et al. 1998). In a small study ($n = 30$) of glucose exposure in non-diabetic middle age and older subjects, decreased general cognitive performance, memory impairment, and hippocampal atrophy was associated with reduced glucose tolerance measured with an i.v. 2-h glucose tolerance test (Convit et al. 2003). Additional research is needed to explore the association of increasing levels of fasting glucose to cognitive impairment.

Severity or duration of disease may modify a diabetic's risk for brain aging. In the SALSA study of older Latinos, compared to subjects with no diabetic complications, diabetics with complications had a greater risk for a 2-year drop in global cognitive functioning (Wu et al. 2003); subjects with untreated diabetes as compared to those with treated diabetes had a higher risk of cognitive decline as well. Among those who were treated, those with more than 5 years of (having the) disease gained more cognitive benefit from treatment than those with less than 5 years duration of disease. Among those with more than 5 years, those receiving a combination of drugs had less cognitive decline than those receiving monotherapy. Similar associations of increased risk for cognitive decline associated with longer duration of disease and no treatment were reported for the Nurses Health Study

(Logroscino et al. 2004). The Rotterdam Study (Ott et al. 1999) found the highest risk for AD in diabetics treated with insulin, suggesting severity of the disease plays a role. Interestingly, in a case control study of older Type 1 diabetics and controls, no differences on MRI characteristics were noted. The authors conclude that these findings suggest changes in brain structure found in Type 2 diabetics do not necessarily reflect only the effects of long-term exposure to hyperglycemia (Brands et al. 2006). Describing and understanding the aging process of Type 1 diabetics will become of increasing importance as more of these patients are able to live longer.

Conclusion

There are an increasing number of population-based studies that provide evidence that hypertension and diabetes increase the risk of premature brain aging and cognitive disorders, either as a direct or indirect result of hyperglycemia and high BP levels, or associated co-morbidities of dyslipidemia and hyperinsulinemia. Current experimental and clinical data support roles for hypertension and diabetes in the development of vascular lesions that can cause cognitive impairment or dementia. In addition, diabetes may have negative consequences separate from a vascular disease. Finally, diabetes, and to a lesser extent hypertension, is associated with Alzheimer's disease. Most of the research on brain outcomes and hypertension and diabetes is based on clinical and epidemiologic observational studies. Interpretation of these studies is limited by the possibility that unmeasured or unknown confounding factors may bias the results. For this reason, randomized trials are needed to ascertain whether changing a risk factor is associated with a change in the outcome of interest. In addition, further research is needed to determine whether specific cognitive functions or brain areas are impaired by these disorders.

References

Amos, A. F., McCarty, D. J., & Zimmet, P. (1997). The rising global burden of diabetes and its complications: Estimates and projections to the year 2010. *Diabetic Medicine, 14*(Suppl 5), S1–S85.

Arvanitakis, Z., Schneider, J. A., Wilson, R. S., Li, Y., Arnold, S. E., Wang, Z., et al. (2006). Diabetes is related to cerebral infarction but not to AD pathology in older persons. *Neurology, 67*(11), 1960–1965.

Arvanitakis, Z., Wilson, R. S., Bienias, J. L., Evans, D. A., & Bennett, D. A. (2004). Diabetes mellitus and risk of Alzheimer disease and decline in cognitive function. *Archives of Neurology, 61*(5), 661–666.

Barber, R., Scheltens, P., Gholkar, A., Ballard, C., McKeith, I., Ince, P., et al. (1999). White matter lesions on magnetic resonance imaging in dementia with Lewy bodies, Alzheimer's disease, vascular dementia, and normal aging. *Journal of Neurology, Neurosurgery, and Psychiatry, 67*(1), 66–72.

Bertram, L., Blacker, D., Mullin, K., Keeney, D., Jones, J., Basu, S., et al. (2000). Evidence for genetic linkage of Alzheimer's disease to chromosome 10q. *Science, 290*(5500), 2302–2303.

Bonora, E., Willeit, J., Kiechl, S., Oberhollenzer, F., Egger, G., Bonadonna, R., et al. (1998). U-shaped and J-shaped relationships between serum insulin and coronary heart disease in the general population. The Bruneck Study. *Diabetes Care, 21*(2), 221–230.

Brands, A. M., Biessels, G. J., de Haan, E. H., Kappelle, L. J., & Kessels, R. P. (2005). The effects of type 1 diabetes on cognitive performance: A meta-analysis. *Diabetes Care, 28*(3), 726–735.

Brands, A. M., Kessels, R. P., Hoogma, R. P., Henselmans, J. M., van der Beek Boter, J. W., Kappelle, L. J., et al. (2006). Cognitive performance, psychological well-being, and brain magnetic resonance imaging in older patients with type 1 diabetes. *Diabetes, 55*(6), 1800–1806.

Coker, L. H., & Shumaker, S. A. (2003). Type 2 diabetes mellitus and cognition: An understudied issue in women's health. *Journal of Psychosomatic Research, 54*(2), 129–139.

Convit, A., Wolf, O. T., Tarshish, C., & de Leon, M. J. (2003). Reduced glucose tolerance is associated with poor memory performance and hippocampal atrophy among normal elderly. *Proceedings of the National Academy of Sciences of the United States of America, 100*(4), 2019–2022.

Cook, D. G., Leverenz, J. B., McMillan, P. J., Kulstad, J. J., Ericksen, S., Roth, R. A., et al. (2003). Reduced hippocampal insulin-degrading enzyme in late-onset Alzheimer's disease is associated with the apolipoprotein E-epsilon4 allele. *The American Journal of Pathology, 162*(1), 313–319.

Craft, S., & Watson, G. S. (2004). Insulin and neurodegenerative disease: Shared and specific mechanisms. *Lancet Neurology, 3*(3), 169–178.

Cukierman, T., Gerstein, H. C., & Williamson, J. D. (2005). Cognitive decline and dementia in diabetes – systematic overview of prospective observational studies. *Diabetologia, 48*(12), 2460–2469.

Cummings, J. L. (1993). Frontal-subcortical circuits and human behavior. *Archives of Neurology, 50*(8), 873–880.

Curb, J. D., Rodriguez, B. L., Abbott, R. D., Petrovitch, H., Ross, G. W., Masaki, K. H., et al. (1999). Longitudinal association of vascular and Alzheimer's dementias, diabetes, and glucose tolerance. *Neurology, 52*(5), 971–975.

DCCT. (1996). Effects of intensive diabetes therapy on neuropsychological function in adults in the diabetes control and complications trial. *Annals of Internal Medicine, 124*(4), 379–388.

DeCarli, C., Fletcher, E., Ramey, V., Harvey, D., & Jagust, W. J. (2005). Anatomical mapping of white matter hyperintensities (WMH): Exploring the relationships between periventricular WMH, deep WMH, and total WMH burden. *Stroke, 36*(1), 50–55.

den Heijer, T., Vermeer, S. E., van Dijk, E. J., Prins, N. D., Koudstaal, P. J., Hofman, A., et al. (2003). Type 2 diabetes and atrophy of medial temporal lobe structures on brain MRI. *Diabetologia, 46*(12), 1604–1610.

Donnan, G. A. (2002). Subcortical stroke. Oxford; New York, Oxford University Press.

Edbauer, D., Willem, M., Lammich, S., Steiner, H., & Haass, C. (2002). Insulin-degrading enzyme rapidly removes the beta-amyloid precursor protein intracellular domain (AICD). *The Journal of Biological Chemistry, 277*(16), 13389–13393.

Elias, M. F., Wolf, P. A., D'Agostino, R. B., Cobb, J., & White, L. R. (1993). Untreated blood pressure level is inversely related to cognitive functioning: The Framingham Study. *American Journal of Epidemiology, 138*(6), 353–364.

Elias, P. K., Elias, M. F., D'Agostino, R. B., Cupples, L. A., Wilson, P. W., Silbershatz, H., et al. (1997). NIDDM and blood pressure as risk factors for poor cognitive performance. The Framingham Study. *Diabetes Care, 20*(9), 1388–1395.

Elmquist, J. K., & Marcus, J. N. (2003). Rethinking the central causes of diabetes. *Nature Medicine, 9*(6), 645–647.

Fazekas, F., Kleinert, R., Offenbacher, H., Schmidt, R., Kleinert, G., Payer, F., et al. (1993). Pathologic correlates of incidental MRI white matter signal hyperintensities. *Neurology, 43*(9), 1683–1689.

Fields, L. E., Burt, V. L., Cutler, J. A., Hughes, J., Roccella, E. J., & Sorlie, P. (2004). The burden of adult hypertension in the United States 1999 to 2000: A rising tide. *Hypertension, 44*(4), 398–404.

Folstein, M. F., Folstein, S. E., & McHugh, P. R. (1975). Mini-mental state. A practical method for grading the cognitive state of patients for the clinician. *Journal of Psychiatric Research, 12*(3), 189–198.

Fontbonne, A., Berr, C., Ducimetiere, P., & Alperovitch, A. (2001). Changes in cognitive abilities over a 4-year period are unfavorably affected in elderly diabetic subjects: Results of the Epidemiology of Vascular Aging Study. *Diabetes Care, 24*(2), 366–370.

Forrester, J. S. (2004). Common ancestors: Chronic progressive diseases have the same pathogenesis. *Clinical Cardiology, 27*(4), 186–190.

Gianaros, P. J., Greer, P. J., Ryan, C. M., & Jennings, J. R. (2006). Higher blood pressure predicts lower regional grey matter volume: Consequences on short-term information processing. Neuroimage, *31*(2), 754–765.

Gispen, W. H., & Biessels, G. J. (2000). Cognition and synaptic plasticity in diabetes mellitus. *Trends in Neurosciences, 23*(11), 542–549.

Goldstein, I. B., Bartzokis, G., Guthrie, D., & Shapiro, D. (2005). Ambulatory blood pressure and the brain: A 5-year follow-up. [see comment]. *Neurology, 64*(11), 1846–1852.

Gregg, E. W., Yaffe, K., Cauley, J. A., Rolka, D. B., Blackwell, T. L., Narayan, K. M., et al. (2000). Is diabetes associated with cognitive impairment and cognitive decline among older women? Study of Osteoporotic Fractures Research Group. *Archives of Internal Medicine, 160*(2), 174–180.

Grodstein, F., Chen, J., Wilson, R. S., Manson, J. E., & Nurses' Health, S. (2001). Type 2 diabetes and cognitive function in community-dwelling elderly women. *Diabetes Care, 24*(6), 1060–1065.

Grossman, H. (2003). Does diabetes protect or provoke Alzheimer's disease? Insights into the pathobiology and future treatment of Alzheimer's disease. *CNS Spectrums, 8*(11), 815–823.

Guo, Z., Fratiglioni, L., Winblad, B., & Viitanen, M. (1997). Blood pressure and performance on the Mini-Mental State Examination in the very old. Cross-sectional and longitudinal data from the Kungsholmen Project. *American Journal of Epidemiology, 145*(12), 1106–1113.

Haan, M. N., Shemanski, L., Jagust, W. J., Manolio, T. A., & Kuller, L. (1999). The role of APOE epsilon4 in modulating effects of other risk factors for cognitive decline in elderly persons. *JAMA, 282*(1), 40–46.

Hachinski, V. C., Potter, P., & Merskey, H. (1987). Leuko-araiosis. *Archives of Neurology, 44*(1), 21–23.

Halter, J. B. (1996). Alzheimer's disease and non-insulin-dependent diabetes mellitus: Common features do not make common bedfellows. *Journal of the American Geriatrics Society, 44*(8), 992–993.

Harris, M. I., Flegal, K. M., Cowie, C. C., Eberhardt, M. S., Goldstein, D. E., Little, R. R., et al. (1998). (1998). Prevalence of diabetes, impaired fasting glucose, and impaired glucose tolerance in U.S. adults. The Third National Health and Nutrition Examination Survey, 1988–1994. *Diabetes Care, 21*(4), 518–524.

Hofman, A., Ott, A., Breteler, M. M., Bots, M. L., Slooter, A. J., van Harskamp, F., et al. (1997). Atherosclerosis, apolipoprotein E, and prevalence of dementia and Alzheimer's disease in the Rotterdam Study.[comment]. *Lancet, 349*(9046), 151–154.

Hong, M., & Lee, V. M. (1997). Insulin and insulin-like growth factor-1 regulate tau phosphorylation in cultured human neurons. *The Journal of Biological Chemistry, 272*(31), 19547–19553.

Hoyer, S. (1998). Is sporadic Alzheimer disease the brain type of non-insulin dependent diabetes mellitus? A challenging hypothesis. *Journal of Neural Transmission, 105*(4–5), 415–422.

Irie, F., Fitzpatrick, A. L., Lopez, O. L., Kuller, L. H., Peila, R., Newman, A. B., Launer, L. J. (2008). Enhanced risk for Alzheimer disease in persons with type 2 diabetes and APOE epsilon4: the Cardiovascular Health Study Cognition Study. Arch Neurol, 65, 89–93.

Isaka, Y., Okamoto, M., Ashida, K., & Imaizumi, M. (1994). Decreased cerebrovascular dilatory capacity in subjects with asymptomatic periventricular hyperintensities. *Stroke, 25*(2), 375–381.

Kalmijn, S., Feskens, E. J., Launer, L. J., & Kromhout, D. (1996). Cerebrovascular disease, the apolipoprotein e4 allele, and cognitive decline in a community-based study of elderly men. *Stroke, 27*(12), 2230–235.

Kalmijn, S., Feskens, E. J., Launer, L. J., Stijnen, T., & Kromhout, D. (1995). Glucose intolerance, hyperinsulinaemia and cognitive function in a general population of elderly men. *Diabetologia, 38*(9), 1096–1102.

Kanaya, A. M., Barrett-Connor, E., Gildengorin, G., & Yaffe, K. (2004). Change in cognitive function by glucose tolerance status in older adults: A 4-year prospective study of the Rancho Bernardo study cohort. *Archives of Internal Medicine, 164*(12), 1327–1333.

Kato, H., Sugawara, Y., Ito, H., & Kogure, K. (1990). White matter lucencies in multi-infarct dementia: A somatosensory evoked potentials and CT study. *Acta Neurologica Scandinavica, 81*(2), 181–183.

Kearney, P. M., Whelton, M., Reynolds, K., Muntner, P., Whelton, P. K., & He, J. (2005). Global burden of hypertension: Analysis of worldwide data. *The Lancet, 365*(9455), 217–223.

Kilander, L., Nyman, H., Boberg, M., Hansson, L., & Lithell, H. (1998). Hypertension is related to cognitive impairment: A 20-year follow-up of 999 men. *Hypertension, 31*(3), 780–786.

Kivipelto, M., Helkala, E. L., Laakso, M. P., Hänninen, T., Hallikainen, M., Alhainen, K., et al. (2001). Midlife vascular risk factors and Alzheimer's disease in later life: longitudinal, population based study. BMJ. 322,1447?51.

Klein, J. P., & Waxman, S. G. (2003). The brain in diabetes: Molecular changes in neurons and their implications for end-organ damage. *Lancet Neurology, 2*(9), 548–554.

Knopman, D. S., Mosley, T. H., Catellier, D. J., & Sharrett, A. R. (2005). Cardiovascular risk factors and cerebral atrophy in a middle-aged cohort. *Neurology, 65*(6), 876–881.

Korf, E. S., White, L. R., Scheltens, P., & Launer, L. J. (2006). Brain aging in very old men with type 2 diabetes: The Honolulu-Asia Aging Study. *Diabetes Care, 29*(10), 2268–2274.

Langan, S. J., Deary, I. J., Hepburn, D. A., & Frier, B. M. (1991). Cumulative cognitive impairment following recurrent severe hypoglycaemia in adult patients with insulin-treated diabetes mellitus. *Diabetologia, 34*(5), 337–344.

Launer, L. J., Andersen, K., Dewey, M. E., Letenneur, L., Ott, A., Amaducci, L. A., et al. (1999). Rates and risk factors for dementia and Alzheimer's disease: Results from EURODEM pooled analyses. EURODEM Incidence Research Group and Work Groups. European Studies of Dementia. *Neurology, 52*(1), 78–84.

Launer, L. J., Ross, G. W., Petrovitch, H., Masaki, K., Foley, D., White, L. R., et al. (2000). Midlife blood pressure and dementia: The Honolulu-Asia Aging Study. *Neurobiology of Aging, 21*(1), 49–55.

Leibson, C. L., Rocca, W. A., Hanson, V. A., Cha, R., Kokmen, E., O'Brien, P. C., et al. (1997). Risk of dementia among persons with diabetes mellitus: A population-based cohort study. *American Journal of Epidemiology, 145*(4), 301–308.

Lobo, A., Launer, L. J., Fratiglioni, L., Andersen, K., Di Carlo, A., Breteler, M. M., et al. (2000). Prevalence of dementia and major subtypes in Europe: A collaborative study of population-based cohorts. Neurologic Diseases in the Elderly Research Group. *Neurology, 54*(11 Suppl 5), S4–S9.

Logroscino, G., Kang, J. H., & Grodstein, F. (2004). Prospective study of type 2 diabetes and cognitive decline in women aged 70–81 years. *BMJ, 328*(7439), 6.

Longstreth, W. T., Jr., Arnold, A. M., Manolio, T. A., Burke, G. L., Bryan, N., Jungreis, C. A., et al. (2000). Clinical correlates of ventricular and sulcal size on cranial magnetic resonance imaging of 3,301 elderly people. The Cardiovascular Health Study. Collaborative Research Group. *Neuroepidemiology, 19*(1), 30–42.

Luchsinger, J. A., Tang, M. X., Stern, Y., Shea, S., & Mayeux, R. (2001). Diabetes mellitus and risk of Alzheimer's disease and dementia with stroke in a multiethnic cohort. *American Journal of Epidemiology, 154*(7), 635–641.

MacMahon, S., Peto, R., Cutler, J., Collins, R., Sorlie, P., Neaton, J., et al. (1990). Blood pressure, stroke, and coronary heart disease. Part 1, Prolonged differences in blood pressure: Prospective observational studies corrected for the regression dilution bias. *Lancet, 335*(8692), 765–774.

Magarinos, A. M., & McEwen, B. S. (2000). Experimental diabetes in rats causes hippocampal dendritic and synaptic reorganization and increased glucocorticoid reactivity to stress. *Proceedings of the National Academy of Sciences of the United States of America, 97*(20), 11056–11061.

McEwen, B. S., Magarinos, A. M., & Reagan, L. P. (2002). Studies of hormone action in the hippocampal formation: Possible relevance to depression and diabetes. *Journal of Psychosomatic Research, 53*(4), 883–890.

McGuinness, B., Todd, S., Passmore, P., & Bullock, R. (2006). Blood pressure lowering on development of cognitive impairment and dementia in patients without apparent prior cardiovascular disease. Cochrane Database Syst Rev, 19(2), CD004034.

Moore, T. L., Killiany, R. J., Rosene, D. L., Prusty, S., Hollander, W., & Moss, M. B. (2002). Impairment of executive function induced by hypertension in the rhesus monkey (Macaca mulatta). *Behavioral Neuroscience, 116*(3), 387–396.

Morris, M. C., Scherr, P. A., Hebert, L. E., Glynn, R. J., Bennett, D. A., & Evans, D. A. (2001). Association of incident Alzheimer disease and blood pressure measured from 13 years before to 2 years after diagnosis in a large community study. *Archives of Neurology, 58*(10), 1640–1646.

Murray, M. D., Lane, K. A., Gao, S., Evans, R. M., Unverzagt, F. W., Hall, K. S., et al. (2002). Preservation of cognitive function With antihypertensive medications: A longitudinal analysis of a community-based sample of African Americans. *Archives Of Internal Medicine, 162*(18), 2090–2096.

Musselman, D. L., Betan, E., Larsen, H., & Phillips, L. S. (2003). Relationship of depression to diabetes types 1 and 2: epidemiology, biology, and treatment. *Biological Psychiatry, 54*(3), 317–329.

Ott, A., Stolk, R. P., van Harskamp, F., Pols, H. A., Hofman, A., & Breteler, M. M. (1999). Diabetes mellitus and the risk of dementia: The Rotterdam Study. *Neurology, 53*(9), 1937–1942.

Panza, F., D'Introno, A., Colacicco, A. M., Capurso, C., Del Parigi, A., Caselli, R. J., et al. (2005). Current epidemiology of mild cognitive impairment and other predementia syndromes. *The American Journal of Geriatric Psychiatry, 13*(8), 633–644.

Peila, R., Rodriguez, B. L., & Launer, L. J. (2002). Type 2 diabetes, APOE gene, and the risk for dementia and related pathologies: The Honolulu-Asia Aging Study. *Diabetes, 51*(4), 1256–1262.

Perez, A., Morelli, L., Cresto, J. C., & Castano, E. M. (2000). Degradation of soluble amyloid beta-peptides 1–40, 1–42, and the Dutch variant 1–40Q by insulin degrading enzyme from Alzheimer disease and control brains. *Neurochemical Research, 25*(2), 247–255.

Perros, P., Deary, I. J., Sellar, R. J., Best, J. J., & Frier, B. M. (1997). Brain abnormalities demonstrated by magnetic resonance imaging in adult IDDM patients with and without a history of recurrent severe hypoglycemia. *Diabetes Care, 20*(6), 1013–1018.

Petrovitch, H., White, L. R., Izmirilian, G., Ross, G. W., Havlik, R. J., Markesbery, W., et al. (2000). Midlife blood pressure and neuritic plaques, neurofibrillary tangles, and brain weight at death: The HAAS. Honolulu-Asia Aging Study. *Neurobiology of Aging, 21*(1), 57–62.

Philippe, P. (2002). Diabetes trends in Europe. *Diabetes/Metabolism Research and Reviews, 18*(S3), S3-S8.

Poirier, J., & Derouesne, C. (1984). Cerebral lacunae. A proposed new classification. *Clinical Neuropathology*, *3*(6), 266.

Posner, H. B., Tang, M. X., Luchsinger, J., Lantigua, R., Stern, Y., & Mayeux, R. (2002). The relationship of hypertension in the elderly to AD, vascular dementia, and cognitive function. *Neurology*, *58*(8), 1175–1181.

Prins, N. D., van Dijk, E. J., den Heijer, T., Vermeer, S. E., Jolles, J., Koudstaal, P. J., et al. (2005). Cerebral small-vessel disease and decline in information processing speed, executive function and memory. *Brain*, *128*(9), 2034–2041.

Qiu, W. Q., Walsh, D. M., Ye, Z., Vekrellis, K., Zhang, J., Podlisny, M. B., et al. (1998). Insulin-degrading enzyme regulates extracellular levels of amyloid beta-protein by degradation. *The Journal Of Biological Chemistry*, *273*(49), 32730–32738.

Resnick, H. E., Harris, M. I., Brock, D. B., & Harris, T. B. (2000). American Diabetes Association diabetes diagnostic criteria, advancing age, and cardiovascular disease risk profiles: Results from the Third National Health and Nutrition Examination Survey. *Diabetes Care*, *23*(2), 176–180.

Sacco, R. L., Anand, K., Lee, H. S., Boden-Albala, B., Stabler, S., Allen, R., et al. (2004). Homocysteine and the risk of ischemic stroke in a triethnic cohort: The Northern Manhattan Study. *Stroke*, *35*(10), 2263–2269.

Sachdev, P. S., Wen, W., Christensen, H., & Jorm, A. F. (2005). White matter hyperintensities are related to physical disability and poor motor function. *Journal of Neurology, Neurosurgery, and Psychiatry*, *76*(3),. 362–367.

Schmidt, R., Launer, L. J., Nilsson, L.-G., Pajak, A., Sans, S., Berger, K., et al. (2004).. Magnetic resonance imaging of the brain in diabetes: The Cardiovascular Determinants of Dementia (CASCADE) Study. *Diabetes*, *53*(3), 687–692.

Schwartz, M. W., Bergman, R. N., Kahn, S. E., Taborsky, G. J., Jr., Fisher, L. D., Sipols, A. J., et al. (1991). Evidence for entry of plasma insulin into cerebrospinal fluid through an intermediate compartment in dogs. Quantitative aspects and implications for transport. The Journal of Clinical Investigation, 88(4), 1272–1281.

Schwartz, M. W., Figlewicz, D. P., Baskin, D. G., Woods, S. C., & Porte, D., Jr. (1992). Insulin in the brain: A hormonal regulator of energy balance. *Endocrine Reviews*, *13*(3), 387–414.

Shibata, K., Osawa, M., & Iwata, M. (2000). Visual evoked potentials in cerebral white matter hyperintensity on MRI. *Acta Neurologica Scandinavica*, *102*(4), 230–235.

Sinclair, A. J., Girling, A. J., & Bayer, A. J. (2000). Cognitive dysfunction in older subjects with diabetes mellitus: Impact on diabetes self-management and use of care services. All Wales Research into

Elderly (AWARE) Study. *Diabetes Research and Clinical Practice*, *50*(3), 203–212.

Singh, P., Heera, P. K., & Kaur, G. (2003). Expression of neuronal plasticity markers in hypoglycemia induced brain injury. *Molecular And Cellular Biochemistry*, *247*(1–2), 69–74.

Singh, R., Barden, A., Mori, T., & Beilin, L. (2001). Advanced glycation end-products: A review. *Diabetologia*, *44*(2), 129–146.

Skoog, I., Lernfelt, B., Landahl, S., Palmertz, B., Andreasson, L. A., Nilsson, L., et al. (1996). 15-year longitudinal study of blood pressure and dementia. *Lancet*, *347*(9009), 1141–1145.

Stewart, R., & Liolitsa, D. (1999). Type 2 diabetes mellitus, cognitive impairment and dementia. *Diabetic Medicine*, *16*(2), 93–112.

Strachan, M. W., Deary, I. J., Ewing, F. M., & Frier, B. M. (1997). Is type II diabetes associated with an increased risk of cognitive dysfunction? A critical review of published studies. *Diabetes Care*, *20*(3), 438–445.

Tanzi, R. E., Moir, R. D., & Wagner, S. L. (2004). Clearance of Alzheimer's Abeta peptide: The many roads to perdition. *Neuron*, *43*(5), 605–608.

Teng, E. L., & Chui, H. C. (1987). The modified mini-mental state (3MS) examination. Journal of Clinical Psychiatry, 48(8), 314–318.

Tullberg, M., Fletcher, E., DeCarli, C., Mungas, D., Reed, B. R., Harvey, D. J., et al. (2004).. White matter lesions impair frontal lobe function regardless of their location. *Neurology*, 246–53, 2004 Jul 27.

Vanhanen, M., Koivisto, K., Kuusisto, J., Mykkanen, L., Helkala, E. L., Hanninen, T., et al. (1998). Cognitive function in an elderly population with persistent impaired glucose tolerance. *Diabetes Care*, *21*(3), 398–402.

Vermeer, S. E., Prins, N. D., den Heijer, T., Hofman, A., Koudstaal, P. J., & Breteler, M. M. (2003). Silent brain infarcts and the risk of dementia and cognitive decline. *New England Journal of Medicine*, *348*(13), 1215–1222.

Wiseman, R. M., Saxby, B. K., Burton, E. J., Barber, R., Ford, G. A., & O'Brien, J. T. (2004). Hippocampal atrophy, whole brain volume, and white matter lesions in older hypertensive subjects. *Neurology*, *63*(10), 1892–1897.

Wu, J. H., Haan, M. N., Liang, J., Ghosh, D., Gonzalez, H. M., & Herman, W. H. (2003). Impact of antidiabetic medications on physical and cognitive functioning of older Mexican Americans with diabetes mellitus: A population-based cohort study. *Annals of Epidemiology*, *13*(5), 369–376.

Yaffe, K., Blackwell, T., Kanaya, A. M., Davidowitz, N., Barrett-Connor, E., & Krueger, K. (2004). Diabetes, impaired fasting glucose, and development of cognitive impairment in older women. *Neurology*, *63*(4), 658–663.

Chapter 15
Neurovascular Consequences of Systemic Disease – Collagen Vascular Disease

Stephen L. Holliday and Robin L. Brey

Introduction

The neurovascular consequences of collagen vascular diseases are due in large part to two major causes: atherosclerosis and prothrombotic effects of antiphospholipid (aPL) antibodies. Patients with systemic lupus erythematosis (SLE) and rheumatoid arthritis (RA) can both develop premature atherosclerosis, and the study of patients with these disorders has been quite informative in understanding the relationship between inflammation, atherosclerosis, and cardio- and cerebrovascular disease outcomes (Manzi et al. 1997; Abou-Raya & Abou-Raya, 2006; Rhew & Ramsey-Goldman, 2006). In this chapter, we will discuss the evidence for the role of inflammation-induced atherosclerosis and aPL antibodies in neurovascular consequences of SLE, a prototypic collagen vascular disease.

Systemic lupus erythematosis is an autoimmune inflammatory disorder affecting multiple organ systems, which affects women nine times more frequently than men (Ward, 2004). The prevalence is approximately 130/100,000 in the United States, with African Americans, Hispanics, and Asians more frequently affected than non-Hispanic Whites (Danchenko, Satia, &

Anthony, 2006). The nervous system is commonly affected in people with SLE (Ainiala, Loukkola, Peltola, Korpela, & Hietaharju, 2001; Brey, Holliday et al., 2002). The American College of Rheumatology ((ACR) established case definitions for 19 CNS and PNS syndromes observed in SLE patients, which collectively are referred to as neuropsychiatric systemic lupus erythematosus (NPSLE) syndromes (Table 1) (The American College of Rheumatology nomenclature and case definitions for neuropsychiatric lupus syndromes, 1999).

Atherosclerosis

Much attention has recently focused on atherosclerosis as an inflammatory disease even in people without collagen vascular diseases (del Zoppo & Hallenbeck, 2000; Stoll & Bendszus, 2006). The earliest stage involves endothelial injury with subsequent adhesion molecule upregulation. This leads to recruitment of activated T-lymphocytes to the site of injury with secretion of proinflammatory cytokines leading to differentiation of monocytes into macrophages. The presence of these cytokines also causes smooth muscle cells to produce collagen and elastin, contributing to fibrous cap formation. Activated macrophages express scavenger receptors for oxidized LDL and become foam cells constituting the lipid core. They also produce collagenases, which

R.L. Brey (✉)
University of Texas Health Science Center at San Antonio, Department of Medicine/Neurology, 7703 Floyd Curl Drive, San Antonio, TX 78228-3900, USA
e-mail: brey@uthscsa.edu

J.R. Festa, R.M. Lazar (eds.), *Neurovascular Neuropsychology*, DOI 10.1007/978-0-387-70715-0_15, © Springer Science+Business Media, LLC 2009

Table 1 Neuropsychiatric manifestations of systemic lupus erythematosus (NPSLE)

NPSLE ASSOCIATED WITH CENTRAL NERVOUS SYSTEM
- Aseptic Meningitis
- Cerebrovascular disease

Stroke

Transient Ischemic Attack

Cerebral Venous Sinus Thrombosis
- Cognitive Disorders

Delirium (Acute confusional state)

Dementia

Mild Cognitive Disorders
- Demyelinating syndrome
- Headaches

Tension Headaches

Migraine Headaches
- Movement disorders (Chorea)
- Psychiatric Disorders

Psychosis

Mood Disorders

Anxiety Disorder
- Seizure Disorders
- Transverse Myelopathy

NPSLE ASSOCIATED WITH PERIPHERAL NERVOUS SYSTEM
- Autonomic Neuropathy
- Myasthenia Gravis
- Peripheral neuropathy
- Sensorineural Hearing Loss

Sudden Onset

Progressive
- Cranial neuropathy

make the fibrous cap fragile and, along with endothelial cells, produce tissue factor which stimulate thrombosis (Stoll & Bendszus, 2006).

We now realize that atherosclerosis is not an irreversible "plumbing problem" caused by slowly progressive narrowing of the arterial lumen, but rather, it is a dynamic process (Stoll & Bendszus, 2006). Both cardiovascular and cerebrovascular diseases are more related to plaque rupture than passive thickening of the vessel wall. Thus, the stability of the atherosclerotic plaque appears to be a key factor in whether or not atherosclerotic plaques become symptomatic (Libby, 2001). Plaque stability is greatly influenced by inflammatory mediators. In an unstable plaque, T-lymphocytes produce

γ-interferon, which inhibits production of structural molecules of the extracellular matric (collagen and elastin) and weakens the fibrous cap (Hallenbeck, Hansson, & Becker, 2005). Clinical data suggest that vulnerable plaques may not show substantial luminal narrowing detectable by angiography (Libby, 2001). This has lead to the search for new biomarkers that predict stroke and myocardial infarction (MI) that may better reflect plaque vulnerability than does anatomic vascular imaging (Wu & Wu, 2006).

Antiphospholipid Antibodies

The antiphospholipid antibody syndrome (APS) is associated with thrombosis; recurrent, unexplained fetal loss; thrombocytopenia; and a variety of neurological manifestations including stroke and cognitive dysfunction (Hughes, 1983). The diagnostic criteria for APS includes arterial or venous thrombosis leading to tissue ischemia or recurrent fetal loss in the presence of aPL antibodies of moderate to high titer that are present on at least two occasions at least 12 weeks apart (Miyakis et al., 2006). There are two types of tests that are commonly used to detect aPL: (1) the presence of a prolongation of phospholipid dependent coagulation tests (called "lupus anticoagulant"); and (2) detection of antibodies to negatively charged phospholipids using a solid phase assay. APS is classified as secondary if it occurs in a patient with SLE, and primary in the absence of SLE (Miyakis et al., 2006).

Although cardiolipin was the initial phospholipid used in antibody testing, there is considerable cross-reactivity to other negatively-charged phospholipids. In 1990, three groups independently reported that beta-2-glycoprotein-1 (β_2GP-1) was needed in the assay system in order to detect most, but not all aPL antibodies (Allegri et al., 1990; Galli et al., 1990; Matsuura, Igarashi, Fujimoto, Ichikawa, & Koike, 1990). Proteins such as prothrombin, annexin V, protein C, protein S, low molecular weight kininogens, and factor XI have also been shown to bind phospholipids, but β_2GP-1 is by far the most common and well characterized protein with this ability (Miyakis, Giannakopoulos, & Krilis, 2004). This suggests that a family of autoantibodies directed toward negatively charged phospholipids or protein-phospholipid complexes including β_2GP-1 could be responsible for APS's clinical manifestations. In addition to the potential for aPL antibodies to lead to thrombotic manifestations, these antibodies have also been linked to atherosclerosis (Matsuura et al., 1990).

Neuropathology/Pathophysiology

The pathogenic etiologies of SLE-related cerebrovascular disease and cognitive dysfunction are likely to be multifactorial and may involve autoantibody production, microangiopathy, and intrathecal production of proinflammatory cytokines and atherosclerosis (Hanly, 2001). Histopathologic studies reveal a wide range of brain abnormalities caused by multifocal microinfarcts, cortical atrophy, gross infarcts, hemorrhage, ischemic demyelination, and patchy multiple-sclerosis-like demyelination in people with SLE (Hanly, Walsh, & Sangalang, 1992). A microvasculopathy is seen which was formerly attributed to deposition of immune complexes but now is suspected to arise from activation of complement, and it appears to be the most common microscopic brain findings in SLE (Belmont, Abramson, & Lie, 1996). However, all of these are non-specific findings since patients without overt NPSLE manifestations also show these changes (Hanly, 2001), and the brain can be pathologically normal in a patient with NPSLE manifestations (Hanly, Walsh et al., 1992).

Vasculopathy in Systemic *Lupus Erythematosis*

Neuropathologic studies in the brains of SLE patients have frequently found a small vessel vasculopathy consisting of proliferative changes of the intima (vascular lining), vascular thickening, and collections of lymphocytes in the space around blood vessels. This small vessel vasculopathy has been seen both in SLE patients with only psychiatric symptoms as well as those with focal nervous system manifestations (Hanly, Walsh et al., 1992). Consistent with these small vessel changes, SPECT, and MR spectroscopy studies suggest that both cerebral atrophy and cognitive dysfunction in SLE patients may be related to chronic diffuse cerebral ischemia (Gonzalez-Crespo et al., 1995; Karassa et al., 2000; Sibbitt, Sibbitt, & Brooks, 1999).

Cytokines

Cytokines appear to have regulatory roles mediating SLE-disease activity and inflammation in target organs including brain (Kelley & Wuthrich, 1999; Shovman, Gilburd, & Shoenfeld, 2006). While many studies suggest that cytokine levels in the CSF may reflect SLE-mediated CNS activity (Alcocer-Varela, Aleman-Hoey, & Alarcon-Segovia, 1992; Jara, Irigoyen, Ortiz, Zazueta, Brarr, & Espinosa, 1998), serum levels (which are easier to measure) also appear to be important in SLE patients with neuropsychiatric manifestations (Kozora, Laudenslager, Lemieux, & West, 2001). In addition, cytokine stimulation of peripheral nerves and sensory receptors also leads to large changes in neural activity, and physiological and behavioral responses in the CNS. The synthesis and release of IL-1α, IL-6, and TNF-α play a prominent role in the mediation of these phenomena (Maier, Goehler, Fleshner, & Watkins, 1998). These pro-inflammatory cytokines do not easily cross the blood-brain barrier, so their effects on neural events are postulated to occur via entry into the CNS using specific transport systems or in areas where the blood-brain barrier is more permeable (e.g., circumventricular organs), or by binding to other receptors on endothelial cells of brain vasculature and stimulating them to release inflammatory mediators into brain parenchyma. Another reasonable alternative is that cytokines act by activating afferent neurons in a paracrine action at the site where they are released, leading to neural events within the CNS in the location where these peripheral afferent neurons terminate. Experimental evidence supports this hypothesis, particularly in the case of the vagus nerve (Maier et al., 1998). In addition, animal models have demonstrated induction of diverse manifestations of "illness behavior" such as fever, fatigue/malaise, decreased pain thresholds, and hippocampal-dependent memory impairment by these mechanisms (Maier et al., 1998).

Adhesion Molecules

Other processes leading to immune-mediated brain dysfunction in SLE probably involve abnormal endothelial-white blood cell interactions that allow proteins or cells access to the central nervous system (CNS). The expression of adhesion proteins on endothelial cells appears to be up-regulated in SLE and facilitates lymphocyte entry in CNS disease (Zaccagni, Fried, Cornell, Padilla, & Brey, 2004). Shedding of the active form of these molecules occurs and soluble levels can be measured in both serum and CSF (Baraczka et al., 1999).Soluble serum levels of ICAM-1 increase with systemic disease activity in patients with SLE (Matsuda, Gohchi, Gotoh, Tsukamoto, & Saitoh, 1994; Sfikakis, Charalambopoulos, Vayiopoulos, Oglesby, Sfikakis, & Tsokso, 1994; Zaccagni et al., 2004) and normalize with remission (Spronk, Bootsma, Huitema, Limburg, & Kallenberg, 1994). In one study, only combined elevation of three adhesion molecules (sCD14, sICAM-1, and sE-selectin) correlated with SLE prognosis (Egerer, Feist, Rohr, Pruss, Burmester, & Dorner, 2000).

Antiphospholipid Antibodies and NPSLE

While the stimulus for aPL production is uncertain, some aPL antibodies may arise due to infection by common viruses and bacteria (A. E. Gharavi & Pierangeli, 1998). Gharavi and colleagues demonstrated that pathogenic aPL and anti-β_2GP-1 antibody production can be induced following immunization with mutant forms of β_2GP-1 containing the aPL binding site alone (A. E. Gharavi, Pierangeli, Colden, Stanfield, Liu, Espinola, & Harris, 1999). These were found to have sequence homology with several common viruses. Normal mice immunized with these viral protein fragments developed aPL antibodies and suffered intrauterine fetal death, spinal cord infarction, and thrombosis (E. E. Gharavi et al., 1999), suggesting that infection may well be the trigger for pathogenic aPL antibody production (A. E. Gharavi & Pierangeli, 1998).

A variety of effects on platelets, coagulation proteins and endothelial cells, including tissue factor up-regulation, have been ascribed to aPL antibodies, making them not only serological markers for APS, but direct contributors to the development of thrombosis and other NPSLE manifestations. There is also evidence that aPL antibody binding to phospholipid complexes on various cells, including platelets and vascular endothelium, also results in their activation through the Fc-gamma receptor (Meroni et al., 1998). Campbell has demonstrated the induction of a dose-dependent increase in the activation and aggregation of human platelets using aPL antibodies from patients with APS (Campbell, Pierangeli, Wellhausen, & Harris, 1995). Evidence also suggests that β_2GP-1 may be involved in lipid metabolism and serve as a growth factor for vascular endothelial cells (Meroni et al., 1998). The majority of evidence favors a prothrombotic mechanism that amplifies thrombosis in certain settings. Pierangeli and Harris demonstrated larger clot size with a longer time to dissolution in mice treated with human aPL antibody compared to control IgG using a pinch clamp injury model (Pierangeli & Harris, 1994). Taken together, these studies provide converging evidence that antibodies to phospholipids and phospholipid-binding proteins like β_2GP-1 can cause thrombosis and other antibody-mediated clinical manifestations such as stroke. As will be discussed more fully below, multiple studies have also shown an association of aPL antibodies with cognitive dysfunction in SLE in the absence of thrombosis, however, the mechanism for this is less clear.

Characteristic Neurobehavioral Syndromes in SLE

Systemic lupus erythematosis is a disease with a fluctuating course and NPSLE manifestations can occur as a single or multiple events at any time during the course of the disease, even during periods in which no non-nervous system SLE disease activity is detected (Rivest et al., 2000; Sibbitt et al., 1999). Approximately 40% of the NPSLE manifestations develop before the onset of SLE or at the time of diagnosis and 63% within the first year after diagnosis (Rivest et al., 2000).

Estimates of the prevalence of NPSLE have ranged from 14% to over 80% (The American College of Rheumatology Nomenclature and Case Definitions for Neuropsychiatric Lupus Syndromes, 1999; Brey, Holliday et al., 2002; Costallat, Bertolo, & Appenzeller, 2001; Hanly, Walsh et al., 1992; Hanly, 2001), and most are based on research conducted before the introduction of the ACR case definitions for NPSLE. At least three studies (Ainiala et al., 2001; Brey, Holliday et al., 2002; Costallat et al., 2001) have reported prevalence of NPSLE based on the ACR 1999 case definitions. The three detected the presence of 14–17 of the 19 syndromes described by the ACR and report identical prevalence of cranial neuropathy (1.5%) and chorea (1%). These studies also report very similar prevalence of five other syndromes: cerebrovascular disease

(2%), total spectrum of headache (56–61%), total spectrum of mood disturbances (69–74%), psychosis (5%), and total range of cognitive disorders (75–80%). Agreement on the prevalence of cognitive, mood, and psychotic manifestations is high in these studies and assessment was based on standardized examination definitions/instruments. This is a significant methodological improvement, as difficulty in defining psychiatric abnormalities and cognitive dysfunction is likely to be a source of discrepant prevalence rates of NPSLE across studies.

In this section, we will consider two NPSLE neurobehavioral syndromes thought to have a potential neurovascular etiology: cerebrovascular disease and cognitive dysfunction.

Cerebrovascular Disease

Cerebrovascular disease is defined as neurological deficits due to arterial insufficiency or occlusion, venous occlusive disease, or hemorrhage with usually focal deficits that may be multifocal in recurrent disease. Cerebral ischemic events may occur early in the course of SLE, or may precede the diagnosis, providing a diagnostic clue of underlying SLE in young patients with stroke that would be otherwise unsuspected (Haas, 1982). The frequency of cerebrovascular disease as a whole has been reported as ranging from 5.3% (Kovacs, Urowitz, & Gladman, 1993) to 19% (Mok, Lau, & Wong, 2001).

Cerebrovascular Disease Related to Atherosclerosis in SLE Patients

Cardio- and cerebrovascular disease is an important clinical problem in people with SLE. Urowitz and colleagues highlighted this in their landmark study in 1976 that showed a bimodal mortality curve over time; early deaths were due to systemic SLE activity or infection and late deaths were due to vascular disease (Urowitz, Bookman, Koehler, Gordon, & Ogryzlo, 1976). More recent studies show that the risk of stroke is increase 6–10-fold in SLE patients as compared to age-matched controls and that stroke is the cause in 15% of SLE deaths (Ward, 1999). Manzi and colleagues found that the risk for MI was increased 50-fold in young women with SLE compared to age-matched women without SLE (Manzi et al., 1997). Using the California Hospital Discharge Database, Ward showed that the risk of stroke is increased 10-fold in women with SLE aged 18–44 years as compared to age-matched controls but equivalent to controls in older women (Ward, 1999).

In an attempt to identify the reason for this increased risk of cardic- and cerebrovascular disease, Esdaile and colleagues studied 263 SLE patients over nearly 9 years for the development of incident MIs and strokes. After controlling for traditional vascular risk factors, they still found a 10-fold increased risk for non-fatal MI and a 7.0-fold increased risk for stroke (Esdaile et al., 2001). This finding that significant risk for vascular events remains unexplained by traditional vascular risk factors has been replicated in several other studies and suggests that some factor(s) related to SLE itself may explain this excess risk. In a multiethnic SLE cohort study, baseline independent predictors of vascular events included the number of traditional vascular risk factors, older age, current smoking status, and abnormally high C-reactive protein levels and aPL antibodies, supporting the idea that inflammation and autoimmunity are important factors underlying vascular disease risk in SLE (Ho et al., 2005). Further, Roman and colleagues reported that the prevalence of carotid atherosclerotic plaque was significantly higher in SLE patients as compared to age-matched controls in the fourth through sixth decades of life. Independent risks for the presence of atherosclerosis in this study included age, hypertension, diabetes, cigarette smoking, high cholesterol, and SLE status. This study also found that SLE patients without atherosclerosis had significantly higher use of prednisone, hydroxychloroquine, and cyclophosphamide than those with plaque, suggesting that aggressive treatment of SLE disease (and possibly more effectively decreasing inflammation) is protective against the development of atherosclerosis (Roman et al., 2003).

Cerebrovascular Disease Related to aPL Antibodies in SLE Patients

Antiphospholipid antibodies are well-established as risk factors in a first ischemic stroke, but their role in recurrent stroke is less clear (Table 2). All (Brey, Hart, Sherman, & Tegeler, 1990; Brey & Stallworth et al., 2002; Nencini, Baruffi, Abbate, Massai, Amaducci, & Inzitari, 1992; Singh, Gaiha, Shome, Gupta, & Anuradha, 2001; Toschi, et.al. 1998) but one (Blohorn et al., 2002) of the case-control and prospective studies that evaluated aPL as a stroke risk factor in young adults (primarily in patients without SLE) showed an increased risk for incident ischemic stroke in young people. The study failing to find an association only tested for aCL antibodies, whereas the other studies evaluated for both aCL antibodies and lupus anticoagulant (LA). The presence and magnitude of the ischemic stroke risk associated with aPL antibodies in older populations is more evenly split between finding an increased risk and no increased risk; however, of the studies where both aCL antibodies and LA were tested, all but one found an increased risk (reviewed in Brey, 2004). This suggests that aPL antibodies may be a more important stroke mechanism in young people, whereas in older populations, other stroke risk factors take on more importance. Alternatively, the presence of LA may be more important in determining stroke risk at any age than aCL antibodies alone. Most of these studies either excluded cardio-embolic disease or did not distinguish between cardio-embolic, artery-to-artery embolic, or thrombotic mechanisms. This is an important point because cardiac

Table 2 Antiphospholipid antibodies and recurrent stroke risk

Author, year	Number of Patients (study includes adults unless otherwise indicated)	Study type	aPL tested	aPL-recurrent stroke risk
Levine, (1990)	48	Prospective case series	aCL; LA	Increased
Nencini, (1992)	55 (<45 years)	Prospective case-control	aCL; LA	Increased
Tohgi, (1994)	184	Prospective Cohort	aCL	Increased
Levine, (1995)	81	Prospective Cohort	aCL; LA	Increased
APASS, (1997)	219	Prospective Cohort	aCL	No Increase
Zielinska, (1999)	194	Prospective case-control	aCL	No Increase
Heinzlef, (2000)	242	Prospective Cohort	aCL	No increase
Tanne, (2002)	300	Prospective Cohort	aCL	No increase
Strater, (2002)	301 children	Prospective Cohort	aPL	No Increase
Lanthier, (2004)	185 children	Prospective Cohort	aCL; LA	No Increase
Van Goor, (2004)	128 (<45 years)	Prospective Cohort	aCL; LA	No Increase

valvular lesions have been reliably associated with aPL antibodies.

Two large studies have evaluated the risk for recurrent stroke and aPL antibodies in young adults (Nencini et al., 1992). One study evaluated both aCL antibodies and LA and found an increase in recurrent stroke risk attributable to aPL antibodies. The other, more recent study, which also evaluated for both aPL and LA found no increased recurrent stroke risk (van Goor, Alblas, Leebeek, Koudstaal, & Dippel, 2004). Two studies done in pediatrics populations, likewise, found no increased stroke risk (Lanthier et al., 2004; Strater et al., 2002).

The Euro-Phospholipid Project Group began a study of the clinical and immunologic manifestations and patterns of disease expression of APS in a cohort of 1,000 patients in 1999 (Cervera et al., 1999). Primary APS was present in 53.1% of patients, APS associated with SLE in 36.2%, APS associated with "lupus-like" disease in 5.9%, and other diseases in 5.9%. At study entry, deep venous thrombosis was the most common thrombotic manifestation occurring in 317 (31.7%) and stroke the most common arterial thrombotic manifestation in 135 (13.1%) patients. Additional cerebrovascular ischemic events were seen as well: transient ischemic attack in 70 (7.0%) and amaurosis fugax in 28 (2.8%) patients. While some clinical differences existed between primary and secondary APS

patients, none of these included thrombotic manifestations. While follow-up information is not yet available for this extremely well-characterized cohort, invaluable information about recurrent stroke and other clinical manifestations will be forth-coming, as 10 years of follow-up is planned.

In another European collaborative study, the European Working Party on SLE, the morbidity and mortality in patients with SLE over a 10-year period was studied in a cohort of 1,000 patients (Cervera et al., 2003). This is the best study of the risk of thrombotic events and aPL antibodies in people with SLE. At the beginning of this study, there were 204 (20.4%) patients with aCL IgG, 108 (10.8%) patients with aCL IgM, and 94 (9.4%) patients with LA. Thromboses were the most common cause of death in the last 5 years of follow-up and were always associated with APS (Cervera et al., 1999). The most common thrombotic events in these patients were strokes (11.8%), followed by MI (7.4%) and pulmonary embolism (5.9%). This suggests an important role for aPL and recurrent thrombosis in patients with SLE.

Cognitive Dysfunction

Multiple studies have shown an association of aPLs with cognitive dysfunction measured by neuropsychological testing in SLE (Denburg, Carbotte, Ginsberg, & Denburg, 1997; Hanly, Hong, Smith, & Fisk, 1999; Leritz, Brandt, Minor, Reis-Jensen, & Petri, 2002; Menon et al., 1999; Mikdashi & Handwerger, 2004). aPL elevations have been associated with several different patterns of cognitive dysfunction in patients with SLE, depending on the study. Verbal memory deficits, decreased psychomotor speed, and decreased cognitive efficiency/ productivity have all been significantly correlated to elevated aPL levels.

Three longitudinal studies have evaluated the relationship between serially obtained aPL levels and cognitive dysfunction in SLE patients (Hanly, Hong et al., 1999; McLaurin, Holliday, Williams, & Brey, 2005; Menon et al., 1999). All studies demonstrated that cognitive dysfunction was significantly associated with persistently positive aPL. Menon and colleagues (1999) reported that SLE patients with persistently elevated IgG aCL levels over a period of 2–3 years performed significantly worse than SLE patients with occasionally elevated or never elevated titers on a variety of neuropsychological tests. These results were not observed with anti-DNA antibody titers or C3 (complement) levels. Attention and concentration, as well as psychomotor speed, were the domains most affected. Hanly, Hong, and colleagues (1999) followed 51 female SLE patients over a 5-year period and found that persistent aCL IgG elevations were associated with decreased psychomotor speed, while persistent aCL IgA elevations were correlated with problems with executive functioning and reasoning abilities. They found no association between cognitive deficits and anti-DNA antibodies. Interestingly, no cross-sectional relationship between cognitive dysfunction and aPL was found in this same population (Hanly, Walsh et al., 1993). Our group prospectively studied the relationship between aCL and anti-β2-glycoprotein 1 antibodies in 123 SLE patients over 3 years (McLaurin et al., 2005). Factors significantly associated with reduced cognitive test scores were persistently positive aPL levels, prednisone use, diabetes, higher

depression scores, and less education. Of four cross-sectional studies, two found a relationship between LA positivity and cognitive dysfunction (Denburg et al., 1997; Leritz et al., 2002), one found no such relationship (Afeltra et al., 2003), and one found no relationship between aCL and cognitive dysfunction (Hanly, Hong et al., 1999).

The etiology of cognitive dysfunction in SLE remains an active research question, but it is becoming clear that it cannot be fully accounted for by strokes, past or current corticosteroid treatment, disease duration, disease activity (SLEDAI) or its associated psychological/emotional distress, or sociodemographic factors (Brey, Holliday et al., 2002; Rivest et al., 2000). The detection of cognitive disorders has been regarded as too time consuming and expensive for routine baseline/follow-up testing. Yet mild to severe cognitive dysfunction remains the most common type of NPSLE manifestation with a prevalence of up to 75% (Ainiala et al., 2001; Brey, Holliday et al., 2002; Costallat et al., 2001). It is most reliably detected and monitored through neuropsychological examination, often revealing a diffuse subcortical syndrome with most prominent compromise in the areas of processing efficiency/speed, attention/concentration, memory function, conceptual reasoning, and cognitive flexibility. Most SLE patients experience only mild levels of diffuse cognitive impairment (about 1 SD below age-peers), but more severe deficits approaching dementia have been reported in 15–25% of SLE patients (Ainiala et al., 2001; Brey & Stallworth et al., 2002).

Cognitive impairment in SLE is not consistently related to psychiatric manifestations and can be detected even in the absence of other current or past overt CNS manifestations (Ainiala et al., 2001). It appears to be selectively linked to aPL but not to anti-ribosomal P antibodies (Brey & Stallworth et al., 2002). Diamond and colleagues demonstrated that a subset of lupus anti-DNA antibodies cross-reacts with the NR2 glutamate receptor in patients with SLE (DeGiorgio,

Konstantinov, Lee, Harden, Volpe, & Diamond, 2001; Gaynor, Patternam, Valadon, Spatz, Scharff, & Diamond, 1997) and that these antibodies are also associated with cognitive dysfunction in animal models of SLE. NR2 glutamate receptors bind the neurotransmitter glutamate and are present on neurons throughout the forebrain (Ozawa, Kamiya, & Tsuzuki, 1998) play a role in learning and memory (Morris, Anderson, Lynch, & Baudry, 1986). Omdal and colleagues (2005) reported an association between anti-NR2 glutamate receptor antibodies and cognitive dysfunction and depression in a group of 57 SLE patients from Norway, supporting the importance the relationship of this autoantibody with cognitive dysfunction and psychiatric disease in SLE, but this finding has not been replicated in another study (Harrison, Ravdin, Volpe, Diamond, & Lockshin, 2004). Diamond and colleagues have recently shown that NR2-immunized mice who have anti-NR2 glutamate receptor antibodies develop neuronal cell loss only when the blood-brain-barrier has been disrupted (Kowal et al., 2004) suggesting that in humans with SLE, blood-brain-barrier disruption may be needed for cognitive dysfunction to occur. Alternatively, persistent levels of anti-NR2 glutamate receptor antibodies may be necessary to lead to cognitive dysfunction as has been seen with aPL.

Supporting Laboratory Studies

There is no single diagnostic test sensitive and specific for SLE-related cerebrovascular disease and cognitive dysfunction. The assessment of individual patients is based on clinical neurologic and rheumatologic evaluation, immunoserologic testing, brain imaging, and psychiatric and neuropsychological assessment. These examinations are used to support or refute the clinical diagnostic impression and rule out alternative explanations and form the basis for prospective monitoring of clinical

evolution and response to treatment interventions. An important consideration in the diagnostic approach to a patient with possible NPSLE manifestations is whether the particular clinical syndrome is due to SLE-mediated organ dysfunction, a secondary phenomenon related to infection, medication side-effects or metabolic abnormalities (e.g. uremia), or is due to an unrelated condition. It cannot be stressed strongly enough that infection is a major cause of CNS syndromes in hospitalized SLE patients (Futrell, Schultz, & Millikan, 1992). Thus, it is always important to suspect infection in patients with SLE and CNS manifestations.

Imaging

Brain magnetic resonance imaging studies in patients with APS (primary or secondary) have revealed small foci of high signal in subcortical white matter scattered throughout the brain (Csepany, Bereczki, Kollar, Sikula, Kiss, & Csiba, 2003; Provenzale et al., 1994; Toubi, Khamashta, Panarra, & Hughes, 1995). This type of pattern is seen in many other disease processes and is therefore non-specific. The correlation between MRI lesions in patients with aPL and clinical nervous system symptoms is reported to be high by some investigators (Csepany et al., 2003; Provenzale, Heines, Ortel, Macik, Charles, & Alberts, 1994; Tietjen et al., 1998; Toubi et al., 1995) and not by others (Sailer et al., 1997; Schmidt, Auer-Grumbach, Fazekas, Offenbacher, & Kapeller, 1995). Appenzeller and colleagues (2005) have demonstrated a reduction in cerebral and corpus callosum volumes SLE patients that are associated with disease duration and cognitive impairment and other CNS manifestations, but not total corticosteroid dose or the presence of aPL.

Sun and colleagues (2003) evaluated Technitium-^{99m} hexamethylpropylene amines oxime (^{99m}Tc HMPAO) to revaluate the effects of anticoagulant therapy on regional cerebral blood flow in patients with primary APS and brain involvement in 16 patients. This was a highly selected group, all with decreased regional blood flow demonstrated on ^{99m}Tc HMPAO prior to anticoagulant therapy. After 1 month of anticoagulant therapy, 11 (68.8%) patients had complete and 5 (32.1%) had partial recovery of regional blood flow. Further studies are needed to determine whether this response is predictive of future clinical events.

Focal neurological and neuropsychological symptoms of SLE-related stroke correlate with structural (MRI) abnormalities. Using structural MRI, the majority (40–80%) of abnormalities in NPSLE are small focal lesions concentrating in periventricular and subcortical white matter (Abreu, Jakosky, Folgecini, Brentol, Xavier, & Kapczinsky, 2005; Sibbitt, Sibbitt, & Brooks, 1999). Cortical atrophy, ventricular dilation, diffuse white matter, and gross infarctions are also common (Sibbitt et al., 1999). MRI reveals multiple discrete white matter lesions in periventricular, cortical/subcortical junction, and frontal lobe more commonly in patients with past NPSLE manifestations, than in SLE patients without history of NPSLE (Abreu et al., 2005; Karassa et al., 2000; Sibbitt et al., 1999).

Visually analysed FDG-PET consistently reveals abnormalities in prefrontal, parietal (inferior and superior), parieto-occipital, posterior temporal, and occipital gray and white matter regions in active and quiescent NPSLE (Otte et al., 1997; Weiner et al., 2000). Prefrontal, anterior cingulate, and inferior parietal white matter abnormalities have been seen during acute NPSLE but not during quiescent NPSLE (Komatsu et al., 1999). The metabolic disturbances in parieto-occipital (peritrigonal) white matter remain an intriguing finding. Approximately 60–80% of active minor and major NPSLE patients consistently show bilateral parieto-occipital white matter FDG-PET hypometabolism in the context of normal conventional MRI and no other PET abnormalities (Otte et al., 1997; Weiner et al., 2000).

More recently, magnetic resonance spectroscopy (MRS) has revealed neurometabolic abnormalities even in white and gray matter that appears normal on conventional MRI. Such abnormalities are thought to reflect neuronal injury or loss and demyelination and have been found during active as well as quiescent periods of NPSLE manifestations (Chinn et al., 1997). Kazora and Colleagues (2006) recently found a correlation between changes in cerebral white matter by MRS and cognitive impairment in SLE patients, even in the absence of overt NPSLE symptoms.

Cerebrospinal Fluid Evaluation

CSF analysis is recommended in some cases of central nervous system NPSLE manifestations; however, lumbar puncture cannot be performed in anticoagulated patients, patients with fewer than 20,000 platelets/mm^3, and patients with a focal mass lesion or edema that would increase risk for herniation. The CSF analysis is essential to the diagnosis of CNS infection, but in the absence of infection may also be helpful in suggesting a CNS SLE flare. When immune-mediated CNS damage is ongoing during an SLE flare, the CSF IgG index or synthesis rate is often elevated and an oligoclonal banding pattern is seen (West, Emlen, Wener, & Kotzin, 1995). In many patients these abnormalities normalize when the flare resolves. Findings of pleocytosis, elevated protein, or hypoglycorrhachia are nonspecific and seen in only about one third of patients (West, Emien, Wener, & Kotzin, 1995).

Autoantibody Testing

Autoantibodies associated with SLE-related cerebrovascular disease include aPL antibodies, and those associated with cognitive dysfunction include aPL and possibly anti-glutamate receptor antibodies. Testing for aPL antibodies is widely available through commercial laboratories, however, testing for anti- NR2 glutamate receptor antibodies is only currently available as a research test.

Neuropsychological Testing

At the ACR Consensus Conference, which defined the clinical manifestations of NPSLE, a group of neuropsychologists active in SLE research proposed a standardized 4-h battery of traditional neuropsycholgical tests thought to be sensitive to the cognitive deficits commonly seen on SLE (The American College of Rheumatology Nomenclature and Case Definitions for Neuropsychiatric Lupus Syndromes, 1999). Kozora and colleagues (2004) validated this battery and a 1-h abbreviated traditional battery in 31 NPSLE patients, 22 non-NPSLE patients, and 25 normal controls tested twice over 1 month. Both batteries successfully discriminated the three study groups and intraclass correlation coefficients between the two testing sessions ranged from 0.40 to 0.90 on the various tests.

Unfortunately, both the ACR battery and briefer batteries of traditional neuropsychological tests may be unsuitable for repeated measures over short intervals due to pronounced test-retest or practice effects. These effects reduce the sensitivity of these tests to detect changes over time and the batteries are too lengthy for frequent repeated testing. In addition, many of the tests in the ACR battery do not have suitable forms or norms to use with illiterate and non-English-speaking subjects. To address these challenges, several groups studying SLE have employed the Automated Neuropsychological Assessment Metrics (ANAM), which is a set of computer-administered cognitive performance tests developed by the US military in the 1970s (Bleiberg, Garmoe, Halpern, Reeves, & Nadler, 1997; Bleiberg, Kane, Reeves, Garmoe, & Halpern, 2000; Holliday et al., 2003; Reeves, Kane, & Winter, 1996). ANAM was

selected from among other computerized neuropsychological tests because it is sensitive to the cognitive deficits documented in SLE, especially cognitive processing speed, complex attention, and visuospatial processing (Holliday et al., 2003). ANAM addresses practice effects by displaying different stimuli for each new administration using a pseudoramndonization paradigm such that test subjects see the same test stimuli for each iteration of ANAM (up to 99 repetitions). Despite these multiple alternative forms, ANAM still shows a robust practice effect over the first several administrations as users become more comfortable with the instrument (Bleiberg et al., 1997). Bleiberg and ANAM's other developers recommend repeating ANAM three times in the initial session to wash out this practice effect. ANAM takes about 30 min to complete, does not require literacy or advanced computer skills, and can be administered to subjects with wide range of languages. Typing skills are not required as subjects only have to press the left or right mouse button to respond to each forced-choice item. The ANAM subtests selected for use in SLE research studies do not require English language fluency as the instructions have been translated into several languages and each ANAM subtest is preceded by a series of practice items so that examiners can ensure subjects understand the task and can respond reliably.

Automated Neuropsychological Assessment Metrics has been validated against traditional neuropsychological test batteries with samples of patients with traumatic brain injuries (Bleiberg & Warden, 2005) and SLE (Holliday et al., 2003; Roebuck-Spencer et al., 2006). These studies found that ANAM correlated reasonably well with traditional neuropsychological tests of memory, working memory, sustained attention, cognitive processing speed, and executive functions; and that weighted combinations of ANAM test scores accounted for over 60% of the variance in the traditional NP tests. ANAM's brevity and repeatability may also help researchers examine performance variability across time, a measure that Bleiberg and colleagues (1997) found promising in differentiating mild traumatic brain injury, another presumably diffuse subcortical process.

Although promising, ANAM's clinical use is limited by a lack of published normative data, although Reeves and colleagues (2006) recently published ANAM norms for a large active duty military sample (limited age/education range). Several longitudinal studies are now ongoing to validate ANAM against traditional neuropsychological test batteries over time and to collect more normative data with repeated administrations.

Disease Course, Treatment, and Prognosis

The general management of patients with NPSLE includes symptomatic and immunosuppressive therapies, but evidence for the efficacy of the treatment modalities commonly used is largely limited to uncontrolled clinical trials and anecdotal experience (Navarrete & Brey, 2000). The key to treatment is to first establish the correct diagnosis by carefully considering all possible etiologies, both SLE-related and those that are not.

Cerebrovascular Disease

Appropriate therapy for cerebrovascular SLE must include the prevention of vasculopathies as well as minimizing the ischemic damage when it occurs. Unless there is evidence of active inflammation, corticosteroids and immunosupression are rarely indicated. Acute therapy consists of limiting the extent of damage to the ischemic tissue includes rest, antiplatelet agents, and appropriate blood pressure management avoiding tight blood pressure control that may result in hypoperfusion (Navarrete & Brey, 2000).

Treatment of the APS can be directed at thrombo-occlusive events using antithrombotic medications or at modulating the immune response with immunotherapy (Brey, 2004). In the case of thrombotic manifestations, both approaches have been used. There are no data that address the use of any specific treatment strategies for primary prevention of aPL-associated stroke. The afore mentioned Euro-Phospholipid Project Group will also have some information that will shed light on the issue of primary prevention, although in that study patients are not randomized to a specific treatment (Cervera et al., 2002), however.

Treatment such as platelet antiaggregant and anticoagulant therapy for secondary stroke prevention have both been used in APS and in cerebrovascular disease associated with aPL immunoreactivity (Crowther et al., 2003; Khamashta et al., 1995; Levine et al., 2004; Rosove & Brewer, 1992). Two groups have retrospective data to suggest that high-intensity warfarin treatment (versus low- or moderate-intensity warfarin or aspirin treatment) is associated with better outcomes in selected cohorts with various types of thrombotic events (Khamashta et al., 1995; Rosove & Brewer, 1992). Patients reported on in these studies did not have repeat aPL testing and would not fulfill current criteria for APS.

Crowther and colleagues performed the first randomized, double-blind, controlled trial of two different intensities of warfarin treatment on the prevention of recurrent thrombotic events in patients with APS (Crowther et al., 2003). There were 114 patients enrolled in the study and followed for an average of 2.7 years. The average INR values in the moderate and high-intensity groups were 2.3 and 3.3, respectively. Recurrent thrombosis occurred in 2/58 (3.4%) patients assigned to moderate-intensity warfarin and in 6/56 (10.7%) patients assigned to receive high-intensity warfarin. There was no difference in recurrent thrombosis or major bleeding rates between the two groups. These results suggest that high-intensity warfarin treatment is *not* more effective than moderate-intensity treatment in preventing recurrent thrombotic events in patients with APS. The study did not specifically address the end-point of stroke.

The APASS Group completed the first prospective study of the role of aPL in recurrent ischemic stroke in collaboration with the WARSS group (Levine et al., 2004). This controlled and blinded study was initiated in 1993 and compared the risk of recurrent stroke and other thrombo-embolic disease over a 2-year follow-up period in patients with ischemic stroke who were randomised to either aspirin therapy (325 mg per day) or warfarin therapy at a dose to maintain the INR between 1.4 and 2.8. The suggested target INR was 2.2. The purpose of the study was to collect information about recurrent stroke rates in aPL positive versus aPL negative patients controlling for treatment. There were 882 patients randomized to warfarin and 890 patients randomized to aspirin who participated in APASS. No increased risk of thrombotic event was associated with the baseline aPL in either the warfarin treated patients (RR 0.97, 95% CI 0.74–1.27, $p = 0.82$), or the aspirin treated patients (RR 0.96, 95% CI 0.71–1.29, $p = 0.77$). Patients with baseline positivity for both LA and aCL antibodies tended to have a higher event rate (31.7%) than patients who were negative on both antibodies (24.0%)—RR 1.36 (95% CI 0.97–1.92, $p = 0.07$). There was no difference in major bleeding complications between treatment groups. Thus it appears that for patients with a positive aPL determination at a single time point at the time of ischemic stroke (including low-titers of aCL and/or IgA aCL) aspirin and warfarin therapy at an INR of approximately 2.0 are equivalent regarding stroke recurrence and major bleeding complications.

Cognitive Dysfunction

Unfortunately, there is no definitive treatment for the diffuse cognitive dysfunction that commonly occurs in patients with SLE at this time. More speculatively, as depression and long-term corticosteriod use have been related to cognitive impairment in SLE patients, appropriate clinical management of depression and use of newer steroid-sparing treatment protocols may be helpful. A recent randomized controlled trial also demonstrated that a cognitive-behavioral stress management group significantly improved pain and psychological well-being in SLE patients, and that these gains were maintained at 9 month follow-up (Greco, Rudy, & Manzi, 2004). A single case study reported by McGrath and colleagues (2005) found that 8 months of low-dose ultraviolet A-1 exposure was associated with normalization of previously high aCL antibodies, normalization of brain PET scans, decreased SLE disease activity, and complete reversal of livedo reticularis. McLaurin and colleagues (2005) reported that SLE patients consistently treated with aspirin had better cognitive performance over 3 years; this association was particularly striking in a subset with diabetes. It is hoped that ongoing research efforts into the underlying pathophysiology of SLE-related cognitive dysfunction will lead to novel and more efficacious therapeutic strategies in the near future.

References

Abou-Raya, A., & Abou-Raya, S. (2006). Inflammation: A pivotal link between autoimmune diseases and atherosclerosis. *Autoimmunity Reviews, 5*(5), 331–337.

Abreu, M. R., Jakosky, A., Folgerini, M., Brenol, J. C., Xavier, R. M., & Kapczinsky, F. (2005). Neuropsychiatric systemic lupus erythematosus: Correlation of brain MR imaging, CT, and SPECT. *Clinical Imaging, 29*(3), 215–221.

Afeltra, A., Garzia, P., Mitterhofer, A. P., Vadacca, M., Galluzzo, S., & Del Porto, F., et al. (2003). Neuropsychiatric lupus syndromes: Relationship with antiphospholipid antibodies. [see comment]. *Neurology, 61*(1), 108–110.

Ainiala, H., Loukkola, J., Peltola, J., Korpela, M., & Hietaharju, A. (2001). The prevalence of neuropsychiatric syndromes in systemic lupus erythematosus. *Neurology, 57*(3), 496–500.

Alcocer-Varela, J., Aleman-Hoey, D., & Alarcon-Segovia, D. (1992). Interleukin-1 and interleukin-6 activities are increased in the cerebrospinal fluid of patients with CNS lupus erythematosus and correlate with local late T-cell activation markers. *Lupus, 1*(2), 111–117.

Allegri, F., Balestrieri, G., Cattaneo, R., Martinelli, M., Tincani, A., & Barcellini, W., et al. (1990). The plasma cofactor and anticardiolipin antibodies. *Clinical & Experimental Rheumatology, 8*(6), 613–615.

Appenzeller S., Rondina J. M., Li L. M., Costallat, T. L., & Cendes F. (2005) Cerebral and corpus callosum atrophy in systemic lupus erythematosus. *Arthritis & Rheumatism, 52*(9), 2783–2789.

The American College of Rheumatology nomenclature and case definitions for neuropsychiatric lupus syndromes (1999). *Arthritis & Rheumatism, 42*(4), 599–608.

Baraczka, K., Pozsonyi, T., Szongoth, M., Nekam, K., Megyeri, A., Balogh, Z., et al. (1999). A study of increased levels of soluble vascular cell adhesion molecule-1 (sVCAM-1) in the cerebrospinal fluid of patients with multiple sclerosis and systemic lupus erythematosus. *Acta Neurologica Scandinavica, 99*(2), 95–99.

Belmont, H. M., Abramson, S. B., & Lie, J. T. (1996). Pathology and pathogenesis of vascular injury in systemic lupus erythematosus. interactions of inflammatory cells and activated endothelium. *Arthritis & Rheumatism, 39*(1), 9–22.

Bleiberg, J., Garmoe, W. S., Halpern, E. L., Reeves, D. L., & Nadler, J. D. (1997). Consistency of within-day and across-day performance after mild brain injury. *Neuropsychiatry, Neuropsychology, & Behavioral Neurology, 10*(4), 247–253.

Bleiberg, J., Kane, R. L., Reeves, D. L., Garmoe, W. S., & Halpern, E. (2000). Factor analysis of computerized and traditional tests used in mild brain injury research. *Clinical Neuropsychologist, 14*(3), 287–294.

Bleiberg, J., & Warden, D. (2005). Duration of cognitive impairment after sports concussion. *Neurosurgery, 56*(5), E1166.

Blohorn, A., Guegan-Massardier, E., Triquenot, A., Onnient, Y., Tron, F., & Borg, J. Y., et al. (2002). Antiphospholipid antibodies in the acute phase of cerebral ischaemia in young adults: A descriptive study of 139 patients. *Cerebrovascular Diseases, 13*(3), 156–162.

Brey, R. L. (2004). Management of the neurological manifestations of APS–what do the trials tell us? *Thrombosis Research, 114*(5–6), 489–499.

Brey, R. L., Hart, R. G., Sherman, D. G., & Tegeler, C. H. (1990). Antiphospholipid antibodies and cerebral ischemia in young people. *Neurology, 40*(8), 1190–1196.

Brey, R. L., Holliday, S. L., Saklad, A. R., Navarrete, M. G., Hermosillo-Romo, D., Stallworth, C. L., et al. (2002). Neuropsychiatric syndromes in lupus: Prevalence using standardized definitions. *Neurology, 58*(8), 1214–1220.

Brey, R. L., Stallworth, C. L., McGlasson, D. L., Wozniak, M. A., Wityk, R. J., Stern, B. J., et al. (2002). Antiphospholipid antibodies and stroke in young women. *Stroke, 33*(10), 2396–2400.

Campbell, A. L., Pierangeli, S. S., Wellhausen, S., & Harris, E. N. (1995). Comparison of the effects of anticardiolipin antibodies from patients with the antiphospholipid syndrome and with syphilis on platelet activation and aggregation. *Thrombosis & Haemostasis, 73*(3), 529–534.

Cervera, R., Khamashta, M. A., Font, J., Sebastiani, G. D., Gil, A., & Lavilla, P., et al. (1999). Morbidity and mortality in systemic lupus erythematosus during a 5-year period. A multicenter prospective study of 1,000 patients. european working party on systemic lupus erythematosus. *Medicine, 78*(3), 167–175.

Cervera, R., Khamashta, M. A., Font, J., Sebastiani, G. D., Gil, A., & Lavilla, P., et al. (2003). Morbidity and mortality in systemic lupus erythematosus during a 10-year period: A comparison of early and late manifestations in a cohort of 1,000 patients. *Medicine, 82*(5), 299–308.

Cervera, R., Piette, J. C., Font, J., Khamashta, M. A., Shoenfeld, Y., & Camps, M. T., et al. (2002). Antiphospholipid syndrome: Clinical and immunologic manifestations and patterns of disease expression in a cohort of 1,000 patients. *Arthritis & Rheumatism, 46*(4), 1019–1027.

Chinn, R. J., Wilkinson, I. D., Hall-Craggs, M. A., Paley, M. N., Shortall, E., Carter, S., et al. (1997). Magnetic resonance imaging of the brain and cerebral proton spectroscopy in patients with systemic lupus erythematosus. *Arthritis & Rheumatism, 40*(1), 36–46.

Costallat, L., Bertolo, M., & Appenzeller, S. (2001). The american college of rheumatology nomenclature and case definitions for neuropsychiatric lupus syndromes: Analysis of 527 patients. *Lupus, 10*(S1), S32.

Crowther, M. A., Ginsberg, J. S., Julian, J., Denburg, J., Hirsh, J., Douketis, J., et al. (2003). A comparison of two intensities of warfarin for the prevention of recurrent thrombosis in patients with the antiphospholipid antibody syndrome. *New England Journal of Medicine, 349*(12), 1133–1138.

Csepany, T., Bereczki, D., Kollar, J., Sikula, J., Kiss, E., & Csiba, L. (2003). MRI findings in central nervous system systemic lupus erythematosus are associated with immunoserological parameters and hypertension. *Journal of Neurology, 250*(11), 1348–1354.

Danchenko, N., Satia, J. A., & Anthony, M. S. (2006). Epidemiology of systemic lupus erythematosus: A comparison of worldwide disease burden. *Lupus, 15*(5), 308–318.

DeGiorgio, L. A., Konstantinov, K. N., Lee, S. C., Hardin, J. A., Volpe, B. T., & Diamond, B. (2001). A subset of lupus anti-DNA antibodies cross-reacts with the NR2 glutamate receptor in systemic lupus erythematosus. *Nature Medicine*, 7(11), 1189–1193.

del Zoppo, G. J., & Hallenbeck, J. M. (2000). Advances in the vascular pathophysiology of ischemic stroke. *Thrombosis Research*, 98(3), 73–81.

Denburg, S. D., Carbotte, R. M., Ginsberg, J. S., & Denburg, J. A. (1997). The relationship of antiphospholipid antibodies to cognitive function in patients with systemic lupus erythematosus. *Journal of the International Neuropsychological Society*, 3(4), 377–386.

Egerer, K., Feist, E., Rohr, U., Pruss, A., Burmester, G. R., & Dorner, T. (2000). Increased serum soluble CD14, ICAM-1 and E-selectin correlate with disease activity and prognosis in systemic lupus erythematosus. *Lupus*, 9(8), 614–621.

Esdaile, J. M., Abrahamowicz, M., Grodzicky, T., Li, Y., Panaritis, C., du Berger, R., et al. (2001). Traditional framingham risk factors fail to fully account for accelerated atherosclerosis in systemic lupus erythematosus. *Arthritis & Rheumatism*, 44(10), 2331–2337.

Futrell, N., Schultz, L. R., & Millikan, C. (1992). Central nervous system disease in patients with systemic lupus erythematosus. *Neurology*, 42(9), 1649–1657.

Galli, M., Comfurius, P., Maassen, C., Hemker, H. C., de Baets, M. H., van Breda-Vriesman, P. J., et al. (1990). Anticardiolipin antibodies (ACA) directed not to cardiolipin but to a plasma protein cofactor. *Lancet*, 335(8705), 1544–1547.

Gaynor, B., Putterman, C., Valadon, P., Spatz, L., Scharff, M. D., & Diamond, B. (1997). Peptide inhibition of glomerular deposition of an anti-DNA antibody. *Proceedings of the National Academy of Sciences of the United States of America*, 94(5), 1955–1960.

Gharavi, A. E., & Pierangeli, S. S. (1998). Origin of antiphospholipid antibodies: Induction of aPL by viral peptides. *Lupus*, 7(Suppl 2), S52–S54.

Gharavi, A. E., Pierangeli, S. S., Colden-Stanfield, M., Liu, X. W., Espinola, R. G., & Harris, E. N. (1999). GDKV-induced antiphospholipid antibodies enhance thrombosis and activate endothelial cells in vivo and in vitro. *Journal of Immunology*, 163(5), 2922–2927.

Gharavi, E. E., Chaimovich, H., Cucurull, E., Celli, C. M., Tang, H., & Wilson, W. A., et al. (1999). Induction of antiphospholipid antibodies by immunization with synthetic viral and bacterial peptides. *Lupus*, 8(6), 449–455.

Gonzalez-Crespo, M. R., Blanco, F. J., Ramos, A., Ciruelo, E., Mateo, I., Lopez Pino, M. A., et al. (1995). Magnetic resonance imaging of the brain in systemic lupus erythematosus. *British Journal of Rheumatology*, 34(11), 1055–1060.

Greco, C. M., Rudy, T. E., & Manzi, S. (2004). Effects of a stress-reduction program on psychological function, pain, and physical function of systemic lupus erythematosus patients: A randomized controlled trial. *Arthritis & Rheumatism*, 51(4), 625–634.

Haas, L. F. (1982). Stroke as an early manifestation of systemic lupus erythematosus. *Journal of Neurology, Neurosurgery & Psychiatry*, 45(6), 554–556.

Hallenbeck, J. M., Hansson, G. K., & Becker, K. J. (2005). Immunology of ischemic vascular disease: Plaque to attack. *Trends in Immunology*, 26(10), 550–556.

Hanly, J. G. (2001). Neuropsychiatric lupus. *Current Rheumatology Reports*, 3(3), 205–212.

Hanly, J. G., Hong, C., Smith, S., & Fisk, J. D. (1999). A prospective analysis of cognitive function and anticardiolipin antibodies in systemic lupus erythematosus. *Arthritis & Rheumatism*, 42(4), 728–734.

Hanly, J. G., Walsh, N. M., Fisk, J. D., Eastwood, B., Hong, C., Sherwood, G., et al. (1993). Cognitive impairment and autoantibodies in systemic lupus erythematosus. *British Journal of Rheumatology*, 32(4), 291–296.

Hanly, J. G., Walsh, N. M., & Sangalang, V. (1992). Brain pathology in systemic lupus erythematosus. *Journal of Rheumatology*, 19(5), 732–741.

Harrison, M., Ravdin, L., Volpe, B., Diamond, B., & Lockshin, M. (2004). Anti-NR2 antibody does not identify cognitive impairment in a general SLE population. *Arthritis and Rheumatism*, 50(9), S596.

Ho, K. T., Ahn, C. W., Alarcon, G. S., Baethge, B. A., Tan, F. K., Roseman, J., et al. (2005). Systemic lupus erythematosus in a multiethnic cohort (LUMINA): XXVIII. factors predictive of thrombotic events. *Rheumatology*, 44(10), 1303–1307.

Holliday, S. L., Navarrete, M. G., Hermosillo-Romo, D., Valdez, C. R., Saklad, A. R., Escalante, A., et al. (2003). Validating a computerized neuropsychological test battery for mixed ethnic lupus patients. *Lupus*, 12(9), 697–703.

Hughes, G. (1983). Thrombosis, abortion, cerebral disease and lupus anticoagulant. *British Medical Journal*, 187, 1088–1089.

Jara, L. J., Irigoyen, L., Ortiz, M. J., Zazueta, B., Bravo, G., & Espinoza, L. R. (1998). Prolactin and interleukin-6 in neuropsychiatric lupus erythematosus. *Clinical Rheumatology*, 17(2), 110–114.

Karassa, F. B., Ioannidis, J. P., Boki, K. A., Touloumi, G., Argyropoulou, M. I., Strigaris, K. A., et al. (2000). Predictors of clinical outcome and radiologic progression in patients with neuropsychiatric manifestations of systemic lupus erythematosus. *American Journal of Medicine*, 109(8), 628–634.

Kelley, V. R., & Wuthrich, R. P. (1999). Cytokines in the pathogenesis of systemic lupus erythematosus. *Seminars in Nephrology*, 19(1), 57–66.

Khamashta, M. A., Cuadrado, M. J., Mujic, F., Taub, N. A., Hunt, B. J., & Hughes, G. R. (1995).

The management of thrombosis in the antiphospholipid-antibody syndrome. *New England Journal of Medicine, 332*(15), 993–997.

Komatsu, N., Kodama, K., Yamanouchi, N., Okada, S., Noda, S., Nawata, Y., et al. (1999). Decreased regional cerebral metabolic rate for glucose in systemic lupus erythematosus patients with psychiatric symptoms. *European Neurology, 42*(1), 41–48.

Kovacs, J. A., Urowitz, M. B., & Gladman, D. D. (1993). Dilemmas in neuropsychiatric lupus. *Rheumatic Diseases Clinics of North America, 19*(4), 795–814.

Kowal, C., DeGiorgio, L. A., Nakaoka, T., Hetherington, H., Huerta, P. T., Diamond, B., et al. (2004). Cognition and immunity; antibody impairs memory. *Immunity, 21*(2), 179–188.

Kozora, E., Laudenslager, M., Lemieux, A., & West, S. (2001). Inflammatory and hormonal measures predict neuropsychological functioning in systemic lupus erythematosus and rheumatoid arthritis patients. *Journal of the International Neuropsychological Society, 7*(6), 745–754.

Kozora E., Ellison MC., & West S. (2004). Reliability and validity of the proposed American College of Rheumatology neuropsychological battery for systemic lupus erythematosus. *Arthritis & Rheumatism, 51*(5), 810–818.

Kozora E., Arciniegas D. B., Filley, C. M., Ellison M. C., West S. G., Brown M. S. & Simon J. H. (2005). Cognition, MRS neurometabolites, and MRI volymetrics in non-neuropsychiatric systemic lupus erythematosis: preliminary data. *Cognitive and Behavioral Neurology, 18,* 159–162.

Lanthier, S., Kirkham, F. J., Mitchell, L. G., Laxer, R. M., Atenafu, E., Male, C., et al. (2004). Increased anticardiolipin antibody IgG titers do not predict recurrent stroke or TIA in children. *Neurology, 62*(2), 194–200.

Leritz, E., Brandt, J., Minor, M., Reis-Jensen, F., & Petri, M. (2002). Neuropsychological functioning and its relationship to antiphospholipid antibodies in patients with systemic lupus erythematosus. *Journal of Clinical & Experimental Neuropsychology: Official Journal of the International Neuropsychological Society, 24*(4), 527–533.

Levine, S. R., Brey, R. L., Tilley, B. C., Thompson, J. L., Sacco, R. L., Sciacca, R. R., et al. (2004). Antiphospholipid antibodies and subsequent thromboocclusive events in patients with ischemic stroke. *JAMA, 291*(5), 576–584.

Libby, P. (2001). Managing the risk of atherosclerosis: The role of high-density lipoprotein. *American Journal of Cardiology, 88*(12A), 3 N–8 N.

Maier, S. F., Goehler, L. E., Fleshner, M., & Watkins, L. R. (1998). The role of the vagus nerve in cytokine-to-brain communication. *Annals of the New York Academy of Sciences, 840,* 289–300.

Manzi, S., Meilahn, E. N., Rairie, J. E., Conte, C. G., Medsger, T. A., Jr, Jansen-McWilliams, L., et al.

(1997). Age-specific incidence rates of myocardial infarction and angina in women with systemic lupus erythematosus: Comparison with the framingham study. *American Journal of Epidemiology, 145*(5), 408–415.

Matsuda, J., Gohchi, K., Gotoh, M., Tsukamoto, M., & Saitoh, N. (1994). Circulating intercellular adhesion molecule-1 and soluble interleukin 2-receptor in patients with systemic lupus erythematosus. *European Journal of Haematology, 52*(5), 302–303.

Matsuura, E., Igarashi, Y., Fujimoto, M., Ichikawa, K., & Koike, T. (1990). Anticardiolipin cofactor(s) and differential diagnosis of autoimmune disease. *Lancet, 336*(8708), 177–178.

McGrath, H., Jr. (2005). Elimination of anticardiolipin antibodies and cessation of cognitive decline in a UV-A1-irradiated sustemic lupus erythematosis patient. *Lupus, 14* (10), 859–861.

McLaurin, E. Y., Holliday, S. L., Williams, P., & Brey, R. L. (2005). Predictors of cognitive dysfunction in patients with systemic lupus erythematosus. *Neurology, 64*(2), 297–303.

Menon, S., Jameson-Shortall, E., Newman, S. P., Hall-Craggs, M. R., Chinn, R., & Isenberg, D. A. (1999). A longitudinal study of anticardiolipin antibody levels and cognitive functioning in systemic lupus erythematosus. *Arthritis & Rheumatism, 42*(4), 735–741.

Meroni, P. L., Del Papa, N., Raschi, E., Panzeri, P., Borghi, M. O., Tincani, A., et al. (1998). Beta2-glycoprotein I as a 'cofactor' for anti-phospholipid reactivity with endothelial cells. *Lupus, 7*(Suppl 2), S44–S47.

Mikdashi, J., & Handwerger, B. (2004). Predictors of neuropsychiatric damage in systemic lupus erythematosus: Data from the maryland lupus cohort. *Rheumatology, 43*(12), 1555–1560.

Miyakis, S., Giannakopoulos, B., & Krilis, S. A. (2004). Beta 2 glycoprotein I–function in health and disease. *Thrombosis Research, 114*(5–6), 335–346.

Miyakis, S., Lockshin, M. D., Atsumi, T., Branch, D. W., Brey, R. L., & Cervera, R., et al. (2006). International consensus statement on an update of the classification criteria for definite antiphospholipid syndrome (APS). *Journal of Thrombosis & Haemostasis, 4*(2), 295–306.

Mok, C. C., Lau, C. S., & Wong, R. W. (2001). Neuropsychiatric manifestations and their clinical associations in southern chinese patients with systemic lupus erythematosus. *Journal of Rheumatology, 28*(4), 766–771.

Morris, R. G., Anderson, E., Lynch, G. S., & Baudry, M. (1986). Selective impairment of learning and blockade of long-term potentiation by an *N*-methyl-D-aspartate receptor antagonist, AP5. *Nature, 319*(6056), 774–776.

Navarrete, G., & Brey, R. (2000). Neuropsychiatric systemic lupus erythematosus. *Current Treatment Options in Neurology, 2*(5), 473–485.

Nencini, P., Baruffi, M. C., Abbate, R., Massai, G., Amaducci, L., & Inzitari, D. (1992). Lupus anticoagulant and anticardiolipin antibodies in young adults with cerebral ischemia. *Stroke*, *23*(2), 189–193.

Omdal, R., Brokstad, K., Waterloo, K., Koldingsnes, W., Jonsson, R., & Mellgren, S. I. (2005). Neuropsychiatric disturbances in SLE are associated with antibodies against NMDA receptors. *European Journal of Neurology*, *12*(5), 392–398.

Otte, A., Weiner, S. M., Peter, H. H., Mueller-Brand, J., Goetze, M., & Moser, E., et al. (1997). Brain glucose utilization in systemic lupus erythematosus with neuropsychiatric symptoms: A controlled positron emission tomography study. *European Journal of Nuclear Medicine*, *24*(7), 787–791.

Ozawa, S., Kamiya, H., & Tsuzuki, K. (1998). Glutamate receptors in the mammalian central nervous system. *Progress in Neurobiology*, *54*, 581–618.

Pierangeli, S. S., & Harris, E. N. (1994). Antiphospholipid antibodies in an in vivo thrombosis model in mice. *Lupus*, *3*(4), 247–251.

Provenzale, J. M., Heinz, E. R., Ortel, T. L., Macik, B. G., Charles, L. A., & Alberts, M. J. (1994). Antiphospholipid antibodies in patients without systemic lupus erythematosus: Neuroradiologic findings. *Radiology*, *192*(2), 531–537.

Reeves, D., Kane, R., & Winter, K. (1996). *Automated neuropsychological assessment metrics (ANAM V3. 11a/96) user's manual: Clinical and neurotoxicology subset (report no. NCRF-SR-96-01)*. San Diego CA: National Cognitive Foundation.

Reeves, D., Vleiberg, J., Roebuck-Spencer, T., Cernich, A., Schwab, K., Ivins, B., Salazar, A., Harvey, S., Brown, F, Warden, D. (2006). Reference values for performance on the Automated Neuropsychological Assessment Metrics V3.0 in an active duty military sample. *Military Medicine*, *171*(10), 982–984.

Rhew, E. Y., & Ramsey-Goldman, R. (2006). Premature atherosclerotic disease in systemic lupus erythematosus–role of inflammatory mechanisms. *Autoimmunity Reviews*, *5*(2), 101–105.

Rivest, C., Lew, R. A., Welsing, P. M., Sangha, O., Wright, E. A., Roberts, W. N., et al. (2000). Association between clinical factors, socioeconomic status, and organ damage in recent onset systemic lupus erythematosus. *Journal of Rheumatology*, *27*(3), 680–684.

Roebuck-Spencer, T. M., Yarboro, C., Nowak, M., Takada, K., Jacobs, G., Lapteva, L., et al. (2006). Use of computerized assessment to predict neuropsychological functioning and emotional distress in patients with systemic lupus erythematosus. *Arthritis & Rheumatism*, *55*(3), 434–441.

Roman, M. J., Shanker, B. A., Davis, A., Lockshin, M. D., Sammaritano, L., Simantov, R., et al. (2003). Prevalence and correlates of accelerated atherosclerosis in systemic lupus erythematosus. *New England Journal of Medicine*, *349*(25), 2399–2406.

Rosove, M. H., & Brewer, P. M. (1992). Antiphospholipid thrombosis: Clinical course after the first thrombotic event in 70 patients. *Annals of Internal Medicine*, *117*(4), 303–308.

Sailer, M., Burchert, W., Ehrenheim, C., Smid, H. G., Haas, J., Wildhagen, K., et al. (1997). Positron emission tomography and magnetic resonance imaging for cerebral involvement in patients with systemic lupus erythematosus. *Journal of Neurology*, *244*(3), 186–193.

Schmidt, R., Auer-Grumbach, P., Fazekas, F., Offenbacher, H., & Kapeller, P. (1995). Anticardiolipin antibodies in normal subjects. neuropsychological correlates and MRI findings. *Stroke*, *26*(5), 749–754.

Sfikakis, P. P., Charalambopoulos, D., Vayiopoulos, G., Oglesby, R., Sfikakis, P., & Tsokos, G. C. (1994). Increased levels of intercellular adhesion molecule-1 in the serum of patients with systemic lupus erythematosus. *Clinical & Experimental Rheumatology*, *12*(1), 5–9.

Shovman, O., Gilburd, B., & Shoenfeld, Y. (2006). The role of inflammatory cytokines in the pathogenesis of systemic lupus erythematosus-related atherosclerosis: A novel target for treatment? *Journal of Rheumatology*, *33*(3), 445–447.

Sibbitt, W. L.,Jr, Sibbitt, R. R., & Brooks, W. M. (1999). Neuroimaging in neuropsychiatric systemic lupus erythematosus. *Arthritis & Rheumatism*, *42*(10), 2026–2038.

Singh, K., Gaiha, M., Shome, D. K., Gupta, V. K., & Anuradha, S. (2001). The association of antiphospholipid antibodies with ischaemic stroke and myocardial infarction in young and their correlation: A preliminary study. *Journal of the Association of Physicians of India*, *49*, 527–529.

Spronk, P. E., Bootsma, H., Huitema, M. G., Limburg, P. C., & Kallenberg, C. G. (1994). Levels of soluble VCAM-1, soluble ICAM-1, and soluble E-selectin during disease exacerbations in patients with systemic lupus erythematosus (SLE); a long term prospective study. *Clinical & Experimental Immunology*, *97*(3), 439–444.

Strater, R., Becker, S., von Eckardstein, A., Heinecke, A., Gutsche, S., Junker, R., et al. (2002). Prospective assessment of risk factors for recurrent stroke during childhood – a 5-year follow-up study. *Lancet*, *360*(9345), 1540–1545.

Stoll, G., & Bendszus, M. (2006). Inflammation and atherosclerosis: Novel insights into plaque formation and destabilization. *Stroke*, *37*(7), 1923–1932.

Sun, S. S., Liu, F. Y., Tsai, J. J., Yen, R. F., Kao, C. H., & Huang, W. S. (2003). Using 99mTc HMPAO brain SPECT to evaluate the effects of anticoagulant therapy on regional cerebral blood flow in primary antiphospholipid antibody syndrome patients with brain involvement-a preliminary report. *Rheumatology International*, *23*(6), 301–304.

Tietjen, G. E., Day, M., Norris, L., Aurora, S., Halvorsen, A., Schultz, L. R., et al. (1998). Role of anticardiolipin antibodies in young persons with migraine and transient focal neurologic events: A prospective study. *Neurology*, *50*(5), 1433–1440.

Toschi, V., Motta, A., Castelli, C., Paracchini, M. L., Zerbi, D., & Gibelli, A. (1998). High prevalence of antiphosphatidylinositol antibodies in young patients with cerebral ischemia of undetermined cause. *Stroke*, *29*(9), 1759–1764.

Toubi, E., Khamashta, M. A., Panarra, A., & Hughes, G. R. (1995). Association of antiphospholipid antibodies with central nervous system disease in systemic lupus erythematosus. *American Journal of Medicine*, *99*(4), 397–401.

Urowitz, M. B., Bookman, A. A., Koehler, B. E., Gordon, D. A., Smythe, H. A., & Ogryzlo, M. A. (1976). The bimodal mortality pattern of systemic lupus erythematosus. *American Journal of Medicine*, *60*(2), 221–225.

van Goor, M. P., Alblas, C. L., Leebeek, F. W., Koudstaal, P. J., & Dippel, D. W. (2004). Do antiphospholipid antibodies increase the long-term risk of thrombotic complications in young patients with a recent TIA or ischemic stroke? *Acta Neurologica Scandinavica*, *109*(6), 410–415.

Ward, M. M. (1999). Premature morbidity from cardiovascular and cerebrovascular diseases in women with systemic lupus erythematosus. *Arthritis & Rheumatism*, *42*(2), 338–346.

Ward, M. M. (2004). Prevalence of physician-diagnosed systemic lupus erythematosus in the united states. *J Women's Health*, *13*(6), 713–718.

Weiner, S. M., Otte, A., Schumacher, M., Klein, R., Gutfleisch, J., Brink, I., et al. (2000). Diagnosis and monitoring of central nervous system involvement in systemic lupus erythematosus: Value of F-18 fluorodeoxyglucose PET. *Annals of the Rheumatic Diseases*, *59*(5), 377–385.

West, S. G., Emlen, W., Wener, M. H., & Kotzin, B. L. (1995). Neuropsychiatric lupus erythematosus: A 10-year prospective study on the value of diagnostic tests. *American Journal of Medicine*, *99*(2), 153–163.

Wu, J. T., & Wu, L. L. (2006). Linking inflammation and atherogenesis: Soluble markers identified for the detection of risk factors and for early risk assessment. *Clinica Chimica Acta*, *366*(1–2), 74–80.

Zaccagni, H., Fried, J., Cornell, J., Padilla, P., & Brey, R. L. (2004). Soluble adhesion molecule levels, neuropsychiatric lupus and lupus-related damage. *Frontiers in Bioscience*, *9*, 1654–1659.

Chapter 16
Neurovascular Disease and Mood Disorders

Maree L. Hackett and Craig S. Anderson

Introduction

Abnormal mood is a common and potentially serious complication of neurovascular disorders. Yet, disorders of mood are generally poorly recognised, under-diagnosed and inadequately managed in clinical practice, although this is typical of most aspects of mental illness around the world (World Health Organization, 2001). Health professionals tend to prioritise management around the physical manifestations of illness (Dew, Dowell, McLeod, Collings, & Bushnell, 2005), but patients place an equally high value on their mental health and well being (Sherbourne, Sturm, & Wells, 1999). A tendency to focus on the physical manifestations of neurovascular disease may divert attention away from the potentially greater problems related to disturbance of mood and behaviour that can impede patients from optimum recovery and readjustment to life with neurovascular disease.

Mood disorders affect people of all ages, ethnicity and socioeconomic status, and are generally characterised by varying degrees of abnormal thinking, emotion, behaviour and relationships with others. Depressive symptoms reduce quality of life (Isacson, Bingefors, & van Knorring, 2005) and are associated with

increased drug and alcohol abuse, use of health-care resources, functional disability and pain than chronic diseases such as diabetes, coronary artery disease and arthritis (Wells et al., 1989). In turn, mood disorders complicate the management of co-morbid conditions by leading to higher complication rates, longer duration of hospital stay, more cardiac deaths, and higher costs per episode of hospital care (Glassman & Shapiro, 1998). Even after recovery of symptoms, people may be unable to return to work or participate in leisure activities due to stigma and discrimination associated with the mental illness (World Health Organization, 2001).

It is important to recognise that the burden of mood disorders often extends into the family. They may experience emotional reactions to the illness, altered relations and stress associated with disturbed behaviour, caregiving and the high costs of treatment. Families may also experience stigma and discrimination. There are high costs to society resulting from dysfunctional families such as absenteeism, decreased productivity, job-related injuries, poorer quality work and high demands on health services (World Health Organization, 2001). With an increase in the prevalence of vascular risk factors in an ageing population, the burden of neurovascular-related mood disorders will inevitably increase for individuals, families, communities and society.

As the profile of mood disorders in the setting of neurovascular disease is best illustrated

M.L. Hackett (✉)
The George Institute for International Health, PO Box M201, Missenden Road, Sydney NSW 2050, Australia
e-mail: mhackett@george.org.au

J.R. Festa, R.M. Lazar (eds.), *Neurovascular Neuropsychology*, DOI 10.1007/978-0-387-70715-0_16,
© Springer Science+Business Media, LLC 2009

by depression (the most common mood disorder) in patients with stroke, depression is the primary focus of this chapter. In order to place these data in context, reference will be made to the prevalence, impact and treatment of mood disorders in the general population.

Neuropathology/Pathophysiology

There is continued controversy as to whether mood disorders associated with stroke are a distinct entity with a biological (related to the location of a lesion and the 'vascular depression' hypothesis), a reactive (a psychological reaction to acute illness and/or subsequent disability), a behavioural (associated with poor health behaviours such as substance misuse) or a psychosocial (consequence of poor social support and resources) explanation. Although mood disorders are common in patients with stroke, we argue that it should not be considered a 'normal' reaction to illness.

The importance of the location of stroke lesion in the left anterior hemisphere, first postulated in 1975 (Robinson, Shoemaker, Schlumpf, Valk, & Bloom, 1975), is traditionally cited as a useful explanation for 'post-stroke depression'. The large number of studies that have focused on developing the 'lesion location' theory have been summarised in three recent systematic reviews (Bhogal, Teasell, Foley, & Speechley, 2004; Carson et al., 2000; Singh, Herrmann, & Black, 1998). Despite these reviews varying in their methodology (for example, different inclusion/exclusion criteria and varying degrees of completeness of search strategies), two reviews found no evidence to support the lesion location theory (Carson et al., 2000; Singh et al., 1998), while the other found only limited evidence: hospital-based patients were more likely to experience depression if they had a lesion in the left hemisphere, whereas population-based patients were more likely to experience depression if they had a lesion in the right hemisphere (Bhogal et al., 2004). The original studies are often criticised

for being small and involving highly selected groups of patients, raising concerns about generalizability, and in some cases, replicability of the findings (Bhogal et al., 2004; Johnson, 1991). We support the general consensus that there is no association between the location of the lesion and the development of depressive symptoms.

'Vascular depression' is a term that is increasingly being used to describe depression in the context of advanced age and where there are also features of cognitive impairment, cerebral white matter disease or 'silent' strokes on neuroimaging. The syndrome is further supported by the high frequency of associated vascular risk factors such as hypertension, diabetes and coronary artery disease (Alexopoulos et al., 1997). The vascular depression hypothesis argues that 'small vessel' cerebrovascular disease, particularly where there is disruption of the frontal-subcortical circuits of the brain, places older people at increased risk of depression (Steffens, Krishnan, Crump, & Burke, 2002). Elderly patients with depression are reported to have high rates of 'silent' stroke (Longstreth et al., 1998), more vascular risk factors and a poorer response to antidepressant treatment compared with people with 'non-vascular' depression (Simpson, Baldwin, Jackson, & Burns, 1998). However, the current literature in support of this hypothesis is primarily associative rather than causal (Baldwin & O'Brien, 2002).

We have recently conducted a systematic literature review to determine what clinical variables had been identified as predictors of the development of depressive symptomatology following stroke (Hackett & Anderson, 2005). The results show a wide variation in the range and significance of factors associated with depression and generally poor use of statistical techniques across studies. Despite the methodological limitations we found that stroke severity, physical disability and cognitive impairment were consistently identified as being positively associated with depression following stroke. Other studies suggest that clinically diagnosed depression following stroke is similar in frequency and nature to depression among older people with other chronic illnesses (Burvill, Johnson, Jamrozik, & Anderson, 1997; Burvill et al., 1996; Sharpe et al., 1990).

The cardiac literature indicates a reciprocal relationship between depressive symptoms and heart disease. Physiologic changes associated with depression including increased platelet activation, excess cortisol and catecholamine levels, increased inflammatory markers and elevated blood pressure (Vieweg et al., 2006) are thought to affect the cardiovascular system and, in turn, increase the risk for (Steptoe, Stroke, Perkins-Porras, McEwan, & Whitehead, 2006) and reduce the prognosis after a cardiac event (Faris, Purcell, Henein, & Coats, 2002; van Melle et al., 2004). However, there does not appear to be a clear relationship between the pathophysiology of depression and neurovascular disease.

Vascular disease alone is as unlikely to be the sole contributor to the development of abnormal mood as abnormal mood is to be the sole contributor to the development of vascular disease (Cole & Dendukuri, 2003). The social and economic environment, age-related factors including disability and bereavement and genetic factors (discussed later in this Chapter) may also play a significant role and exhibit an additive or even multiplicative effect on depression risk. Unfortunately, the persistent focus on potential pathophysiological pathways is likely to detract from the need for improved recognition and treatment of mood disorder in people with vascular disease.

Diagnostic Criteria

In clinical practice, a similar approach is used to identify and diagnose mood disorders as is used for physical illnesses, including taking a detailed personal and family history, conducting a clinical examination and in some instances having the person undergo further tests and investigations. However, unlike other areas of medicine, psychiatric diagnoses lack external validating criteria such as confirmatory laboratory or imaging tests. Considerable efforts have been made to standardise criteria used in the diagnosis of mood disorders that can be consistently replicated among clinicians. The term 'case' is often used to indicate a person with a diagnosis that meets certain criteria such as the International Classification of Diseases (ICD) (World Health Organization, 1992), or Diagnostic and Statistical Manual of Mental Disorders (DSM) (American Psychiatric Association, 1994) criteria. These criteria dominate official classification and coding systems in most countries and are often referred to as the gold standards for psychiatric classification. There are moderate similarities between these criteria but they are not identical (Paykel, 2002).

The term 'depression' is used to describe a variety of mood states that range from mild to life-threatening psychiatric illness. In a typical depressive episode, a person suffers from a lowering of mood, and/or a marked reduction in the performance of everyday activities over a 2-week period (referred to as core symptoms). In addition, five or more of the following symptoms should also be present: insomnia or hypersomnia; psychomotor agitation or retardation; changes in appetite; fatigue or loss of energy nearly every day; feelings of worthlessness or inappropriate guilt; diminished ability to think or concentrate or indecisiveness; and suicidal ideation or recurrent thoughts of death. For 'moderate' depressive disorder, three or four of these symptoms need to be present (for 'minor' depression, two symptoms) with at least one core symptom (American Psychiatric Association, 1994). Depressive symptomatology refers to the presence of depressive symptoms in the absence of core symptoms, considered clinically significant when symptoms interfere with normal activities (Peveler, Carson, & Rodin, 2002).

There are several caveats to the diagnosis of mood disorders in people with stroke. First, there is considerable overlap in the symptomatology associated with different mood disorders and it is not uncommon for two or more mood disorders to occur together. Moreover, mild impairment of cognitive functioning is often associated with depression, particularly in older people, while grief, demoralisation and apathy often accompanies dementia (*The Global Burden of Disease: A Comprehensive Assessment of Mortality and Disability from Diseases, Injuries and Risk Factors in 1990 and Projected to 2020*, 1996), making it difficult to distinguish depressive symptomatolgy from an early dementia syndrome (Viners et al., 2005). Mixed depression and anxiety is the most common form of abnormal mood associated with physical illness. Symptoms of anxiety (muscle tension, worry, shortness of breath, rapid heartbeat and dizziness) may precede, or occur together with, symptoms of depression (Reiger, Narrow, & Rae, 1990). Whereas loss is often associated with depression, threatening events (for example, stroke) are more likely to be associated with anxiety disorders. Chronic anxiety may result in a reduction in social contacts outside of the family and withdrawal from normal social interaction (Åström, 1996). Social isolation may, in turn, exacerbate symptoms of depression and anxiety.

Emotionalism is a specific mood disorder that is associated with other forms of neurovascular disease more specific to stroke. Although there is no widely accepted standardised definition or set of diagnostic criteria for emotionalism, it can be characterised as an increase in sudden and uncontrollable emotional behaviour which results in socially inappropriate emotional expression that is often embarrassing (House, 1987). The most prominent feature is easy crying (and rarely an increase in laughter), which makes it difficult to distinguish from depression. In most cases the disorder is mild and transient, though, when severe, emotionalism may cause distress and embarrassment to the patient, their family and friends, which may lead to the avoidance of social contacts (Horrocks, Hackett, Anderson, & House, 2004).

Other major mood disorders associated with stroke include, but are not limited to, the 'catastrophic' and 'indifference' reactions. A catastrophic reaction may occur in response to a request to perform certain tasks, or where failure to complete a task seems imminent. It may be difficult to distinguish from emotionalism, but is typically characterised by anxiety, tears and sometimes aggressive behaviour (A. House, 1987). An indifference reaction is characterised by morbid apathy, lack of motivation and often an absence of concern regarding disabilities and the effect this is having on others (A. House, 1987). Given the overlapping nature of the symptoms of most mood disorders associated with neurovascular disease and the stigma associated with making a diagnosis, health professionals may overlook or avoid the use of specific diagnoses in clinical practice.

Mood Disorder Assessment

Few health professionals would experience difficulty diagnosing a mood disorder in a young, healthy patient with predominant complaints of feeling sad, hopeless or depressed in the presence of insomnia and loss of appetite. In the setting of stroke and other disabling illnesses, the assessment of mood is complex and there is little agreement among clinicians and researchers about the most appropriate method of assessment (Gupta, Pansari, & Shetty, 2002).

Broadly speaking there are three standardised methods of identifying caseness. These include conducting a full or semi-structured psychiatric interview, completing a rating scale of observed behaviour and using mood rating scales, either patient-completed or interviewer-administered. Each method has advantages and disadvantages for both clinical practice and research. The informal opinion of a patient, family member, close friend or health professional is considered the least reliable assessment method due to the possible lack of distinction between normal distress and diagnosable disorders (Patten, 2003). The subjective reporting of symptoms requires some judgement by the individual about what they are experiencing, some willingness to communicate it, and an appreciation of the context in which the symptoms occur. In a semi-structured interview, the interviewer participates in such judgements, whereas during a fully-structured interview or when completing self-completed questionnaires the respondent is asked to make the judgement themselves.

The Structured Clinical Interview for DSM-IV (SCID), a semi-structured interview, is often considered to be the gold standard method of obtaining a reliable DSM psychiatric diagnosis (Spitzer, Williams, Gibbon, & First, 1990). The SCID provides structure to the questions being asked but requires the interviewer to make clinical judgments as to whether a patient's answers meet diagnostic criteria, or whether further questions need to be asked. This is particularly important in the setting of stroke as the somatic symptoms of psychomotor retardation, fatigue, sleep and appetite disturbances may all be a consequence of the disease itself rather than an underlying symptom of a depressive disorder meeting DSM diagnostic criteria (American Psychiatric Association, 1994; Swartzman, Gibson, & Armstrong, 1998). In contrast, disturbances in behaviour, facial expression and verbal communication resulting from a stroke may mask or mimic symptoms of depression. In addition, the DSM diagnostic criteria require modification for use in the setting of stroke. The requirement for symptoms of dysthymia (or mild depression) to be present for at least 2 years and the presence of the concurrent medical condition must be overlooked. Furthermore, structured interviews are heavily weighted towards verbal responses, making the assessment of aphasic patients particularly difficult, if not impossible.

An alternative approach is to use the Composite International Diagnostic Interview (CIDI), a fully structured interview or questionnaire that does not require clinical judgement (World Health Organization, 1993). Since the CIDI may be administered by lay interviewers, it provides a useful diagnostic tool for research purposes. In the United Kingdom, the Present State Examination (PSE), a semi-structured interview sampling a broad range of psychiatric symptoms, is the method of choice for research (Patten, 2003). The PSE approach is different from the CIDI and the SCID in that it does not focus on either DSM or ICD diagnostic criteria.

Structured interviews enable a diagnosis to be made that meets standardised diagnostic criteria. However, they only provide a limited amount of information regarding the spectrum and severity of a disorder and the interview process requires training and is time-consuming to undertake. Therefore, simple standardised mood scales or questionnaires are the most valuable case-finding tool. There are a large number of mood rating scales available. Two such scales that are readily completed by a clinician following observation and interview are the Hamilton Depression Rating Scale (HDRS) (Hamilton, 1960) and the Montgomery-Åsberg Depression Rating Scale (MADRS) (Montgomery & Åsberg, 1979), although these were designed principally for psychiatric use in the grading of established depressive illness. Other rating scales that were designed to be self- or interviewer-administered include the Beck Depression Inventory (BDI) (Beck, Ward, Mendelson, Mock, & Erbaugh, 1961), the Geriatric Depression Scale (GDS) (Yesavage et al., 1983) and the General Health Questionnaire (GHQ), which also includes a subscale for major depression (Goldberg, 1972).

The BDI is probably the most widely used self-administered screening instrument for depressive symptoms. It is a 21-item scale designed to be self- or interviewer-administered that relies on responses to verbal or written information, and starts with the assumption that the patient is clinically depressed and asks 'how depressed?'(Rogers, Adler, Bungay, & Wilson, 2005). However, the scale's authors did not provide cut points for caseness (the suggested score on a scale that is said to indicate the best trade-off between sensitivity and specificity for identification of a disorder) for the classification of depression. The BDI-II was published in 1996 (Beck, Steer, & Brown, 1996) with changes to some of the original items and a change to the frame of reference from 'now' to 'the last two weeks' to better reflect DSM-IV criteria. The BDI for Primary Care for use in patients with medical problems was published in 1997 (Beck, Guth, Steer, & Ball, 1997). Despite these advances, it would appear that most research on mood disorders in patients with stroke has been undertaken with the original 21-item BDI.

Although responses on a mood scale cannot be used to directly derive a DSM or ICD diagnosis of depression, a high score does indicate the presence of greater depressive symptom burden and, in clinical practice, indicates that the subject requires a clinical interview to establish whether or not there are clinically significant symptoms and an underlying disorder meeting diagnostic criteria. However, there is considerable variability over what cut points are recommended to determine caseness for many of the standardised scales (Hackett, Anderson, & House, 2004) and experts often view these cut points with scepticism (Bowling, 1995). Further, a simple total score derived from a scale does not allow the easy separation of emotional disturbance from somatic symptoms attributed to physical illness (House et al., 1991).

In general, the diagnoses and symptom profiles derived using mood scales are considered inferior to those obtained from structured interviews. Conversely, clinical research is often criticised for relying too heavily on broad diagnostic criteria, resulting in a lack of distinction between abnormal mood symptoms elicited from standardised questionnaires and diagnosable mood disorders elicited from semi-structured psychiatric interviews (Hibbard, Gordon, Stein, Grober, & Sliwinski, 1993). The diagnostic criteria used in making psychiatric diagnoses have been criticised for being too complex (Paykel, 2002), unnatural,

influenced by the pharmaceutical industry for regulatory purposes and of questionable clinical relevance, especially with regard to the distinction between depressive and anxiety disorders (Shorter & Tyrer, 2003). Therefore, we consider the use of a broad category of 'abnormal mood' or 'symptom burden' in research better reflects the situation in clinical practice and allows consideration of the broad range of mood disorders that may be experienced in neurovascular disease. In clinical practice, a stepped diagnostic process seems reasonable, with referral of suspected 'cases' on to have a semi-structured interview by a psychiatrist, psychologist or other similar qualified health professional.

As a direct result of the under-diagnosis of mood disorders by healthcare professionals there are regular calls for compulsory screening of all patients to assist with the detection of symptoms. While this appears, at face value, to provide a simple solution, the evidence shows that such screening is unlikely to be clinically effective, cost effective or to improve patient outcomes (Gilbody, Sheldon, & Wessely, 2006). Even when patients' depression scores (irrespective of severity) were provided to clinicians, the rate of recognition of anxiety and depression did not increase (Gilbody, House, & Sheldon, 2001).

If one accepts that the gold standard for a diagnosis of depression is really a gold standard of 'convenience' rather than a robust diagnosis, then there cannot be a valid study of any diagnostic test for a mood disorder. Despite this, a number of standardised mood scales claim to have been 'validated for use' in patients with stroke, however, concerns remain with the use of self- and interviewer-administered scales in this clinical setting. Arguably most obvious is a patient's ability to complete any of the scales in the context of aphasia and other disorders that complicate communication, including impairments that affect writing and vision (Catapano & Galderisi, 1990). In these instances, an interviewer may read aloud a self-report scale or use an observer-rated scale. Self- and interviewer-administered scales have been shown to yield very similar results in identifying cases, despite respondents being likely to provide more socially acceptable answers with an interviewer (Okamoto et al., 2002).

There will always be the possibility that higher cut points are required to detect caseness in patients with stroke, as has been suggested with assessment of mood in the elderly (Zung, 1967). However, the concurrent presence of a neurovascular condition does not make the diagnosis or treatment of depressive symptoms less important (*The Global Burden of Disease: A Comprehensive Assessment of Mortality and Disability from Diseases, Injuries and Risk Factors in 1990 and Projected to 2020*, 1996). While anxiety, sadness and somatic discomfort are part of the normal psychological response to medical illness, clinicians must be aware that persistent low mood and lack of interest and pleasure in life cannot be accounted for by physical illness alone. Even if patients recognize symptoms of abnormal mood, they may feel that it is a consequence of illness or recovery. Of course, major depressive illness may lead a patient to think that their condition is beyond help, while people with the more common mild depression may be afraid to seek help because of potential stigma associated with such action and any subsequent treatment received.

When mood disorders are present in older people, they are often missed or attributed to other factors (Mulsant & Ganguli, 1999; Simon, Goldberg, Tiemens, & Ustun, 1999). It is important to emphasize two erroneous assumptions: that diagnostic criteria for mood disorders are expected to apply to older adults in the same way they apply to younger adults (Sneed, Roose, & Sackeim, 2006) and that symptoms have the same etiology across the life span (Alexopoulos, 2006). While there may be some common predisposing factors, these mistaken assumptions ignore the physical and psychosocial changes that are associated with aging, which may influence the course and presentation of abnormal mood symptoms. Despite older people having a higher prevalence

of physical illness, being at greater risk of bereavement (Cole & Dendukuri, 2003), more likely to be female (Beekman, Copeland, & Prince, 1999) and living alone, depression should not be regarded as a natural consequence of aging.

Natural History

Mental illness is extremely common. More than one in four people experience at least one mental or behavioural disorder in their lifetime. At any one time, one in ten adults, an estimated 450 million worldwide, are affected by mental disorder, which accounts for about 12.3% of the global burden of disease (World Health Organization, 2001). Major depression is ranked as the second leading cause of disease burden in developed countries and is expected to show a rising trend over the next 20 years (*The Global Burden of Disease: A Comprehensive Assessment of mortality and Disability from Diseases, Injuries and Risk Factors in 1990 and Projected to 2020*, 1996). The incidence of depression in the general population is highest between the ages of 25 and 44 years (Fawcett, 2003), with the average age for a first episode being in the mid-20s (National Institute for Clinical Excellence, 2004), and with higher rates for women than men in all countries (Weissman et al., 1996).

Depression is not an illness with discrete episodes but rather a chronic relapsing disorder (Judd, Schettler, & Akiskal, 2002) that if untreated, lasts on average between 6–9 months (Royal Australian and New Zealand College of Psychiatrists Clinical Practice Guidelines Team for Depression, 2004). Following effective treatment, a high likelihood of relapse may be indicated if the patient has had two or more episodes of depression within the last 5 years (Peveler et al., 2002). The risk of relapse is greatest during the first several months after remission and declines slowly thereafter (Keller, 2003), but after a second and third episode, the risk of further relapse increases to 70–90%

respectively (Kupfer, 1991). In 5–10% of cases, major depressive episodes persist for 2 years or longer (American Psychiatric Association, 2000). Up to one in four cases have only partial recovery with persistent symptoms and diminished interpersonal, social and occupational function. Unfortunately, only a minority of people receive treatment (Kleinman, 2004). In an American study, less than one quarter of cases received adequate treatment (Kessler et al., 2003), and many people are the target of stigma and discrimination (Fawcett, 2003).

A wide range of factors have been associated with the prevalence, onset and course of depression. Mood disorders tend to occur in families (Weissman et al., 2005) and major depression is up to three times more common among first-degree biological relatives of individuals with depression than among the general population (American Psychiatric Association, 2000; Klein & Santiago, 2003). It is estimated that 50–80% of those with a personal history of depression, including those who have attempted suicide, will eventually experience another depressive episode (Fawcett, 2003).

Depression is consistently found to be twice as common in women than men (Weissman et al., 1996). Women are more likely to provide care for mentally or physically ill family members and are exposed to higher rates of domestic violence and sexual abuse, a common consequence of which are depressive and anxiety disorders (World Health Organization, 2001). However, it must also be acknowledged that most of the methods used for the assessment of depression are biased towards detecting symptoms in women because many of the items reflect feelings and behaviours that are more readily reported and acceptable in women (e.g., crying) (Weissman & Klerman, 1977).

Poor social support appears to be an important determinant of depressive disorders. This includes those who are socially isolated (Michalak et al., 2002), are without a close personal confidant and are either divorced or separated, especially men (Weissman et al., 1996). However, social isolation may become self perpetuating, with depressed individuals shunning personal relationships, and thereby increasing their level of loneliness and risk of further depression (Charney et al., 2003).

In practically all studies, associations have been found between depression and indicators of socioeconomic status (Gilman, Kawachi, Fitzmaurice, & Buka, 2002; Lorant et al., 2003). This includes poor housing, crowding, low education, employment status (Michalak et al., 2002) and low or no income (Harris et al., 2003). This association is found for all age groups and for both men and women (Beekman et al., 1999). Stressful life events (Michalak et al., 2002) including abuse, divorce and premature parental loss are also considered to be predisposing factors (Kendler, Karkowski, & Prescott, 1999). It must also be acknowledged, though, that most cases of depression arise in the absence of such traumatic events (Fawcett, 2003).

Major depression in later life is associated with high levels of dysfunction (Lenze et al., 2005), reduced quality of life, including falls (Turcu et al., 2004), increased rates of drug and alcohol abuse, increased use of healthcare resources (Charney et al., 2003, Frasure-Smith, 2000), greater functional disability and greater number of physical symptoms. Large scale epidemiological studies demonstrate that while some older people may have unresolved psychological difficulties, cognitive decline over time is better explained by early dementia rather than a positive family or personal history of depression (Alexopoulos et al., 2002). Most, but not all, associations between depressive symptoms and cognitive impairment in the elderly have been found in clinic-based and cross-sectional studies of patients with major depression where the direction of causality is unknown (Barnes, Alexopoulos, Lopez, Williamson, & Yaffe, 2006; Ganguli, Du, Dodge, Ratcliff, & Chang, 2006). While it seems increasingly likely that cognitive impairment is the precursor to depressive symptoms (Vinkers, Gussekloo, Stek, Westendorp, & van der Mast, 2004), in-depth studies of the relationship between cognitive impairment and abnormal mood are just beginning (Ebmeier, Donaghey, & Steele, 2006).

It is common, especially with advancing age, for co-morbid physical conditions to occur with depression, and clinically significant depressive symptoms are detectable in 12–36% of patients with any active medical disorder (*The Global Burden of Disease: A Comprehensive Assessment of Mortality and Disability from Diseases, Injuries and Risk Factors in 1990 and Projected to 2020*, 1996). Depression occurs in up to a third of physically-ill hospital inpatients, but is even more common among ambulatory patients with chronic (Verhaak, Heijmans, Peters, & Rijken, 2005) or life-threatening illness (Martin, 2001), those receiving unpleasant and demanding treatment, those with low social support (Bisschop, Kriegsman, Beekman, & Deeg, 2004), those with a history of depression, alcoholism and substance misuse and in those patients who are receiving medication with depression as one of the side effects (Peveler et al., 2002). Whereas the association between depression and stroke may be explained by the degree of physical limitations, this is not the case for all forms of neurovascular diseases, cardiac disease, arthritis, cancer or respiratory disease (Bisschop, Kriegsman, Deeg, Beekman, & van Tilburg, 2004).

Older neurovascular populations are different from other mood-disordered groups. Older neurovascular patients are more likely to be recovering from an acute life threatening health event, attempting recommended lifestyle changes such as smoking cessation, diet and exercise to reduce risk factors for subsequent disease, adjusting to the prospect of chronic vascular disease and at an increased risk of cardiovascular mortality. The majority will be discharged from the hospital on a variety of medications they will be expected to take for the rest of their lives. A substantial minority will also be adjusting to losses in physical and cognitive functioning and will require assistance with activities of daily living where they had previously been independent. The combination of increased age and vascular disease (severe stroke, atrial fibrillation and dementia) further increases the risk of dependency and shortens long-term survival

(Appelros, Nydevik, & Viitanen, 2003). While late-onset depression tends to occur in those with high-level premorbid psychosocial functioning, the response to treatment appears limited in comparison with other mood disordered groups (Taylor, Steffens, & Krishnan, 2006).

The frequency of depression following vascular disease varies enormously across individual studies depending on the characteristics of the populations studied and methods used for the diagnosis and classification of depression. A systematic review of the observational studies indicates that about one in three patients will experience significant depressive symptoms at some time point following stroke and approximately 20% will experience major depression (Hackett, Yapa, Parag, & Anderson, 2005). A similar frequency of depression is seen in cardiovascular disease (Dobbels et al., 2002), including 15–25% of patients with major depression and approximately 27% with minor depression after acute myocardial infarction (Burg & Abrams, 2001) with approximately 40% remaining depressed in the year following discharge (Koenig, 1998).

Studies have reached conflicting conclusions regarding the complex interactions of many of these predisposing factors and causality is likely to be bi-directional. People with lower socioeconomic status are subject to more stressful life events, have less social support and have poorer health behaviours. Smoking, hypertension, diabetes, hypercholesterolemia and obesity all increase the risk of cardiovascular disease. Depressed patients may be more likely to have one or more of these risk vascular factors and the link between depression and neurovascular disease may be due to the clustering of risk factors (Joynt, Whellan, & O'Connor, 2003). Cardiovascular patients with depressive symptoms may be non-compliant with recommendations for risk-factor reducing lifestyle modification, which may in turn influence the development and course of cardiovascular disease (Joynt et al., 2003). In spite of epidemiological evidence of the association between depression and vascular disease, the exact nature of the relationship remains unclear (Kaufman, 2003).

Few studies have collected or reported data on the frequency of anxiety or emotionalism following neurovascular disease. Stroke studies with specific questions about crying, reported much variation in the frequency of emotionalism, with estimates ranging from 8% (Burvill et al., 1995) in one population-based study to 32% in a rehabilitation-based study (Morris, Robinson, & Raphael, 1990). Where standardised diagnostic criteria have been used the frequency of anxiety disorders after stroke range from 0% in a population-based study (House, Dennis, Molyneux, Warlow, & Hawton, 1989) to 31% in a rehabilitation-based study. Anxiety disorders have also been found in up to 20% of patients following MI (Thornton, Bundred, Tytherleigh, & Davies, 2006) and in up to 45% of chronic heart failure patients (Friedmann et al., 2006).

The Impact of Mood Disorders

Among people with physical illness, the diagnosis and management of mood disorders is paramount given the adverse effect of mood on recovery and rehabilitation, patient self-management and long-term survival (Martin, 2001). Depression also complicates the medical management of co-morbid conditions leading to higher complications, decreased adherence to medications and medical recommendations, including poor control of vascular risk factors through lifestyle modification (Joynt et al., 2003), longer length of hospital stay, higher costs per episode and more cardiac deaths. In cardiac patients it has been postulated that depression leads to an increased awareness of chest symptoms may, in part, account for an increase in healthcare usage, however, increases in visits to physicians for non-cardiac reasons also occur (Frasure-Smith et al., 2000). Depressed cardiovascular patients are less likely to comply with recommended daily aspirin therapy (Carney, Freedland, Eisen, Rich, &

Jaffe, 1995; Rieckmann et al., 2006), hypertension treatment (Wang et al., 2002), or adhere to rehabilitation programs after MI (Glazer, Emery, Frid, & Banyasz, 2002) and depression may even diminish the functional benefits of coronary artery bypass graft surgery (Mallik et al., 2005). Therefore, it is not unexpected that depression following MI is associated with more than double the risk of cardiac mortality and new cardiovascular events (van Melle et al., 2004).

Depression has important negative effects on longer-term outcomes after stroke, particularly impairing physical functioning (Pohjasvaara, Vataja, Leppaevuori, Kaste, & Erkinjuntti, 2001; van de Weg, Kuik, & Lankhorst, 1999) possibly by reducing progress through rehabilitation (Parikh et al., 1990), impairing cognitive functioning (Robinson, Bolla-Wilson, Kaplan, Lipsey, & Price, 1986), increasing suicidal ideation (Pohjasvaara, Vataja, Leppavuori, Kaste, & Erkinjuntti, 2001) and increasing the risk of premature death (Morris, Robinson, Andrzejewski, Samuels, & Price, 1993). Higher healthcare use and costs are also seen in depressed stroke patients (Jia et al., 2006). Although the onset of major depression within the first few months of stroke may impair cognition at 1 year (Kotila, Numminen, Waltimo, & Kaste, 1999), depressive symptoms per se do not appear to increase the risk of dementia (Vinkers et al., 2004). In fact, patients showing improvements in major depression after stroke experienced greater recovery in cognitive function than those patients whose major depression did not improve (Murata, Kimura, & Robinson, 2000).

Health-related quality of life (HRQoL) refers to the subjective impact of health on the ability to live a fulfilling life and incorporates concepts of functioning and well-being (Bullinger, Anderson, Cella, & Aaronson, 1993). The HRQoL of survivors of stroke is consistently lower than that of age- and sex-matched, non-stroke controls in the first few years after onset (Bays, 2001), with physical function being the most affected component (Anderson, Laubscher, & Burns, 1996; Carod-Artal, Egido, Gonzalez, & Varela de Seijas,

2000; Hackett, Duncan, Anderson, Broad, & Bonita, 2000; Viitanen, Fugl-Meyer, Bernspang, & Fugl-Meyer, 1988). A substantial proportion of stroke survivors have 'very poor' levels of HRQoL 2 years after stroke, with 8% rating their HRQoL as 'worse than death' in one study where depression and anxiety along with age, disability and physical impairment were found to be important determinants of handicap (Sturm et al., 2004). Depression and anxiety 6 months after first MI, but not premorbid depression and anxiety have also been shown to predict impairment in the physical aspects of HRQoL at 12 months (Dickens et al., 2006). It is important to note that as most commonly employed generic HRQoL measures were not designed to evaluate patients with neurovascular disease, they may miss key aspects of health (e.g., self care, language or communication ability) that are selectively influenced by neurovascular disease (Golomb, Vickrey, & Hays, 2001; Williams, 1998) and these measures are likely to provide conservative estimates.

Treatment

The principle aims of treatment are to reduce depressive symptoms, improve mood and quality of life, reduce the risk of medical complications including relapse and facilitate the appropriate use of healthcare resources (Alexopoulos et al., 2002; Peveler et al., 2002). The optimal outcome of treatment is full remission and staying well long-term. Although there is no universal definition of remission, in clinical practice it is generally considered to be minimal or no symptoms of depression and a return to normal functioning. The management of depressive symptoms and disorders requires consideration of medication (or pharmacotherapy), psychotherapy (World Health Organization, 2001) and electroconvulsive therapy (ECT) in those with severe depressive illness (*Depression: Management of Depression in Primary and Secondary Care*, 2004).

Unfortunately the majority of patients with depression and vascular disease do not receive effective treatment (Hackett, Anderson, & Group, 2006; Insel, 2006; Koenig, 2006).

Pharmacotherapy

In an otherwise well population, antidepressants are an effective treatment for most moderate and severe grades of depressive disorder and are generally not indicated for milder states because the balance of benefits and risks is poor (*Depression: Management of Depression in Primary and Secondary Care*, 2004). Antidepressant treatment is intended to reduce or control depressive symptoms and to prevent relapse (World Health Organization, 2001). While newer drugs may have fewer side effects (*Depression: Management of Depression in Primary and Secondary Care*, 2004), current data do not support the efficacy of one antidepressant over another (American Psychiatric Association, 2000; Royal Australian and New Zealand College of Psychiatrists Clinical Practice Guidelines Team for Depression, 2004; World Health Organization, 2001). The potential adverse effects of antidepressants have become a contentious issue. Consideration must be given to what side-effects are mild and tolerable in exchange for the medication's intended beneficial effect (Marano, 2003). Unfortunately, antidepressants are often prescribed at inadequate doses and for shorter durations than is recommended (Peveler et al., 2002), with 30% of patients not responding to the first antidepressant tried (Marano, 2003).

Current guidelines indicate that antidepressants should be offered before psychological interventions to those with moderate to severe depression (American Psychiatric Association, 2000; *Depression: Management of Depression in Primary and Secondary Care*, 2004; National Institute for Clinical Excellence, 2004), and be continued for at least 4–6 weeks, in the first instance, at the dose recommended by the manufacturer. If the response to treatment is unsatisfactory after this time, the clinician should first determine whether the patient adhered to the treatment plan. If there is no improvement in or reduction of symptoms, then an alternative antidepressant should be selected or psychotherapy added. Once an effective type and dose of antidepressant has been identified, treatment should be continued for 9–12 months (*Guidelines for the Treatment and Management of Depression by Primary Healthcare Professionals*; Royal Australian and New Zealand College of Psychiatrists Clinical Practice Guidelines Team for Depression, 2004; World Health Organization, 2001). Consideration may then be given to maintenance therapy for at least 6 months to reduce the risk of relapse. However, concerns have been raised regarding the gap between the level of efficacy of antidepressants demonstrated in randomised trials and the lower effectiveness in real world settings (Charney et al., 2003).

The American Heart Association (AHA) has not published guidelines specifically for the management of mood disorders following stroke. The guidelines for the early management of patients with ischaemic stroke state simply that treatment of depression can be started when appropriate, after a patient has stabilised (Adams et al., 2003). In 2005, clinical practice guidelines for the management of adult stroke rehabilitation care were published by the Veterans Affairs/Department of Defense and endorsed by the AHA, which recommend treatment with psychotherapy or pharmacotherapy (SSRIs) to stabilise mood and improve the ability to participate in therapies (Bates et al., 2005). However, the recommendations do not indicate the severity of depression that requires treatment nor the guidelines for cessation of therapy. AHA guidelines for the management of patients with heart disease are similarly vague. Other AHA endorsed guidelines discuss the potential for arrhythmias and overdose toxicity caused by tricyclic antidepressants (TCAs) but the guidelines allow the use of TCAs in patients with structural heart disease (European Heart Rhythm Association et al., 2006) and valvular heart disease (American College of Cardiology/American Heart Association Task Force on Practice Guidelines et al., 2006). The guidelines for the management of patients with ST-elevation MI suggest SSRI treatment in combination with cognitive-behavioural therapy (Antman et al., 2005). The Sertraline Anti-Depressant Heart Attack Trial (SADHART) (Glassman et al., 2002) is the largest placebo-controlled study of antidepressant treatment in patients with ischaemic heart disease and depression to date. The trial found sertraline (a SSRI) was safe in that it did not cause change in left ventricular ejection fraction, increase in premature ventricular contractions or prolongation of the QT interval, but it was no more effective than placebo in treating depression in this patient group.

Individual trials for treatment of depression after stroke suggest a benefit of antidepressants, not only in terms of remission of abnormal mood, but also in terms of cognitive impairment and, possibly, improved long-term survival (Marano, 2003). However, case selection and small sample size associated with many of these studies limits the external validity of the data. We conducted two systematic reviews, using Cochrane Review methodology, of randomised controlled trials of pharmacological agents used either selectively for treatment or more generally for prevention, of depression following stroke (Anderson, Hackett, & House, 2004; Hackett et al., 2004). We identified seven treatment trials with 615 patients at entry and nine prevention trials with 479 patients at entry. (Further details of these reviews are presented in the Cochrane Library.)

Most trials included patients between the mean ages of 56–73 years recruited within 1 month of stroke onset, however, the time from stroke onset to entry into a trial ranged from 'within a few days' to 195 days. Most trials excluded patients with communication or cognitive difficulties or other co-existing conditions that would interfere with the assessments or adherence to the treatment. Other common exclusion criteria were a history of depression, recent or current use of antidepressant medication and concurrent psychiatric disorders or deterioration. Seven trials used an SSRI, two used a serotonin antagonist and reuptake inhibitor (SARI) and other agents with antidepressant effects were used in the remaining trials. Treatment duration was generally short, but ranged from 2 weeks to 12 months.

We were unable to show that pharmacotherapy was definitely effective in either producing a remission or preventing the onset of a 'diagnosable' depressive illness in stroke patients. However, overall there was a reduction (improvement) in mood scores as defined by the rating scales used in the treatment studies, but this was not seen in the prevention trials. A major challenge in undertaking this review, though, was in addressing the considerable methodological heterogeneity both across and within studies, including variation in patient characteristics, methods of diagnosis and assessment of depression, multiple endpoints and the frequent absence of a clearly defined, a priori, measurable primary outcome. While there was no evidence of harm associated with antidepressant treatment as evident by the reporting of adverse events, such adverse event data were seldom collected or reported adequately.

Although antidepressant treatment may, on average, be more effective than placebo in reducing depressive symptoms in stroke patients, the clinical significance of such modest changes in mood scores is uncertain. It is also important to note that up to a half of all potentially eligible stroke patients were excluded from these trials due to communication problems, cognitive loss or previous psychiatric illness. Also, given that a key requirement of effective pharmacological treatment is that patients achieve a therapeutic dose of medication for an adequate period of time, treatments in most studies may have been provided for an inadequate duration.

We conducted an additional systematic review, using Cochrane Review methodology, of randomised controlled trials of pharmaceutical agents used to treat emotionalism following stroke (House, Hackett, Anderson, & Horrocks, 2004). We identified five trials with 104 patients at entry. (Further details are presented in the Cochrane Library version of these reviews.) As two trials were of crossover design, we reported data from three trials that recruited patients within 6 days to 13 years after stroke. These trials showed that antidepressant treatment produced a 50% reduction in emotionalism, and reduced self-reported tearfulness. However, the confidence intervals were wide around the point estimates suggesting that the positive benefits observed may have been very small, or even negative in one trial.

On the basis of the limited direct evidence demonstrating antidepressant's benefits in stroke patients, and the considerable randomised evidence in other clinical situations, we recommend that antidepressant treatment be given in patients with an overt major depressive episode of moderate to severe degree, and continued for 4–6 weeks in the first instance. Psychological interventions could be added in resistant cases according to availability and costs relevant to the health care setting. Special care should be taken in the treatment of patients with co-morbid conditions and of contributing to polypharmacy in older, frailer patients as no systematic reviews are available in this area. The complex inter-relationships of depressive symptoms with disability, one or more co-morbid disorders, treatment adherence, increased sensitivity to medication side effects (*The Global Burden of Disease: A Comprehensive Assessment of Mortality and Disability from Diseases, Injuries and Risk Factors in 1990 and projected to 2020*, 1996) and other psychosocial factors may complicate the care of depressed older adults (Alexopoulos et al., 2002).

Psychotherapy

Some form of psychological therapy is preferable in the treatment of mild mood disorders. Psychotherapy is a general term that refers to the treatment of psychological disorders using planned and structured interventions aimed at influencing behaviour, mood and emotional patterns of reacting. There are a variety of psychotherapeutic methods, some of which are cognitive behavioural therapy (CBT), problem solving therapy (PST) and interpersonal therapy (IPT): CBT focuses on changing cognitive and behavioural patterns in order to improve a patient's emotional state; PST targets depression by systematically teaching patients skills for improving their ability to deal with their own specific everyday problems and life crises, rather than developing generic skills; and IPT is a short-term psychotherapy that was developed specifically for the treatment of major depression, and focuses on correcting current social dysfunction, focusing primarily on the 'here and now' factors that directly interfere with social relationships (World Health Organization, 2001).

Psychotherapy should be provided by trained health professionals, usually psychiatrists, psychologists, psychotherapists or qualified counsellors (*The Global Burden of Disease: A Comprehensive Assessment of Mortality and Disability from Diseases, Injuries and Risk Factors in 1990 and Projected to 2020*, 1996). In most cases, approximately 6–8 sessions need to be provided over a 10- to 12-week period (*Depression: Management of Depression in Primary and Secondary Care*, 2004), although there is no evidence to guide the optimal frequency of treatment (American Psychiatric Association, 2000). Most people experience an improvement in mood and a reduction in symptoms after 2 months of therapy, so that the response to therapy can be reviewed after eight sessions (American Psychiatric Association, 2000). If a person has multiple issues, or severe co-morbidity, therapy may be extended for a further 6 months (*Depression: Management of Depression in Primary and Secondary Care*, 2004).

Using Cochrane Review methodology, we conducted two systematic reviews of randomised controlled trials of psychotherapy used either selectively for treatment or more generally for prevention of depression following stroke (Anderson et al., 2004; Hackett et al.,

2004). We identified one treatment trial with 121 patients at entry (Lincoln & Flannaghan, 2003), and three prevention trials with 745 patients at entry (Forster & Young, 1996; Goldberg, Segal, Berk, Schall, & Gershkoff, 1997; House, 2000). (Further details are presented in the Cochrane Library version of these reviews.) Patients ranged in mean age from 66 to 74 years and were recruited up to 6 months after stroke onset, however, one trial did not specify the time from stroke onset to entry into the trial (Forster & Young, 1996). Most trials only excluded patients who were unable to partake in the intervention due to communication or cognitive difficulties with one trial also excluding patients who received treatment for depression in the previous 5 years. Two trials explicitly specified that the intervention was PST, one provided CBT and one provided an intervention that was more broadly defined. The interventions were delivered by a variety of trained professionals including specialist nurses and a mixed team of therapists (Forster & Young, 1996; House, 2000; Lincoln & Flannaghan, 2003). Therapy averaged 5–12 sessions and continued for up to 1 year after randomization.

In this review, we did not find evidence that psychotherapy was effective in producing a remission of diagnosable depressive illness in stroke patients, although a small, significant improvement (reduction) in psychological distress was seen in the prevention trials. However, once again there was much heterogeneity both across and within studies, including variation in patient characteristics, methods of diagnosis and assessment of depression and multiple endpoints. While there was also no evidence of harm through the reporting of adverse events, once again, adverse event data were seldom collected or reported adequately.

Early discontinuation of pharmacotherapy or psychotherapy leads to a high relapse rate. CBT is the psychotherapy of choice for depressive disorders, with PST and IPT as further treatment options if the patient indicates a preference for these methods (*Depression:*

Management of Depression in Primary and Secondary Care, 2004). Almost all antidepressants and psychotherapies are equally effective for moderate depression, but CBT in combination with antidepressants appears to give better results than either treatment on its own. For severe depression, psychotherapy may be used in addition to initial treatment with antidepressants to reduce residual symptoms and the risk of relapse (Royal Australian and New Zealand College of Psychiatrists Clinical Practice Guidelines Team for Depression, 2004), or in those with moderate or severe depression who refuse antidepressant treatment (*Depression: Management of Depression in Primary and Secondary Care*, 2004).

The Enhancing Recovery In Coronary Heart Disease (ENRICHED) trial, the largest trial of individually tailored CBT therapy versus usual care following MI, found that CBT improved depression and social support, but had no impact on event-free survival (Writing Committee for the ENRICHED Investigators, 2003). This is in line with a Cochrane systematic review in coronary heart disease which concludes that small reductions in anxiety and depression from psychological therapies do not impact on total or cardiac mortality (Rees, Bennett, West, Davey, & Ebrahim, 2006), however, no randomised controlled trials of psychological therapy have been conducted to treat depression in patients with heart failure (Lane, Chong, & Lip, 2006).

Electroconvulsive Therapy

Electroconvulsive therapy involves the brief passage of an electrical current through the brain to induce a generalized seizure. The primary indication is severe depressive illness, or when a disorder, or its symptoms, are considered potentially life threatening and an urgent response is required. ECT must be administered by appropriately trained health professionals under accredited guidelines (Anderson et al., 2005), and should only be used to achieve rapid and short-term improvement of severe symptoms after other treatments have proven ineffective (*Depression: management of depression in primary and secondary care*, 2004). As the longer term benefits and risks of ECT are unequivocal, and there are no double-blind, randomized controlled trials of ECT for the treatment of depression in patients with stroke, it is not recommended as a maintenance therapy for depression. However, case series indicate that the presence of stroke does not increase the risk of ECT treatment in patients with severe depression (Anderson et al., 2005).

Access to Treatment

Promoting effective treatment and understanding the barriers to treatment access is becoming a more significant problem than developing new and more effective treatments. Only a small proportion of people access effective medical or psychological treatment for their depression and most receive no treatment for a variety of reasons. Approximately half of those with depression do not see a health professional due to stigma, fear about drugs, misinformation about antidepressants and the consequences of being diagnosed with a psychological disorder (Hickie, Davenport, & Scott, 2003). Others may seek help but their disorder remains undiagnosed and untreated (Dew et al., 2005). This may be due to an unwillingness to communicate what they are experiencing, poor recognition of symptoms by health professionals, unwillingness by health professionals to provide a diagnosis 'label', lack of access to preferred treatments, especially psychological therapies, and a patient's unwillingness to take antidepressants. As previously mentioned, many of those diagnosed with symptoms are prescribed antidepressants at inadequate doses and for shorter durations than is recommended by manufacturers (Peveler et al., 2002).

General practitioners manage up to 75% of those who seek care (Hickie et al., 2003). In an international study of pharmacotherapy for depression in primary care, the proportion of patients receiving potentially effective treatment varied from 1% to 40%, with cost and concern about adverse effects of medication being the two most commonly reported barriers to treatment (Simon, Fleck, Lucas, & Bushnell, 2004). Approximately 40% of those with a major depressive disorder are non-compliant with their treatment (Charney et al., 2003), and depressed medical patients are three times more likely to be non-compliant than non-depressed ones (Charney et al., 2003). Patients who do not follow treatment advice do so for many different reasons, including stigma associated with antidepressants, inadequate education and support, adverse effects, drug interactions, complexity of dosing regimens, and lack of awareness about the sequelae and chronicity of mood disorders. Older adults may also lack appropriate social support and increased forgetfulness may make them less likely to take their medication (*The Global Burden of Disease: A Comprehensive Assessment of Mortality and Disability from Diseases, Injuries and Risk Factors in 1990 and Projected to 2020*, 1996). Compliance with a particular treatment may also be influenced by the relationship between therapist and patient (Royal Australian and New Zealand College of Psychiatrists Clinical Practice Guidelines Team for Depression, 2004).

Special attention is required to overcome the many barriers to obtaining and adhering to treatment for mood disorders. All treatment should be tailored to individual needs taking into consideration the severity and duration of the disorder as well as patient preferences including cost, accessibility and availability (Fawcett, 2003). Effective treatment will generally include the involvement of spouses or partners, family and other support networks. In all circumstances recommendations include monitoring a patient presenting with depression at least weekly for the first 6 weeks to assess the patient's mood, suicidal thinking, physical safety and social situation as well as any side effects of drugs that have been prescribed. Education about the depressive disorder should also be provided in short sessions and lifestyle changes may be recommended including stress management, reducing drug and alcohol use, improving sleep patterns, maintaining a balanced diet and partaking in physical exercise (*The Global Burden of Disease: A Comprehensive Assessment of Mortality and Disability from Diseases, Injuries and Risk Factors in 1990 and Projected to 2020*, 1996).

Future Directions

Clinical practice is not limited to the treatment of patients with acute illness but rather, also includes the maintenance of health for all patients with neurovascular disease. The presence of depression in addition to physical and cognitive impairment in neurovascular patients should be of particular concern to physicians. It is likely that depression reduces desire and capacity to participate in rehabilitation. Moreover, affected people are less inclined to socialise. Social isolation may be complicated by the stigma associated with acknowledging a mental health problem: some people 'mask' symptoms so family members and health professionals may be unaware of an underlying problem. Depression and social isolation may put people at a greater risk of adverse health behaviours, such as poor adherence to medications and increased alcohol and drug intake (Kessler et al., 2003; Weissman et al., 1996).

There is insufficient evidence from trials in stroke patients to support the routine use of prescription antidepressants or psychotherapy to treat depression and improve recovery after stroke. While antidepressants appear to produce lower scores on mood rating scales, there may be a concomitant increase in symptoms of anxiety. The current use of antidepressant therapy following stroke can only be justified by making reference to the wider literature on antidepressant effectiveness in the general population, specifically in older people. Despite the high use of antidepressants in the community, it is probably wise to use these agents with caution in those with a persistent depressive disorder following stroke, given the paucity of knowledge regarding the risks especially of seizures, falls and delirium.

There is also inadequate evidence to support the routine use of antidepressants, psychostimulants or other drugs to prevent depression and improve recovery following stroke. The small positive benefit of psychological strategies demonstrated in prevention trials may endorse the use of more structured approaches in education targeting emotional recovery and adjustment to the effects of stroke. However, the evidence to support the routine use of psychological approaches in stroke rehabilitation and the availability of, and access to, these approaches is limited.

Healthcare professionals should inform patients, their families and carers that approximately one in three patients experience some form of mood disorder after the onset of physical illness. People with a history of depression and severe disability as a consequence of neurovascular illness and those who are socially isolated may benefit from a closer level of contact after discharge from the hospital. Access to and availability of therapy should be discussed with the patient and their family and any potential barriers to the uptake of therapy should be identified and addressed prior to discharge. Whether a patient is prescribed a talking therapy or an antidepressant, regular follow-up is required to assess adherence and efficacy of therapy and to enable tailoring of the dosage or alteration of therapy where necessary.

References

Adams, H. P., Jr., Adams, R. J., Brott, T., del Zoppo, G. J., Furlan, A., Goldstein, L. B., et al. (2003). Guidelines for the early management of patients with ischemic stroke: A scientific statement from the Stroke Council of the American Stroke Association. *Stroke, 34*, 1056–1083.

Alexopoulos, G. S. (2006). The vascular depression hypothesis: 10 years later. *Biological Psychiatry, 60*, 1304–1305.

Alexopoulos, G. S., Buckwalter, K., Olin, J., Martinez, R., Wainscott, C., & Krishnan, K. R. R. (2002). Comorbidity of late life depression: An opportunity for research on mechanisms and treatment. *Biological Psychiatry, 52*, 543–558.

Alexopoulos, G. S., Meyers, B. S., Young, R. C., Campbell, S., Silbersweig, D., & Charlson, M. (1997). The "vascular depression" hypothesis. *Archives of General Psychiatry, 54*(10), 915–922.

American College of Cardiology/American Heart Association Task Force on Practice Guidelines, Society of Cardiovascular Anesthesiologists, Society for Cardiovascular Angiography Interventions, Society of Thoracic Surgeons, Bonow, R. O., Carabello, B. A., Chatterjee, K., de Leon, A. C. Jr, Faxon, D. P., Freed, M. D., et al. (2006). ACC/AHA 2006 guidelines for the management of patients with valvular heart disease: a report of the American College of Cardiology/American Heart Association Task Force on Practice Guidelines (writing committee to revise the 1998 Guidelines for the Management of Patients With Valvular Heart Disease): developed in collaboration with the Society of Cardiovascular Anesthesiologists: endorsed by the Society for Cardiovascular Angiography and Interventions and the Society of Thoracic Surgeons. *Circulation, 114*(5), e84–e231.

American Psychiatric Association. (1994). *Diagnostic and Statistical Manual of Mental Disorders: DSM-IV.* Washington DC: Author.

American Psychiatric Association. (2000). Practice guideline for the treatment of patients with major depression. *American Journal of Psychiatry, 157*, 15–18.

Anderson, C., Laubscher, S., & Burns, R. (1996). Validation of the Short Form 36 (SF-36) health survey questionnaire among stroke patients. *Stroke, 27*(10), 1812–1816.

Anderson, C., Skegg, P., Wilson, R., Hackett, M., Snelling, J., & Grover, A. (2005). *Use of electroconvulsive therapy (ECT) in New Zealand: a review of efficacy, safety and regulatory controls (PDF, 219 kB).* Wellington: Ministry of Health, New Zealand.

Anderson, C. S., Hackett, M. L., & House, A. O. (2004). Interventions for preventing depression after stroke (Cochrane review). In *The Cochrane Library, Issue 2*, Oxford: Update Software.

Antman, E. M., Anbe, D. T., Armstrong, P. W., Bates, E. R., Green, L. A., Hand, M., et al. (2005). ACC/AHA guidelines for the management of patients with ST-elevation myocardial infarction: executive summary. A report of the American College of Cardiology/American Heart Association Task Force on Practice Guidelines (Writing Committee to revise the 1999 guidelines for the management of patients with acute myocardial infarction). *Journal of the American College of Cardiology, 45*(8), 671–719.

Appelros, P., Nydevik, I., & Viitanen, M. (2003). Poor outcome after first-ever stroke: predictors for death, dependency, and recurrent stroke within the first year. *Stroke, 34*(1), 122–126.

Åström, M. (1996). Generalized anxiety disorder in stroke patients. A 3-year longitudinal study. *Stroke, 27*(2), 270–275.

Baldwin, R. C., & O'Brien, J. (2002). Vascular basis of late-onset depressive disorder. *British Journal of Psychiatry, 180*(2), 157–160.

Barnes, D. E., Alexopoulos, G. S., Lopez, O. L., Williamson, J. D., & Yaffe, K. (2006). Depressive symptoms, vascular disease and mild cognitive impairment: findings from the Cardivascular Health Study. *Archives of General Psychiatry, 63*, 273–280.

Bates, B., Choi, J. Y., Duncan, P. W., Glasberg, J. J., Graham, G. D., Katz, R. C., et al. (2005). Veterans Affairs/Department of Defence Clinical Practice Guideline for the Management of Adult Stroke Rehabilitation Care: executive summary. *Stroke, 36*, 2049–2056.

Bays, C. L. (2001). Quality of life of stroke survivors: a research synthesis. *Journal of Neuroscience Nursing, 33*(6), 310–316.

Beck, A. T., Guth, D., Steer, R. A., & Ball, R. (1997). Screening for major depression disorders in medical inpatients with the Beck Depression Inventory for Primary Care. *Behaviour Research and Therapy, 35*, 785–791.

Beck, A. T., Steer, R. A., & Brown, G. K. (1996). *BDI-II Manual* (Second ed.). New York: Psychological Corporation.

Beck, A. T., Ward, C. H., Mendelson, M., Mock, J., & Erbaugh, J. (1961). An inventory for measuring depression. *Archives of General Psychiatry, 1*, 561–571.

Beekman, A. T. F., Copeland, J. R. M., & Prince, M. J. (1999). Review of community prevalence of depression in later life. *British Journal of Psychiatry, 174*, 307–311.

Bhogal, S. K., Teasell, R., Foley, N., & Speechley, M. (2004). Lesion location and poststroke depression: systematic review of the methodological limitations in the literature. *Stroke, 35*, 794–802.

Bisschop, M. I., Kriegsman, D. M. W., Beekman, A. T. F., & Deeg, D. J. H. (2004). Chronic diseases and depression: the modifying role of psychosocial resources. *Social Science & Medicine, 59*, 721–733.

Bisschop, M. I., Kriegsman, D. M. W., Deeg, D. J. H., Beekman, A. T. F., & van Tilburg, W. (2004). The longitudinal relation between chronic diseases and depression in older persons in the community: the Longitudinal Aging Study Amsterdam. *Journal of Clinical Epidemiology, 57*, 187–194.

Bowling, A. (1995). *Measuring Disease*. Buckingham: Open University Press.

Bullinger, M., Anderson, R., Cella, D., & Aaronson, N. (1993). Developing and evaluating cross-cultural instruments from minimum requirements to optimal models. *Quality of Life Research, 2*, 451–459.

Burg, M. M., & Abrams, D. (2001). Depression in Chronic Medical Illness: The Case of Coronary Heart Disease. *In Session: Psychotherapy in Practice, 57*(11), 1323–1337.

Burvill, P., Johnson, G., Jamrozik, A. K., & Anderson, C. (1997). Risk factors for post-stroke depression. *International Journal of Geriatric Psychiatry, 12*, 219–226.

Burvill, P. W., Johnson, G. A., Chakera, T. M. H., Stewart-Wynne, E. G., Anderson, C. S., & Jamrozik, K. D. (1996). The place of site of lesion in the aetiology of post-stroke depression. *Cerebrovascular Diseases, 6*, 208–215.

Burvill, P. W., Johnson, G. A., Jamrozik, K. D., Anderson, C. S., Stewart-Wynne, E. G., & Chakera, T. M. (1995). Anxiety disorders after stroke: results from the Perth Community Stroke Study. *British Journal of Psychiatry, 166*, 328–332.

Carney, R. M., Freedland, K. E., Eisen, S. A., Rich, M. W., & Jaffe, A. S. (1995). Major depression and medication adherence in elderly patients with coronary artery disease. *Health Psychology, 14*, 88–90.

Carod-Artal, J., Egido, J. A., Gonzalez, J. L., & Varela de Seijas, E. (2000). Quality of life among stroke survivors evaluated 1 year after stroke: experience of a stroke unit. *Stroke., 31*, 2995–3000.

Carson, A. J., MacHale, S., Allen, K., Lawrie, S. M., Dennis, M., House, A., et al. (2000). Depression after stroke and lesion location: a systematic review. *Lancet, 356*, 122–126.

Catapano, F., & Galderisi, S. (1990). Depression and cerebral stroke. *Journal of Clinical Psychiatry, 51* (Suppl) Sep 1990, 9–12.

Charney, D. S., Reynolds, C. F., III, Lewis, L., Lebowitz, B. D., Sunderland, T., Alexopoulos, G. S., et al. (2003). Depression and Bipolar Support Alliance consensus statement on the unmet needs in diagnosis and treatment of mood disorders in late life. *Archives of General Psychiatry., 60*, 664–672.

Cole, M. G., & Dendukuri, N. (2003). Risk factors for depression among elderly community subjects: a systematic review and meta-analysis. *American Journal of Psychiatry, 160*, 1147–1156.

Depression: management of depression in primary and secondary care. (2004). http://www.nice.org.uk/page.aspx?o = 235213

Dew, K., Dowell, A., McLeod, D., Collings, S., & Bushnell, J. (2005). "This glorious twilight zone of uncertainty": mental health consultations in general practice in New Zealand. *Social Science & Medicine, 61*, 1189–1200.

Dickens, C. M., McGowan, L., Percival, C., Tomenson, B., Cotter, L., Heagerty, A., et al. (2006). Contribution of depression and anxiety to impaired health-related quality of life following ifrst myocardial infarction. *British Journal of Psychiatry, 289*, 367–372.

Dobbels, F., De Geest, S., Vanhees, L., Schepens, K., Fagard, R., & Vanhaecke, J. (2002). Depression and the heart: a systematic overview of definition, measurement, consequences and treatment of depression in cardiovascular disease. *European Journal of Cardiovascular Nursing, 1*, 45–55.

Ebmeier, K. P., Donaghey, C., & Steele, J. D. (2006). Recent developments and current controversies in depression. *Lancet, 367*, 153–167.

European Heart Rhythm Association., Heart Rhythm Society., Zipes, D. P., Camm, A. J., Borggrefe, M., Buxton, A. E., et al. (2006). ACC/AHA/ESC 2006 guidelines for management of patients with ventricular arrhythmias and the prevention of sudden cardiac death: a report of the American College of Cardiology/American Heart Association Task Force and the European Society of Cardiology Committee for Practice Guidelines (Writing Committee to Develop Guidelines for Management of Patients With Ventricular Arrhythmias and the Prevention of Sudden Cardiac Death). *Journal of the American College of Cardiology, 48*(5), e247-e346.

Faris, R., Purcell, H., Henein, M. Y., & Coats, A. J. S. (2002). Clinical depression is common and significantly associated with reduced survival in patients with non-ischaemic heart failure. *The European Journal of Heart Failure, 4*, 541–551.

Fawcett, J. (2003, October 15). *Depression*. Retrieved 7/07/2004, from http://merck.micromedex.com/index.asp? page = bpm_brief&article_id = BPM01PS19

Forster, A., & Young, J. (1996). Specialist nurse support for patients with stroke in the community: a randomised controlled trial. *British Medical Journal, 312*, 1642–1646.

Frasure-Smith, N., Lesperance, F., Gravel, G., Masson, A., Juneau, M., Talajic, M., et al. (2000). Depression and health-care costs during the first year following myocardial infarction. *Journal of Psychosomatic Research, 48*, 471–478.

Friedmann, E., Thomas, S. A., Liu, F., Morton, P. G., Chapa, D., Gottlieb, S. S., et al. (2006). Relationship of depression, anxiety, and social isolation to chronic heart failure outpatient mortality. *American Heart Journal, 152*, 940.e941-e940.e948.

Ganguli, M., Du, Y., Dodge, H. H., Ratcliff, G. G., & Chang, C. H. (2006). Depressive symptoms and cognitive decline in late life: a prospective epidemiological study. *Archives of General Psychiatry, 63*, 153–160.

Gilbody, S., Sheldon, T., & Wessely, S. (2006). Should we screen for depression? *British Medical Journal, 332*, 1027–1030.

Gilbody, S. M., House, A. O., & Sheldon, T. A. (2001). Routinely administered questionnaires for depression and anxiety: Systematic review. *British Medical Journal, 322*(7283), 406–409.

Gilman, S. E., Kawachi, I., Fitzmaurice, G. M., & Buka, S. L. (2002). Socioeconomic status in childhood and the lifetime risk of major depression. *International Journal of Epidemiology, 31*(2), 359–367.

Glassman, A. H., O'Connor, C. M., Califf, R. M., Swedberg, K., Schwartz, P., Bigger, J. T., et al. (2002). Sertraline treatment of major depression in patients with acute MI or unstable angina. *Journal of the American Medical Association, 288*, 701–709.

Glassman, A. H., & Shapiro, P. A. (1998). Depression and the course of coronary artery disease. *American Journal of Psychiatry, 155*, 4–11.

Glazer, K. M., Emery, C. F., Frid, D. J., & Banyasz, R. E. (2002). Psychological predictors of adherence and outcomes among patients in cardiac rehabilitation. *Journal of Cardiopulmonary Rehabilitation, 22*, 40–46.

The Global Burden of Disease: A comprehensive assessment of mortality and disability from diseases, injuries and risk factors in 1990 and projected to 2020. (1996). Boston: Harvard School of Public Health.

Goldberg, D. P. (1972). *The detection of psychiatric illness by questionnaire* (Vol. Maudsley Monograph No. 21). Oxford: Oxford University Press.

Goldberg, G., Segal, M. E., Berk, S. N., Schall, R. R., & Gershkoff, A. M. (1997). Stroke transition after inpatient rehabilitation. *Topics in Stroke Rehabilitation, 4*, 64–79.

Golomb, B. A., Vickrey, B. G., & Hays, R. D. (2001). A review of health-related quality-of-life measures in stroke. *Pharmacoeconomics, 19*(2), 155–185.

Guidelines for the treatment and management of depression by primary healthcare professionals. (1996). Wellington: National Health Committee.

Gupta, A., Pansari, K., & Shetty, H. (2002). Poststroke depression. *International Journal of Clinical Practice, 56*(7), 531–537.

Hackett, M. L., Anderson, C. A., & Group., o. b. o. t. A. R. C. S. A. S. (2006). Frequency, management and predictors of abnormal mood after stroke: the Auckland Regional Community Stroke (ARCOS) study 2002–2003. *Stroke, 37*, 2123–2128.

Hackett, M. L., & Anderson, C. S. (2005). Predictors of depression following stroke: a systematic review of observational studies. *Stroke, 36*, 2296–2301.

Hackett, M. L., Anderson, C. S., & House, A. O. (2004). Interventions for treating depression after stroke (Cochrane review). *In: The Cochrane Library, Issue 3*, Oxford: Update Software.

Hackett, M. L., Duncan, J. R., Anderson, C. S., Broad, J. B., & Bonita, R. (2000). Health-related quality of life among long-term survivors of stroke: results from the Auckland Stroke Study, 1991–1992. *Stroke, 31*, 440–447.

Hackett, M. L., Yapa, C., Parag, V., & Anderson, C. S. (2005). The frequency of depression after stroke: a systematic review of observational studies. *Stroke, 36*, 1330–1340.

Hamilton, M. (1960). Rating scale for depression. *Journal of Neurology, Neurosurgery & Psychiatry, 23*, 56–62.

Harris, T., Cook, D. G., Victor, C., Rink, E., Mann, A. H., Shah, S., et al. (2003). Predictors of depressive symptoms in older people - a survey of two general practice populations. *Age & Ageing, 32*(5), 510–518.

Hibbard, M. R., Gordon, W. A., Stein, P. N., Grober, S., & Sliwinski, M. (1993). A multimodal approach to the diagnosis of post-stroke depression. In W. A. Gordon (Ed.), *Advances in stroke rehabilitation* (pp. 185–214). Stoneham, MA: Butterworth-Heinemann.

Hickie, I., Davenport, T., & Scott, E. (2003). *Depression: out of the shadows*: ACP Publishing Pty Ltd & Media 21 Publishing Pty Ltd.

Horrocks, J. A., Hackett, M. L., Anderson, C. S., & House, A. O. (2004). Pharmaceutical interventions for emotionalism after stroke. *Stroke, 35*, 2610–2611.

House, A. (1987). Mood disorders after stroke: a review of the evidence. *International Journal of Geriatric Psychiatry, 2*, 211–221.

House, A. (2000). The treatment of depression after stroke. *Journal of Psychosomatic Research, 48*, 235.

House, A., Dennis, M., Mogridge, L., Warlow, C., Hawton, K., & Jones, L. (1991). Mood disorders in the year after first stroke. *British Journal of Psychiatry, 158*, 83–92.

House, A., Dennis, M., Molyneux, A., Warlow, C., & Hawton, K. (1989). Emotionalism after stroke. *British Medical Journal, 298*, 991–994.

House, A. O., Hackett, M. L., Anderson, C. S., & Horrocks, J. A. (2004). Interventions for emotionalism after stroke (Cochrane review). *In: The Cochrane Library, Issue 2*, Oxford: Update Software.

Insel, T. R. (2006). Beyond efficacy: the STAR*D trial. *American Journal of Psychiatry, 163*, 5–7.

Isacson, D., Bingefors, K., & van Knorring, L. (2005). The impact of depression is unevenly distributed in the population. *European Psychiatry, 20*, 205–212.

Jia, H., Damush, T. M., Qin, H., Ried, L. D., Wang, X., Young, L. J., et al. (2006). The impact of poststroke depression on healthcare use by veterans with acute stroke. *Stroke, 37*, 2796–2801.

Johnson, G. A. (1991). Research into psychiatric disorder after stroke: the need for further studies. [comment]. *Australian & New Zealand Journal of Psychiatry., 25*, 358–370.

Joynt, K. E., Whellan, D. J., & O'Connor, C. M. (2003). Depression and cardiovascular disease: mechanisms of interaction. *Biological Psychiatry, 54*, 248–261.

Judd, L. L., Schettler, P. J., & Akiskal, H. S. (2002). The prevalence, clinical relevance, and public health significance of depressions. *Psychiatric Clinics of North America, 25*, 685–698.

Kaufman, P. G. (2003). Depression in cardiovascular disease: can the risk be reduced. *Biological Psychiatry, 54*, 187–190.

Keller, M. B. (2003). Past, present, and future directions for defining optimal treatment outcome in depression: remission and beyond. *Journal of the American Medical Association, 289*, 3152–3160.

Kendler, K. S., Karkowski, L. M., & Prescott, C. A. (1999). Causal relationship between stressful life events and the onset of major depression. *American Journal of Psychiatry, 156*, 837–841.

Kessler, R. C., Berglund, P., Demler, O., Jin, R., Koretz, D., Merikangas, K. R., et al. (2003). The epidemiology of major depressive episodes: Results from the National Comorbidity Survey Replication (NCS-R). *Journal of the American Medical Association, 289*, 3095–3105.

Klein, D. N., & Santiago, N. J. (2003). Dysthymia and chronic depression: Introduction, classification, risk factors, and course. *Journal of Clinical Psychology, 59*, 807–816.

Kleinman, A. (2004). Culture and depression. *New England Journal of Medicine, 351*(10), 951–953.

Koenig, H. G. (1998). Depression in hospitalized older patients with congestive heart failure. *General Hospital Psychiatry, 20*, 29–43.

Koenig, H. G. (2006). Depression outcome in inpatients with congestive heart failure. *Archives of Internal Medicine, 166*, 991–996.

Kotila, M., Numminen, H., Waltimo, O., & Kaste, M. (1999). Post-stroke depression and functional recovery in a population-based stroke register. The Finnstroke study. *European Journal of Neurology, 6*, 309–312.

Kupfer, D. J. (1991). Long-term treatment of depression. *Journal of Clinical Psychiatry, 52*(Suppl. 5), 28–34.

Lane, D. A., Chong, A. Y., & Lip, G. Y. H. (2006). Psychological interventions for depression in heart failure (Cochrane review). *In: The Cochrane Library*(Issue 4), Oxford: Update Software.

Lenze, E. J., Schulz, R., Martire, L. M., Zdaniuk, B., Glass, T., Kop, W. J., et al. (2005). The course of functional decline in older people with persistently elevated depressive symptoms: longitudinal findings from the Cardiovascular Health Study. *Journal of the American Geriatrics Society, 53*(4), 569–575.

Lincoln, N. B., & Flannaghan, T. (2003). Cognitive behavioral psychotherapy for depression following stroke. A randomized controlled trial. *Stroke, 34*, 111–115.

Longstreth, W. T., Bernick, C., Manolio, T. A., Bryan, N., Jungreis, C. A., & Price, T. R. (1998). Lacunar infarcts defined by magnetic resonance imaging of 3660 elderly people: The Cardiovascular Heatlh Study. *Archives of Neurology, 55*, 1217–1225.

Lorant, V., Deliege, D., Eaton, W., Robert, A., Philippot, P., & Ansseau, M. (2003). Socioeconomic inequalities in depression: a meta-analysis. [comment]. *American Journal of Epidemiology., 157*(2), 98–112.

Mallik, S., Krumholz, H. M., Lin, Z. Q., Kasl, S. V., Mattera, J. A., Roumanis, S. A., et al. (2005). Patients with depressive symptoms have lower health status benefits after coronary artery bypass surgery. *Circulation, 111*, 271–277.

Marano, E. (2003). How to take an antidepressant. *Psychology Today, January/February*, 58–95.

Martin, F. (2001). Co-morbidity of depression with physical illnesses: a review of the literature. *Mental Health Care, 4*(12), 405–408.

Michalak, E. E., Wilkinson, C., Hood, K., Srinivasan, J., Dowrick, C., Dunn, G., et al. (2002). Prevalence and risk factors for depression in a rural setting. Results from the North Wales arm of the ODIN project. *Social Psychiatry & Psychiatric Epidemiology., 37*(12), 567–571.

Montgomery, S. A., & Åsberg, M. (1979). A new depression scale designed to be sensitive to change. *British Journal of Psychiatry, 134*, 382–389.

Morris, P. L., Robinson, R. G., Andrzejewski, P., Samuels, J., & Price, T. R. (1993). Association of depression with 10-year poststroke mortality. *American Journal of Psychiatry, 150*, 124–129.

Morris, P. L. P., Robinson, R. G., & Raphael, B. (1990). Prevalence and course of depressive disorders in hospitalized stroke patients. *International Journal of Psychiatry in Medicine, 20*, 349–364.

Mulsant, B. H., & Ganguli, M. (1999). Epidemiology and diagnosis of depression in late life. *Journal of Clinical Psychiatry, 60*, 9–15.

Murata, Y., Kimura, M., & Robinson, R. G. (2000). Does cognitive impairment cause poststroke depression? *American Journal of Geriatric Psychiatry, 8*(4), 310–317.

National Institute for Clinical Excellence. (2004). *Depression: management of depression in primary and secondary care*. Retrieved July 2005, www.nice.org.uk/CG023

Okamoto, K., Ohsuka, K., Shiraishi, T., Hukazawa, E., Wakasugi, S., & Furuta, K. (2002). Comparability of epidemiological information between self- and interviewer-administered questionnaires. *Journal of Clinical Epidemiology, 55*(5), 505–511.

Parikh, R. M., Robinson, R. G., Lipsey, J. R., Starkstein, S. E., Fedoroff, J. P., & Price, T. R. (1990). The impact of poststroke depression on recovery in activities of daily living over a 2-year follow-up. *Archives of Neurology, 47*, 785–789.

Patten, S. B. (2003). International differences in major depression prevalence: what do they mean? *Journal of Clinical Epidemiology., 56*(8), 711–716.

Paykel, E. S. (2002). Mood disorders: review of current diagnostic systems. *Psychopathology., 35*(2–3), 94–99.

Peveler, R., Carson, A., & Rodin, G. (2002). Depression in medical patients. *British Medical Journal, 325*, 149–152.

Pohjasvaara, T., Vataja, R., Leppaevuori, A., Kaste, M., & Erkinjuntti, T. (2001). Depression is an independent predictor of poor long-term functional outcome poststroke. *European Journal of Neurology, 8*, 315–319.

Pohjasvaara, T., Vataja, R., Leppavuori, A., Kaste, M., & Erkinjuntti, T. (2001). Suicidal ideas in stroke patients 3 and 15 months after stroke. *Cerebrovascular Diseases, 12*, 21–26.

Rees, K., Bennett, P., West, R., Davey, S. G., & Ebrahim, S. (2006). Psychological interventions for coronary heart disease (Cochrane review). *In: The Cochrane Library*(Issue 4), Oxford: Update Software.

Reiger, D. A., Narrow, W. E., & Rae, D. S. (1990). The epidemiology of anxiety disorders: the Epidemiologic Catchment Area (ECA) experience. *Journal of Psychiatric Research., 24*, 3–14.

Rieckmann, M., Kronish, I. M., Haas, D., Gerin, W., Chaplin, W. F., Burg, M. M., et al. (2006). Persistent depressive symptoms lower aspirin adherence after acute coronary syndromes. *American Heart Journal, 152*, 922–927.

Robinson, R. G., Bolla-Wilson, K., Kaplan, E., Lipsey, J. R., & Price, T. R. (1986). Depression influences intellectual impairment in stroke patients. *British Journal of Psychiatry., 148*, 541–547.

Robinson, R. G., Shoemaker, W. J., Schlumpf, M., Valk, T., & Bloom, F. E. (1975). Effect of experimental cerebral infarction in rat brain on catecholamines and behaviour. *Nature, 255*, 332–334.

Rogers, W. H., Adler, D. A., Bungay, K. M., & Wilson, I. B. (2005). Depression screening instruments made good severity measures in a cross-sectional analysis. *Journal of Clinical Epidemiology, 58*(4), 370–377.

Royal Australian and New Zealand College of Psychiatrists Clinical Practice Guidelines Team for Depression. (2004). Australian and New Zealand clinical practice guidelines for the treatment of depression. *Australian & New Zealand Journal of Psychiatry, 38*, 389–407.

Sharpe, M., Hawton, K., House, A., Molyneux, A., Sandercock, P., Bamford, J., et al. (1990). Mood disorder in long-term survivors of stroke: associations with brain lesion location and volume. *Psychological Medicine, 20*, 815–828.

Sherbourne, C. D., Sturm, R., & Wells, K. B. (1999). What outcomes matter to patients? *Journal of General Internal Medicine, 14*(6), 357–363.

Shorter, E., & Tyrer, P. (2003). Separation of anxiety and depressive disorders: blind alley in psychopharmacology and classification of disease. *British Medical Journal, 327*, 158–160.

Simon, G. E., Fleck, M., Lucas, R., & Bushnell, D. M. (2004). Prevalence and predictors of depression treatment in an international primary care study. *American Journal of Psychiatry, 161*(9), 1626–1634.

Simon, G. E., Goldberg, D., Tiemens, B. G., & Ustun, T. B. (1999). Outcomes of recognized and unrecognized depression in an international primary care study. *General Hospital Psychiatry., 21*(2), 97–105.

Simpson, S., Baldwin, R. C., Jackson, A., & Burns, A. S. (1998). Is subcortical disease associated with a poor response to antidepressants? Neurological, neuropsychological and neuroradiological finds in late-life depression. *Psychological Medicine, 28*, 1015–1026.

Singh, A., Herrmann, N., & Black, S. E. (1998). The importance of lesion location in poststroke depression: A critical review. *Canadian Journal of Psychiatry-Revue Canadienne De Psychiatrie, 43*, 921–927.

Sneed, J. R., Roose, S. P., & Sackeim, H. A. (2006). Vascular depression: a distinct diagnostic subtype? *Biological Psychiatry, 60*, 1295–1298.

Spitzer, R. L., Williams, J. B. W., Gibbon, M., & First, M. B. (1990). *User's guide for the structured clinical interview for DSM-III-R: SCID.* Washington, DC, US: American Psychiatric Association.

Steffens, D. C., Krishnan, K. R. R., Crump, C., & Burke, G. L. (2002). Cerebrovascular disease and evolution of depressive symptoms in the cardiovascular health study. *Stroke, 33*(6), 1636–1644.

Steptoe, A., Stroke, P. C., Perkins-Porras, L., McEwan, J. R., & Whitehead, D. L. (2006). Acute depressed mood as a trigger of acute coronary syndromes. *Biological Psychiatry, 60*, 837–842.

Sturm, J. W., Donnan, G. A., Dewey, H. M., Macdonell, R. A. L., Gilligan, A. K., Srikanth, V., et al. (2004). Quality of life after stroke: the North East Melbourne Stroke Incidence Study (NEMESIS). *Stroke, 35*, 2340–2345.

Swartzman, L. C., Gibson, M. C., & Armstrong, T. L. (1998). Psychosocial consideration in adjustment to stroke. *Physical Medicine and Rehabilitation, 12*, 519–541.

Taylor, W. D., Steffens, D. C., & Krishnan, K. R. (2006). Psychiatric disease in the twenty-first century: the case for subcortical ischemic depression. *Biological Psychiatry, 60*, 1299–1303.

Thornton, E. W., Bundred, P., Tytherleigh, M., & Davies, A. D. M. (2006). Anxiety, depression and myocardial infarction: a survey of their impact on consultation rates before and after an acute primary episode. *British Journal of Cardiology, 13*, 220–224.

Turcu, A., Toubin, S., Mourey, F., D'Athis, P., Manckoundia, P., & Pfitzenmeyer, P. (2004). Falls and depression in older people. *Gerontology, 50*(5), 303–308.

van de Weg, F. B., Kuik, D. J., & Lankhorst, G. J. (1999). Post-stroke depression and functional outcome: a cohort study investigating the influence of depression on functional recovery from stroke. *Clinical Rehabilitation, 13*, 268–272.

van Melle, J. P., de Jonge, P., Spijkerman, T. A., Tijssen, J. G. P., Ormel, J., van Veldhuisen, D. J., et al. (2004). Prognostic association of depression following myocardial infarction with mortality and cardiovascular events: a meta-analysis. *Psychosomatic Medicine, 66*, 814–822.

Verhaak, P. F. M., Heijmans, J. W. M., Peters, L., & Rijken, M. (2005). Chronic disease and mental disorder. *Social Science & Medicine, 60*, 789–797.

Vieweg, W. V. R., Julius, D. A., Fernandez, A., Wulsin, L. R., Mohanty, P. K., Beatty-Brooks, M., et al. (2006). Treatment of depression in patients with coronary heart disease. *The American Journal of Medicine, 119*, 567–573.

Viitanen, M., Fugl-Meyer, K. S., Bernspang, B., & Fugl-Meyer, A. (1988). Life satisfaction in long-term survivors after stroke. *Scandinavian Journal of Rehabilitation Medicine, 20*, 17–24.

Viners, D. J., Stek, M. L., van der Mast, R. C., de Craen, A. J. M., Le Cessie, S., Jolles, J., et al. (2005). Generalized atherosclerosis, cognitive decline, and depressive symptoms in old age. *Neurology, 65*, 107–112.

Vinkers, D. J., Gussekloo, J., Stek, M. L., Westendorp, R. G. J., & van der Mast, R. C. (2004). Temporal relation between depression and cognitive impairment in old age: prospective population based study. *British Medical Journal, 329*, 881.

Wang, P. S., Bohn, R. L., Knight, E., Glynn, R. J., Mogun, H., & Avorn, J. (2002). Noncompliance with antihypertensive medications: the impact of depressive symptoms and psychosocial factors. *Journal of General Internal Medicine, 17*, 504–511.

Weissman, M. M., Bland, R. C., Canino, G. J., Faravelli, C., Greenwald, S., Hwu, H. G., et al. (1996). Cross-national epidemiology of major depression and bipolar disorder. *Journal of the American Medical Association, 276*, 293–199.

Weissman, M. M., & Klerman, G. L. (1977). Sex differences and the epidemiology of depression. *Archives of General Psychiatry, 34*, 99–111.

Weissman, M. M., Wickramaratne, P., Nomura, Y., Warner, V., Verdeli, H., Pilowsky, D. J., et al. (2005). Families at high and low risk for depression: a 3-generaltion study. *Archives of General Psychiatry, 62*, 29–36.

Wells, K. B., Stewart, A., Hays, R. D., Burman, A., Rogers, W., Daniels, M., et al. (1989). The functioning and well-being of depressed patients. *Journal of the American Medical Association, 262*(7), 914–919.

Williams, L. S. (1998). Health-related quality of life outcomes in stroke. *Neuroepidemiology, 17*(3), 116–120.

World Health Organization. (1992). *The ICD-10 classification of mental and behavioural disorders: clinical descriptions and diagnostic guidelines.* Geneva: Author.

World Health Organization. (1993). Composite International Diagnostic Interview (Version 1.1). Geneva: Author.

World Health Organization. (2001). *The World Health Report 2001: Mental health: new understanding, new hope.* Geneva: Author.

Writing Committee for the ENRICHED Investigators. (2003). The effects of treating depression and low perceived social support on clinical events after myocardial infarction: the Enhancing Recovery in Coronary Heart Disease Patients (ENRICHED) Randomized Trial. *JAMA, 289*, 3106–3116.

Yesavage, J. A., Brink, T. L., Rose, T. L., Lum, O., Huang, V., Adey, M. B., et al. (1983). Development and validation of a geriatric depression screening scale: A preliminary report. *Journal of Psychiatric Research., 17*, 37–49.

Zung, W. W. K. (1967). Depression in the normal aged. *Psychosomatics, 8*, 287–292.

Chapter 17
Functional Imaging in Stroke Recovery

R.S. Marshall

Introduction

Functional neuroimaging is a general term for techniques that image brain activity, above and beyond the structural anatomy information that is derived from standard imaging. The functional imaging techniques, which include positron emission tomography (PET), magnetic encephalography (MEG), single photon emission computed tomography (SPECT), and functional magnetic imaging (fMRI) have contributed greatly to our understanding of the mechanisms of recovery. The techniques generally work by having the patient perform a physical or mental task during scanning and then deriving a statistical map of the regional activation that correlates with that task.

The most commonly used signal to demonstrate task-related, focal neuronal activity with fMRI is the blood oxygen level dependent (BOLD) signal, which is generated by the paramagnetic characteristics of increased oxygenated blood flow that follows the increase in local neuronal metabolic activity (Logothetis, 2002). The BOLD response is felt to be reliable in animal models and humans (Logothetis & Wandell, 2004), and has been used widely in

functional activation studies, including stroke (Cao, Vikingstad, George, Johnson, & Welch, 1999; Cramer et al., 1997; Dijkhuizen et al., 2003; Feydy et al., 2002; Foltys et al., 2003; Marshall et al., 2000; Rijntjes & Weiller, 2002; Small, Hlustik, Noll, Genovese, & Solodkin, 2002; Ward, Brown, Thompson, & Frackowiak, 2003a). High-resolution mapping of various neurological functions has thus become possible.

In motor function, for example, opening and closing the hand is associated with activation primarily in the sensorimotor cortex contralateral to the hand being moved (Alkadhi et al., 2002; Remy, Zilbovicius, Leroy-Willig, Syrota, & Samson, 1994). Language tasks tend to be represented more broadly and bilaterally in normal subjects, but activate predominantly the dominant hemisphere. Naming of pictured objects, for example, has been shown to activate the left greater than right inferior frontal gyrus, temporo-parietal (auditory association area), and temporo-occipital (visual association area) regions (Deblaere et al., 2002; Smith et al., 1996).

In pathological states such as stroke, functional imaging allows us to identify the degree to which a patient's brain activity differs from that in normal subjects. It is generally thought that any patterns of regional brain activity not typical of normal activations represent recruitment of alternative regions and pathways that may play a role in recovery or support the performance of the task in the pre-recovered

R. Marshall (✉)
Stroke Division, Department of Neurology, Neurological Institute, New York Presbyterian Hospital, Columbia University, College of Physicians & Surgeons, New York, NY, USA
e-mail: rsm2@columbia.edu

J.R. Festa, R.M. Lazar (eds.), *Neurovascular Neuropsychology*, DOI 10.1007/978-0-387-70715-0_17, © Springer Science+Business Media, LLC 2009 state. As a complement to functional imaging, newer physiological probes such as transcranial magnetic stimulation (TMS) and imaging modalities such as diffusion tensor imaging (DTI) are also being used to assess the integrity of existing axonal projection pathways and to test hypotheses about alterations in physiology that occur as a consequence of the injury. This chapter will review the existing knowledge about acute and chronic changes that occur after stroke, and address the ways in which functional imaging may be helpful in predicting recovery and in understanding the variables that induce reorganization after injury. A series of fMRI tasks performed in normal subjects is shown in Fig. 1.

Impact of Stroke on Functional Networks

In the acute state, stroke produces a widely-distributed effect on brain metabolism that extends far beyond the bounds of the infarct itself, including in the opposite hemisphere (Attig, Capon, Demeurisse, & Verhas, 1990; Cappa et al., 1997; Metter et al., 1990; Weiller, Chollet, Friston, Wise, & Frackowiak, 1992). The impact includes both effects on resting metabolism, termed "diaschisis" (Feeney & Baron, 1986), as well as on regional patterns of activity during performance of motor, language, and visual-spatial tasks (Byrnes et al., 1998; Nudo & Milliken, 1996; Cao, D'Olhaberriague

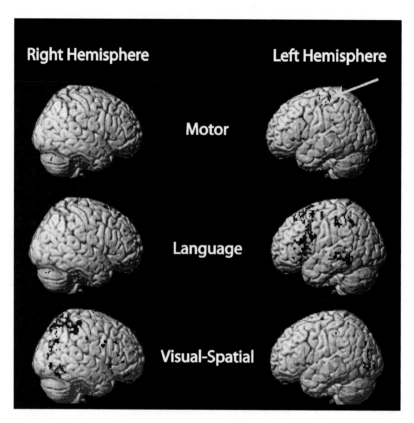

Fig. 1 Functional activation pattern in a group of normal subjects performing (a) a simple hand motor task with the right hand, demonstrating highly focal activation in the hand knob area of the left primary motor cortex, (b) a language task requiring a yes/no response, showing activation in the dominant (left) hemisphere prefrontal, posterior temporal, and posterior parietal cortex, and (c) a visual-spatial task requiring judgment of the midpoint of a horizontal line showing activation in the parieto-occipital and temporo-occipital cortex of the non-dominant (right) hemisphere

Vikingstad, Levine, & Welch, 1998; Dancause et al., 2005). Taken together, these results suggest that focal injury can lead to substantial effects on functional neural networks.

Several questions arise regarding reorganization that are well-suited to be explored with functional neuroimaging. First, how extensive can brain reorganization be? From clinical observations, one dramatic example of the extent of reorganization is that patients with childhood hemispherectomy can function normally with only one hemisphere, suggesting that a remarkable amount of reorganization is possible (Rutten, Ramsey, van Rijen, Franssen, & van Veelen, 2002; Villemure & Rasmussen, 1993). Another question concerns how rapidly reorganization can occur. Although most post-stroke functional imaging has been done in the subacute and chronic periods, investigators perturbing the system experimentally have demonstrated that brain reorganization can occur within minutes of induction of a virtual brain injury with a disruptive transcranial magnetic stimulus (Strens, Fogelson, Shanahan, Rothwell, & Brown, 2003) or by the induction of an anesthetic syndrome by inflating a blood pressure cuff (Brasil-Neto et al., 1993). In these studies, cortical disinhibition in the contralesional hemisphere emerged within minutes of the virtual lesion. Finally, one may ask what is the minimal stimulus required to induce a reorganization. Certainly structural injury such as stroke may produce the changes, but in a recent set of investigations, blockage in a carotid artery producing hypoperfusion in one hemisphere but no stroke was shown to alter the motor networks even in the absence of structural brain injury (Krakauer et al., 2004; Marshall et al., 2004). Thus, relatively subtle changes in the physiological environment seem to be sufficient to induce reorganization. Given the wide range of circumstances that can produce brain reorganization, it should be no surprise that brain reorganization is an integral part of brain recovery after injury. Because brain reorganization after stroke may involve both adjacent and remote regions, imaging techniques capable of surveying simultaneous whole-brain activity are necessary to fully characterize the brain's reaction to injury and the potential for restoration of neurological function (Chen, Cohen, & Hallett, 2002; Rijntjes & Weiller, 2002; Weiller, 1998).

Imaging Stroke Recovery

There is unexplained variability in how patients recover after stroke. Infarct size and initial stroke severity are two variables that have been shown to partially predict clinical outcome at 3 months, but among studies tracking motor impairment and recovery, only 30–50% of the variance of recovery is explained (Duncan, Goldstein, Matchar, Divine, & Feussner, 1992; Feys et al., 2000; Lyden, Lu, Levine, Brott, & Broderick, 2001). Some patients with large strokes and severe deficits recover rapidly and completely, and others with small strokes and relatively moderate deficits recover slowly, incompletely, or not at all. Through functional imaging, we are beginning to gain insight into the mechanisms of brain reorganization and recovery.

One way to investigate the reorganization is to perform functional imaging studies in patients who have recovered fully from their stroke deficits, and compare their activation patterns while performing a particular task in which they once had deficits with activation patterns in individuals who have never had stroke. In recovered stroke patients, in fact, additional regions of activity have been demonstrated. In patients recovered completely from hemiparesis, for example, PET studies have shown that simple sequential finger opposition movements in the formerly paretic hand produced activation in the ipsilateral (contralesional) primary sensorimotor and premotor cortex, as well as in the inferior parietal and cingulate gyri and in typical motor areas in the ipsilesional hemisphere (Chollet et al., 1991; Weiller et al., 1992). A Broca's aphasic patient who had recovered fully demonstrated fMRI activity in the right hemisphere in regions homologous to Broca's area (Thulborn, Carpenter, & Just, 1999). The existence of such atypical activity suggests that after recovery from stroke, the brain recruits alternative areas to achieve the same performance as normal controls. The new regional activity is not randomly distributed, but related to the neurological function being tested: the pattern of activity in recovered hemiparetics, for example, involves typical motor regions in the ipsilesional hemisphere, as well as parts of the "motor network" that are represented to a much lesser degree in normal controls in the opposite hemisphere. Likewise, regional activity in recovered aphasics is shown to occur both in expected language regions in the ipsilesional hemisphere as well as in homologous "language" regions in the contralesional hemisphere (Thulborn et al., 1999). Whereas these early studies in well-recovered patients contributed to our knowledge of the end result in some patients, additional approaches have been attempted in order to track the evolution of functionally-related spatial patterns during the course of recovery, prior to the patient's final clinical state.

Two general approaches to date have been used to investigate the functional reorganization that occurs over the course of recovery—a cross-sectional comparison of those who recover poorly with those who recover well, and a longitudinal approach in which multiple scans are obtained over time to track changes in activation pattern as the patient recovers.

Cross-sectional Studies. The cross-sectional comparison design has demonstrated contralesional activity in patients in varying states of recovery from motor (Cao et al., 1998; Cramer et al., 1997), language, and visual-spatial deficits (Calvert et al., 2000; Cao et al., 1999; Karbe et al., 1998; Ohyama et al., 1996; Pizzamiglio, Galati, & Committeri, 2001; Thulborn et al., 1999; Warburton, Price, Swinburn, & Wise, 1999). The general conclusion from these studies was that in the chronic phase after stroke, good recoverers tend to have relatively greater activity in typical, ipsilesional regions. Because these studies included patients whose function had not

returned to normal, however, one cannot be sure that differences in imaging results at a single time point were not due to incomplete recovery among the "poorly recovered" patients (i.e., the patient was still in the process of recovering) or to differences in how well patients were performing the task. In other words, the differences in pattern of activity could reflect a difference in the way the still-impaired patients were performing the task compared to the recovered patients' performance, and not to a true difference in pattern of brain activity between the two types of patients had they been performing the task exactly the same way (Krakauer, 2007). In order to achieve adequate similarity of performance, the fMRI task must be designed so that all patients can achieve a similar performance. Even if the performance appears the same based on observation, for example, hand closure synchronized to a metronome beat, the effort with which patients versus controls actually perform the task cannot be controlled for simultaneously, introducing another element of performance confound. A recent cross-sectional study by Ward et al. controlling at least for in-scanner rate of movement, demonstrated a *negative* correlation between the degree of activation in contralesional primary and secondary motor regions and degree of recovery (Ward, Brown, Thompson, & Frackowiak, 2003b). This study like many others, however, was performed in the chronic period, between 3 months and 6 years after stroke, raising the possibility that early contralesional activity has different significance from late, performance-related, contralesional activity.

Longitudinal Studies. The longitudinal approach to functional imaging of stroke recovery has added support for the notion that the adult human brain is capable of reorganizing over time, although these studies still fall short of answering the question of the functional significance of the activation pattern in the acute stroke period. Marshall et al. published a prospective study, tracking fMRI patterns during recovery of hemiparesis, and showed that contralesional brain activity appeared as early as 24 h after stroke onset, followed by a later shift back toward the ipsilesional hemisphere as the patients recovered function (Marshall et al., 2000). Dijkhuizen et al. extended the finding of the shift from contralesional to ipsilesional activity over time in an experimental animal model of MCA occlusion (Dijkhuizen et al., 2001, 2003). Four other longitudinal studies correlated motor performance with functional activation. Feydy et al. found that among 14 patients with variable recovery from 1 to 6 months after stroke, two patterns of reorganization occurred: "focusing," in which contralesional activity appeared early on and then reverted to a more typical ipsilesional predominance, and "persistent recruitment," in which the contralesional activity persisted late after the injury. Neither of these patterns was shown to be associated with recovery (Feydy et al., 2002). The number of subjects, however, was small in that study. Calautti et al. found that among five hemiparetic patients with subcortical stroke, poorer recovery from 2 months to 7 months after stroke was associated with a shift of activity toward the contralesional hemisphere. Small et al. found that among six hemiparetic stroke patients who recovered poorly and six who recovered well over 1–6 months, only increased activity in the ipsilesional cerebellum, part of the ipsilesional motor network, correlated with better recovery. Finally, Ward et al. showed that progressive decreases in activity in motor and non-motor regions, bilaterally, occurred as patients recovered from motor deficits (Ward et al., 2003a). Thus, although these dynamic shifts of activity pattern are clearly demonstrable, there is conflicting evidence regarding the functional significance with regard to recovery.

Among the stroke studies of aphasic patients, the most evidence supports a return to ipsilesional activation as being associated with good performance in the chronic phase. In a PET study of 12 aphasic patients with strokes in the left MCA territory, unique activation during a word-repetition task was seen at 3–4 weeks after stroke in the right supplementary motor area

(SMA) that was not seen in ten roughly age-matched controls. In follow-up PET scans done at 18 months after stroke, return of left superior temporal (Wernicke's area) activity was associated with good performance on an auditory comprehension task, suggesting that it was the return of left hemisphere function over time that was important for better performance. Persistence of the right SMA activity was *inversely* correlated with performance on the language comprehension task, and persistence of right temporal activation was inversely correlated with return of left temporal activity. In a follow-up study by the same investigators, 23 aphasic patients with cortical or subcortical strokes had PET imaging at 1 week and 8 weeks after stroke (Heiss, Kessler, Thiel, Ghaemi, & Karbe, 1999). Unique activation was seen in the right inferior frontal region at the 1-week time point. Good language performance correlated with activity in the left superior temporal region at 1 week and/or 8 weeks, and a disappearance of the right hemisphere activation over that time period. Stroke patients whose index infarct destroyed the left superior temporal region had worse ultimate performance, perhaps because Wernicke's area could not be re-incorporated back into a language network. As in the motor studies, these early language recovery studies had little to say about the functional significance of the right hemisphere activity. More recent evidence from fMRI demonstrated that there may be a subacute period 1–2 weeks after aphasic stroke in which the non-dominant hemisphere, in particular the non-dominant hemisphere Broca's area homologue and the SMA, plays a critical supportive role in language function (Saur et al., 2006).

Mechanisms of Recovery

Although it seems increasingly likely that there is alternative brain activity in the contralesional hemisphere that appears early after stroke, it has been difficult to prove whether the activity is functionally significant. Does an early appearance of activity in the contralesional hemisphere mean that alternative networks are being recruited and the prognosis is good, or does it mean that the normal networks are dysfunctional and therefore the prognosis is poor? It would seem important to show that the early regional activity represents recruitment of functionally important networks that assume a temporary role in performing a lost function, and/or play a role in the restorative process leading toward more "normal" networks that were lost when the stroke occurred. Certain physiological consequences of the infarct may promote the reorganization process. The ischemia may create a more plasticity-conducive environment by reducing global inhibition via decreases in gamma-aminobutyric acid related (GABAergic) activity (Buchkremer-Ratzmann, August, Hagemann, & Witte, 1996; Neumann-Haefelin et al., 1998). Two recent animal studies showed that without reduction of GABA, recovery did not occur (Hernandez & Schallert, 1988; Schallert, Hernandez, & Barth, 1986). An alternative explanation would be that early alternative activation sites appear only as an epiphenomenon of the brain injury, so that activity in regions surrounding the infarct or in the opposite, uninjured hemisphere could be a result of infarction-induced disinhibition, locally or across the corpus callosum, and therefore appear activated on an fMRI scan without having a functional role (Liepert, Hamzei, & Weiller, 2000; Meyer, Roricht, Grafin von Einsiedel, Kruggel, & Weindl, 1995; Shimizu et al., 2002). Early alternative activity has also been postulated to reflect a non-specific increase in effort or attention because the given task has become more difficult for the post-stroke patient to perform (Binkofski et al., 2002; Johansen-Berg et al., 2002).

Another potentially confounding factor concerns whether the fMRI signal, the BOLD response (Ogawa et al., 1993), is a valid index of the local neuronal activity in stroke patients. In certain cerebrovascular conditions, the BOLD response has been shown to be reduced. For example, in patients with small vessel disease (Pineiro, Pendlebury, Johansen-Berg, & Matthews, 2002) and in some cases of large vessel stenosis or occlusion (Bilecen et al., 2002), particularly when the hemodynamic state of ipsilesional hemisphere is compromised (Powers, Fox, & Raichle, 1988), there is a lower than expected BOLD signal. In one study of patients with carotid occlusion and impaired hemodynamic status, task-related activity was shown to be present by MEG (which does not require blood flow to identify activity) but absent on fMRI BOLD scanning (Rossini et al., 2004). The results were not consistent across patients, however, and included some patients with a well-coupled neuronal-vascular response even when blood flow was impaired. In addition, the time point after stroke of fMRI has been a concern. Because acute stroke may alter local autoregulation even in the absence of large vessel disease (Dawson, Blake, Panerai, & Potter, 2000; Eames, Blake, Dawson, Panerai, & Potter, 2002), some have suggested that the BOLD signal could be blunted or absent in the region of a fresh infarct where important information regarding stroke recovery may be located. However, there is little direct information on this matter. In one human (Marshall et al., 2000) and two animal studies (Dijkhuizen et al., 2001, 2003), the BOLD signal in the ipsilesional hemisphere was low in the acute stroke period and increased later after the stroke. The lower ipsilesional signal early after stroke could be due to the physiological suppression of the hemodynamic response, but it is also possible that there was neuronally mediated reduction in activity in that hemisphere. The BOLD response in that case could be a valid representation of reduced neuronal activity, reflecting a direct effect of the infarct on anatomically connected neuronal populations. Overall, most studies support the assertion that stroke-induced alterations in BOLD signal changes are neuronally mediated, truly reflecting an altered functional network early after injury.

One technique that has been helpful to validate a functional role of atypical activity is "functional deactivation" using transcranial magnetic stimulation (TMS), akin to the knock-out model used commonly in animal studies. In TMS, a train of magnetic pulses can be administered to a focal region of cortex, temporarily disrupting function in that area. One combined fMRI-TMS study demonstrated the functional significance of contralesional activity during motor tasks early after recovery in hemiparetic patients. In this study, a finger reaction-time task was associated with fMRI activation in primary motor and premotor regions, bilaterally, both in hemiparetic stroke patients and in controls (Johansen-Berg et al., 2002). The application of TMS over the contralesional premotor cortex 100 ms after the "GO" signal significantly slowed the reaction time in patients but not in controls, suggesting that the contralesional premotor cortex was, in fact, playing a new role in performing that task after stroke. Using TMS in another approach, Strens et al. induced a "functional stroke" in the motor cortex by delivering a train of repetitive TMS stimuli at 5 Hz (Strens et al., 2003). The stimulus was weak enough so as not to elicit motor activity at rest, but during a hand dexterity task (controlling the amount of force during finger tapping), a second stimulus to the "contralesional" cortex produced a degradation in performance that correlated with a delayed and temporary reduction in excitability in the contralesional cortex. The change in excitability appeared in a time-dependent way, at 1–2 min after the induction of the disruptive train, suggesting that the "contralesional" hemisphere begins to play a functional role immediately after stroke onset. Two other recent studies have also demonstrated that remapping of cortical motor areas occurs within minutes after perturbation of the system, either by disruptive TMS stimulation (Lee et al., 2003) or tumor resection (Duffau, 2001). The accumulated evidence from these studies seems to demonstrate that the presence of alternative regional activation occurs even in the hyperacute state, although proof of its functional significance still remains elusive.

Perhaps a contributing reason for the difficulty in establishing the functional significance of early alternative activation in imaging studies lies in a flaw in experimental design. A distinction has not been made in most studies between *performance* (behavior measured at a given time point) and *recovery* (change in behavior over time). As discussed above, cross-sectional studies comparing "good" recovery versus "poor" recovery can, at best, only analyze imaging information with reference to the patient's task performance at that time, along with historical clinical information. Longitudinal studies, tracking the progression of functional activity as the patient is recovering, show differences in activity that relate to the patient's changing clinical status, although not the brain's potential for future recovery. If one wishes to address the question, "*What brain processes in the acute period are important for the later restoration of neurological function?*," a different experimental design is necessary. One must correlate the pattern of brain activity at a baseline time point (T_0) with the change in clinical performance from T_0 to a future point in time (T_1). Such a design has been applied recently to a functional-recovery study in 14 patients with fMRI at T_0 in the first 24–48 h after stroke (Krakauer, Zarahn, Lazar, & Marshall, 2007). A multivariate regression was used to correlate acute functional imaging data with a measure of motor recovery defined as the change in upper arm Fugl-Meyer score (Fugl-Meyer, 1980) from 24–48 h to 3 months later. A pattern of early brain activation was identified, distributed predominantly outside of motor and premotor cortex, whose degree of expression correlated with subsequent motor recovery: greater degrees of expression of this activation at T_0 was associated with better motor recovery at T_1. These results suggested that there are determinants of the recovery process identifiable very early after stroke that play a role in the subsequent course of recovery.

Functional neuroimaging has helped move forward in our understanding of the time course, anatomical substrate, and physiological mechanisms of stroke recovery. Further technical advances and development of new analytical methods promise to further our grasp of the complex set of events the brain puts in motion in response to focal injury.

References

Alkadhi, H., Crelier, G. R., Boendermaker, S. H., Golay, X., Hepp-Reymond, M. C., & Kollias, S. S. (2002). Reproducibility of primary motor cortex somatotopy under controlled conditions. *AJNR American Journal of Neuroradiology, 23*(9), 1524–1532.

Attig, E., Capon, A., Demeurisse, G., & Verhas, M. (1990). Remote effect of deep-seated vascular brain lesions on cerebral blood flow. *Stroke, 21*(11), 1555–1561.

Bilecen, D., Radu, E. W., Schulte, A. C., Hennig, J., Scheffler, K., & Seifritz, E. (2002). fMRI of the auditory cortex in patients with unilateral carotid artery steno-occlusive disease. *Journal of Magnetic Resonance Imaging, 15*(6), 621–627.

Binkofski, F., Fink, G. R., Geyer, S., Buccino, G., Gruber, O., Shah, N. J., et al. (2002). Neural activity in human primary motor cortex areas 4a and 4p is modulated differentially by attention to action. *Journal of Neurophysiology, 88*(1), 514–519.

Brasil-Neto, J. P., Valls-Sole, J., Pascual-Leone, A., Cammarota, A., Amassian, V. E., Cracco, R., et al. (1993). Rapid modulation of human cortical motor outputs following ischaemic nerve block. *Brain, 116 (Pt 3),* 511–525.

Buchkremer-Ratzmann, I., August, M., Hagemann, G., & Witte, O. W. (1996). Electrophysiological transcortical diaschisis after cortical photothrombosis in rat brain. *Stroke, 27*(6), 1105–1109; discussion 1109–1111.

Byrnes, M. L., Thickbroom, G. W., Wilson, S. A., Sacco, P., Shipman, J. M., Stell, R., et al. (1998). The corticomotor representation of upper limb muscles in writer's cramp and changes following botulinum toxin injection. *Brain, 121 (Pt 5),* 977–988.

Calvert, G. A., Brammer, M. J., Morris, R. G., Williams, S. C., King, N., & Matthews, P. M. (2000). Using fMRI to study recovery from acquired dysphasia. *Brain Language, 71*(3), 391–399.

Cao, Y., D'Olhaberriague, L., Vikingstad, E. M., Levine, S. R., & Welch, K. M. (1998). Pilot study of functional MRI to assess cerebral activation of motor function after poststroke hemiparesis. *Stroke, 29*(1), 112–122.

Cao, Y., Vikingstad, E. M., George, K. P., Johnson, A. F., & Welch, K. M. (1999). Cortical language

activation in stroke patients recovering from aphasia with functional MRI. *Stroke, 30*(11), 2331–2340.

Cappa, S. F., Perani, D., Grassi, F., Bressi, S., Alberoni, M., Franceschi, M., et al. (1997). A PET follow-up study of recovery after stroke in acute aphasics. *Brain Lang, 56*(1), 55–67.

Chen, R., Cohen, L. G., & Hallett, M. (2002). Nervous system reorganization following injury. *Neuroscience, 111*(4), 761–773.

Chollet, F., DiPiero, V., Wise, R. J., Brooks, D. J., Dolan, R. J., & Frackowiak, R. S. (1991). The functional anatomy of motor recovery after stroke in humans: a study with positron emission tomography. *Annals of Neurology, 29*(1), 63–71.

Cramer, S. C., Nelles, G., Benson, R. R., Kaplan, J. D., Parker, R. A., Kwong, K. K., et al. (1997). A functional MRI study of subjects recovered from hemiparetic stroke. *Stroke, 28*(12), 2518–2527.

Dancause, N., Barbay, S., Frost, S. B., Plautz, E. J., Chen, D., Zoubina, E. V., et al. (2005). Extensive cortical rewiring after brain injury. *Journal of Neuroscience, 25*(44), 10167–10179.

Dawson, S. L., Blake, M. J., Panerai, R. B., & Potter, J. F. (2000). Dynamic but not static cerebral autoregulation is impaired in acute ischaemic stroke. *Cerebrovascular Diseases, 10*(2), 126–132.

Deblaere, K., Backes, W. H., Hofman, P., Vandemaele, P., Boon, P. A., Vonck, K., et al. (2002). Developing a comprehensive presurgical functional MRI protocol for patients with intractable temporal lobe epilepsy: a pilot study. *Neuroradiology, 44*(8), 667–673.

Dijkhuizen, R. M., Ren, J., Mandeville, J. B., Wu, O., Ozdag, F. M., Moskowitz, M. A., et al. (2001). Functional magnetic resonance imaging of reorganization in rat brain after stroke. *Proceedings of the National Academy of Sciences of the United States of America, 98*(22), 12766–12771.

Dijkhuizen, R. M., Singhal, A. B., Mandeville, J. B., Wu, O., Halpern, E. F., Finklestein, S. P., et al. (2003). Correlation between brain reorganization, ischemic damage, and neurologic status after transient focal cerebral ischemia in rats: a functional magnetic resonance imaging study. *Journal of Neuroscience, 23*(2), 510–517.

Duffau, H. (2001). Acute functional reorganisation of the human motor cortex during resection of central lesions: a study using intraoperative brain mapping. *Journal of Neurology, Neurosurgery, and Psychiatry, 70*(4), 506–513.

Duncan, P. W., Goldstein, L. B., Matchar, D., Divine, G. W., & Feussner, J. (1992). Measurement of motor recovery after stroke. Outcome assessment and sample size requirements. *Stroke, 23*(8), 1084–1089.

Eames, P. J., Blake, M. J., Dawson, S. L., Panerai, R. B., & Potter, J. F. (2002). Dynamic cerebral autoregulation and beat to beat blood pressure control are impaired in acute ischaemic stroke. *Journal of Neurology, Neurosurgery, and Psychiatry, 72*(4), 467–472.

Feeney, D. M., & Baron, J. C. (1986). Diaschisis. *Stroke, 17*(5), 817–830.

Feydy, A., Carlier, R., Roby-Brami, A., Bussel, B., Cazalis, F., Pierot, L., et al. (2002). Longitudinal study of motor recovery after stroke: recruitment and focusing of brain activation. *Stroke, 33*(6), 1610–1617.

Feys, H., De Weerdt, W., Nuyens, G., van de Winckel, A., Selz, B., & Kiekens, C. (2000). Predicting motor recovery of the upper limb after stroke rehabilitation: value of a clinical examination. *Physiotherapy Research International, 5*(1), 1–18.

Foltys, H., Krings, T., Meister, I. G., Sparing, R., Boroojerdi, B., Thron, A., et al. (2003). Motor representation in patients rapidly recovering after stroke: a functional magnetic resonance imaging and transcranial magnetic stimulation study. *Clinical Neurophysiology, 114*(12), 2404–2415.

Fugl-Meyer, A. R. (1980). Post-stroke hemiplegia assessment of physical properties. *Scandinavian Journal of Rehabilitation Medicine. Supplement, 7,* 85–93.

Heiss, W. D., Kessler, J., Thiel, A., Ghaemi, M., & Karbe, H. (1999). Differential capacity of left and right hemispheric areas for compensation of post-stroke aphasia. *Annals of Neurology, 45*(4), 430–438.

Hernandez, T. D., & Schallert, T. (1988). Seizures and recovery from experimental brain damage. *Experimental Neurology, 102*(3), 318–324.

Johansen-Berg, H., Rushworth, M. F., Bogdanovic, M. D., Kischka, U., Wimalaratna, S., & Matthews, P. M. (2002). The role of ipsilateral premotor cortex in hand movement after stroke. *Proceedings of the National Academy of Sciences of the United States of America, 99*(22), 14518–14523.

Karbe, H., Thiel, A., Weber-Luxenburger, G., Herholz, K., Kessler, J., & Heiss, W. D. (1998). Brain plasticity in poststroke aphasia: what is the contribution of the right hemisphere? *Brain Language, 64*(2), 215–230.

Krakauer, J. W. (2007). Avoiding performance and task confounds: multimodal investigation of brain reorganization after stroke rehabilitation. *Experimental Neurology, 204*(2), 491–495.

Krakauer, J. W., Radoeva, P. D., Zarahn, E., Wydra, J., Lazar, R. M., Hirsch, J., et al. (2004). Hypoperfusion without stroke alters motor activation in the opposite hemisphere. *Annals of Neurology, 56*(6), 796–802.

Krakauer, J. W., Zarahn E, Lazar RM, & Marshall RS. (2007). Imaging "Likelihood to Recover" in Acute Stroke. *Stroke 38,* 520 (abs).

Lee, L., Siebner, H. R., Rowe, J. B., Rizzo, V., Rothwell, J. C., Frackowiak, R. S., et al. (2003). Acute remapping within the motor system induced

by low-frequency repetitive transcranial magnetic stimulation. *Journal of Neuroscience, 23*(12), 5308–5318.

Liepert, J., Hamzei, F., & Weiller, C. (2000). Motor cortex disinhibition of the unaffected hemisphere after acute stroke. *Muscle Nerve, 23*(11), 1761–1763.

Logothetis, N. K. (2002). The neural basis of the blood-oxygen-level-dependent functional magnetic resonance imaging signal. *Philosophical Transactions of the Royal Society of London. Series B, Biological Sciences, 357*(1424), 1003–1037.

Logothetis, N. K., & Wandell, B. A. (2004). Interpreting the BOLD signal. *Annual Review of Physiology, 66,* 735–769.

Lyden, P. D., Lu, M., Levine, S. R., Brott, T. G., & Broderick, J. (2001). A modified National Institutes of Health Stroke Scale for use in stroke clinical trials: preliminary reliability and validity. *Stroke, 32*(6), 1310–1317.

Marshall, R. S., Krakauer, J. W., Radoeva, P. D., Wydra, J., Lazar, R. M., & Hirsch, J. (2004). Hemispheric hemodynamic impairment in the absence of stroke induces fMRI activation in the opposite hemisphere. *Neurology, 62*(7), A541.

Marshall, R. S., Perera, G. M., Lazar, R. M., Krakauer, J. W., Constantine, R. C., & DeLaPaz, R. L. (2000). Evolution of cortical activation during recovery from corticospinal tract infarction. *Stroke, 31*(3), 656–661.

Metter, E. J., Hanson, W. R., Jackson, C. A., Kempler, D., van Lancker, D., Mazziotta, J. C., et al. (1990). Temporoparietal cortex in aphasia. Evidence from positron emission tomography. *Archives of Neurology, 47*(11), 1235–1238.

Meyer, B. U., Roricht, S., Grafin von Einsiedel, H., Kruggel, F., & Weindl, A. (1995). Inhibitory and excitatory interhemispheric transfers between motor cortical areas in normal humans and patients with abnormalities of the corpus callosum. *Brain, 118 (Pt 2),* 429–440.

Neumann-Haefelin, T., Staiger, J. F., Redecker, C., Zilles, K., Fritschy, J. M., Mohler, H., et al. (1998). Immunohistochemical evidence for dysregulation of the GABAergic system ipsilateral to photochemically induced cortical infarcts in rats. *Neuroscience, 87*(4), 871–879.

Nudo, R. J., & Milliken, G. W. (1996). Reorganization of movement representations in primary motor cortex following focal ischemic infarcts in adult squirrel monkeys. *Journal of Neurophysiology, 75*(5), 2144–2149.

Ogawa, S., Menon, R. S., Tank, D. W., Kim, S. G., Merkle, H., Ellermann, J. M., et al. (1993). Functional brain mapping by blood oxygenation level-dependent contrast magnetic resonance imaging. A comparison of signal characteristics with a biophysical model. *Biophys J, 64*(3), 803–812.

Ohyama, M., Senda, M., Kitamura, S., Ishii, K., Mishina, M., & Terashi, A. (1996). Role of the nondominant hemisphere and undamaged area during word repetition in poststroke aphasics. A PET activation study. *Stroke, 27*(5), 897–903.

Pineiro, R., Pendlebury, S., Johansen-Berg, H., & Matthews, P. M. (2002). Altered hemodynamic responses in patients after subcortical stroke measured by functional MRI. *Stroke, 33*(1), 103–109.

Pizzamiglio, L., Galati, G., & Committeri, G. (2001). The contribution of functional neuroimaging to recovery after brain damage: a review. *Cortex, 37*(1), 11–31.

Powers, W. J., Fox, P. T., & Raichle, M. E. (1988). The effect of carotid artery disease on the cerebrovascular response to physiologic stimulation. *Neurology, 38*(9), 1475–1478.

Remy, P., Zilbovicius, M., Leroy-Willig, A., Syrota, A., & Samson, Y. (1994). Movement- and task-related activations of motor cortical areas: a positron emission tomographic study. *Annals of Neurology, 36*(1), 19–26.

Rijntjes, M., & Weiller, C. (2002). Recovery of motor and language abilities after stroke: the contribution of functional imaging. *Prog Neurobiol, 66*(2), 109–122.

Rossini, P. M., Altamura, C., Ferretti, A., Vernieri, F., Zappasodi, F., Caulo, M., et al. (2004). Does cerebrovascular disease affect the coupling between neuronal activity and local haemodynamics? *Brain, 127*(Pt 1), 99–110.

Rutten, G. J., Ramsey, N. F., van Rijen, P. C., Franssen, H., & van Veelen, C. W. (2002). Interhemispheric reorganization of motor hand function to the primary motor cortex predicted with functional magnetic resonance imaging and transcranial magnetic stimulation. *Journal of Child Neurology, 17*(4), 292–297.

Saur, D., Lange, R., Baumgaertner, A., Schraknepper, V., Willmes, K., Rijntjes, M., et al. (2006). Dynamics of language reorganization after stroke. *Brain, 129*(Pt 6), 1371–1384.

Schallert, T., Hernandez, T. D., & Barth, T. M. (1986). Recovery of function after brain damage: severe and chronic disruption by diazepam. *Brain Research, 379*(1), 104–111.

Shimizu, T., Hosaki, A., Hino, T., Sato, M., Komori, T., Hirai, S., et al. (2002). Motor cortical disinhibition in the unaffected hemisphere after unilateral cortical stroke. *Brain, 125*(Pt 8), 1896–1907.

Small, S. L., Hlustik, P., Noll, D. C., Genovese, C., & Solodkin, A. (2002). Cerebellar hemispheric activation ipsilateral to the paretic hand correlates with functional recovery after stroke. *Brain, 125*(Pt 7), 1544–1557.

Smith, C. D., Andersen, A. H., Chen, Q., Blonder, L. X., Kirsch, J. E., & Avison, M. J. (1996). Cortical activation in confrontation naming. *Neuroreport, 7*(3), 781–785.

Strens, L. H., Fogelson, N., Shanahan, P., Rothwell, J. C., & Brown, P. (2003). The ipsilateral human motor cortex can functionally compensate for acute contralateral motor cortex dysfunction. *Current Biology, 13*(14), 1201–1205.

Thulborn, K. R., Carpenter, P. A., & Just, M. A. (1999). Plasticity of language-related brain function during recovery from stroke. *Stroke, 30*(4), 749–754.

Villemure, J. G., & Rasmussen, T. (1993). Functional hemispherectomy in children. *Neuropediatrics, 24*(1), 53–55.

Warburton, E., Price, C. J., Swinburn, K., & Wise, R. J. (1999). Mechanisms of recovery from aphasia: evidence from positron emission tomography studies. *Journal of Neurology, Neurosurgery, and Psychiatry, 66*(2), 155–161.

Ward, N. S., Brown, M. M., Thompson, A. J., & Frackowiak, R. S. (2003a). Neural correlates of motor recovery after stroke: a longitudinal fMRI study. *Brain, 126*(Pt 11), 2476–2496.

Ward, N. S., Brown, M. M., Thompson, A. J., & Frackowiak, R. S. (2003b). Neural correlates of outcome after stroke: a cross-sectional fMRI study. *Brain, 126*(Pt 6), 1430–1448.

Weiller, C. (1998). Imaging recovery from stroke. *Experimental Brain Research, 123*(1–2), 13–17.

Weiller, C., Chollet, F., Friston, K. J., Wise, R. J., & Frackowiak, R. S. (1992). Functional reorganization of the brain in recovery from striatocapsular infarction in man. *Annals of Neurology, 31*(5), 463–472.

Chapter 18
Pharmacological Treatment for Cognitive Disorders of Neurovascular Origin

Steven Flanagan and Wayne A. Gordon

Introduction

Neurovascular disease is the most common cause of adult disability, resulting in both physical and cognitive impairments as well as behavioral disturbances. Physical problems, such as hemiplegia have an obvious impact on mobility and ability to participate in activities of daily living. However, cognitive impairments, while often less obvious on superficial examination, have a tremendous impact on the same skills. In fact, in the absence of physical impairments, cognitive dysfunction often results in an inability to participate in desired roles. Traditional rehabilitation efforts to ameliorate these impairments are varied and often require prolonged periods of time to achieve desired outcomes. While rehabilitation interventions are widely used and are felt to be effective in restoring functional skills, individuals are often left with residual disability. Enhancing traditional rehabilitation techniques with pharmacological interventions has been an area of interest and research for several decades. Ideally, pharmacological intervention following stroke should speed the rehabilitation process, in addition to improving overall outcomes. This is becoming increasingly important now that modern health care systems have placed increasing emphasis on both shorter hospitalizations and more efficient treatments.

Unfortunately, there is a paucity of evidence-based clinical guidelines for the use of pharmacological agents to enhance the recovery of functional skills after stroke. This is the result of limited research and poor study design, which minimizes the validity and clinical utility of the outcomes. In addition, the precise cognitive skill being assessed was frequently not adequately described in most studies. For example, studies examining the impact of drugs on attention often failed to account for the range of skills that comprise attention, such as vigilance, resistance to distraction, processing speed, and ability to direct attention across competing environmental stimuli. Also, the assessment of the impact of any intervention on outcomes is often limited in scope, so that studies typically examine the impact on impairment as defined by changes on specific tests, with little concern for the impact on activity or participation in societal roles. Furthermore, relatively little was known until recently about the normal anatomy and physiology of cognitive, motor, and behavioral processes. However, recent insights regarding the neurophysiological and neuroanatomical basis of human behavior have improved the ability of scientists to understand how neurotransmitters interact with receptors in various regions of the brain. This has led to a more focused approach to studying how drugs

S. Flanagan (✉)
New York University School of Medicine, Rusk
Institute of Rehabilitation Medicine, NYU-Langone
Medical Center, New York, NY, USA
e-mail: Steven.Flanagan@nyumc.org

J.R. Festa, R.M. Lazar (eds.), *Neurovascular Neuropsychology*, DOI 10.1007/978-0-387-70715-0_18,   255
© Springer Science+Business Media, LLC 2009

impact behavior and cognition, which will likely result in the future development of comprehensive evidence-based standards of care to enhance recovery.

Despite recent advances in knowledge pertaining to brain physiology, prescribing medications to improve functional recovery following stroke remains confusing to many clinicians. To date, there are no standards of care in this area because of the paucity of Class I studies. As a result, there are only a few practice guidelines and options for using selected drugs to enhance various cognitive skills following traumatic brain injury (TBI) (Neurobehavioral Guidelines Working Group et al., 2006), and none for stroke. Therefore, clinicians who choose to prescribe medications to improve recovery after brain injury must critically assess and judiciously use available information to logically approach treatment (Simon, 1981). This includes having a basic understanding of the currently known neurophysiological and neuroanatomical basis of cognition, as well as the results of clinical trials examining this issue in humans. However, given the marked paucity of Class I data, clinicians choosing to prescribe medications to enhance recovery of function do so, understanding that use remains off-label.

Cognition

Although there are many neurotransmitters, norepinephrine, dopamine, serotonin, acetylcholine, and glutamate are the ones that have been most often implicated in cognitive function, including but not limited to attention, concentration, learning, executive function, memory, language, motivation, and arousal. Diseases or injury impacting theses neurotransmitter systems are typically associated with either impairments in various cognitive skills or affective disorders and have provided clues to their role in normal behavior. Many cognitive skills are mediated by specific levels

of neurotransmitters acting on specific receptor subtypes in specific regions of the brain. Not surprisingly, the mechanisms by which drugs impact cognition also depends on numerous factors, including their actions on specific receptors and the predominance of these receptor in specific regions of the brain. A further complication is the fact that many available drugs for human use lack receptor-type specificity, limiting their ability to pharmacologically fine-tune cognitive function. It is also important to note that a cognitive skill maybe impacted by a complex interaction among several neurotransmitters, making difficult attempts to modify them. Therefore, clinicians who use drugs to improve cognition must consider the complexity of the deficit being targeted for intervention, the general lack of receptor-type specificity of most currently available drugs, and the assessment of its desired and potentially undesired actions.

If clinicians choose to use drugs to enhance recovery, several recommendations should be considered. Ideally, a specific impairment or function targeted for improvement should be identified prior to choosing a drug. Drug selection should be based on available knowledge of the underlying pathology of the individual to be treated, as well as an understanding of the physiologic mechanism underlying the specific skill to be addressed. Objective assessment of that function or skill should be made prior to and during active treatment, as well as after each dose adjustment, in order to evaluate its effectiveness. In general, the lowest effective dose without undesired side effects should be used. When making assessments of drug effectiveness, however, one needs to consider the confounding role of spontaneous recovery, particularly following acute injury when improvements are likely to occur regardless of drug intervention. When a drug intervention is considered to be effective, an important issue is how long the treatment should continue. While there are no standard guidelines, it is reasonable to withdraw drugs periodically to determine whether their use is still beneficial. Finally, drug treatment alone is typically ineffective in improving rehabilitation outcomes. Therefore, nearly all pharmacological interventions need to be accompanied by more traditional rehabilitation interventions, such cognitive remediation, physical, occupational or speech therapies.

Many cognitive skills share overlapping characteristics, often making specific taxonomies used to classify them seem arbitrary or incorrect. For example, while many consider working memory an executive skill, others consider it in the domain of attention. While there is some controversy regarding the categorization of cognitive skills, the following discussion will discuss certain skills within the broad headings of executive skills, attention, memory, and language for the sake of clarity and organization. Also, a considerable amount of information regarding pharmacological treatment has been obtained from populations of individuals with brain injuries of various etiologies, which will also be discussed, since they provide potential insights into stroke treatment.

Catecholamine Role in Cognitive Function

Catecholamines have widespread activity in the brain, impacting multiple cognitive functions. A more thorough understanding of the role catecholamines play in cognition has emerged from studies examining the prefrontal cortex (PFC), hippocampus, and amygdala. The PFC is involved in working memory, response inhibition, sustained attention, and executive skills, whereas the hippocampus and amygdala are involved in memory, learning, and retention. The circuits responsible for their normal execution can be disrupted by ischemia and trauma. Interestingly, it is often these cognitive impairments that prevent effective function following injury, rather than their associated physical impairment. It has long been known that catecholamines are critical modulators of cognitive function in both the PFC and hippocampus, demonstrated by the similarity of cognitive impairments resulting from their enzymatic depletion in the PFC compared to total resection of the frontal lobes (Simon, 1981; Collins, Roberts, Dias, Everitt, & Robbins, 1998). However, the relationship between catecholamine action and cognitive performance is extremely complex and depends on many factors. For example, differing synaptic concentrations of neurotransmitters or receptor type, as well as the action of any single transmitter on various receptor subtypes can have dramatically different effects on cognitive performance. An individual's catecholamine concentration is, in part, determined by their genotype as well as by the presence of certain disease states such as stroke, which impacts not only behavior, but also the response a drug will have on that behavior. Additionally, behavior is modulated by the firing pattern of catecholaminergic neurons, which, in turn, is modified by various receptor subtypes and the impact of other neurotransmitters (Rao, Williams, & Goldman-Rakic, 2000). Furthermore, activation of postsynaptic receptors results in activation or inhibition of second messengers that impacts performance and behavior. Such complexity has provided researchers several venues in their attempts to pharmacologically modify cognitive performance. For example, synaptic concentration of endogenous neurotransmitters may be altered by inhibiting or promoting their presynaptic release, modifying their catabolism, inhibiting their reuptake into the presynpatic terminal, or by potentiating the action of endogenous neurotransmitters. Alternatively, exogenous agents may be administered that act either at receptor sites or by altering the activation of second messengers. However, it is important to note that the impact of any single agent is dependent on many factors, including the baseline cognitive performance of an individual, specific disease states, and the specific genotype of an individual.

Norepinephrine Anatomy and Physiology

Norepinephrine (NE) containing cell bodies in the central nervous system are predominantly located in the locus coeruleus, which has multiple projections to the PFC, cerebellum, limbic system, and brain stem, thereby impacting a host of physiological and cognitive functions such as attention, motor control, emotion, and cardiovascular tone. Reported CNS effects of NE include enhancing signal-to-noise ratio, promoting long-term potentiation in the amygdala and hippocampus, and regulation of both working memory and attention (Ramos, Colgan, Nou, & Arnsten, 2007).

Synaptic NE is inactivated by several mechanisms. NE is actively returned to the presynaptic terminal by the norepinephrine transport system (NET). Enzymatic deactivation is mediated by monoamine oxidase (MAO) and catechol-O-methyltransferase (COMT). It is important to note that the level of COMT activity is at least partially dependent on individual genotype. The gene coding for COMT exists in three isoforms, val/val, val/met, and met/met, each causing either a relative increase or decrease in enzymatic activity resulting in various levels of synaptic NE. The val/val genotype codes for increased COMT activity, followed in descending order by the val/met and met/met isoforms. The val/val genotypes is associated with the greatest degree of COMT activity causing decreased levels of synaptic NE and has been associated with poorer cognitive abilities in both healthy individuals (Roussos, Giakoumaki, Pavlakis, & Bitsios, 2008) and those with brain injury (Lipsky et al., 2005).

Functional MRI (fMRI) data support the findings that COMT polymorphism affects cognitive performance. Activation patterns on fMRI observed during a working-memory task varied in both healthy individuals and on those with TBI, depending on COMT genotype (McAllister et al., 2004). Interestingly, the presence or absence of a val allele results in different activation patterns following ingestion of a catecholaminergic agent in the same populations, suggesting that individual genotype has the potential to impact the effect some drugs have on cognition (McAllister et al., 2004).

Postsynaptic cerebral NE receptors are classified as alpha or beta, which are further subdivided into alpha-1, alpha-2, beta-1, and beta-2 receptors. Alpha-2 receptors are also found on the presynaptic membrane and when activated serve to inhibit the release of NE. Postsynaptic alpha-2 receptors have the highest affinity for NE in the PFC, followed in descending order by alpha-1 and beta. Alpha-2 receptors act on G_i proteins, which when activated inhibit adenylyl cyclase/cAMP pathways, promoting cognitive function within the PFC. This has been demonstrated by studies resulting in impaired PFC function by activation of adenylyl cyclase/cAMP pathways (Duman & Dalley, 2000).

Under non-stressful conditions, cognitive functions mediated by the PFC are activated by moderate levels of synaptic NE that act primarily on alpha-2 receptors. Studies on non-human primates have demonstrated that selective alpha-2 stimulation greatly improves working memory in animals that have depleted levels of catecholamines (Arnsten & Goldman-Rakic, 1985; Cai, Ma, Xu, & Hu, 1993; Rama, Linnankoski, Tanila, Pertovaara, & Carlson, 1996). Similar results were also obtained with direct alpha-2 stimulation in animals with normal, age-related depletion of catecholamines (Arnsten & Goldman-Rakic, 1985; Arnsten, Cai, & Goldman-Rakic, 1988). However, increased levels of NE in the PFC, which occurs during times of stress, results in sufficient alpha-1 receptor stimulation that effectively overrides its action on alpha-2 receptors, resulting in impaired PFC function and impaired cognitive performance. Therefore, observed behaviors resulting from the action of NE in the PFC are dependent on specific NE concentration, and can be represented by an inverted "U" shaped curve, where either too little or too much NE results in impaired cognitive performance while optimal function occurs only with moderate levels.

Alpha-1 receptor stimulation activates phosphotidyl inositol/PKC pathways through G_q proteins (Duman & Dalley, 2000), which impair PFC function. However, inhibiting the phosphotidyl/PKC cascade can block the adverse cognitive impairments resulting from excessive alpha-1 stimulation (Runyan, Moore, & Dash, 2005). Although alpha-1 stimulation in the PFC impairs performance, it plays an important modulating role in memory by its action in the amygdala.

Noradrenergic beta stimulation plays an important role in long-term memory consolidation (Cahill & McGaugh, 1996; Roullet & Sara, 1998), long-term potentiation (Lacaille & Harley, 1985; Chaulk & Harley, 1998), and retention (Ferry & McGaugh, 1999). Beta-1 and beta-2 receptors have specific roles that are at least partly dependent on synaptic NE concentration as well as on which brain region the receptors lay, and are impacted by other neurotransmitters. For example, increased beta-1 stimulation, which typically occurs during times of stress, impairs working memory in a fashion similar to the action of alpha-1 stimulation previously-mentioned under the same conditions. Not surprisingly, infusion of beta-1 antagonists directly into the PFC improves cognitive functioning (Ramos et al., 2005). However, within the hippocampus, beta-1 stimulation plays an important role in memory retrieval. Beta-2 stimulation has been shown to improve memory function when infused into the amygdala of rats (Introini-Collison, Miyazaki, & McGaugh, 1991) and has also enhanced working memory in aged animals (Ramos et al., 2007). Beta stimulation, whether through beta-1 or beta-2 receptors, is coupled to G_s proteins, which in turn increases cAMP levels. Although alpha-1 receptors do not directly impact cAMP activity, evidence suggests that they can potentiate it indirectly by enhancing beta-2 stimulation in the basolateral amygdala (BLA) of rats (Ferry, Roozendaal, & McGaugh, 1999). cAMP appears to be involved in the memory-enhancing effects of beta stimulation in the BLA as demonstrated the effects of beta-2 agonism, which increases cAMP. Alpha-1 stimulation has also increased cAMP activity, but only in the presence of properly functioning beta-2 receptors, suggesting alpha-1 receptors modulate the role of beta receptors in memory function (Ferry et al., 1999).

Dopamine (DA)

There are several dopaminergic pathways in the brain. The meoslimbic pathway originates from the ventral tegmentum and projects to the limbic system, including the nucleus accumbens, amygdala, and anterior cingulate cortex. Overactivity of this system is believed to be associated with symptoms of schizophrenia as well as with aggression and hostility. The mesocortical pathway arises from cells in close proximity to those of the mesolimbic system within the ventral tegmentum, but projects to the cortex, particularly in the limbic area where DA activity is thought to mediate various cognitive functions. The nigrostriatal dopaminergic system maintains its cell bodies within the substantia nigra with projections to the basal ganglia. Diseases or injury of the nigrostriatal system are implicated in various motor disorders including Parkinson's disease, chorea, tics, and dyskinesias. The tuberoinfundibular dopaminergic pathway originates in the hypothalamus where its fiber tracts project to the anterior pituitary. DA acts here to inhibit prolactin release. In post-partum women, DA is inhibited, resulting in increased prolactin release causing lactation.

There are numerous DA receptors (D1–D5), with the D2 receptor the most-widely studied because of its role in schizophrenia and Parkinson's disease. D5 receptors share considerable homology with D1 receptors and are often collectively referred to as D1-like receptors. Similarly, D3 and D4 receptors share considerable homology with D2 receptors, and are often collectively referred to as D2-like receptors. Presynaptic DA receptors act in a similar manner as presynaptic alpha-2 NE receptors in that they inhibit release of DA when activated. DA release can also be inhibited by serotonin through activation of the 5HT2A receptor located on DA neurons. Synaptic DA is inactivated by the same enzymes as NE, namely MAO and COMT, and is also impacted by COMT polymorphism in the same manner as NE. Last, DA is actively transported back into the presynpatic terminal by the dopamine axonal transport system (DAT) in a manner similar to NET.

Similar to NE, there is a high concentration of DA receptors within the PFC where they play an important role in cognition, particularly regarding executive skills, including working memory, set shifting, and decision-making. As stated previously, the PFC receives DA input via the mesocortical pathway, which has been implicated in contributing to impaired cognition in various disease states when functioning suboptimally. These conditions are also associated with impairments in executive skills, providing clues to both the normal and impaired anatomy and physiology of executive functions. For example, impaired executive skills has been associated with increased COMT activity (Egan et al., 2001), suggesting that decreased synaptic DA resulting from its increased catabolism impairs cognition. Evidence also suggests that the DA blockade impairs executive skills (Luciana & Collins, 1997), while DA agonists improve them (Luciana, Depue, Arbisi, & Leon, 1992; Bartholomeusz, Box, Van Rooy, & Nathan, 2003).

However, particular executive skills appear to be subserved by specific DA receptor subtypes. Working memory, which is best described as a collection of various cognitive skills working synergistically to retain information that is quickly encoded and manipulated, appears to be modulated predominantly by D1 receptors in animals (Williams & Goldman-Rakic, 1995; Floresco & Phillips, 2001), although D2 receptors have been shown to be involved as well in human trials (Roesch-Ely et al., 2005). Similarly, set shifting

(the ability to alter behaviors or strategies in response to changing environmental cues or conditions) appears to be modulated by both D1 and D2 receptors, although each receptor appears to have a specific role. More specifically, D1 receptor activation is felt to be responsible for stabilizing the novel strategies needed to manipulate environmental cues and information. D2 activation appears to permit processing of multiple stimulations and representations necessary to change strategies when it is appropriate to do so (Floresco & Magyar, 2006; Seamans & Yang, 2004). Various aspects of decision-making are impacted by the actions of D1, D2, and D4 receptors in specific ways. D1 and D2 receptors modulate impulsive decision, as noted by studies showing D1 blockade increases impulsivity, while and D2 activation inhibits it (van Gaalen, van Koten, Schoffelmeer, & Vanderschuren, 2006). Furthermore, D2 activation appears to mediate the formation of associations between specific actions and their consequences (Floresco & Magyar, 2006). D4 receptor activation is felt to inhibit actions associated with adverse stimulation, thereby impacting decision-making (Floresco & Magyar, 2006; Laviolette, Lipski, & Grace, 2005). PFC D1 receptors also appear to be involved in attention performance, since specific D1 blockade impairs attention in animals with high levels of baseline performance, whereas D2 blockade has no effect (Granon et al., 2000).

The overall effect DA receptor activation has on cognitive performance depends on many individualized factors, making prediction of who will respond favorably to dopaminergic intervention nearly impossible at the present time. Similar to NE, optimal levels of synaptic DA are required for normal cognition. For example, optimal working memory function requires moderate levels of DA receptor activation in the PFC, whereas either reduced or higher levels of activation result in impaired performance (Williams & Goldman-Rakic, 1995; Cai & Arnsten, 1997; Arnsten, Cai, Murphy, & Goldman-Rakic, 1994; Zahrt, Taylor, Mathew, & Arnsten, 1997)

This type of response is best represented by the same inverted "U" shaped curve described for optimal manifestation of skills mediated by NE in which there is a specific range of synaptic DA concentration that optimizes cognitive function, with either too little or too much impairing performance.

Baseline cognitive function on specific cognitive tasks also impacts the overall effect exogenously administered receptor agonists have on performance. For example, several studies have shown that individuals manifesting impaired working memory generally benefit from DA agonism while those performing optimally at baseline experience impaired function with similar drugs (Granon et al., 2000; Mehta et al., 2000; Kimberg, D'Esposito, & Farah, 1997). This may in part be the result of COMT polymorphism. As described previously, individuals with the val/val genotype manifest higher levels of COMT as compared to either val/met or met/met genotypes, resulting in lower synaptic concentration of DA, which has been associated with poorer baseline cognitive skills. Taken together, these findings support the notion of the inverted "U" shaped curve and suggest that only selected population of individuals will benefit from an intervention that promotes DA agonism; for example, those with poorer baseline performance, those with less than optimal levels of DA, or those with the val/val genotype. Variable response to DA agonist administration in other studies may also be explained by the timing the drug was administered in relation to when outcome measures were obtained (Kimberg & D'Esposito, 2003), so that the impact a drug has on performance is likely related to its plasma concentration at the time the cognitive skill is assessed. Based on the inverted "U" shape response, differing drug concentrations should be expected to have varying effects on cognitive performance, which in part depends on when it has reached maximal concentration in the brain. In many studies, medications are provided as a single dose, with plasma concentrations varying significantly over the course of time, rather than allowing it to reach a relatively steady state, the latter occurring only with a more chronic dosing schedule. Therefore, the time post-administration a single drug dose will have on outcome measures is critically important when assessing study results. Also, variable doses may have other unexpected effects that may inadvertently alter outcomes in an indirect manner. For example, it has been suggested that higher doses of certain drugs may cause nausea, thereby masking an improvement in cognitive performance (Luciana & Collins, 1997). Finally, normal aging results in alterations of DA concentrations, which based on the above discussion, should be expected to factor into how a specific drug will impact cognition (Reeves, Bench, & Howard, 2002).

Serotonin

Cell bodies containing serotonin (5HT) are located in the raphe nuclei in the brain stem with projections to the frontal cortex, basal ganglia, limbic area, hypothalamus, brain stem, and spinal cord. It mediates a variety of functions including affect, motor control, appetite, sleep, and sexual responses. 5HT activity is terminated by either MAO or by presynaptic reuptake in a manner similar to both NE and DA. There are several 5HT receptors. Postsynaptic receptors include 5HT1A, 5HT1D, 5HT2A, 5HT2C, 5HT3, and 5HT4 subtypes. 5HT1A and 5HT1D receptors are also found on the presynaptic membrane and serve to inhibit 5HT release when activated. Serotonin neurons also have alpha-1 and alpha-2 NE receptors that when activated serve to either increase or decrease 5HT release, respectively.

5HT2A receptors are also located on DA neurons, which when activated, serve to inhibit DA release. Conversely, blocking 5HT2A receptors on DA neurons results in increased DA release. This property is exploited by the atypical anti-psychotics, which manifest both D2 and 5HT2A antagonism. The balance of each receptor type in each of the DA pathways theoretically inhibits sufficient D2 activity in the mesolimbic system to control behavioral problems while preserving DA activity in the other systems preventing the side effects of pure D2 blockade.

Acetylcholine (ACh)

The major acetylcholine-containing nucleus with widespread brain projection is the nucleus basalis of Meynert, located in the basal forebrain. Its projections reach the hippocampus, amygdala, and neocortex and are involved in several cognitive processes including memory, learning, problem solving, attention, and judgment. Other ACh systems in the brain, such as those arising from the lateral tegmental area, are likely not involved in cognitive function. Cerebral ACh is predominantly inactivated by acetylcholinesterase (AchE), although butyrylcholinesterase (BuChE) performs the same function, with its CNS action more concentrated in glial cells. The major ACh receptors are generally classified as either muscarinic (M) or nicotinic (N), with each further subtyped. The M1 receptor is felt to mediate memory function although other receptors may also play a role.

Glutamate

Glutamate is a ubiquitous excitatory neurotransmitter found throughout the brain that impacts a host of physiological functions, cognitive skills, and the activity of other neurotransmitter systems. It acts on several receptor subtypes, each classified by their affinity for specific chemical compounds that exert their effects by either opening ion channels or by initiating an enzymatic cascade. N-methyl-D-aspartate (NMDA) and α-amino-3-hydroxy-5-methyl-4-isoxalepropanoic acid (AMPA) are two of the most studied glutamate receptors. When activated, NMDA receptors permit calcium entry into the neuron.

This flow of calcium has been postulated to play an important role in neurotoxicity, particularly when present in high concentrations in the extracellular space. The excitotoxic properties of glutamate have been implicated in the development of several neurodegenerative conditions such as Alzheimer's disease (AD) and Parkinson's disease, as well as stroke and TBI. However, they also play a vital role in normal cerebral function. Activation of AMPA receptors permits sodium entry into the cells that mediates fast excitatory post-synaptic currents and appears to play an important role in long-term potentiation.

When activated, AMPA receptors are physically altered. This alteration opens a channel that permits the passage of sodium through the post-synaptic membrane. Channel closure, causing the cessation of current flow, occurs by one of two mechanisms. The receptor can be deactivated by the removal of glutamate from the binding site. Alternatively, the site can become desensitized, manifested by channel closure despite the persistent presence of bound glutamate within the binding site. Various pharmacological agents have been developed to inhibit either deactivation or desensitization, resulting in prolonged glutamate-induced excitation. Prolonged activation of AMPA receptors have been shown to increase the release of ACh (Giovannini, Rakovska, Della Corte, Bianchi, & Pepeu, 1998), DA, 5HT (Maione, Biggs, Rossi, Fowler, & Whitton, 1995; Tao, Ma, & Auerbach, 1997), and NE (Lockhart, Iop, Closier, & Lestage, 2000), indicating these drugs have the potential to impact a host of physiological as well as cognitive processes. Furthermore, enhancing excitatory neurotransmission has been associated with increased production of neurotrophic growth factors, such as brain-derived neurotrophic factor (BDNF) (Lauterborn et al., 2003; Mackowiak, O'Neill, Hicks, Bleakman, & Skolnick, 2002). BDNF appears to have a role in maintaining hippocampal function as well as mnemonic performance (Hariri et al., 2003), suggesting another potential benefit of moderate glutamate transmission. Ampakines are drugs that are being examined as a means to enhance cognitive function, although no agents are currently clinically available.

Enhancement of Specific Cognitive Skills

Executive Skills

Pharmacological enhancement of executive skills has focused primarily on methylphenidate and dextroamphetamine, with more recent examinations of gaunfacine, atomoxetine, modafinil, COMT inhibitors, and ampakines.

Evidence supporting the use of catecholaminergic agents that impact cognitive performance varies. There are several potential reasons that may account for these conflicting reports. Unlike drugs used in animal studies, many pharmacological agents available for humans typically act by non-selective presynaptic release or reuptake blockade, rather than by specific receptor subtype activation, resulting in a variety of effects, some desired and some not. Many human studies have examined the impact of drug enhancement in young healthy adults while many of the animal studies examined elderly, non-human primates, who unlike their younger counterparts likely had normal age-related reductions in DA and NE function and were therefore more likely to benefit from pharmacological enhancement.

Table 1 describes the mechanism of action and reported effects on cognition of some catecholaminergic agents.

Several studies have examined the impact of catecholaminergic agonists on various executive skills in both healthy subjects and those with brain injury or disease. Amphethamines such as methylphenidate or dextroamphetamine, which non-selectively increase synaptic NE and DA as well as gaunfacine, one of only a few receptor specific agents (in this case an alpha-2 receptor agonist) have been shown to improve performance on tests of spatial working memory (Elliott et al., 1997; Jakala et al., 1999; Mattay et al., 2000; Mintzer & Griffiths, 2003) Atomoxetine, a selective NE reuptake blocker, has also been shown to improve working memory in adults with ADHD (Elliott et al., 1997). Methylphenidate also appears to work in part by improving efficiency of cognitive processing as noted by decrease regional blood flow to the PFC during a working memory task (Mehta et al., 2000). Bromocriptine, a selective D2 receptor agonist also improved spatial working memory in healthy adults (Luciana et al., 1992; Mehta, Swainson, Ogilvie, Sahakian, & Robbins, 2001). However, results of other studies using either NE or DA agonists contradict these findings, showing either a decrement in function or no change in executive skills (Jakala et al., 1999; Kimberg et al., 1997; U. Muller, von Cramon, & Pollmann, 1998; Roesch-Ely et al., 2005). These conflicting findings may be due to a host of issues, which

Table 1 Catecholaminergic agents

Agent	Mechanism of action	Reported cognitive effects
Methylphenidate	Non-selective blockade of NE and DA reuptake	↑speed of cognitive processing, ↑working memory, ↑cognitive efficiency, ↑attention
Dextroamphetamine	Enhances NE and DA	↑working memory, ↑attention
Guanfacine	α2 receptor agonist	↑working memory, ↑attention
Atomoxetine	Selective NE reuptake blocker	↑working memory, ↑attention,
Bromocriptine	D2 receptor agonist	↑↓working memory (variable results reported), ↑mental flexibility
Tolcapone	COMT inhibitor	↑executive skills, ↑verbal memory, ↑attention, ↓ apraxia
Modafinil	Unknown. Increases synaptic NE, DA, 5T, glutamate, GABA	↑working memory, ↑sustained attention, ↑ set shifting, ↑recall

are detailed in previous sections of this chapter.

Studies have also examined whether the use of catecholaminergic enhancement in various disease states improves working memory. Subjects with Parkinson's disease untreated by medications have been shown to have impairments in working memory (Owen, Iddon, Hodges, Summers, & Robbins, 1997). L-dopa administration in subjects with Parkinson's disease has resulted in improved working memory in several studies (Fournet, Moreaud, Roulin, Naegele, & Pellat, 2000; Malapani, Pillon, Dubois, & Agid, 1994; Owen et al., 1997). Bromocriptine was also found to improve mental flexibility and tasks involving initiation in subjects with severe TBI in a double-blind, placebo-controlled crossover trial (McDowell, Whyte, & D'Esposito, 1998) and its use has been recommended as a guideline to improve executive skills in patients with severe TBI (Neurobehavioral Guidelines Working Group et al., 2006; Neurobehavioral Guidelines Working Group et al., 2006).

The effects of these drugs are also impacted by several other factors, including baseline cognitive performance and genotype. Dextroamphetamine improved working memory capacity when given to healthy volunteers, but only in those who were more impaired, i.e., those with relatively poorer baseline capacity. Consistent with the inverted U-shaped curve described previously, catecholinergic agonist administration resulted in impaired cognitive function in those with relatively high baseline working memory skills (Mattay et al., 2000). Thus it appears that those who benefit most are those with poorer baseline capacity, whereas those who are highly skilled do worse (Kimberg et al., 1997; Mattay et al., 2000). However, this relationship is likely more complex, as recent evidence suggest that when decision-making is dependent on emotional feedback, lower levels of PFC DA is more beneficial than higher levels (Roussos et al., 2008).

Accordingly and as mentioned previously, genotype may also impact the utility of pharmacological enhancement, particularly for those skills mediated by the PFC. Both NE and DA are enzymatically deactivated by COMT. Animal studies have shown that COMT-mediated deactivation of DA is greater in the mesocortical system compared to the mesolimbic and nigrostriatal systems, indicating that specific COMT polymorphisms likely have a greater impact on cognitive functions subserved by the PFC (Gogos et al., 1998; Huotari et al., 2002; Malhotra et al., 2002). Furthermore, human studies reveal that DAT activity is lower in the PFC as compared to other cerebral regions, again indicating that COMT activity is the primary means of DA deactivation in this region (Ciliax et al., 1999). Not surprisingly, individuals with a val allele have been shown to have poorer baseline cognitive performance (Goldberg et al., 2003) and should theoretically be more likely to benefit from catecholaminergic agonism. Researchers have taken advantage of COMT activity by developing compounds that inhibit it in order to enhance PFC activity.

Tolcapone is a COMT inhibitor that has been shown to increase DA in the PFC with an associated improvement in set-shifting ability in mice (Tunbridge, Bannerman, Sharp, & Harrison, 2004). When given to healthy human subjects, improvements were noted in executive skills and verbal episodic memory, although only in those subjects with the val/val genotype (Apud et al., 2007). In the same study, those with the met/met genotype performed more poorly under the drug's influence, in accordance with other studies suggesting maximal cognitive performance requires optimal synaptic catecholamine concentrations. In another human study examining individuals with advanced Parkinson's disease, the combination of tolcapone and L-dopa resulted in significant improvements in attention tasks, auditory verbal short-term memory, visuo-spatial recall, and constructional apraxia (Gasparini, Fabrizio, Bonifati, & Meco, 1997). However, tolcapone can be hepatotoxic, limiting its widespread use. Despite this, COMT inhibition remains a potentially attractive means to improve cognitive skills in individuals with cognitive impairments and/or with specific genotypes. Although routine genotyping is not currently practical for patients, it may become commonplace in the future in order to direct specific treatment modalities to those most likely to benefit.

Modafinil is an agent currently approved for the treatment of narcolepsy. Its wake-promoting effects have led some to speculate that it may also have a favorable impact on various cognitive functions, including executive skills and attention. Its mechanism of action is not well delineated but it appears to be distinctly different from the amphetamines, marked by its lower abuse potential and as well as its more favorable cardiovascular side-effect profile. Recent studies suggest that it increases cerebral concentrations of several neurotransmitters, including but not limited to DA, NE, 5HT, glutamate, and GABA. PET studies on non-human primates indicate that modafinil impacts both DAT and NET (Madras et al., 2006), with other studies indicating it increases extracellular concentrations of both DA and NE in the PFC of rats (de Saint Hilaire, Orosco, Rouch, Blanc, & Nicolaidis, 2001). Human studies examining the cognitive-enhancing potential of modafinil have demonstrated improvements in working memory and sustained attention in healthy adults (U. Muller, Steffenhagen, Regenthal, & Bublak, 2004; Randall et al., 2005; Turner et al., 2003). Other studies suggests it improved set shifting, attention, delayed visual recognition (Turner et al., 2004), and working memory (Spence, Green, Wilkinson, & Hunter, 2005). Its cognitive-enhancing effects following vascular brain injury have not yet been explored, although it represents a potential mechanism to improve a host of deficits. Just as catecholaminergic agonism improves cognitive skills, it is important to limit NE and DA antagonism in clinical practice following stroke whenever possible. Impaired cognitive functioning has been associated with antipsychotic medication, particularly by those that are potent D2 blockers. Studies on healthy subjects without brain injury or psychiatric

diseases have shown that non-selective D2 blockade with haloperidol impairs cognitive skills assessed by both objective (Luciana & Collins, 1997; Saeedi, Remington, & Christensen, 2006) and subjective measures (Artaloytia et al., 2006). Their use has also been associated with impaired cognitive performance following brain injury (Stanislav, 1997) as well as decreased rate of recovery following TBI (Mysiw et al., 2006). Additionally, the adverse effect of NE and DA blockade on other brain-injury related impairments, such as motor and language function, must also be considered. Retrospective evidence in humans suggests that commonly-used drugs impair both motor and functional recovery following stroke in patients who receive one of several detrimental drugs, including α1 antagonists, presynaptic α2 agonists, benzodiazepines, phenytoin, and phenobarbital, in addition to DA receptor antagonists (Goldstein, 1995a). Despite the evidence that these drugs impair recovery, they are frequently prescribed to patients with brain injury (Goldstein, 1995b; Goldstein & Davis, 1988).

Dopamine antagonism also presents a dilemma when treating individuals with both behavioral problems and impaired cognition. Impaired behavior following brain injury, including stroke, may be manifested in several ways, including verbal and physical agitation or frank aggression. While DA antagonism may effectively control agitated or aggressive behavior, most likely by acting on the mesolimbic system, they also impair cognitive performance, most likely by their action within the mesocortical system. While controlling behavioral disturbances is clearly a treatment goal for some patients with stroke, impairing cognitive performance is not, considering that many have reduced cognitive skills as a result of their injury. The atypical anti-pyschotics were developed in part to address this problem. As discussed previously, 5HT2A receptors are found on DA neurons. When this receptor is activated it inhibits DA release. The atypical antipsychotics manifest both D2 and 5HT2A receptor antagonism properties. While activation on 5HT2A receptors inhibits DA release, their blockade will enhance its release. Because different concentrations of receptors exist in the various DA systems, the net effect of atypical anti-psychotics is to control agitated behavior by its D2 blocking action on the mesolimbic system, with a more potent 5HT2A blockade in the mesocortical and nigrostriatal system. This tends to spare cognitive skills and lessens the likelihood of D2 blockade-induced motor impairments typically associated with the use of the older anti-psychotic medications.

Attention

Problems of attention are extremely common following vascular injury. NE is thought to impact attention through its action on the PFC, where it appears to maintain alertness. However, attention is multifaceted, encompassing a host of cognitive processes such as vigilance, susceptibility to distraction, speed of processing, and ability to direct or allocate attention to specific environmental stimuli. Attentional processes can also be divided into other components, including sustained attention, divided attention, alertness, and focused attention. Not surprisingly, impairments in these various attentional components can have detrimental effects on other cognitive functions such as memory and executive skills. Normal attention is mediated in frontal-parietal lobe networks by ascending catecholaminergic and cholinergic pathways (Coull, 1998). Therefore, pharmacological enhancement of attention has focused on the utility of both catecholaminergic agents, predominantly amphetamine drugs, as well as cholinergic drugs. The majority of these studies have examined subjects with ADHD, a condition primarily characterized by impaired attention. Amphetamines have consistently been shown to improve attention in both children and adults with ADHD (Boonstra, Kooij, Oosterlaan, Sergeant, & Buitelaar, 2005;

Turner, Blackwell, Dowson, McLean, & Sahakian, 2005), leading to many studies examining their impact on attention deficits caused by other conditions.

The most commonly studied amphetamine for treatment of impaired attention is methylphenidate. In studies examining its impact following TBI, it has been found most consistently effective in improving processing speed (Gualtieri & Evans, 1988; Mahalick et al., 1998; Whyte et al., 1997). In a well-designed study to better assess the impact of medications on the various components of attention, it was shown to reliably improve speed of cognitive processing that was separate from its effect on motor speed (Whyte et al., 2004). In this crossover study, subjects' caregivers, who were blinded to drug/placebo timing, reported improvements in attention during the active phase of treatment, indicating that improvements in processing speed have beneficial impacts on other aspects of daily life. Although many other studies have also found that methylphenidate improved TBI-related impaired attention (Kim, Ko, Na, Park, & Kim, 2006); Plenger et al., 1996), its impact on vigilance, sustained attention, and distractibility has not been consistently demonstrated (Speech, Rao, Osmon, & Sperry, 1993; Whyte et al., 1997). Despite this, methylphenidate use has been recommended as a guideline for the treatment of TBI-related attention impairments, particularly to enhance both speed of cognitive processing and sustained attention (Neurobehavioral Guidelines Working Group et al., 2006). Methylphenidate has also been used in other neurological conditions associated with impaired attention. In an open-label trial, it was found to be both safe and effective in ameliorating impaired attention, concentration, and memory in subjects with epilepsy (Moore, McAuley, Long, & Bornstein, 2002). Atomoxetine, a selective NE reuptake inhibitor, is also approved for the treatment of ADHD, but it has not yet been well studied in other neurologically-impaired populations.

Although typically used to enhance memory function, there is evidence to suggest that acetylcholinergic agonists also have the potential to improve attention in various neurological conditions. Rivastigmine was found to significantly improve several measures of cognition in a large sample of subjects with Parkinson's disease (Wesnes, McKeith, Edgar, Emre, & Lane, 2005), while donepezil (Khateb, Ammann, Annoni, & Diserens, 2005; Tenovuo, 2005; Zhang, Plotkin, Wang, Sandel, & Lee, 2004), galantamine (Tenovuo, 2005), rivastigmine (Tenovuo, 2005), and physostigmine (Levin et al., 1986) have been shown to improve various aspects of attention in subjects with TBI. In one cross-over design study, the beneficial effects of donepezil on both attention and memory persisted during the placebo phase (Zhang et al., 2004). Donepezil-use following TBI has been recommended as a guideline for treating TBI-related impaired attention (Neurobehavioral Guidelines Working Group et al., 2006).

Hemi-spatial neglect is a specific form of impaired attention in which individuals with injuries to their non-dominant cerebral hemisphere neglect or are inattentive to the environment contralateral to their lesion, including ischemic and hemorrhagic stroke. A few studies have examined pharmacological interventions to improve attention to the neglected space. A small double-blind cross over trial demonstrated that guanfacine improved attention to the neglected space in two of three subjects in a computerized exploration task. The one subject who did not respond had a lesion involving the right PFC, suggesting that location of lesion may be an important factor in predicting response to medication intervention (Malhotra et al., 2002). Although similar results have been noted in other small trials (Mukand et al., 2001) and case reports utilizing catecholaminergic agonists (Fleet, Valenstein, Watson, & Heilman, 1987; Hurford, Stringer, & Jann, 1998), others have reported worsening neglect, perhaps because of more potent enhancement of attention to the non-neglected hemispace (Barrett, Crucian, Schwartz, & Heilman, 1999).

Memory

Memory impairments are among the most common complaints after brain injury. It is a complex cognitive skill that is composed of sequential processes, including acquisition, consolidation, and both short- and long-term retrieval. Its normal function is dependent on several neurotransmitters and is impacted by other cognitive processes such as executive function and attention. Many neurotransmitters are involved in normal memory function, including ACh (Zafonte, Elovic, Mysiw, O'Dell, & Watanabe, 1999), glutamate, and catecholamines, as expected given the complexity of this skill.

Acetylcholine has long been implicated in normal learning and memory (Hagan, Alpert, Morris, & Iversen, 1983), with dysfunction of this neurotransmitter system demonstrated in several disease states manifested by impaired memory. Additional evidence supporting ACh's role in cognition comes from studies examining the adverse effects of anticholinergic agents, which have been shown to cause sedation, confusion, delirium, cognitive decline, and psychotic symptoms in individuals with AD (Lu & Tune, 2003). In healthy adults, anticholinergic administration has been associated with impaired cognitive skills that are involved in both declarative and procedural memory (Rammsayer, Rodewald, & Groh, 2000), while in older adults they have been associated with decrements in several cognitive skills, including visual scanning, attention, and cognitive flexibility, all of which potentially impair ADL functioning (Bottiggi et al., 2006).

The majority of research examining the utility of ACh agonism to enhance memory function exists for AD. The use of acetylcholinesterase inhibitors (AChEI) were initially developed based on the theory that the memory disturbance in AD was caused by the degeneration of acetylcholinergic neurons (Bartus, Dean, Beer, & Lippa, 1982). This was supported by post-mortem examinations revealing evidence of markedly reduced ACh transmission in patients with AD. AChEI were developed to treat the cognitive impairments associated with AD, primarily memory and attention, with several drugs now approved for that purpose. Interestingly, some new lines of evidence now suggests the possibility that the AChEIs also alter the disease process by potentially increasing cerebral blood flow to critical areas involved in various cognitive processes, slowing the rate of hippocampus volume loss as well as the decline in glucose utilization (Relkin, 2007).

Norepinephrine also plays an important role in memory function. As mentioned previously, memory is dependent on both attention and executive skills, two cognitive processes that are strongly impacted by NE activity. In addition to that, the hippocampus receives considerable adrenergic input from the locus coeruleus (Bergles, Doze, Madison, & Smith, 1996; Devauges & Sara, 1991; Murchison et al., 2004), which is activated by environment stimuli (Aston-Jones, Rajkowski, & Kubiak, 1997; Aston-Jones, Rajkowski, & Cohen, 2000; Hagan et al., 1983), causing an increase in NE turnover within the hippocampus by acting primarilyon beta-1 receptors. It is suspected that NE is involved in the retrieval of memories that are in the intermediate phase of consolidation (Hagan et al.; Murchison et al., 2004). This is potentially an important fact when one considers that beta-blockade is often a first-line treatment for hypertension. Given the staggering prevalence of hypertension and the potential risk beta-blockers pose regarding memory impairments, clinicians may worry that hypertension treatment with these agents may impair cognitive function. However, in hypertensive adults with normal cognitive skills, it appears that beta-blockade does not impair memory function (Perez-Stable et al., 2000). Conversely, those individuals with cognitive impairments do appear to be susceptible to lipophilic beta-blockers that have the potential to pass the blood-brain barrier and impair memory, presumably by blocking beta-1 receptors in the hippocampus (Gliebus & Lippa, 2007). Although clinicians

may consider this when prescribing antihypertensive medications, controlling elevated blood pressure is a primary means of decreasing the risk of stroke and thereby the risk of cognitive decline as well.

Vascular Dementia

Impairments in cognition resulting from cerebrovascular disease are very common and likely to increase as the population ages. Various terminologies have been proposed to classify cerebrovascular disease-induced cognitive changes. Vascular dementia generally refers to individuals who have impaired cognition that must include memory dysfunction, presumed to be caused by neurovascular-induced lesions that are observed on imaging studies. However, cognitive impairments often occur in the presence of relatively preserved memory, but also in the setting of neurovascular disease. Therefore, an alternative term, vascular cognitive impairment (VCI), has been proposed and refers to any cognitive dysfunction "associated and presumed to be caused by cerebrovascular disease" (O'Brien et al., 2003). Regardless of the terminology, these conditions have been associated with reduced levels of ACh activity in the brain, suggesting that the cognitive impairments may be amenable to AChEI intervention.

A Cochrane review examining the effects of donepezil for VCI revealed that it improved both cognitive function and ADL skills (Malouf & Birks, 2004). A similar review of galantamine suggested that it has a beneficial role in cognition, including executive skills, although evidence was not consistent across studies. This may have been due to differing inclusion criteria in the reviewed studies (Craig & Birks, 2006). Others studies examining donepezil and galantamine revealed a small but beneficial effect on cognitive skills at low and high dosages, while only high doses resulted in improved ADL function. However, both drugs were associated with a higher incidence of gastrointestinal side effects, particularly at high dosages, that caused many subjects to withdraw from participation. In general, these results suggest that while AChEIs likely improve cognitive function in individuals with VCI, the effect is small and often associated with unacceptable side effects (Birks & Flicker, 2007).

Glutamate has also been implicated in VCI, with evidence suggesting that neuronal loss may be in part due to increased sensitivity to or increased levels of glutamate (Cacabelos, Takeda, & Winblad, 1999). Excessive glutamate stimulation can be caused by ischemia and may therefore be a mechanism of neuronal demise following stroke (Lancelot & Beal, 1998), contributing to impaired cognition and memory. Memantine, an antagonist to the NMDA receptor, may therefore improve cognitive skills in VCI. Preliminary studies have indicated that it is both safe and effective in improving cognition skills in VCI (Orgogozo, Rigaud, Stoffler, Mobius, & Forette, 2002; Wilcock, Mobius, Stoffler, & MMM 500 group, 2002), supporting the theory that glutamate hypersensitivity plays a role in VCI (Wilcock et al., 2002).

Language

Aphasia afflicts between 21 and 38% of individuals with acute stroke (Kauhanen et al., 2000; Pedersen, Jorgensen, Nakayama, Raaschou, & Olsen, 1995; Pedersen, Vinter, & Olsen, 2004; Wade, Hewer, David, & Enderby, 1986). Similar to other cognitive impairments, it frequently prevents effective participation in pre-injury roles. Although the mainstay of aphasia treatment is speech-language therapy, reports of its efficacy are conflicting (Basso, Capitani, & Vignolo, 1979; Bhogal, Teasell, & Speechley, 2003; Bhogal, Teasell, Foley, & Speechley, 2003; David, Enderby, & Bainton, 1982; Greener, Enderby, & Whurr, 2000; Laska, Hellblom, Murray, Kahan, & Von Arbin, 2001; Robey, 1994; Robey, 1998; Taylor Sarno, 1998; Wertz

et al., 1986). Accordingly, several researchers have evaluated the potential role of pharmacological enhancement of language function after stroke. Various drugs, including piracetam, catecholiminergic and DA agonists, serotonergic agents, and cholinergic drugs have been studied regarding their potential role in treating aphasia. However, like many other studies examining the effectiveness of drug treatment on post-stroke outcomes, no standards of care are yet available because of limited data and inadequately designed and powered studies.

When evaluating studies examining the effectiveness of drug treatment for aphasia, it is important to consider whether there were adequate controls for several parameters, including lesion size, etiology, and time post-stroke. Measures should be taken to control for subject age, handedness, education level, and mood as well as aphasia severity and type (de Boissezon, Peran, de Boysson, & Demonet, 2007). Additionally, the type and intensity of speech therapy provided during the study period is extremely important, since drug therapy alone is felt to be ineffective in treating aphasia (de Boissezon et al., 2007; Small, 1994). Although many studies have examined drug treatment for aphasia, there is no consensus regarding its effectiveness. A Cochrane review published in 2001 that assessed ten randomized studies examining various drug treatment, including piracetam, bifenalane, piribedil, bromocriptine, idebenon, and Dextran 40 concluded that there was only weak evidence to support piracetam (Greener, Enderby, & Whurr, 2001).

Piracetam is a drug that has been used to improve various cognitive skills, including learning, memory, and language following brain injury. It is not approved for use in the United States, although it is available in many other countries. It is a derivative of GABA that crosses the blood brain barrier and concentrates in the cerebral cortex (Vernon & Sorkin, 1991), and was the first of a class of drugs known as nootropics. The precise mechanism by which the drug exerts a positive effect on cognition is not well delineated, although proposed means include increasing oxygen and glucose utilization through ATP pathways, inhibition of platelet aggregation, prevention of capillary vasospasm, improved deformability of red blood cells, and enhancement of cholinergic (Oyaizu & Narahashi, 1999; Pepeu & Spignoli, 1989) and glutaminergic (Pittaluga et al., 1999) neurotransmission.

Several studies have examined piracetam as a potential means to ameliorate aphasia (Enderby, Broeckx, Hospers, Schildermans, & Deberdt, 1994; Huber, Willmes, Poeck, Van Vleymen, & Deberdt, 1997; Orgogozo, 1999; Szelies, Mielke, Kessler, & Heiss, 2001), with results suggesting it may improve certain aspects of language acutely following stroke. In one randomized, double-blind, placebo-controlled trial of acute stroke subjects with aphasia, all of whom received speech therapy, piracetam was found to significantly improve language skills in the spheres of written language, naming, comprehension, spontaneous speech, and semantic structure, as opposed to only written language in the control group (Kessler, Thiel, Karbe, & Heiss, 2000). This study also assessed changes in cerebral activations on H_2O^{15} labeled PET scans at rest and during a word-repetition task. Subjects receiving piracetam had significantly increased activation in the left transverse temporal gyrus, left superior temporal gyrus (Wernicke's area), and the triangular part of the left frontal gyrus (Broca's area) (Kessler et al., 2000) while the placebo group had increased activation only in the left precentral gyrus. The significance of the PET changes are unclear, although the authors suggested it may be due to piracetam's effect on transmitter release and function (Coq & Xerri, 1999; W. E. Muller, Hartman, Koch, Scheuer, & Stoll, 1994) as well as its impact on compromised tissue in the immediate post-stroke period that assisted it in reintegrating into a functional network (Kessler et al., 2000; W. E. Muller et al., 1994). Piracetam treatment has also been associated with both electroencephalographic

changes and improved language skills in aphasic stroke subjects (Szelies B et al., 2001).

Dopamine agonist have also been proposed as a means to treat aphasia, based on the rationale that certain features of aphasia are thought to result from disruption of mesocortical and mesolimbic pathways, impacting the basal ganglia and supplementary motor areas (Albert, 1998). Several early case series examining predominantly subjects with transcortical motor aphasia reported promising results (Albert, Bachman, Morgan, & Helm-Estabrooks, 1988; Gold, VanDam, & Silliman, 2000), although these were not confirmed in later studies of subjects with more varied types of aphasia (Hughes, Jacobs, & Heilman, 2000; Ozeren, Sarica, Mavi, & Demirkiran, 1995). Several other randomized, controlled trials using bromocriptine have reported mixed results (Bragoni et al., 2000; Gupta, Mlcoch, Scolaro, & Moritz, 1995; Sabe, Salvarezza, Garcia Cuerva, Leiguarda, & Starkstein, 1995), including a recent randomized double-blind, placebo-controlled study in subjects with non-fluent aphasia acutely post-stroke that failed to reveal a difference between the treatment and placebo groups (Ashtary, Janghorbani, Chitsaz, Reisi, & Bahrami, 2006). Taking these studies together, the effectiveness of bromocriptine in treating aphasia remains unanswered. This may be because specific types of aphasia result from lesions in different cerebral structures and pathways. For example, individuals with Broca's or global aphasia often have large lesions involving the anterior persisylvian cortex, where DA agonism alone would likely be insufficient to improve language function (Raymer, 2003). However, where lesions involve predominantly subcortical structures, particularly discrete lesions in the mesocortical DA system or frontal lobe, DA agonism may be more effective (Raymer, 2003).

Several lines of reasoning suggest that cholinergic agonism may also positively impact language function after stroke. Cholinergic depletion is associated with language impairments (Mesulam, Siddique, & Cohen, 2003; Tanaka, Miyazaki, & Albert, 1997) and cholinergic pathways arising from the nucleus basalis of Meynert are frequently disrupted by ischemic lesions (Selden, Gitelman, Salamon-Murayama, Parrish, & Mesulam, 1998). A few small trials have demonstrated a potential benefit of donepezil when paired with speech therapy in subjects with either acute or chronic stroke (Berthier, Hinojosa, Martin Mdel, & Fernandez, 2003; Berthier et al., 2006). In both studies, the beneficial effects on language were lost when the drug was discontinued, indicating that if donepezil is proven as an effective means to improve language skills, it will need to be provided on a long-term basis.

Post-Stroke Depression and Cognition

The association between depression and impaired cognition has long been known in several populations (Austin et al., 1992; Caine, 1981; KILOH, 1961; Rabins, 1981; Rabins, Merchant, & Nestadt, 1984), including individuals with stroke (Andersen, Vestergaard, Riis, & Ingeman-Nielsen, 1996); Lipsey, Robinson, Pearlson, Rao, & Price, 1984; Robinson et al., 2000). The relationship between depression and cognitive skills following stroke has been debated, with some suggesting that depression impairs cognition (Kimura, Robinson, & Kosier, 2000), while others argue that impaired cognition results in depression (Andersen et al., 1996). Regardless of the answer to this question, cognitive impairments of varying severity afflicts between 13.6 and 35.2% of individuals with stroke (Censori et al., 1996; Desmond et al., 2000; Inzitari et al., 1998; Pohjasvaara et al., 1998; Tatemichi et al., 1992; Tatemichi et al., 1994), prompting several researchers to examine whether anti-depressant medications can effectively treat both stroke-related depression and impaired cognition.

Evidence arising from studies examining this issue has been mixed, although the predominance of data support the notion that ameliorating depression is associated with improved cognition. The impact of several anti-depressant medications, including nortriptyline, fluoxetine, and citalopram have been investigated, with most studies indicating that as depression fades, cognitive skills improve (Kimura et al., 2000; Narushima, Paradiso, Moser, Jorge, & Robinson, 2007; Simis & Nitrini, 2006). The effect of improved cognition appears to be long lasting, with several studies demonstrating maintenance of gains for up to 2 years post-treatment (Narushima, Chan, Kosier, & Robinson, 2003; Narushima et al., 2007). Several studies seem to contradict these findings (Andersen et al., 1996; Lipsey et al., 1984; Robinson et al., 2000; Robinson et al., 2000), although some of these examined too few subjects to detect significant changes (Andersen et al., 1996; Lipsey et al., 1984; Robinson et al., 2000) or used global cognitive assessment measures, such as the Mini Mental State Examination that are insensitive to changes in specific cognitive domains (Robinson et al., 2000).

It is important to tease out the effect improved mood has on cognitive performance from the direct effect an anti-depressant medication has on cognition independent of mood. Using various designs and/or multiple linear regression analysis, results of several studies indicate that improved mood results in improved cognition rather than the drug directly impacting cognition (Kimura et al., 2000; Narushima et al., 2003; Narushima et al., 2007). For instance, non-depressed subjects provided nortriptyline failed to show improved cognition (Narushima et al., 2003), while subjects whose mood improved without medications did experience enhanced cognition (Kimura et al., 2000).

Summary

Traditional rehabilitation techniques are effective in reducing disability, although the impairments and the associated restrictions in participation resulting from neurovascular diseases are often permanent. Pharmacological intervention, when used as an adjuvant in rehabilitation, is prescribed by some clinicians in an attempt to more effectively treat individuals with post-stroke cognitive impairments. However, there is currently insufficient evidence to develop standards of care for using pharmacological agents to ameliorate these impairments. Accurately identifying which patient will benefit from drugs as well as which drugs to use and for how long remain unanswered questions, leaving clinicians with the dilemma of whether to pursue this line of treatment. Thus physicians who prescribe these medications must acknowledge that their use remains off-label. For those who choose to use drugs to enhance recovery following stroke, it is important to identify a specific impairment for intervention, assess the effectiveness of the drug at different dosages, and periodically withdraw the drug to evaluate its continued utility. Furthermore, a solid knowledge-base of both the specific disease process associated with the impairment and the physiological basis of the behavior to which treatment is directed is required in order to embark on the most reasonable path possible. As scientists continue their quest to better understand the physiological basis of behavior, it is anticipated that better designed studies will ultimately result in better guidelines for using pharmacological agents to reduce disability.

References

Albert, M. L. (1998). Treatment of aphasia. *Archives of Neurology*, *55*(11), 1417–1419.

Albert, M. L., Bachman, D. L., Morgan, A., & Helm-Estabrooks, N. (1988). Pharmacotherapy for aphasia. *Neurology*, *38*(6), 877–879.

Andersen, G., Vestergaard, K., Riis, J. O., & Ingeman-Nielsen, M. (1996). Dementia of depression or depression of dementia in stroke? *Acta Psychiatrica Scandinavica*, *94*(4), 272–278.

Apud, J. A., Mattay, V., Chen, J., Kolachana, B. S., Callicott, J. H., Rasetti, R., et al. (2007). Tolcapone improves cognition and cortical information processing in normal human subjects. *Neuropsycho-pharmacology : Official Publication of the American College of Neuropsychopharmacology*, *32*(5), 1011–1020.

Arnsten, A. F., Cai, J. X., & Goldman-Rakic, P. S. (1988). The alpha-2 adrenergic agonist guanfacine improves memory in aged monkeys without sedative or hypotensive side effects: Evidence for alpha-2 receptor subtypes. *The Journal of Neuroscience : The Official Journal of the Society for Neuroscience*, *8*(11), 4287–4298.

Arnsten, A. F., Cai, J. X., Murphy, B. L., & Goldman-Rakic, P. S. (1994). Dopamine D1 receptor mechanisms in the cognitive performance of young adult and aged monkeys. *Psychopharmacology*, *116*(2), 143–151.

Arnsten, A. F., & Goldman-Rakic, P. S. (1985). Alpha 2-adrenergic mechanisms in prefrontal cortex associated with cognitive decline in aged nonhuman primates. *Science (New York, N.Y.)*, *230*(4731), 1273–1276.

Artaloytia, J. F., Arango, C., Lahti, A., Sanz, J., Pascual, A., Cubero, P., et al. (2006). Negative signs and symptoms secondary to antipsychotics: A double-blind, randomized trial of a single dose of placebo, haloperidol, and risperidone in healthy volunteers. *The American Journal of Psychiatry*, *163*(3), 488–493.

Ashtary, F., Janghorbani, M., Chitsaz, A., Reisi, M., & Bahrami, A. (2006). A randomized, double-blind trial of bromocriptine efficacy in nonfluent aphasia after stroke. *Neurology*, *66*(6), 914–916.

Aston-Jones, G., Rajkowski, J., & Cohen, J. (2000). Locus coeruleus and regulation of behavioral flexibility and attention. *Progress in Brain Research*, *126*, 165–182.

Aston-Jones, G., Rajkowski, J., & Kubiak, P. (1997). Conditioned responses of monkey locus coeruleus neurons anticipate acquisition of discriminative behavior in a vigilance task. *Neuroscience*, *80*(3), 697–715.

Austin, M. P., Ross, M., Murray, C., O'Carroll, R. E., Ebmeier, K. P., & Goodwin, G. M. (1992). Cognitive function in major depression. *Journal of Affective Disorders*, *25*(1), 21–29.

Barrett, A. M., Crucian, G. P., Schwartz, R. L., & Heilman, K. M. (1999). Adverse effect of dopamine agonist therapy in a patient with motor-intentional neglect. *Archives of Physical Medicine and Rehabilitation*, *80*(5), 600–603.

Bartholomeusz, C. F., Box, G., Van Rooy, C., & Nathan, P. J. (2003). The modulatory effects of dopamine D1 and D2 receptor function on object working memory in humans. *Journal of Psychopharmacology (Oxford, England)*, *17*(1), 9–15.

Bartus, R. T., Dean, R. L., III, Beer, B., & Lippa, A. S. (1982). The cholinergic hypothesis of geriatric memory dysfunction. *Science (New York, N.Y.)*, *217*(4558), 408–414.

Basso, A., Capitani, E., & Vignolo, L. A. (1979). Influence of rehabilitation on language skills in aphasic patients. A controlled study. *Archives of Neurology*, *36*(4), 190–196.

Bergles, D. E., Doze, V. A., Madison, D. V., & Smith, S. J. (1996). Excitatory actions of norepinephrine on multiple classes of hippocampal CA1 interneurons. *The Journal of Neuroscience : The Official Journal of the Society for Neuroscience*, *16*(2), 572–585.

Berthier, M. L., Green, C., Higueras, C., Fernandez, I., Hinojosa, J., & Martin, M. C. (2006). A randomized, placebo-controlled study of donepezil in poststroke aphasia. *Neurology, 67*(9), 1687–1689.

Berthier, M. L., Hinojosa, J., Martin Mdel, C., & Fernandez, I. (2003). Open-label study of donepezil in chronic poststroke aphasia. *Neurology, 60*(7), 1218–1219.

Bhogal, S. K., Teasell, R., & Speechley, M. (2003). Intensity of aphasia therapy, impact on recovery. *Stroke; a Journal of Cerebral Circulation, 34*(4), 987–993.

Bhogal, S. K., Teasell, R. W., Foley, N. C., & Speechley, M. R. (2003). Rehabilitation of aphasia: More is better. *Topics in Stroke Rehabilitation, 10*(2), 66–76.

Birks, J., & Flicker, L. (2007). Investigational treatment for vascular cognitive impairment. *Expert Opinion on Investigational Drugs, 16*(5), 647–658.

Boonstra, A. M., Kooij, J. J., Oosterlaan, J., Sergeant, J. A., & Buitelaar, J. K. (2005). Does methylphenidate improve inhibition and other cognitive abilities in adults with childhood-onset ADHD? *Journal of Clinical and Experimental Neuropsychology : Official Journal of the International Neuropsychological Society, 27*(3), 278–298.

Bottiggi, K. A., Salazar, J. C., Yu, L., Caban-Holt, A. M., Ryan, M., Mendiondo, M. S., et al. (2006). Long-term cognitive impact of anticholinergic medications in older adults. *The American Journal of Geriatric Psychiatry : Official Journal of the American Association for Geriatric Psychiatry, 14*(11), 980–984.

Bragoni, M., Altieri, M., Di Piero, V., Padovani, A., Mostardini, C., & Lenzi, G. L. (2000). Bromocriptine and speech therapy in non-fluent chronic aphasia after stroke. *Neurological Sciences : Official Journal of the Italian Neurological Society and of the Italian Society of Clinical Neurophysiology, 21*(1), 19–22.

Cacabelos, R., Takeda, M., & Winblad, B. (1999). The glutamatergic system and neurodegeneration in dementia: Preventive strategies in Alzheimer's disease. *International Journal of Geriatric Psychiatry, 14*(1), 3–47.

Cahill, L., & McGaugh, J. L. (1996). Modulation of memory storage. *Current Opinion in Neurobiology, 6*(2), 237–242.

Cai, J. X., & Arnsten, A. F. (1997). Dose-dependent effects of the dopamine D1 receptor agonists A77636 or SKF81297 on spatial working memory in aged monkeys. *The Journal of Pharmacology and Experimental Therapeutics, 283*(1), 183–189.

Cai, J. X., Ma, Y. Y., Xu, L., & Hu, X. T. (1993). Reserpine impairs spatial working memory performance in monkeys: Reversal by the alpha 2-adrenergic agonist clonidine. *Brain Research, 614*(1–2), 191–196.

Caine, E. D. (1981). Pseudodementia. current concepts and future directions. *Archives of General Psychiatry, 38*(12), 1359–1364.

Censori, B., Manara, O., Agostinis, C., Camerlingo, M., Casto, L., Galavotti, B., et al. (1996). Dementia after first stroke. *Stroke; a Journal of Cerebral Circulation, 27*(7), 1205–1210.

Chaulk, P. C., & Harley, C. W. (1998). Intracerebroventricular norepinephrine potentiation of the perforant path-evoked potential in dentate gyrus of anesthetized and awake rats: A role for both alpha- and beta-adrenoceptor activation. *Brain Research, 787*(1), 59–70.

Ciliax, B. J., Drash, G. W., Staley, J. K., Haber, S., Mobley, C. J., Miller, G. W., et al. (1999). Immunocytochemical localization of the dopamine transporter in human brain. *The Journal of Comparative Neurology, 409*(1), 38–56.

Collins, P., Roberts, A. C., Dias, R., Everitt, B. J., & Robbins, T. W. (1998). Perseveration and strategy in a novel spatial self-ordered sequencing task for nonhuman primates: Effects of excitotoxic lesions and dopamine depletions of the prefrontal cortex. *Journal of Cognitive Neuroscience, 10*(3), 332–354.

Coq, J. O., & Xerri, C. (1999). Acute reorganization of the forepaw representation in the rat SI cortex after focal cortical injury: Neuroprotective effects of piracetam treatment. *The European Journal of Neuroscience, 11*(8), 2597–2608.

Coull, J. T. (1998). Neural correlates of attention and arousal: Insights from electrophysiology, functional neuroimaging and psychopharmacology. *Progress in Neurobiology, 55*(4), 343–361.

Craig, D., & Birks, J. (2006). Galantamine for vascular cognitive impairment. *Cochrane Database of Systematic Reviews (Online), (1)* (1), CD004746.

David, R., Enderby, P., & Bainton, D. (1982). Treatment of acquired aphasia: Speech therapists and volunteers compared. *Journal of Neurology, Neurosurgery, and Psychiatry, 45*(11), 957–961.

de Boissezon, X., Peran, P., de Boysson, C., & Demonet, J. F. (2007). Pharmacotherapy of aphasia: Myth or reality *Brain and Language, 102*(1), 114–125.

de Saint Hilaire, Z., Orosco, M., Rouch, C., Blanc, G., & Nicolaidis, S. (2001). Variations in extracellular monoamines in the prefrontal cortex and medial hypothalamus after modafinil administration: A microdialysis study in rats. *Neuroreport, 12*(16), 3533–3537.

Desmond, D. W., Moroney, J. T., Paik, M. C., Sano, M., Mohr, J. P., Aboumatar, S., et al. (2000). Frequency and clinical determinants of dementia after ischemic stroke. *Neurology, 54*(5), 1124–1131.

Devauges, V., & Sara, S. J. (1991). Memory retrieval enhancement by locus coeruleus stimulation: Evidence for mediation by beta-receptors. *Behavioural Brain Research, 43*(1), 93–97.

Duman, R. S., & Dalley, J. W. (2000). Signal transduction patways for catecholamine receptors. In F. E. Bloom, & D. L. Hupfer (Eds.), *Psychopharmacology: The fourth generaion of progress* (pp. 303–320). New York: Raven Press.

Egan, M. F., Goldberg, T. E., Kolachana, B. S., Callicott, J. H., Mazzanti, C. M., Straub, R. E., et al. (2001). Effect of COMT Val108/158 met genotype on frontal lobe function and risk for schizophrenia. *Proceedings of the National Academy of Sciences of the United States of America, 98*(12), 6917–6922.

Elliott, R., Sahakian, B. J., Matthews, K., Bannerjea, A., Rimmer, J., & Robbins, T. W. (1997). Effects of methylphenidate on spatial working memory and planning in healthy young adults. *Psychopharmacology, 131*(2), 196–206.

Enderby, P., Broeckx, J., Hospers, W., Schildermans, F., & Deberdt, W. (1994). Effect of piracetam on recovery and rehabilitation after stroke: A double-blind, placebo-controlled study. *Clinical Neuropharmacology, 17*(4), 320–331.

Ferry, B., & McGaugh, J. L. (1999). Clenbuterol administration into the basolateral amygdala post-training enhances retention in an inhibitory avoidance task. *Neurobiology of Learning and Memory, 72*(1), 8–12.

Ferry, B., Roozendaal, B., & McGaugh, J. L. (1999). Basolateral amygdala noradrenergic influences on memory storage are mediated by an interaction between beta- and alpha1-adrenoceptors. *The Journal of Neuroscience : The Official Journal of the Society for Neuroscience, 19*(12), 5119–5123.

Fleet, W. S., Valenstein, E., Watson, R. T., & Heilman, K. M. (1987). Dopamine agonist therapy for neglect in humans. *Neurology, 37*(11), 1765–1770.

Floresco, S. B., & Magyar, O. (2006). Mesocortical dopamine modulation of executive functions: Beyond working memory. *Psychopharmacology, 188*(4), 567–585.

Floresco, S. B., & Phillips, A. G. (2001). Delay-dependent modulation of memory retrieval by infusion of a dopamine D1 agonist into the rat medial prefrontal cortex. *Behavioral Neuroscience, 115*(4), 934–939.

Fournet, N., Moreaud, O., Roulin, J. L., Naegele, B., & Pellat, J. (2000). Working memory functioning in medicated parkinson's disease patients and the effect of withdrawal of dopaminergic medication. *Neuropsychology, 14*(2), 247–253.

Gasparini, M., Fabrizio, E., Bonifati, V., & Meco, G. (1997). Cognitive improvement during tolcapone treatment in parkinson's disease. *Journal of Neural Transmission (Vienna, Austria : 1996), 104*(8–9), 887–894.

Giovannini, M. G., Rakovska, A., Della Corte, L., Bianchi, L., & Pepeu, G. (1998). Activation of non-NMDA receptors stimulates acetylcholine and GABA release from dorsal hippocampus: A microdialysis study in the rat. *Neuroscience Letters, 243*(1–3), 152–156.

Gliebus, G., & Lippa, C. F. (2007). The influence of beta-blockers on delayed memory function in people with cognitive impairment. *American Journal of Alzheimer's Disease and Other Dementias, 22*(1), 57–61.

Gogos, J. A., Morgan, M., Luine, V., Santha, M., Ogawa, S., Pfaff, D., et al. (1998). Catechol-O-methyltransferase-deficient mice exhibit sexually dimorphic changes in catecholamine levels and behavior. *Proceedings of the National Academy of Sciences of the United States of America, 95*(17), 9991–9996.

Gold, M., VanDam, D., & Silliman, E. R. (2000). An open-label trial of bromocriptine in nonfluent aphasia: A qualitative analysis of word storage and retrieval. *Brain and Language, 74*(2), 141–156.

Goldberg, T. E., Egan, M. F., Gscheidle, T., Coppola, R., Weickert, T., Kolachana, B. S., et al. (2003). Executive subprocesses in working memory: Relationship to catechol-O-methyltransferase Val158Met genotype and schizophrenia. *Archives of General Psychiatry, 60*(9), 889–896.

Goldstein, L. B. (1995a). Common drugs may influence motor recovery after stroke. the sygen in acute stroke study investigators. *Neurology, 45*(5), 865–871.

Goldstein, L. B. (1995b). Prescribing of potentially harmful drugs to patients admitted to hospital after head injury. *Journal of Neurology, Neurosurgery, and Psychiatry, 58*(6), 753–755.

Goldstein, L. B., & Davis, J. N. (1988). Physician prescribing patterns following hospital admission for ischemic cerebrovascular disease. *Neurology, 38*(11), 1806–1809.

Granon, S., Passetti, F., Thomas, K. L., Dalley, J. W., Everitt, B. J., & Robbins, T. W. (2000). Enhanced and impaired attentional performance after infusion of D1 dopaminergic receptor agents into rat prefrontal cortex. *The Journal of Neuroscience : The Official Journal of the Society for Neuroscience, 20*(3), 1208–1215.

Greener, J., Enderby, P., & Whurr, R. (2000). Speech and language therapy for aphasia following stroke. *Cochrane Database of Systematic Reviews (Online), (2)*(2), CD000425.

Greener, J., Enderby, P., & Whurr, R. (2001). Pharmacological treatment for aphasia following stroke. *Cochrane Database of Systematic Reviews (Online), (4)*(4), CD000424.

Gualtieri, C. T., & Evans, R. W. (1988). Stimulant treatment for the neurobehavioural sequelae of traumatic brain injury. *Brain Injury : [BI]*, *2*(4), 273–290.

Gupta, S. R., Mlcoch, A. G., Scolaro, C., & Moritz, T. (1995). Bromocriptine treatment of nonfluent aphasia. *Neurology*, *45*(12), 2170–2173.

Hagan, J. J., Alpert, J. E., Morris, R. G., & Iversen, S. D. (1983). The effects of central catecholamine depletions on spatial learning in rats. *Behavioural Brain Research*, *9*(1), 83–104.

Hariri, A. R., Goldberg, T. E., Mattay, V. S., Kolachana, B. S., Callicott, J. H., Egan, M. F., et al. (2003). Brain-derived neurotrophic factor val66met polymorphism affects human memory-related hippocampal activity and predicts memory performance. *The Journal of Neuroscience : The Official Journal of the Society for Neuroscience*, *23*(17), 6690–6694.

Huber, W., Willmes, K., Poeck, K., Van Vleymen, B., & Deberdt, W. (1997). Piracetam as an adjuvant to language therapy for aphasia: A randomized double-blind placebo-controlled pilot study. *Archives of Physical Medicine and Rehabilitation*, *78*(3), 245–250.

Hughes, J. D., Jacobs, D. H., & Heilman, K. M. (2000). Neuropharmacology and linguistic neuroplasticity. *Brain and Language*, *71*(1), 96–101.

Huotari, M., Gogos, J. A., Karayiorgou, M., Koponen, O., Forsberg, M., Raasmaja, A., et al. (2002). Brain catecholamine metabolism in catechol-*O*-methyltransferase (COMT)-deficient mice. *The European Journal of Neuroscience*, *15*(2), 246–256.

Hurford, P., Stringer, A. Y., & Jann, B. (1998). Neuropharmacologic treatment of hemineglect: A case report comparing bromocriptine and methylphenidate. *Archives of Physical Medicine and Rehabilitation*, *79*(3), 346–349.

Introini-Collison, I. B., Miyazaki, B., & McGaugh, J. L. (1991). Involvement of the amygdala in the memory-enhancing effects of clenbuterol. *Psychopharmacology*, *104*(4), 541–544.

Inzitari, D., Di Carlo, A., Pracucci, G., Lamassa, M., Vanni, P., Romanelli, M., et al. (1998). Incidence and determinants of poststroke dementia as defined by an informant interview method in a hospital-based stroke registry. *Stroke; a Journal of Cerebral Circulation*, *29*(10), 2087–2093.

Jakala, P., Sirvio, J., Riekkinen, M., Koivisto, E., Kejonen, K., Vanhanen, M., et al. (1999). Guanfacine and clonidine, alpha 2-agonists, improve paired associates learning, but not delayed matching to sample, in humans. *Neuropsychopharmacology : Official Publication of the American College of Neuropsychopharmacology*, *20*(2), 119–130.

Kauhanen, M. L., Korpelainen, J. T., Hiltunen, P., Maatta, R., Mononen, H., Brusin, E., et al. (2000). Aphasia, depression, and non-verbal cognitive impairment in ischaemic stroke. *Cerebrovascular Diseases (Basel, Switzerland)*, *10*(6), 455–461.

Kessler, J., Thiel, A., Karbe, H., & Heiss, W. D. (2000). Piracetam improves activated blood flow and facilitates rehabilitation of poststroke aphasic patients. *Stroke; a Journal of Cerebral Circulation*, *31*(9), 2112–2116.

Khateb, A., Ammann, J., Annoni, J. M., & Diserens, K. (2005). Cognition-enhancing effects of donepezil in traumatic brain injury. *European Neurology*, *54*(1), 39–45.

KILOH, L. G. (1961). Pseudo-dementia. *Acta Psychiatrica Scandinavica*, *37*, 336–351.

Kim, Y. H., Ko, M. H., Na, S. Y., Park, S. H., & Kim, K. W. (2006). Effects of single-dose methylphenidate on cognitive performance in patients with traumatic brain injury: A double-blind placebo-controlled study. *Clinical Rehabilitation*, *20*(1), 24–30.

Kimberg, D. Y., & D'Esposito, M. (2003). Cognitive effects of the dopamine receptor agonist pergolide. *Neuropsychologia*, *41*(8), 1020–1027.

Kimberg, D. Y., D'Esposito, M., & Farah, M. J. (1997). Effects of bromocriptine on human subjects depend on working memory capacity. *Neuroreport*, *8*(16), 3581–3585.

Kimura, M., Robinson, R. G., & Kosier, J. T. (2000). Treatment of cognitive impairment after poststroke depression : A double-blind treatment trial. *Stroke; a Journal of Cerebral Circulation*, *31*(7), 1482–1486.

Lacaille, J. C., & Harley, C. W. (1985). The action of norepinephrine in the dentate gyrus: Beta-mediated facilitation of evoked potentials in vitro. *Brain Research*, *358*(1–2), 210–220.

Lancelot, E., & Beal, M. F. (1998). Glutamate toxicity in chronic neurodegenerative disease. *Progress in Brain Research*, *116*, 331–347.

Laska, A. C., Hellblom, A., Murray, V., Kahan, T., & Von Arbin, M. (2001). Aphasia in acute stroke and relation to outcome. *Journal of Internal Medicine*, *249*(5), 413–422.

Lauterborn, J. C., Truong, G. S., Baudry, M., Bi, X., Lynch, G., & Gall, C. M. (2003). Chronic elevation of brain-derived neurotrophic factor by ampakines. *The Journal of Pharmacology and Experimental Therapeutics*, *307*(1), 297–305.

Laviolette, S. R., Lipski, W. J., & Grace, A. A. (2005). A subpopulation of neurons in the medial prefrontal cortex encodes emotional learning with burst and frequency codes through a dopamine D4 receptor-dependent basolateral amygdala input. *The Journal of Neuroscience : The Official Journal of the Society for Neuroscience*, *25*(26), 6066–6075.

Levin, H. S., Peters, B. H., Kalisky, Z., High, W. M.,Jr, von Laufen, A., Eisenberg, H. M., et al. (1986). Effects of oral physostigmine and lecithin on memory and attention in closed head-injured patients.

Central Nervous System Trauma : Journal of the American Paralysis Association, 3(4), 333–342.

Lipsey, J. R., Robinson, R. G., Pearlson, G. D., Rao, K., & Price, T. R. (1984). Nortriptyline treatment of post-stroke depression: A double-blind study. *Lancet, 1*(8372), 297–300.

Lipsky, R. H., Sparling, M. B., Ryan, L. M., Xu, K., Salazar, A. M., Goldman, D., et al. (2005). Association of COMT Val158Met genotype with executive functioning following traumatic brain injury. *The Journal of Neuropsychiatry and Clinical Neurosciences, 17*(4), 465–471.

Lockhart, B., Iop, F., Closier, M., & Lestage, P. (2000). (S)-2,3-dihydro-[3,4]cyclopentano-1,2,4-benzothiadiazine-1,1-dioxide: (S18986-1) a positive modulator of AMPA receptors enhances (S)-AMPA-mediated [3H]noradrenaline release from rat hippocampal and frontal cortex slices. *European Journal of Pharmacology, 401*(2), 145–153.

Lu, C. J., & Tune, L. E. (2003). Chronic exposure to anticholinergic medications adversely affects the course of alzheimer disease. *The American Journal of Geriatric Psychiatry : Official Journal of the American Association for Geriatric Psychiatry, 11*(4), 458–461.

Luciana, M., & Collins, P. F. (1997). Dopaminergic modulation of working memory for spatial but not object cues in normal volunteers. *J.Cogn.Neurosci., 4*, 330–347.

Luciana, M., Depue, R. A., Arbisi, P., & Leon, A. (1992). Facilitation of working memory in humans by a D2 dopamine receptor. *Journal of Cognitive Neuroscience, 4*, 58–67.

Mackowiak, M., O'Neill, M. J., Hicks, C. A., Bleakman, D., & Skolnick, P. (2002). An AMPA receptor potentiator modulates hippocampal expression of BDNF: An in vivo study. *Neuropharmacology, 43*(1), 1–10.

Madras, B. K., Xie, Z., Lin, Z., Jassen, A., Panas, H., Lynch, L., et al. (2006). Modafinil occupies dopamine and norepinephrine transporters in vivo and modulates the transporters and trace amine activity in vitro. *The Journal of Pharmacology and Experimental Therapeutics, 319*(2), 561–569.

Mahalick, D. M., Carmel, P. W., Greenberg, J. P., Molofsky, W., Brown, J. A., Heary, R. F., et al. (1998). Psychopharmacologic treatment of acquired attention disorders in children with brain injury. *Pediatric Neurosurgery, 29*(3), 121–126.

Maione, S., Biggs, C. S., Rossi, F., Fowler, L. J., & Whitton, P. S. (1995). Alpha-amino-3-hydroxy-5-methyl-4-isoxazolepropionate receptors modulate dopamine release in rat hippocampus and striatum. *Neuroscience Letters, 193*(3), 181–184.

Malapani, C., Pillon, B., Dubois, B., & Agid, Y. (1994). Impaired simultaneous cognitive task performance in parkinson's disease: A dopamine-related dysfunction. *Neurology, 44*(2), 319–326.

Malhotra, A. K., Kestler, L. J., Mazzanti, C., Bates, J. A., Goldberg, T., & Goldman, D. (2002). A functional polymorphism in the COMT gene and performance on a test of prefrontal cognition. *The American Journal of Psychiatry, 159*(4), 652–654.

Malouf, R., & Birks, J. (2004). Donepezil for vascular cognitive impairment. *Cochrane Database of Systematic Reviews (Online), (1)*(1), CD004395.

Mattay, V. S., Callicott, J. H., Bertolino, A., Heaton, I., Frank, J. A., Coppola, R., et al. (2000). Effects of dextroamphetamine on cognitive performance and cortical activation. *NeuroImage, 12*(3), 268–275.

McAllister, T. W., McDonald, B. C., Flashman, L. A., Rhodes, C. H., Shaw, P. K., Ferrell, R., et al. (2004). Differential effect of COMT allele status on frontal activation associated with a dopaminergic agonist. *The Journal of Neuropsychiatry and Clinical Neurosciences, 16*(2), 240.

McDowell, S., Whyte, J., & D'Esposito, M. (1998). Differential effect of a dopaminergic agonist on prefrontal function in traumatic brain injury patients. *Brain : A Journal of Neurology, 121* (Pt 6)(Pt 6), 1155–1164.

Mehta, M. A., Owen, A. M., Sahakian, B. J., Mavaddat, N., Pickard, J. D., & Robbins, T. W. (2000). Methylphenidate enhances working memory by modulating discrete frontal and parietal lobe regions in the human brain. *The Journal of Neuroscience : The Official Journal of the Society for Neuroscience, 20*(6), RC65.

Mehta, M. A., Swainson, R., Ogilvie, A. D., Sahakian, J., & Robbins, T. W. (2001). Improved short-term spatial memory but impaired reversal learning following the dopamine D(2) agonist bromocriptine in human volunteers. *Psychopharmacology, 159*(1), 10–20.

Mesulam, M., Siddique, T., & Cohen, B. (2003). Cholinergic denervation in a pure multi-infarct state: Observations on CADASIL. *Neurology, 60*(7), 1183–1185.

Mintzer, M. Z., & Griffiths, R. R. (2003). Triazolam-amphetamine interaction: Dissociation of effects on memory versus arousal. *Journal of Psychopharmacology (Oxford, England), 17*(1), 17–29.

Moore, J. L., McAuley, J. W., Long, L., & Bornstein, R. (2002). An evaluation of the effects of methylphenidate on outcomes in adult epilepsy patients. *Epilepsy & Behavior : E&B, 3*(1), 92–95.

Mukand, J. A., Guilmette, T. J., Allen, D. G., Brown, L. K., Brown, S. L., Tober, K. L., et al. (2001). Dopaminergic therapy with carbidopa L-dopa for left neglect after stroke: A case series. *Archives of Physical Medicine and Rehabilitation, 82*(9), 1279–1282.

Muller, W. E., Hartman, H., Koch, S., Scheuer, K., & Stoll, S. (1994). Neurotransmission in aging: Therapeutic aspects. In N. Racagni, N. Brunello & S. Langer (Eds.), *Recent advances in the treatment of neurodegenerative disorders and cognitive dysfunction* (pp. 166–173). Basel, Switzerland: Karger.

Muller, U., Steffenhagen, N., Regenthal, R., & Bublak, P. (2004). Effects of modafinil on working memory processes in humans. *Psychopharmacology, 177*(1–2), 161–169.

Muller, U., von Cramon, D. Y., & Pollmann, S. (1998). D1- versus D2-receptor modulation of visuospatial working memory in humans. *The Journal of Neuroscience : The Official Journal of the Society for Neuroscience, 18*(7), 2720–2728.

Murchison, C. F., Zhang, X. Y., Zhang, W. P., Ouyang, M., Lee, A., & Thomas, S. A. (2004). A distinct role for norepinephrine in memory retrieval. *Cell, 117*(1), 131–143.

Mysiw, W. J., Bogner, J. A., Corrigan, J. D., Fugate, L. P., Clinchot, D. M., & Kadyan, V. (2006). The impact of acute care medications on rehabilitation outcome after traumatic brain injury. *Brain Injury : [BI], 20*(9), 905–911.

Narushima, K., Chan, K. L., Kosier, J. T., & Robinson, R. G. (2003). Does cognitive recovery after treatment of poststroke depression last? A 2-year follow-up of cognitive function associated with poststroke depression. *The American Journal of Psychiatry, 160*(6), 1157–1162.

Narushima, K., Paradiso, S., Moser, D. J., Jorge, R., & Robinson, R. G. (2007). Effect of antidepressant therapy on executive function after stroke. *British Journal of Psychiatry, 190*, 260–265.

Neurobehavioral Guidelines Working Group, Warden, D. L., Gordon, B., McAllister, T. W., Silver, J. M., Barth, J. T., et al. (2006). Guidelines for the pharmacologic treatment of neurobehavioral sequelae of traumatic brain injury. *Journal of Neurotrauma, 23*(10), 1468–1501.

O'Brien, J. T., Erkinjuntti, T., Reisberg, B., Roman, G., Sawada, T., Pantoni, L., et al. (2003). Vascular cognitive impairment. *Lancet Neurology, 2*(2), 89–98.

Orgogozo, J. M. (1999). Piracetam in the treatment of acute stroke. *Pharmacopsychiatry, 32* Suppl 1, 25–32.

Orgogozo, J. M., Rigaud, A. S., Stoffler, A., Mobius, H. J., & Forette, F. (2002). Efficacy and safety of memantine in patients with mild to moderate vascular dementia: A randomized, placebo-controlled trial (MMM 300). *Stroke; a Journal of Cerebral Circulation, 33*(7), 1834–1839.

Owen, A. M., Iddon, J. L., Hodges, J. R., Summers, B. A., & Robbins, T. W. (1997). Spatial and non-spatial working memory at different stages of parkinson's disease. *Neuropsychologia, 35*(4), 519–532.

Oyaizu, M., & Narahashi, T. (1999). Modulation of the neuronal nicotinic acetylcholine receptor-channel by the nootropic drug nefiracetam. *Brain Research, 822*(1–2), 72–79.

Ozeren, A., Sarica, Y., Mavi, H., & Demirkiran, M. (1995). Bromocriptine is ineffective in the treatment of chronic nonfluent aphasia. *Acta Neurologica Belgica, 95*(4), 235–238.

Pedersen, P. M., Jorgensen, H. S., Nakayama, H., Raaschou, H. O., & Olsen, T. S. (1995). Aphasia in acute stroke: Incidence, determinants, and recovery. *Annals of Neurology, 38*(4), 659–666.

Pedersen, P. M., Vinter, K., & Olsen, T. S. (2004). Aphasia after stroke: Type, severity and prognosis. the copenhagen aphasia study. *Cerebrovascular Diseases (Basel, Switzerland), 17*(1), 35–43.

Pepeu, G., & Spignoli, G. (1989). Nootropic drugs and brain cholinergic mechanisms. *Progress in Neuro-Psychopharmacology & Biological Psychiatry, 13* Suppl, S77–S88.

Perez-Stable, E. J., Halliday, R., Gardiner, P. S., Baron, R. B., Hauck, W. W., Acree, M., et al. (2000). The effects of propranolol on cognitive function and quality of life: A randomized trial among patients with diastolic hypertension. *The American Journal of Medicine, 108*(5), 359–365.

Pittaluga, A., Pattarini, R., Andrioli, G. C., Viola, C., Munari, C., & Raiteri, M. (1999). Activity of putative cognition enhancers in kynurenate test performed with human neocortex slices. *The Journal of Pharmacology and Experimental Therapeutics, 290*(1), 423–428.

Plenger, P. M., Dixon, C. E., Castillo, R. M., Frankowski, R. F., Yablon, S. A., & Levin, H. S. (1996). Subacute methylphenidate treatment for moderate to moderately severe traumatic brain injury: A preliminary double-blind placebo-controlled study. *Archives of Physical Medicine and Rehabilitation, 77*(6), 536–540.

Pohjasvaara, T., Erkinjuntti, T., Ylikoski, R., Hietanen, M., Vataja, R., & Kaste, M. (1998). Clinical determinants of poststroke dementia. *Stroke; a Journal of Cerebral Circulation, 29*(1), 75–81.

Rabins, P. V. (1981). The prevalence of reversible dementia in a psychiatric hospital. *Hospital & Community Psychiatry, 32*(7), 490–492.

Rabins, P. V., Merchant, A., & Nestadt, G. (1984). Criteria for diagnosing reversible dementia caused by depression: Validation by 2-year follow-up. *The British Journal of Psychiatry : The Journal of Mental Science, 144*, 488–492.

Rama, P., Linnankoski, I., Tanila, H., Pertovaara, A., & Carlson, S. (1996). Medetomidine, atipamezole, and guanfacine in delayed response performance of aged monkeys. *Pharmacology, Biochemistry, and Behavior, 55*(3), 415–422.

Rammsayer, T. H., Rodewald, S., & Groh, D. (2000). Dopamine-antagonistic, anticholinergic, and GABAergic effects on declarative and procedural memory functions. *Brain Research.Cognitive Brain Research, 9*(1), 61–71.

Ramos, B. P., Colgan, L., Nou, E., Ovadia, S., Wilson, S. R., & Arnsten, A. F. (2005). The beta-1 adrenergic antagonist, betaxolol, improves working memory performance in rats and monkeys. *Biological Psychiatry*, *58*(11), 894–900.

Ramos, B. P., Colgan, L. A., Nou, E., & Arnsten, A. F. (2007). Beta2 adrenergic agonist, clenbuterol, enhances working memory performance in aging animals. *Neurobiology of Aging*,

Randall, D. C., Viswanath, A., Bharania, P., Elsabagh, S. M., Hartley, D. E., Shneerson, J. M., et al. (2005). Does modafinil enhance cognitive performance in young volunteers who are not sleep-deprived? *Journal of Clinical Psychopharmacology*, *25*(2), 175–179.

Rao, S. G., Williams, G. V., & Goldman-Rakic, P. S. (2000). Destruction and creation of spatial tuning by disinhibition: GABA(A) blockade of prefrontal cortical neurons engaged by working memory. *The Journal of Neuroscience : The Official Journal of the Society for Neuroscience*, *20*(1), 485–494.

Raymer, A. M. (2003). Treatment of adynamia in aphasia. *Frontiers in Bioscience : A Journal and Virtual Library*, *8*, s845–s51.

Reeves, S., Bench, C., & Howard, R. (2002). Ageing and the nigrostriatal dopaminergic system. *International Journal of Geriatric Psychiatry*, *17*(4), 359–370.

Relkin, N. R. (2007). Beyond symptomatic therapy: A re-examination of acetylcholinesterase inhibitors in Alzheimer's disease. *Expert Review of Neurotherapeutics*, *7*(6), 735–748.

Robey, R. R. (1994). The efficacy of treatment for aphasic persons: A meta-analysis. *Brain and Language*, *47*(4), 582–608.

Robey, R. R. (1998). A meta-analysis of clinical outcomes in the treatment of aphasia. *Journal of Speech, Language, and Hearing Research : JSLHR*, *41*(1), 172–187.

Robinson, R. G., Schultz, S. K., Castillo, C., Kopel, T., Kosier, J. T., Newman, R. M., et al. (2000). Nortriptyline versus fluoxetine in the treatment of depression and in short-term recovery after stroke: A placebo-controlled, double-blind study. *The American Journal of Psychiatry*, *157*(3), 351–359.

Roesch-Ely, D., Scheffel, H., Weiland, S., Schwaninger, M., Hundemer, H. P., Kolter, T., et al. (2005). Differential dopaminergic modulation of executive control in healthy subjects. *Psychopharmacology*, *178*(4), 420–430.

Roullet, P., & Sara, S. (1998). Consolidation of memory after its reactivation: Involvement of beta noradrenergic receptors in the late phase. *Neural Plasticity*, *6*(3), 63–68.

Roussos, P., Giakoumaki, S. G., Pavlakis, S., & Bitsios, P. (2008). Planning, decision-making and the COMT rs4818 polymorphism in healthy males. *Neuropsychologia*, *46*(2), 757–763.

Runyan, J. D., Moore, A. N., & Dash, P. K. (2005). A role for prefrontal calcium-sensitive protein phosphatase and kinase activities in working memory.

Learning & Memory (Cold Spring Harbor, N.Y.), *12*(2), 103–110.

Sabe, L., Salvarezza, F., Garcia Cuerva, A., Leiguarda, R., & Starkstein, S. (1995). A randomized, double-blind, placebo-controlled study of bromocriptine in nonfluent aphasia. *Neurology*, *45*(12), 2272–2274.

Saeedi, H., Remington, G., & Christensen, B. K. (2006). Impact of haloperidol, a dopamine D2 antagonist, on cognition and mood. *Schizophrenia Research*, *85*(1–3), 222–231.

Seamans, J. K., & Yang, C. R. (2004). The principal features and mechanisms of dopamine modulation in the prefrontal cortex. *Progress in Neurobiology*, *74*(1), 1–58.

Selden, N. R., Gitelman, D. R., Salamon-Murayama, N., Parrish, T. B., & Mesulam, M. M. (1998). Trajectories of cholinergic pathways within the cerebral hemispheres of the human brain. *Brain : A Journal of Neurology*, *121* (Pt 12) (Pt 12), 2249–2257.

Simis, S., & Nitrini, R. (2006). Cognitive improvement after treatment of depressive symptoms in the acute phase of stroke. *Arquivos De Neuro-Psiquiatria*, *64*(2B), 412–417.

Simon, H. (1981). Dopaminergic A10 neurons and frontal system (author's transl). [Neurones dopaminergiques A10 et systeme frontal] *Journal De Physiologie*, *77*(1), 81–95.

Small, S. L. (1994). Pharmacotherapy of aphasia. A critical review. *Stroke; a Journal of Cerebral Circulation*, *25*(6), 1282–1289.

Speech, T. J., Rao, S. M., Osmon, D. C., & Sperry, L. T. (1993). A double-blind controlled study of methylphenidate treatment in closed head injury. *Brain Injury : [BI]*, *7*(4), 333–338.

Spence, S. A., Green, R. D., Wilkinson, I. D., & Hunter, M. D. (2005). Modafinil modulates anterior cingulate function in chronic schizophrenia. *The British Journal of Psychiatry : The Journal of Mental Science*, *187*, 55–61.

Stanislav, S. W. (1997). Cognitive effects of antipsychotic agents in persons with traumatic brain injury. *Brain Injury : [BI]*, *11*(5), 335–341.

Szelies, B., Mielke, R., Kessler, J., & Heiss, W. D. (2001). Restitution of alpha-topography by piracetam in post-stroke aphasia. *International Journal of Clinical Pharmacology and Therapeutics*, *39*(4), 152–157.

Tanaka, Y., Miyazaki, M., & Albert, M. L. (1997). Effects of increased cholinergic activity on naming in aphasia. *Lancet*, *350*(9071), 116–117.

Tao, R., Ma, Z., & Auerbach, S. B. (1997). Influence of AMPA/kainate receptors on extracellular 5-hydroxytryptamine in rat midbrain raphe and forebrain. *British Journal of Pharmacology*, *121*(8), 1707–1715.

Tatemichi, T. K., Desmond, D. W., Mayeux, R., Paik, M., Stern, Y., Sano, M., et al. (1992). Dementia after stroke: Baseline frequency, risks, and clinical features in a hospitalized cohort. *Neurology*, *42*(6), 1185–1193.

Tatemichi, T. K., Desmond, D. W., Stern, Y., Paik, M., Sano, M., & Bagiella, E. (1994). Cognitive impairment after stroke: Frequency, patterns, and relationship to functional abilities. *Journal of Neurology, Neurosurgery, and Psychiatry, 57*(2), 202–207.

Taylor Sarno, M. (1998). Recovery and rehabilitation in aphasia. In M. Taylor Sarno (Ed.), *Acquired aphsia* (3rd ed., pp. 595–631). San Diego: Academic Press.

Tenovuo, O. (2005). Central acetylcholinesterase inhibitors in the treatment of chronic traumatic brain injury-clinical experience in 111 patients. *Progress in Neuro-Psychopharmacology & Biological Psychiatry, 29*(1), 61–67.

Tunbridge, E. M., Bannerman, D. M., Sharp, T., & Harrison, P. J. (2004). Catechol-o-methyltransferase inhibition improves set-shifting performance and elevates stimulated dopamine release in the rat prefrontal cortex. *The Journal of Neuroscience: The Official Journal of the Society for Neuroscience, 24*(23), 5331–5335.

Turner, D. C., Blackwell, A. D., Dowson, J. H., McLean, A., & Sahakian, B. J. (2005). Neurocognitive effects of methylphenidate in adult attention-deficit/hyperactivity disorder. *Psychopharmacology, 178*(2–3), 286–295.

Turner, D. C., Clark, L., Pomarol-Clotet, E., McKenna, P., Robbins, T. W., & Sahakian, B. J. (2004). Modafinil improves cognition and attentional set shifting in patients with chronic schizophrenia. *Neuropsychopharmacology: Official Publication of the American College of Neuropsychopharmacology, 29*(7), 1363–1373.

Turner, D. C., Robbins, T. W., Clark, L., Aron, A. R., Dowson, J., & Sahakian, B. J. (2003). Cognitive enhancing effects of modafinil in healthy volunteers. *Psychopharmacology, 165*(3), 260–269.

van Gaalen, M. M., van Koten, R., Schoffelmeer, A. N., & Vanderschuren, L. J. (2006). Critical involvement of dopaminergic neurotransmission in impulsive decision making. *Biological Psychiatry, 60*(1), 66–73.

Vernon, M. W., & Sorkin, E. M. (1991). Piracetam. an overview of its pharmacological properties and a review of its therapeutic use in senile cognitive disorders. *Drugs & Aging, 1*(1), 17–35.

Wade, D. T., Hewer, R. L., David, R. M., & Enderby, P. M. (1986). Aphasia after stroke: Natural history and associated deficits. *Journal of Neurology, Neurosurgery, and Psychiatry, 49*(1), 11–16.

Wertz, R. T., Weiss, D. G., Aten, J. L., Brookshire, R. H., Garcia-Bunuel, L., Holland, A. L., et al. (1986). Comparison of clinic, home, and deferred language treatment for aphasia. A veterans administration cooperative study. *Archives of Neurology, 43*(7), 653–658.

Wesnes, K. A., McKeith, I., Edgar, C., Emre, M., & Lane, R. (2005). Benefits of rivastigmine on attention in dementia associated with parkinson disease. *Neurology, 65*(10), 1654–1656.

Whyte, J., Hart, T., Schuster, K., Fleming, M., Polansky, M., & Coslett, H. B. (1997). Effects of methylphenidate on attentional function after traumatic brain injury. A randomized, placebo-controlled trial. *American Journal of Physical Medicine & Rehabilitation / Association of Academic Physiatrists, 76*(6), 440–450.

Whyte, J., Hart, T., Vaccaro, M., Grieb-Neff, P., Risser, A., Polansky, M., et al. (2004). Effects of methylphenidate on attention deficits after traumatic brain injury: A multidimensional, randomized, controlled trial. *American Journal of Physical Medicine & Rehabilitation/ Association of Academic Physiatrists, 83*(6), 401–420.

Wilcock, G., Mobius, H. J., Stoffler, A., & MMM 500 group. (2002). A double-blind, placebo-controlled multicentre study of memantine in mild to moderate vascular dementia (MMM500). *International Clinical Psychopharmacology, 17*(6), 297–305.

Williams, G. V., & Goldman-Rakic, P. S. (1995). Modulation of memory fields by dopamine D1 receptors in prefrontal cortex. *Nature, 376*(6541), 572–575.

Zafonte, R. D., Elovic, E., Mysiw, W. J., O'Dell, M., & Watanabe, T. (1999). Pharmacology in traumatic brain injury: Fundamentals and treatment strategies. In M. Rosenthal, J. S. Kreutzer, E. R. Griffith & B. Pentland (Eds.), *Rehabilitation of the adult and child with traumatic brain injury* (3rd ed., pp. 536–555). Philadelphia: FA Davis.

Zahrt, J., Taylor, J. R., Mathew, R. G., & Arnsten, A. F. (1997). Supranormal stimulation of D1 dopamine receptors in the rodent prefrontal cortex impairs spatial working memory performance. *The Journal of Neuroscience : The Official Journal of the Society for Neuroscience, 17*(21), 8528–8535.

Zhang, L., Plotkin, R. C., Wang, G., Sandel, M. E., & Lee, S. (2004). Cholinergic augmentation with donepezil enhances recovery in short-term memory and sustained attention after traumatic brain injury. *Archives of Physical Medicine and Rehabilitation, 85*(7), 1050–1055.

Chapter 19
Neuropsychological Rehabilitation

Gail A. Eskes and Anna M. Barrett

Introduction

Cognitive impairment after stroke is common and can significantly impact on recovery of function and return to functional activities and roles. The term "vascular cognitive impairment" encompasses the continuum of vascular changes in brain cognition, ranging from mild impairment (no impact on functional abilities) to frank vascular dementia (see Chapter 7). Management of individuals with attentional, conative (the translation of knowledge and emotion to behavior), and cognitive impairment varies, depending upon the severity of the deficits and their functional consequences. Review of the evidence for rehabilitation of individuals with cognitive deficits post-stroke (without dementia) will be the focus of this chapter. In this chapter, we define cognitive function broadly as multiple modular mental systems either containing and/or acting on domain-specific knowledge representations (e.g. language, spatial function, calculations).

What is cognitive rehabilitation? Most definitions converge on the idea that cognitive rehabilitation is a systematic, therapeutic process designed to remediate, alleviate, or manage cognitive deficits in order to improve daily functioning (Cicerone et al., 2000; Sohlberg & Mateer 2001a, Wilson 2002). Cognitive and other mental processes frequently affected by stroke include attention and memory, visuo-perceptual abilities, and executive function. In this chapter we will provide an overview of the evidence for the efficacy of procedures targeted toward rehabilitation of these cognitive disorders after stroke. While each cognitive domain is discussed in separate sections, we recognize that cognitive functions frequently interact, and stroke survivors commonly have multiple deficits; the potential behavior and response to intervention may interact. In addition, the presence of affective disorders (as dealt with in Chapter 16) also modifies response to treatment and should be included as part of a care plan, but will not be discussed in this chapter.

Impact of Cognitive Deficits Post-Stroke

While a comprehensive review of post-stroke cognitive deficits is outside the scope of this chapter (see Chapter 2), we will first briefly summarize the impact of common deficits on stroke recovery and outcome. Post-stroke deficits in executive function, attention and memory, language, visuo-spatial processing,

G.A. Eskes (✉)
Departments of Psychiatry, Psychology and Medicine (Neurology), Brain Repair Centre, Dalhousie University, Halifax, Nova Scotia, Canada
e-mail: Gail.Eskes@Dal.Ca

J.R. Festa, R.M. Lazar (eds.), *Neurovascular Neuropsychology*, DOI 10.1007/978-0-387-70715-0_19, and speed of processing are common both in the acute and rehabilitation phases (Azouvi et al., 2002; Ballard et al., 2003; Hochstenbach, Mulder, van Limbeek, Donders, & Schoonwaldt, 1998; Hochstenbach, Prigatano, & Mulder 2005; Hoffmann 2001; Riepe, Riss, Bittner, & Huber, 2004; Stone, Halligan, & Greenwood, 1993); reviewed in Barker-Collo & Feigin, 2006; Gillespie Bowen, & Foster, 2006) and remain prevalent in the long term (Ferro & Crespo 1988; Nys, Van Zandvoort, De Kort, Jansen et al., 2005, Patel Coshall, Rudd, & Wolfe, 2003; Rasquin, Lodder, Ponds, Winkens, Jolles et al., 2004; Tham Auchus, Thong, Goh, Chang et al., 2002. For example, Hoffmann (2001) examined the frequency of cognitive and mental impairment based on bedside neurologic testing in 1,000 patients within the first month after stroke. Higher cortical function abnormality was detected in 63.5% of patients and included aphasia, apraxia, amnesia, and executive dysfunction. Ballard et al. (2003) found 32% of 150 stroke survivors met criteria for global cognitive impairment, with up to 73% impaired in information processing speed at least 3 months post-stroke. Cognitive impairment as detected by a neuropsychological battery was also common in another group of 237 patients 3 months post-stroke (Madureira Guerreiro, & Ferro, 2001). The most frequent deficits were memory and orientation, and aspects of language. In a similar study, Hochstenbach, Mulder, et al. (1998) reported that 70% of 229 patients assessed with a neuropsychological battery 2–3 months post-stroke had impaired information processing speed, and at least 40% had difficulty within a variety of domains, including memory, visuo-spatial and constructional abilities, language, and arithmetic.

Deficits persist in chronic post-stroke recovery: at 27.7 months, a representative sub-group was restudied in Hochstenbach et al. (2003). While a small minority showed significant improvement, particularly in areas of attention, language, and visuo-spatial skills, most patients showed no improvement or

declined (Hochstenbach, den Otter, & Mulder et al., 2003). Likewise, Tatemichi, Desmond, Stern, Paik, Sano, et al. (1994) found that 35% of a group of 227 patients showed cognitive impairment on multiple tests at 3 months post-stroke, with improvement seen in only 19 of 151 patients in memory, orientation, visuospatial function and attention in yearly follow-ups (Desmond Moroney, Sano, & Stern, 1996). Thus, in screening, post-stroke cognitive and mental deficits are common, they are potentially chronic, and they span a range of cognitive domains.

The impact of cognitive impairment on rehabilitation and long-term functional outcome has also been documented widely. The presence of cognitive impairment in general is associated with increased functional disability (Claesson, Linden, Skoog, & Blomstrand, 2005; Tatemichi et al., 1994; Zinn et al., 2004). Poor outcome has been associated with a number of cognitive variables, including the presence of spatial neglect and related symptoms, such as anosognosia (Appelros et al., 2003; Buxbaum et al., 2004; Fullerton et al., 1988; Gillen et al., 2005; Mark 1993; Paolucci et al., 2001), attention deficits (Hyndman & Ashburn 2003; McDowd, Filion, Pohl, Richards, & Stiers 2003; Nys, Van Zandvoort, de Kort, van der Worp et al., 2005b), working memory (Malouin, Belleville, Richards, Desrosiers, & Doyon, 2004), verbal memory (Wade, Parker, & Hewer, 1986), and executive dysfunction (Mok Wong, Lam, Fan, & Tang, 2004; Stephens et al., 2005). While the role of good cognitive skills in many instrumental activities of daily living such as following a recipe, driving, or going to work seems obvious, cognitive deficits also adversely affect physical disability via reduced response to rehabilitation in other domains based on learning, e.g., motor skill reacquisition. For example, Cirstea, Ptito, and Levin (2006) found that arm motor-skills training progress as measured by precision and variability of performance was correlated with memory and planning skills. In addition, working memory skills were related to learning of locomotor-related skills using combined mental and physical practice in standing up and sitting down (Malouin et al., 2004). Finally, Robertson, Ridgeway, Greenfield, and Parr (1997) reported that measures of sustained attention at 2 months post-stroke could predict motor recovery at 2 years as measured by the Rivermead Mobility Test and the 9-Hole Peg Test. Thus, the presence of cognitive impairment has wide-reaching impact and deserves early intervention even when initial rehabilitation goals are focused on physical recovery.

Framework for Rehabilitation

Our approach to rehabilitation of cognitive disorders post-stroke is based on several principles (see Table 1). First, a comprehensive assessment of the cognitive profile of the individual is needed to identify strengths and weaknesses. A thorough understanding of the deficit(s), as well as identification of the preserved functions, is critical to the selection of rehabilitation techniques. This step will improve the likelihood of successful outcome and also provide important information about cause-and-effect relationships between patients, therapies, and outcomes for continued improvement of interventions. Neuropsychologists and other specialists trained in brain-behavior assessment can

play a key role in this first step, providing detailed assessments of affected and intact aspects of cognition and mental function. Knowledge of the associations of behavioral/cognitive functions with particular brain regions is also important for determining what cognitive and neural mechanisms might be available for recruitment in a rehabilitation program. Thus, knowledge of both the neuropsychological function and neuroanatomical involvement can provide clinicians with the information needed to decide which rehabilitation program might be most effective.

A second principle is that the choice of intervention should be evidence-based when possible, ideally grounded on the theoretical underpinnings of the targeted cognitive system(s). Our level of understanding of the underlying mechanisms and effectiveness of rehabilitation processes varies by cognitive domain, but we are clearly in the early stages of cognitive rehabilitation as a science-based discipline. The inclusion of theory-based interventions, well-controlled studies and focus on relevant outcomes are highlighted as important goals for continued scientific progress in the field.

A third principle for success is that the ultimate focus of the intervention should be on patient-relevant functional goals, identified in collaboration with the stroke survivor and family. While clinical rehabilitation goals

Table 1 Factors affecting rehabilitation of cognitive function

Factors	Cognitive profile	Other psychological factors	Physical health	Environmental factors
Definition	Strengths and weaknesses that interact to produce level of functioning in a cognitive domain. Domains can include attention, memory, speech and language, visuo-spatial and perceptual function, executive function and limb praxis.	Factors related to awareness of deficits and motivation for change (e.g., anosognosia, anxiety, and depression), disorders of conation, drive.	Co-morbidities and physical issues that can impact on cognitive function, e.g., pain, fatigue, sleep disorders, delirium, sensory deficits (hearing, vision)	Physical and social contexts that can influence cognitive recovery, e.g., noise and distraction, presence of signs, cuing and feedback by spouse

normally target daily functioning, it is important to keep in mind that outcomes have been measured at a number of levels in the rehabilitation literature. Most efficacy studies have focused on changes in training performance, or on different measures of the impaired domain itself (e.g., psychometric measures of cognitive abilities or neurophysiological changes such as EEG, or other measures of functional brain activity). While obtaining evidence for generalization of training to other tests of the same domain is a first step, the question of whether the intervention improves daily functioning is critical for ultimate evaluation of efficacy/effectiveness, and unfortunately, limited information about the impact of rehabilitative techniques on everyday activities (e.g., self care, cooking, driving) or quality of life is available. Thus, it is unclear if training outcomes simply represent improvements in a specific skill (e.g., due to practice in taking a reaction time test) versus improved cognitive

function per se (Park, Proulx, & Towers, 1999). Considering generalization to dissimilar tasks as well as functional abilities is critical to our understanding of rehabilitation effects as well as improving potential clinical outcomes.

A final principle is that rehabilitation of cognitive deficits must take place in context; effective management of persons with cognitive deficits takes into account a variety of personal and environmental factors potentially influencing cognitive function. Potential factors that can interact to influence cognitive functioning are presented in Table 1. While the focus of this chapter is on rehabilitation of the cognitive components, recognition and amelioration of the impact of these other factors within a multi-disciplinary setting will optimize the intervention and improve functional outcomes.

Cognitive rehabilitation processes can be grouped into one of five approaches (see Table 2): (1) remediation or restoration of the

Table 2 Summary of rehabilitation approaches

Rehabilitation approach	Methods/goals	Strengths & weaknesses
Restoration of damaged function—targets impairment	Intensive and repetitive practice and drills/exercises to improve damaged cognitive function directly.	If successful, could lead to most generalizable effects. Currently limited by atheoretical approaches, poor generalization and lack of understanding of neurocognitive mechanisms underlying plasticity/regeneration
Optimization of residual function—targets impairment	Teaching of compensatory strategies to improve remaining function	Can apply to a wide range of patients and goals. Currently needs better theoretical approach and better focus on generalization; not applicable with severe deficits
Compensation through substitution of remaining intact skills—targets functional goals	Uses alternative domain-specific processes to achieve a functional goal	Focus on functional outcome is a strength. Depends upon careful assessment of cognitive strengths and weaknesses
Compensation through use of environmental supports or external aids—targets functional goals	Uses a range of devices and environmental supports to achieve functional goal	Wide applicability, even with severe deficits. Can require extensive training and support.
Vicariation though recruitment of functionally or structurally related behavioral processes which may directly increase activation and impaired processes	Uses training techniques, exercise devices	Strengths similar to compensatory approaches; requires knowledge of cognitive and behavioral theory often not available to clinicians.

damaged skill; (2) optimization of residual function; (3) compensation through substitution of remaining intact skills; (4) compensation through use of environmental supports or external aids; and (5) vicariation through recruitment of functionally or structurally-related, brain-behavior systems. The first two approaches focus on attempting to improve the underlying impairment, with the hope of general enhancement of the damaged function. Compensatory approaches, in contrast, focus on training processes that can substitute for the damaged function—either another intact cognitive domain or by use of external devices that substitute for the function. Like compensation, vicariation engages intact cognitive processes, but unlike compensation, vicariation may engage processes not directly related to the impaired function or task. Instead, intact cognitive processes, structurally or functionally related to the impaired brain-behavior systems, are activated so as to secondarily activate and support the impaired processes. This may occur at an implicit or procedural level, inaccessible to conventional treatment or training. A number of vicariative approaches are being researched (e.g., intention treatment in non-fluent aphasia; Crosson et al., 2007). However, since more information is available on the use of remediation and compensation in clinical practice, our presentation will emphasize these approaches.

Use of remediation and compensation is not mutually exclusive, and therapies may use a combination of the above approaches. While many rehabilitation techniques focus on compensation by internal or external means, there is some evidence supporting the possibility of actual restoration or optimizing of residual functions (e.g., Lillie, 2006). A number of recent "evidence-based" reviews of cognitive rehabilitation studies in acquired brain injury are available (Cappa et al. 2003; Cicerone et al. 2000; Cicerone et al. 2005; Lincoln et al. 2002; Majid et al. 2000) and summaries with periodic updates are also accessible on the worldwide web (Evidence-Based Review of Stroke Rehabilitation; www.ebrsr.com). Overall, more well-controlled research is needed to identify optimal cognitive rehabilitation methods. One major issue is the choice of outcome measures to evaluate generalizability, as discussed above. Other issues not yet resolved include the best time to begin rehabilitation, its duration, and optimal intensity (Bayley et al., 2007). In addition, while we attempt here to focus on evidence derived from studies of stroke survivors, more stroke-specific studies are needed. We thus included literature dealing with acquired brain injury at times, when relevant.

Focal Cognitive/Perceptual Deficit Syndromes

Attention

Pathophysiology and Mechanisms

Attention is the faculty by which we select among various possible inputs those stimuli that will receive further processing. Posner and colleagues have developed an influential model of attention highlighting three basic functions: vigilance (mediated by the right hemisphere and involved in achieving and maintaining an alert state); orienting (mediated by the posterior attention network with role of searching and selection of sensory information); and executive control (mediated by the anterior attention system and involved in the orchestration of complex computations, or allocation of resources in a limited capacity system) (Fernandez-Duque & Posner 2001; Posner & Petersen 1990). Other well-known clinical models of attention also include functions related to sustaining attention over time (vigilance), selection of information, and need for control due to competing or conflicting demands (see Table 3) and two particular models (Sohlberg & Mateer, 1989b; Sturm, Willmes, Orgass, & Hartje 1997) formed the basis for the development and testing of theoretically driven rehabilitation protocols for impaired attention.

Disorders of attention are common in stroke, and impaired attention may be an important independent factor for stroke

Table 3 Relationship of components of attention in 3 models

Posner et al.	Sturm et al. (1997)	Sohlberg et al.	Deficit
Alerting—achieving and maintaining an alert state	Alertness (phasic): enhancement of response readiness following a warning stimulus	Focused attention: basic responding to specific stimuli	Reduced arousal; diminished response to input
	Vigilance: sustained maintenance of alertness for rare events in monotonous situations	Sustained attention: The ability to maintain a consistent behavioral response during continuous or repetitive activity (includes components of vigilance and mental control)	Distractibility; difficulty in maintaining focus; attention lapses
Orienting—selection of information from sensory input	Selective attention: ability to focus on certain features of a task and at the same time to suppress voluntarily responses to irrelevant features	Selective attention: the ability to maintain a cognitive set in the face of distracting or competing stimuli	Spatial neglect; distractibility
Executive control—resolving conflict among responses	Divided attention: Dividing attention between two or several sources of information	Alternating attention: the capacity for mental flexibility which allows for moving between tasks having different cognitive requirements. Divided attention: The ability to simultaneously respond to multiple tasks or demands	Difficulty with interference, allocation of resources, inhibition

recovery (McDowd et al., 2003; Robertson et al., 1997; Stapleton et al., 2001; Tatemichi et al., 1994). Depending upon the brain region affected, attentional deficits may occur in one or more components identified by Posner and colleagues (Fernandez-Duque & Posner 2001; Posner & Petersen 1990). Deficits in spatial attention (neglect) and non-spatial attention will be dealt with separately. There have been a number of reviews focused on the effectiveness of intervention for attentional impairments (Lincoln, Majid, & Weyman 2000; Michel & Mateer 2006; Park & Ingles 1999).

Current Research

Direct Remediation of Non-Spatial Attention

Published studies indicate that vigilance, selection and executive functioning can be improved with direct remediation. Sturm and colleagues performed the most extensive set of stroke rehabilitation studies, based on their model of attention components (Table 3) and using a computer-assisted attention training program (AIXTENT, recently programmed for the PC) for each of four domains (Sturm, Hartje, Orgass, & Willmes, 1993). In several studies of stroke survivors at 3 months to 13 years post event, they reported that attention improves most from deficit specific training (e.g., vigilance training for vigilance deficits, selective attention training for selective attention deficits), while non-specific training may even adversely affect attention functions (Sturm, Fimm et al., 2002; Sturm & Willmes, 1991; Sturm, Willmes, Orgass et al., 1997). Training was delivered in 30–60 min sessions for 14 sessions over 3–4 weeks, and involved training one domain at a time. Outcome measures have been limited to similar computerized tests, or psychometric tasks of attention (e.g., d2 Test). This training program was also reported to be effective for improving attention in multiple sclerosis (Plohmann et al., 1998) and associated with improvement in self-reported everyday attention difficulties. More research on the generalizability of this training program to functional improvements is clearly warranted.

A second attention training program based on a similar conceptual model of attentional functions is the Attention Process Training (APT) (Table 3) (Sohlberg, M. & Mateer, C. 1989a). The APT program consists of hierarchically organized tasks that exercise different components of attention, at increasing levels of complexity and task demands; examples include listening for number sequences, alphabetizing words heard in a sentence, detecting targets in the presence of distractor noise, or switching between complex semantic categorization tasks (Sohlberg, McLaughlin et al., 2000). Although published research with this tool focused on individuals with traumatic brain injury, the program is conceptually similar to the Sturm approach, and thus theoretically may benefit stroke survivors. Solhlberg, Mateer, and colleagues (Sohlberg & Mateer 1987; Sohlberg, McLaughlin et al., 2000) reported that APT training with brain-injured individuals in chronic recovery phases (1 year or more) experienced greater improvements in psychometric tests of attention (PASAT, Stroop, Trail Making, Location memory) compared to a control baseline or control group receiving brain injury education. While the specific effects of the different attention training components in the APT have not been examined, the primary effects of APT overall were obtained on executive control and working memory tasks, while no training effects were seen on vigilance or orienting (Sohlberg, McLaughlin et al., 2000). APT training in the home environment was evaluated in a study of chronic stroke recovery (at least 9 months post onset). While performance improved on training tasks, as well memory testing, no effects were seen on functional activities or self-rated quality of life. Thus, whether this training targets specific skills or a generalized cognitive function is still unresolved (for a discussion and meta-analysis, see Park & Ingles 2001).

Mazur et al. (2003) evaluated computer-assisted training using a visual-attention measure, the Useful Field of View (UFOV) test, to improve attention and success in an on-road driving evaluation in survivors ≤ 6 months post-stroke. The UFOV measures and trains three visual attention functions: processing speed, selective attention, and divided attention. Twenty 30–60 min sessions took place 2–4 times per week, with results compared to a group receiving non-specific visuoperceptual training (computer games). Subjects with right hemisphere stroke benefited most, experiencing an almost twofold increase in success of on-roadside evaluation driving (52.4% versus 28.6%). There were, however, no other significant differences between the groups on tests of attention or driving performance. The specific effect for right brain stroke survivors, however, suggests a more targeted approach with specific deficits might be more beneficial.

Compensatory Strategies for Non-Spatial Attention Deficits

Sohlberg and Mateer (2001b) note that compensatory strategies can include environmental modifications (e.g., to reduce distraction), external aids (e.g., use of organizers), or self-regulatory strategies (e.g., orienting, pacing, key ideas log). Unfortunately, no studies directly examine the use of compensatory strategies in subjects after stroke, although a number of studies included strategy training with direct-attention remediation and reported positive results (Boman, Lindstedt, Hemmingsson, & Bartfai 2004; Cicerone 2002; Niemann Ruff, & Baser, 1990; Park, Proulx et al., 1999; Sohlberg & Mateer 1987). Fasotti et al. examined the effects of teaching specific time-pressure management (TPM) strategies versus concentration training in a group of subjects in chronic recovery stages of severe brain injury (Fasotti, Kovacs, Eling, & Brouwer, 2000). Both groups improved on tasks of speeded information processing, although the TPM group improved more and also showed more generalization in benefit to psychometric tests of attention and memory. Since a non-intervention group was not included in this study, however, the benefits of strategy training, per se, cannot be evaluated, and specific effects of compensatory attentional strategy treating warrant further study.

Clinical Applications and Future Directions

As discussed above, consistent with recommendations of previous cognitive rehabilitation reviews for treatment of stroke and acquired brain injury (Cappa et al., 2003, 2005; Cicerone et al., 2000, 2005; Lincoln et al., 2000; Teasell et al., 2006) remediation of attention deficits may be efficacious. Computer-assisted treatment or Attention Process Training (APT) of domain-specific attention may particularly benefit specific attention functions, although generalization to everyday functioning needs further investigation.   Effective training includes a theory-based approach, with gradually increasing levels of difficulty and complexity, and feedback and reinforcement. Attentional strategy training also appears to be helpful and should be included.

Spatial Neglect

Pathophysiology and Mechanisms

Spatial neglect, a failure to report, respond, or orient to stimuli in contralesional space after brain injury (Heilman, 1979) associated with functional disability (Barrett and Burkholder, 2006) is a "class common" disorder demonstrated in mammals from rats to primates (see Payne and Rushmore, 2004 for a review). Neglect symptoms are present in up to 82% of patients in the acute phase and 48% in the early rehabilitation phase (Bowen et al., 1999; Buxbaum et al., 2004; Stone et al., 1998). The presence of spatial neglect is clinically important because in acute and chronic stages it is

associated with poorer rehabilitation outcomes and worse independence in everyday life tasks such as dressing, bathing, eating and mobility (Appelros et al., 2003; Cherney et al., 2001; Fullerton et al., 1988; Gillen et al., 2005; Henley et al., 1985; Katz et al., 1999; Paolucci et al., 2001). Although there are several theories on the mechanisms of the spatial cognitive deficit in this syndrome, two distinct behavioral-physiologic processes may contribute to recovery of post-stroke spatial neglect. The key components may be described as (1) a "where" capacity to respond to environmental information during spatial training, and (2) a motor-intentional "aiming" capacity that enables appropriate initiation and direction of movement in training.

Evidence for separating "where" (also termed "sensory perceptual" or "perceptual attentional") and "aiming" (also termed "motor intentional" or "premotor") recovery components comes from substantial cognitive neuroscience literature comprising both human and animal studies. In our previous work (Barrett et al., 2001; Barrett & Burkholder, 2006) and that of others (Schwartz et al., 1999; Na et al., 1999; Na et al., 1998; Nico, 1996; Làdavas, 1994; Bisiach et al., 1990; Tegner & Levander, 1991; Coslett et al., 1990), stroke survivors with spatial neglect demonstrated perceptual-attentional or representational right-brain "where" dysfunction, hypothesized to be highly feedback-dependent. These behaviors include detection errors such as extinction of left-sided sensory stimuli in the presence of a matched right-sided stimulus; in other words, unawareness of left-sided events.

A separable motor-intentional "aiming" component of spatial neglect recovery was demonstrated in animal studies supporting a critical contribution of subcortical dopaminergic activation to spatial orienting (Ungerstedt, 1976; Marshall et al., 1979; Schneider et al., 1984; see review in Schwarting & Huston, 1996; Schneider et al., 1992; Eslamboli et al., 2003; Milton et al., 2004). In these studies, unilaterally depleting dopaminergic activity— e.g., via unilateral lesions of ascending dopaminergic pathways, even in animals without cortical lesions—induced symptoms characteristic of the spatial-neglect syndrome in humans. Animals demonstrated profound ipsilesional movement and orienting bias in the presence of sensory stimulation. In these animals, contralesional spatial attention and orienting could be pharmacologically manipulated (see Schwarting & Huston, 1996, for a review). Human "aiming" spatial deficit, or motor neglect, could include (1) failure to move the left side of the body spontaneously, despite intact ability to move the limb to confrontation, or (2) failure to move an unaffected limb effectively leftward, although the arm moves well in a rightward direction. Other types of motor-intentional "aiming" deficit have also been reported (Heilman, 2004).

Other components or "subtypes" of neglect that may affect recovery and response to rehabilitation have also been reported. Neglect severity can vary depending upon the reference space where it is tested (e.g. personal versus near peripersonal versus far extrapersonal; Berti & Frassinetti 2000; Barrett et al., 2000; Butler et al., 2004; Cowey et al., 1999; Halligan & Marshall 1991; Vuilleumier et al., 1998), or for object- versus body- or environment-centered frames (Bisiach, 1993; Coslett, 1997). The reliability and validity of these subtypes and standard measurement tools have not yet been identified. Unfortunately, it is not yet known if "where" and "aiming" deficits measurable in individual patients or groups of patients correlate with overall severity of functional deficit or recovery profile. Specific research is needed to investigate whether "where" and "aiming" performance measures may be used to stratify stroke survivors to predict neglect recovery or assign best treatments.

Current Research

Direct Remediation of Spatial Neglect

Pharmacological treatment of the spatial neglect syndrome has been attempted via dopamine-agonist treatment and reported to improve symptoms (Fleet et al., 1987; Mukand et al., 2001). However, its influence may be selective to certain symptoms (Barrett et al., 1999; Geminiani et al., 1998). Paradoxical worsening of spatial bias may also occur with dopamine-agonist therapy (Barrett et al., 1999; Grujic et al., 1998). Barrett et al. (1999) proposed that this may occur when the only receptors available to respond to medication treatment are those dopamine receptors in the intact (left) hemisphere.

Remediative behavioral treatment of spatial neglect might be more effective if clinicians could selectively target dysfunctional "where" and "aiming" recovery processes. Current literature, however, does not reflect direct attempts to examine this aim. Single-subject and group studies, case series, and expert-opinion review articles/chapters are available describing current spatial-neglect treatments, but very few discuss how patient characteristics of any kind influence treatment candidacy.

Nine recent "evidence-based" reviews summarize the relevant literature on behavioral treatment of spatial neglect: Bowen and Lincoln (2007) (twelve studies reviewed); the Evidence-Based Review of Stroke Rehabilitation, eighth edition, Module 13, Teasell et al. (2007a) (73 studies reviewed); StrokEngine: Systematic stroke rehabilitation and intervention reviews (Teasell et al., 2007b) (63 studies reviewed); Luauté et al. (2006) (54 studies reviewed); Lincoln and Bowen, (2006) (twenty-five studies reviewed); Cappa et al., (2005) (35 studies reviewed); Cicerone et al. (2005) (11 studies reviewed); Jutai et al. (2003) (61 studies reviewed); Bowen et al. (2002) (15 studies reviewed).

Bowen et al. (2002), Lincoln & Bowen (2006), and Bowen and Lincoln (2007) noted the paucity of studies employing functional-based outcomes, concluding that there is insufficient evidence to confirm or exclude an effect of rehabilitation on actual daily activities. Intensive visual-scanning training was the remediative treatment which came closest to receiving general endorsement (Weinberg et al., 1977; Weinberg et al., 1979; daily 1-h sessions for 4 weeks). This method was classified as having "strong or moderate evidence of effectiveness" in Teasell et al., 2007a; Lincoln and Bowen, 2006; Cappa et al., 2005; and Cicerone et al., 2005); it was not unanimously supported.

There are a number of factors that make it difficult to evaluate existing spatial neglect treatment studies and "evidence-based" reviews. Except for the work of Cicerone et al. (2000) and (2005), which suggested scanning training is highly useful in patients with severe symptoms, the "evidence-based" review articles did not consider subject heterogeneity. Only some of the above papers acknowledged that efficacy might differ by intervention or considered efficacy of different types of treatment separately (Jutai et al., 2003; Teasell et al., 2007a, 2007b; Cappa et al., 2005).

Approaches that do not consider targeted treatment leave open the question that if a treatment did not reach criteria for efficacy, it may have been potentially effective but targeted inappropriately, to patients whose symptoms may not have been likely to benefit. For example, a treatment specifically targeting "where," perceptual-attention abilities, may lack effect if most subjects recruited to receive treatment demonstrate primarily "aiming," motor-intentional pathology.

The evidence-based reviews above yield three limited conclusions. First, there is consensus that treatment (of many types) may improve spatial-neglect symptoms but may not improve daily function. The range of potential treatments that have been investigated are listed in Table 4 and have included methods to increase phasic arousal (e.g. Robertson et al., 1998), visual scanning training (e.g. Webster et al., 1984; Webster et al., 2001), adaptation to rightward-deviating prisms (prism adaptation; e.g. Berberovic & Mattingly, 2003; Berberovic et al., 2004; Rossetti et al., 1998), passive and active left limb movements (limb activation; e.g. Eskes & Butler, 2006; Kalra, 1994; Làdavas et al., 1997; Robertson & North, 1993; Robertson

& North, 1992; Robertson et al., 1992), and monocular patching (e.g. Barrett & Burkholder, 2006; Walker et al., 1996). Second, visual-scanning training is judged by several reviews to be supported as a treatment to improve symptoms and function, even severe spatial neglect, although there is also contradictory evidence (Gordon et al., 1985; Gouvier et al., 1987; Robertson et al., 1993; Wagenaar et al., 1992). Third, while the existence of separable components in spatial neglect has been widely acknowledged, few clinical studies take individual symptom patterns into account, and most fail to consider how treatment matching to subject characteristics or deficits might change treatment response. A translational approach in which known neural components of a recovery process are identified and addressed with treatments of known neural action, is needed.

Compensatory Strategies for Spatial Neglect

Unfortunately, management and compensation for spatial neglect is still not supported by specific prospective studies. Consensus documents published through professional organizations that summarize expert recommendations for management and compensation, or comprehensive needs assessments based on family and caregiver research are greatly needed.

Family counseling is standard and may be helpful to reduce caregiver stress and burden. The stroke survivor's abnormal spatial behaviors, and associated anosognosia or anosodiaphoria (lack of awareness or lack of concern about spatial errors or motoric or other deficits) may alarm and frustrate the survivor's caregivers and family. Not having concepts for the specific functions of the damaged right cerebral hemisphere, family members may attribute problems to psychological or personality factors—concluding that the person is "lazy," "in denial," or "hallucinating."

Environmental manipulations, such as placing the stroke survivor's bed on the good side of the room so that she or he will "need to look" to the neglected side, or standing on the stroke survivor's bad side so as to "draw attention" to that direction, have been examined only in an inpatient study of bed placement and found no beneficial effect (Kelly & Ostreicher, 1985). This supports the possibility that environmental manipulation either exerts only a small effect or that subgroups of patients with spatial neglect may respond differently to the same environmental change. For example, although a patient with primary motor-intentional "aiming" deficit may perform better with the room on the neglected side, a patient with a primary perceptual "where" deficit may become disoriented in that situation due to sensory deprivation.

Clinical Applications and Future Directions

Scientific translational treatment of spatial neglect may ideally be composed of three steps: First, the clinician hypothetically categorizes observed spatial neglect behaviors, noting whether the behavior is likely to be the result of specific components underlying neglect symptoms, e.g. primary "where" perceptual-attentional, or "aiming" motor-intentional failure. Symptoms for treatment are then ranked in priority based upon their potential interference with short-term and long-term goals set by the client-therapy team.

Lastly, a stepwise, rational approach to rehabilitation of spatial neglect tailors a treatment for a specific impaired behavior to that deficit. Thus, a treatment primarily acting in increasing stimulus detection might improve a primary "where" deficit (e.g., eye patching might improve extinction), while a motor treatment (dopaminergic medication) might improve a primary "aiming" deficit. The translational stepwise approach needs to be systematically evaluated to determine whether evidence of its effectiveness can be obtained. It should also be noted that the approach must be applied as objectively as possible in every patient in order to yield information of clinical value. One possible method of classification of available spatial neglect treatments is summarized in Table 4, to stimulate further discussion and research.

Some practitioners object to using the above approach, since in some cases it may lead to choosing relatively under-investigated treatments over treatments subjected to randomized controlled trials. However, previous RCTs did not stratify patients by potentially affected brain-behavior networks. The clinical rehabilitation standard is individualized therapy, and single subject investigations with high internal validity indicate that dissociated effects of specific treatments occur (e.g., Schwartz et al., 1999). It is true, however, that in some settings

Table 4 Potential treatments for spatial neglect

Treatment possibly affecting perceptual "where" system function	Treatment possibly affecting representational/imagery "where" systems
Devices, medications increasing arousal – "Phasic alerting" self-cuing – Transdermal Electrical Nerve Stimulation (TENS)	Exposure or adaptation with right-shifting prisms (may enhance rightward processing) Caloric stimulation Galvanic stimulation/Neck vibration Optikinetic stimulation
Induced asymmetry/selective sensory deprivation – Scanning training – Environmental manipulation – Monocular patching/right visual field occlusion – Constraint-Induced Movement Therapy	Mirror therapy (Virtual reality?) **Treatment possibly affecting motor-intentional action planning "aiming" systems:**
Medications increasing signal/noise ratio?	Adaptation to right-shifting prisms (may increase bias leftward) Dopaminergic medications Limb activation therapy Constraint-Induced Movement Therapy Tool-use movement therapy (Scanning training?)

patients cannot be reliably examined by skilled practitioners trained to analyze symptoms of spatial neglect. In these situations, broad use of a single treatment of proven benefit is unlikely to cause worsening (e.g., intensive visual scanning training or limb activation therapy) and may be appropriate.

Memory

Pathophysiology and Mechanisms

Memory (the ability to process, store, and retrieve experiences) is not a unitary function, but consists of various interacting components and underlying neuro-cognitive mechanisms. Studies of normal subjects and individuals after brain damage suggest a distinction between explicit or declarative memory (memory that is accessed consciously and deliberately retrieved; tested by direct methods such as recognition and free recall paradigms) and implicit or non-declarative memory (memory that results in behavioral or performance changes without awareness, tested by indirect methods such as priming or procedural learning paradigms) (Gabrieli 1998; Squire 1986; Tulving & Schacter, 1990). Stroke and/or brain injury frequently results in memory disturbance, with the most obvious deficits and complaints related to difficulties with deliberate information retrieval, i.e., explicit memory. The degree and type of impairment depends upon the location and extent of stroke (Gillespie et al., 2006; Ott & Saver 1993; Stewart et al., 1996). Since known memory processes may consist of encoding (acquisition), storage (consolidation), and retrieval (recall or recognition), memory rehabilitation techniques frequently focus on optimizing and compensatory strategies to improve encoding or retrieval steps. These strategies include teaching mechanisms to optimize remaining memory abilities such as teaching effective encoding and rehearsal strategies, or mnemonics (e.g., imagery), semantic processing,

massed practice, and spaced retrieval. External aids and environmental supports, such as alarm watches, memory notebooks, and pagers, have also been used with benefit in individuals with a broad range of memory deficit severity. In cases of severe amnesia, efforts have been focused on teaching direct, functional skills through the use of the normally preserved procedural implicit system. Reviews of the efficacy of rehabilitation for memory deficits after stroke are available (Majid, Lincoln, & Weyman, 2000; Teasell et al., 2006).

Current Research

Direct Remediation of Memory Function

Most current evidence suggests that repetitive exercises and practice drills to restore lost information in memory are unlikely to be successful. This approach usually involves intensive, repetitive practice with learning digits, words, locations, etc., in the hopes that these exercises will (1) reinforce representations of the trained information and (2) generalize to everyday memory function. These studies indicated that, while individual subjects improve on test performance with the practiced material (albeit sometimes only with extensive practice), improvements rarely generalize to new material or to other contexts (Berg et al., 1991; Doornhein & De Haan 1998; Glisky et al., 1986; Godfrey & Knight 1985; Towle et al., 1988; Wilson 1997). The lack of a theoretical model and limited understanding of the underlying mechanisms for neural plasticity related to these exercises also limits this approach (Wilson 1997).

Compensatory Strategies for Improving Memory Function

There are limited number of studies examining compensatory strategies used to optimize residual memory function in stroke survivors. These techniques can include semantic processing (e.g., relating material to information already known), imagery (forming unique visual images to link information), distributed practice (using several short periods over time for practice), and spaced retrieval (retrieving and rehearsing material over gradually increasing time intervals). These studies have, in general, indicated that teaching of internal strategies can improve performance on objective memory tests relative to control procedures in individuals with mild to moderate memory deficits due to stroke (Gasparrini & Satz 1979; Gianutsos & Gianutsos 1979). It should be noted, however, that even some control procedures (e.g., psychoeducation about memory strategies, memory drills, and practice) can lead to benefits on both objective and subjective measures (Doornhein & De Haan 1998; Hildebrandt et al., 2006) and the critical aspects of the strategy training have yet to be identified. Intensity of training and practice may be one relevant variable: Hildebrandt et al. (2006) found that 20 h of practice and teaching of strategies (including massed practice, semantic processing, spaced retrieval learning, and coping with interference) produced more benefits for a group of individuals with mild-moderate learning difficulties (mostly due to stroke), on objective memory testing than a psychoeducational approach or only 7 h of training in total. Generalization to untrained materials and/or everyday functioning has also been found in some studies (Hildebrandt et al., 2006; Kaschel et al., 2000), but not all (Doornhein & De Haan 1998; Gasparrini & Satz 1979; Gianutsos & Gianutsos 1979). Strategy use may be more successful when directed at specific problems in everyday functioning as identified by the individual. Identifying an appropriate strategy also depends upon careful assessment of cognitive deficits and remaining strengths (e.g., verbal versus visual strategies). Since a strategy approach assumes some residual function, individuals with mild to moderate memory deficits will most likely benefit from this training, particularly if focused on specific, everyday needs.

Use of external devices to compensate for memory deficits, such as memory notebooks, and electronic reminders has been investigated mostly in individuals with acquired head injury (Cicerone et al., 2000, 2005). Findings suggest these devices may be applicable to individuals with a wide range of memory deficit. The choice of a device will depend upon matching the required level of involvement with the device to the cognitive abilities of the individual. Some devices require minimal training (e.g., electronic pagers), while others require considerable client involvement (e.g., memory notebooks, palmheld calendars/alarms). Wilson, Emslie, Quirk, & Evans (2001) reported on the use of a portable paging system (NeuroPage) in a group of 143 individuals with acquired brain injury (~25% due to stroke) who were randomized to a controlled, crossover design with pager and wait-list conditions. Individual outcomes were developed for relevant tasks that needed reminders (e.g., remembering to take medications). The number of memory successes was significantly increased for the pager conditions compared to baseline and in total 85% of participants were more successful with the pager compared to the baseline condition. Those noted most likely to benefit included individuals with some insight into memory difficulties, sufficient vision to read the screen, and a lifestyle that needed independence in tasks (Wilson et al., 2001). Of relevance to the current review, no difference was noted due to etiology of memory deficit. The advantage of this type of device is that it requires less training as long as someone is available to enter the necessary information, and thus it is applicable to a wider population.

Memory notebook training has been studied in individuals with mild memory deficits (Schmitter-Edgecombe, Fahy, Whelan, and Long, 1995). Participants ($n = 8$) were randomly assigned to notebook training or supportive therapy and received 16 h of treatment over 8 weeks. Group notebook training resulted in significantly fewer reports of everyday memory failures at post treatment, although the group difference was not significant at 6 months follow-up. Effective use of a memory notebook may require extensive training and role playing in a variety of situations, depending upon the individual's cognitive profile (Sohlberg & Mateer 2001a). Several case studies also indicated that memory notebooks can be effective with extensive training in individuals with severe memory impairment due to TBI (Burke et al., 1994; Sohlberg, M. & Mateer, C. 1989a) or stroke (Squires et al., 1996).

Errorless learning and vanishing cue techniques may be central to training specific tasks such as a memory notebook, or teaching domain-specific information (e.g., caregiver names, computer operations) in individuals with severe amnesia. This approach presumably draws upon a preserved implicit-memory system (Baddeley & Wilson 1994; Glisky et al., 1985). The errorless learning method was used successfully to teach a memory-notebook strategy to an individual at 8 months post-stroke (Squires et al., 1996). Since there is no transfer to other untrained tasks, use of these techniques requires considerable time investment and the identification of specific functional goals.

Clinical Application and Future Research

Specific drills and practice to restore memory function have not yet shown clinical benefit. For individuals with mild to moderate memory deficit, restitutive or compensatory strategies including mnemonics (e.g., semantic elaboration, imagery, spaced retrieval) or external devices (e.g., diaries, electronic pagers, hand-held calendars/alarms) can be of value. In their updated review, Cicerone et al. (2005) judged the evidence extensive enough to rate the use of both the memory strategy training and external devices as a practice standard for those with mild memory impairment. In addition, those devices requiring less extensive training can be applied to functional goals with

individuals with moderate to severe memory deficits as well, using specialized training techniques to bypass the damaged explicit memory system (recommended as a practice guideline; Cicerone et al., 2005). Specific evidence for individuals post-stroke is very limited, however, and more research is required to understand the impact of interventions in this group, as well as relevant factors for stratification for treatment selection (Cappa et al., 2005).

Executive Function

Pathophysiology and Mechanisms

Executive function is not a unitary concept, but encompasses a range of processes that are needed to integrate information from sensory and memory systems, and organize goal-directed response behaviors. The range of executive functions has been hard to define, and a variety of models of executive function have been proposed. One model suggests four functional categories that follow anatomical and evolutionary development: (1) executive cognitive functions; (2) behavioral self-regulation; (3) activation regulation; and (4) metacognitive process (Stuss, 2007). These domains relate to different anatomical regions and systems in the frontal lobe that can be differentially affected by brain injury, although more than one domain is often involved. An understanding of these different functions is thus relevant to the development of theory-driven rehabilitation programs.

Executive cognitive functions include the control and orchestration of basic cognitive functions, such as memory, that involve such processes as planning, sequencing, monitoring, switching, and inhibiting. The dorsolateral prefrontal cortex is primarily responsible for executive control; damage to this system can lead to difficulties with control of many cognitive operations, despite intact basic skills, and issues with problem-solving, decision-making, and distractibility can arise. Behavioral self-regulatory functions include those processes involved in emotional processing, reward, and adaptive responding. The ventral medial frontal regions support this function; damage to these regions can result in difficulties with inappropriate emotional responding and regulation. Activation regulation involves appropriate initiative and energizing behaviors to apply to goals. Pathology of the medial frontal areas can lead to apathy or abulia. Finally, the frontal poles may criticaly integrate metacognitve processes, such as self-awareness, insight, and social cognition. Damage to this domain can lead to lack of insight into deficits and loss of awareness of social contexts.

The complexity and interaction among these domains are difficult to assess and objectively characterize, and neuropsychological assessment is critical to identify both affected and preserved domains in order to plan and direct treatment. The very nature of executive function impairments may make it difficult for a stroke survivor to learn and assume responsibility for using a compensatory strategy in learned or novel situations. Impaired insight can also be a mediating issue (Cicerone, Levin, Malec, Stuss, & Whyte 2006). The complexity of these issues and potentially affected domains has led to a wide range of proposed interventions, including specific skill training with behavioral methods in a functional context, methods to teach internal compensatory strategies for initiation and self-monitoring, and the use of external devices to cue and support learned strategies. Research on most interventions target more than one domain, and thus make it difficult to identify the specific, effective processes that lead to any treatment effect. The majority of the evidence to date is also derived from studies of individuals with traumatic brain injury rather than stroke. We emphasize here the few studies including stroke survivors, the majority of whom had anterior communication artery (ACoA) aneurysm rupture/surgical repair.

Current Research

Direct Skill Training

Stablum et al. (2000) used a dual-task paradigm to provide training in the ability to coordinate two actions to a group with closed head injury as well as a group with ACoA surgery, and matched controls. Stroke survivors were 2–7 months post injury and had a number of executive function deficits. Training consisted of extensive practice (1,080 trials) with a dual task in 5 weekly sessions. Before training, the ACoA group had significantly more dual-task reaction-time cost than the matched controls. Both brain-injured groups improved over training sessions, and performed comparably to controls (who received no training) at 3-months follow-up testing. Some dual task cost benefit was lost at 12 months, but performance was still superior to pre-training. Improvement was also seen at 3 and 12 months on other executive-function tests (e.g., PASAT, CPT) compared to initial assessment. Given the lack of placebo/control patient groups, however, it is unclear whether any of this improvement can be attributed to training or to spontaneous recovery in the first year. Problem-solving training (PST) has also been investigated by von Cramon et al. (1991) in a mixed, acquired brain-injury group (n=37, 13 stroke survivors) with problem solving deficits at 6 months post injury. Patients were assigned to a PST training procedure, or a memory training (MT) control procedure each given for an average of 25 sessions for 6 weeks. The PST program provided individualized training with a range of everyday tasks in either group or individual sessions emphasizing five aspects of problem-solving: problem orientation, definition, generating alternatives, decision-making, and solution verification. The MT group concentrated on strategies to improve memory (e.g., visual imagery). The PST group improved on a variety of tests, including tests of conceptual reasoning and planning, while the MT group improved more on tests of learning and memory. Improvement in problem-solving in the PST group was confirmed in behavioral ratings by the clinical team, thus suggesting some generalization to every-day activities. A stepwise, structured approach to teaching self-regulation in an unstructured situation is also seen in studies of goal management training (GMT) by Levine et al. (2000), based on Duncan's suggestion that goal neglect underlies disorganized behavior seen in patients with frontal-lobe lesions (Duncan et al., 1996). Strategy training to treat problem-solving and other self-regulation deficits in acquired brain injury and/or stroke patients is also supported in case and small group studies (Cicerone & Wood 1987; Honda 1999; Ownsworth et al., 2000; Rath et al., 2003); reviewed in (Cicerone et al., 2006, 2000, 2005).

External Compensatory Strategies to Treat Executive Function Impairments

External aids or environmental support also may be useful for rehabilitation of executive problems. Evans et al. (1998) successfully used a radio paging system (Neuropage®), and a paper and pencil checklist to prompt everyday actions (e.g., taking medication, watering plants) in a case-study design with a patient after stroke related to ACoA aneurysm repair. Another study examined the effects of periodic auditory alerts to improve performance on an executive-function task that required self-monitoring, switching and maintenance of intention (Manly et al., 2002). Alerts improved the performance of a group of 10 acquired brain injury patients (including one with stroke) compared to no alerts, to a level comparable to matched controls. The authors suggested that the alerts may have refocused attention away from the task at hand and back to the overall goal, although other explanations (e.g., increased arousal or responsivity) may also have influenced treatment benefit (Manly et al., 2002).

Clinical Application and Future Research

Approaches to treat problem-solving and strategy-use deficits in individuals with executive dysfunction after stroke appear a fruitful line of research that remains to be developed. While significant benefits have been obtained with small studies and structured techniques, the effectiveness of these approaches in clinical practice remains unclear. Examination of the literature on treatment of executive deficits in other populations does suggest that training of problem-solving strategies may be a useful intervention, and future studies examining these techniques in individuals after stroke is warranted.

Language and Communication Disorders

Pathophysiology and Mechanism

Language can be broadly defined as the set of visual or spoken symbols and rules by which we think and communicate about our internal and external world. Language function is localized to the left hemisphere in most individuals, and strokes involving left-sided vascular territories have identified a number of component abilities as defined by aphasia subtypes. In terms of spoken and written communication, aphasia syndromes can be divided into two broad categories: non-fluent and fluent aphasias. Fluent speech depends upon the ability to produce the correct motor patterns in the correct order. Lesions in anterior left brain (e.g. Broca's area, Brodmann area 44, 45) may produce non-fluent aphasia, characterized by some or all of the following symptoms: anomia, reduced phrase length, disrupted articulation or programming of motor speech, impaired rhythm and/or agrammatic sentence production. Single word comprehension and understanding of simple phrases in natural conversation may be relatively preserved. In contrast, damage to more posterior areas, e.g., Wernicke's area (Brodmann area 22) produces a fluent aphasia, characterized by relatively preserved and melodic spontaneous speech, but with neologisms (jargon) and reduced content, associated with poor comprehension of written and spoken language, including reduced awareness of one's own errors (anosognosia). There are eight classical perisylvian and extrasylvian aphasia syndromes, and other aphasia subtypes are also proposed as variants of these patterns (Bookheimer, 2007; Hillis 2007). In normal practice, classic subtypes are rare, and the impaired and preserved functions usually contain a mixture of fluent and nonfluent characteristics.

A variety of aphasia treatment approaches have been used over the last 130 years, ranging from generic mental stimulation, to theoretically-driven treatment of specific cognitive-linguistic deficits in a case-study approach (e.g., letter-by-letter alexia). Evidence-based reviews (Bhogal, Teasell, Foley et al., 2003, Cicerone et al., 2005; Greener et al., 1999; Robey 1998), mainly conclude that treatment is effective, although well-controlled group studies are limited in number, and further studies are recommended, including controls for spontaneous recovery, random assignment and blinded outcome measurement. In addition, many group studies report an individualized approach to therapy, but have limited description of the actual therapy conducted; it is thus hard to evaluate specific components that may be critical to overall efficacy.

Current Research

According to Cicerone et al. (2000) and (2005), several early Class I studies support the cognitive linguistic therapies as a practice standard during acute and postacute rehabilitation for left hemisphere stroke survivors with aphasia. Conflicting opinions exist, however, regarding this practice standard. A Cochrane review of the aphasia therapy literature (Greener et al., 1999) reported that the current evidence did not provide support for the efficacy of speech therapy, citing the need for better quality studies. In contrast, a meta-analysis of clinical outcomes of the aphasia treatment literature by Robey (1998) provided effects sizes for treatment and found that treatment in the acute phase overall produced a moderate to large effect size (compared to no treatment), while treatment in the subacute or chronic phase produced a small effect size compared to no treatment. Other moderators of the effect included intensity/amount of treatment (>2 h/week was better) and severity of aphasia.

Intensity of treatment appears to be a critical variable and may explain some of the discrepancy in findings by the above reviews. Intensity was highlighted in recent reviews by Bhogal, Teasell, and Speechley (2003) and Bhogal, Teasell, Foley, et al. (2003), who reviewed the literature up to 2002 and evaluated outcomes based on intensity of therapy in ten trials of 864 individual patients. They found that the five studies demonstrating a significant effect compared to controls provided an average of 7.8 h of therapy/week for 18 weeks, versus five negative studies that only provided approximately 2.4 h per week for 22.9 weeks. Average total therapy time was also greater in the positive studies (108 h) compared to negative ones (43.6 h) (Bhogal et al., 2003). The importance of intensity was also supported in a study of the effects of aphasia therapy based on constraint-induced (CI) therapy principles for extremity movement (Pulvermuller et al., 2001). CI therapy involves the massing or concentration of practice, and constraint of undesirable behaviors or responses, and has been used successfully in the motor rehabilitation of post-stroke hemiparesis (Taub et al., 1999). These principles have recently been applied to other domains such as speech therapy (Taub et al., 2006). Stroke survivors with chronic aphasia, who had previously reached an apparent maximum in recovery of language function, received constraint-induced aphasia therapy for 3 h each weekday over 2 weeks. Significant improvement on both standardized tests and everyday communication was found in the CI group in comparison to more limited change found in control patients receiving the same number of treatment hours spread over a longer 4 week period (Pulvermuller et al. 2001). These gains were replicated in a follow-up study and appeared to remain stable for at least 6 months (Meinzer, Djundja, Barthel, Elbert, & Rockstroh, 2005). Intensity has also been reported as an important factor in several other studies of individuals with chronic stroke and/or TBI (Cicerone et al., 2005).

Group therapy or community therapy are reported to be beneficial when involving trained laypersons. In one study, group therapy was found to improve both linguistic and communication skills in individuals with chronic stroke in comparison to a deferred-treatment group and progress was maintained at 4–6 weeks follow-up (Elman & Bernstein-Ellis 1999). The advantages of group-based therapy for improving not only impairment measures but functional communication skills have been emphasized (Marshall 2005). The involvement of trained laypersons in the community has also received some support and appears to be a useful method for enhancing professional delivery of services (Teasell et al., 2006). Clients may also find lay-administered therapies appealing, as feelings of self-efficacy or empowerment may be enhanced when stroke survivors practice language skills with a lay partner perceived as a social equal.

While group studies usually lack a comprehensive description of the aphasia therapy approach with individual subjects, the effects of specific cognitive-linguistic remediation techniques for specified linguistic deficits (e.g., anomia, alexia) have been evaluated in a wide variety of studies. As reviewed by Cicerone et al. (2000) and (2005), the evidence suggests that cognitive-linguistic techniques directed at specific deficits in individuals with chronic aphasia can be beneficial, although the issues of generalization and effectiveness of such approaches clearly need more evaluation.

Evidence-based reviews traditionally do not consider results of case studies and small group studies, and often also do not include large studies using quasi-experimental method rather than placebo-controlled group assignment. This difference in criteria may account for differences in conclusions regarding aphasia therapy efficacy. We (Barrett & Rothi, 2006; Rothi & Barrett, 2006) strongly suggest that "evidence" should be defined with criteria extending beyond those employed in phase III pharmaceutical clinical trials (randomized placebo-control between-subjects studies). In earlier stages of translational science, defining treatment effect characteristics is the priority. If researchers rush to perform overvalued placebo-comparison studies, incomplete understanding of the appropriate dose, subject selection criteria, or time post-event reduces the likelihood of treatment benefit, and negative results may not reflect the real value of the treatment under consideration. Additionally, in the rehabilitation setting, ethical considerations about withholding treatment, multiple-subject strata relevant to treatment assignment, and inter-hospital differences make newer methodologies with high internal validity, such as growth curve modeling attractive (Singer & Willet 2003). These techniques have superior rigor to parametric methods when a changing baseline for group performance is expected (e.g. natural stroke recovery).

Clinical Application and Future Research

There is general agreement that, overall, aphasia therapy is efficacious for individuals after stroke (Cappa et al., 2003, 2005; Teasell et al., 2006), and it is recommended as a practice standard.

While overall language interventions appear effective, more information is needed about the specific techniques and parameters that relate to effectiveness, including specific cognitive-linguistic techniques, intensity of therapy, the role of group, and community therapy. Results of combinations of aphasia interventions, attention to functional outcomes and long-term follow-up would also be of benefit.

Conclusions

The field of rehabilitation of cognitive deficits post stroke is newly emerging, with more questions than answers for interested clinicians. Clearly it is an area of great possible benefit for individuals after stroke and one that deserves more development using well-designed, theoretically driven and eventually multi-centre approaches. The heterogeneity of behavioural, cognitive and physical symptoms after stroke presents a challenging opportunity to clinicians and researchers and requires innovative approaches that take into account individual differences due to the variety of lesion sizes and sites, complex constellations of symptoms, and environmental mileau. Use of single subject designs, innovative treatment targeted to specific, well-defined deficits, with a focus on long-term functional outcomes is needed for advances at this stage of the field in most areas of cognitive treatment. Larger controlled group studies will be most useful when the specifics of treatment efficacy at the individual level are well-defined. It is hoped that this chapter has provided useful starting points for both clinicians and researchers dealing with the complex issues related to treatment of vascular cognitive impairment.

References

Appelros, P., Karlsson, G. M., Seiger, A., & Nydevik, I. (2003) Prognosis for patients with neglect and anosognosia with special reference to cognitive impairment. *Journal of Rehabilitation Medicine 35*: 254–258

Azouvi, P., Samuel, C., Louis-Dreyfus, T., Bernati, T., Bartolomeo, P., Beis. J. M. et al. (2002) Sensitivity of clinical and behavioral tests of spatial neglect after right hemisphere stroke. *Journal of Neurology, Neurosurgery and Psychiatry 73*: 160–166

Baddeley, A., & Wilson, B. A. (1994) When implicit learning fails: Amnesia and the problem of error elimination. *Neuropsychologia 32*: 53–68

Ballard, C., Stephens, S., Kenny, R. A., Kalaria, R. N., Tovee, M., & O'Brien, J. (2003) Profile of neuropsychological deficits in older stroke survivors without dementia. *Dementia and Geriatric Cognitive Disorders 16*: 52–56

Barker-Collo, S., & Feigin, V. (2006) The impact of neuropsychological deficits on functional stroke outcomes. *Neuropsychology Review 16*: 53–64

Barrett, A. M., Crucian, G. P., Schwartz, R. L., & Heilman, K. M. (1999) Adverse effect of dopamine agonist therapy in a patient with motor-intentional neglect. *Archives of Physical Medicine and Rehabilitation 80*: 600–603

Barrett, A. M., Schwartz, R. L., Crucian, G. P., Kim, M. H., & Heilman, K. M. (2000) Attentional grasp in far extrapersonal space after thalamic infarction. *Neuropsychologia 38*(6): 778–784

Barrett, A. M., Crucian, G. P., Beversdorf, D. Q., & Heilman, K. M. (2001) Monocular patching may worsen sensory–attentional neglect: A case report. *Archives of Physical Medicine and Rehabilitation 82*: 516–518

Barrett, A. M., & Burkholder, S. (2006) Monocular patching in subjects with right-hemisphere stroke affects perceptual-attentional Bias. *Journal of Rehabilitation Research and Development 43*: 337–346

Barrett, A. M., & Rothi, L. J. G. (2006) Treatment innovation in behavioral rehabilitation of stroke: Removing limits on recovery. *Journal of Rehabilitation Research and Development 43*(3): vii–ix

Bayley, M. T., Hurdowar, A., Teasell, R., Wood-Dauphinee, S., Korner-Bitensky, N., et al. (2007) Priorities for stroke rehabilitation and research: Results of a 2003 Canadian stroke network consensus conference. *Archives of Physical Medicine and Rehabilitation 88*: 526–528

Berberovic, N., & Mattingley, J. (2003) Effects of prismatic adaptation on judgements of spatial extent in peripersonal and extrapersonal space. *Neuropsychologia 41*: 493–503

Berberovic, N., Pisella, L., Morris, A. P., & Mattingley, J. B. (2004) Prismatic adaptation reduces biased temporal order judgments in spatial neglect. *Neuroreport 15*: 1199–1204

Berg, I. J., Koning-Haanstra, M., & Deelman, B. G. (1991) Long-term effects of memory rehabilitation: a controlled study. *Neuropsychological Rehabilitation1*: 97–111

Berti, A., & Frassinetti, F. (2000) When far becomes near: Remapping of space by tool use. *Journal of Cognitive Neuroscience 12*: 415–420

Bhogal, S. K., Teasell, R., & Speechley, M. (2003) Intensity of aphasia therapy, impact on recovery. *Stroke 34*: 987–993

Bhogal, S. K., Teasell, R. W., Foley, N. C., & Speechley, M. R. (2003) Rehabilitation of aphasia: More is better. *Topics in Stroke Rehabilitation 10*: 66–76

Bisiach, E., Geminiani, G., Berti, A., & Rusconi, M. L. (1990) Perceptual and premotor factors of unilateral neglect. *Neurology 40*: 1278–1281

Bisiach, E. (1993) Mental representation in unilateral neglect and related disorders: The twentieth Bartlett memorial lecture. *The Quarterly Journal of Experimental Psychology 46*A: 435–461

Boman, I. L., Lindstedt, M., Hemmingsson, H., & Bartfai, A. (2004) Cognitive training in home environment. *Brain Injury 18*: 985–995

Bookheimer, S. (2007) Pre-surgical language mapping with functional magnetic resonance imaging. *Neuropsychology Review 17*: 145–155

Bowen, A., McKenna, K., & Tallis, R. C. (1999) Reasons for variability in the reported rate of occurrence of unilateral spatial neglect after stroke. *Stroke 30*: 1196–1202

Bowen, A., Lincoln, N. B., & Dewey, M. (2002) Cognitive rehabilitation for spatial neglect following stroke (Cochrane Review). In *The Cochrane Library, Issue 3*. Oxford: Update Software

Bowen, A., & Lincoln, N. B. (2007) Cognitive rehabilitation for spatial neglect following stroke. *Cochrane Database of Systematic Reviews* Issue 2. Art. No.: CD003586. DOI: 10.1002/14651858.CD003586.pub2

Burke, J. M., Danick, J. A., Bemis, B., & Durgin, C. J. (1994) A process approach to memory book training for neurological patients. *Brain Injury 8*: 71–81

Butler, B. C., Eskes, G. A., & Vandorpe, R. A. (2004) Gradients of detection in neglect: comparison of peripersonal and extrapersonal space. *Neuropsychologia 42*: 346–358

Buxbaum, L. J., Ferraro, M. K., Veramonti, T., Farne, A., Whyte, J., Làdavas, E., et al. (2004) Hemispatial neglect: subtypes, neuroanatomy, and disability. *Neurology 62*: 749–756

Cappa, S. F., Benke, T., Clarke, S., Rossi, B., Stemmer, B., & van Heugten, C. M. (2003) EFNS guidelines on cognitive rehabilitation: report of an EFNS task force. *European Journal of Neurology 10*: 11–23

Cappa, S. F., Benke, T., Clarke, S., Rossi, B., Stemmer, B., & van Heugten, C. M. (2005) EFNS guidelines on cognitive rehabilitation: report of an EFNS task force. *European Journal of Neurology 12*: 665–680

Cherney, L. R., Halper, A. S., Kwasnica, C. M., Harvey, R. L., & Zhang, M. (2001) Recovery of functional status after right hemisphere stroke: Relationship with unilateral neglect. *Archives of Physical Medicine and Rehabilitation 82*: 322–328

Cicerone, K., Levin, H., Malec, J., Stuss, D., & Whyte, J. 2006. Cognitive rehabilitation interventions for executive function: moving from bench to bedside in patients with traumatic brain injury. *Journal of Cognitive Neuroscience 18*: 1212–1222

Cicerone, K. D. 2002. Remediation of 'working attention' in mild traumatic brain injury. *Brain Injury 16*: 185–195

Cicerone, K. D., Dahlberg, C., Kalmar, K., Langenbahn, D. M., Malec, J. F., et al. (2000) Evidence-based cognitive rehabilitation: Recommendations for clinical practice. *Archives of Physical Medicine and Rehabilitation 81*: 1596–1615

Cicerone, K. D., Dahlberg, C., Malec, J. F., Langenbahn, D. M., Felicetti, T., Kneipp, S. et al. (2005) Evidence-based cognitive rehabilitation: Updated review of the literature from 1998 through 2002. *Archives of Physical Medicine and Rehabilitation 86*: 1681–1692

Cicerone, K. D., & Wood, J. C. (1987) Planning disorder after closed head injury: A case study. *Archives of Physical Medicine and Rehabilitation 68*: 111–115

Cirstea, C. M., Ptito, A., & Levin, M. F. (2006) Feedback and cognition in arm motor skill reacquisition after stroke. *Stroke 37*: 1237–1242

Claesson, L., Linden, T., Skoog, I, & Blomstrand, C. (2005) Cognitive impairment after stroke – Impact on activities of daily living and costs of care for elderly people. *Cerebrovascular Diseases 19*: 102–109

Coslett, H. B., Bowers, D., Fitzpatrick, E., Haws, B., & Heilman, K. M. (1990) Directional hypokinesia and hemispatial inattention in neglect. *Brain 113*: 475–486

Coslett, H. B. (1997) Neglect in vision and visual imagery: A double dissociation. *Brain 120*: 1163–1171

Cowey, A., Small, M., & Ellis, S. (1999) No abrupt change in visual hemineglect from near to far space. *Neuropsychologia 17*: 1–6

Crosson, B., Fabrizio, K. S., Singletary, F., Cato, M. A., Wierenga, C. E., Parkinson, R. B., et al. (2007) Treatment of naming in nonfluent aphasia through manipulation of intention and attention: a phase 1 comparison of two novel treatments. *J Int Neuropsychol Soc. 13*(4): 582–594

Desmond, D. W., Moroney, J. T., Sano, M., & Stern, Y. (1996) Recovery of cognitive function after stroke. *Stroke 27*: 1798–1803

Doornhein, K., & De Haan, E. H. F. (1998) Cognitive training for memory deficits in stroke patients. *Neuropsychological Rehabilitation 8*: 393–400

Duncan, J., Emslie, H., Williams, P., Johnson, R., & Freer, C. (1996) Intelligence and the frontal lobe: The organization of goal-directed behavior. *Cognitive Psychology 30*: 257–303

Elman, R. J., & Bernstein-Ellis, E. 1999. The efficacy of group communication treatment in adults with chronic aphasia. *Journal of Speech, Language and Hearing Research 42*: 411–419

Eskes, G. A., & Butler, B. (2006) Using limb movements to improve neglect: The role of functional electrical stimulation. *Restorative Neurology and Neuroscience 24*: 385–398

Eslamboli, A., Baker, H. F., Ridley, R. M., & Annett, L. E. (2003) Sensorimotor deficits in a unilateral intrastriatal 6-OHDA partial lesion model of Parkinson's disease in marmoset monkeys. *Experimental Neurology 183*: 418–419

Evans, J. J., Emslie, H., & Wilson, B. A. (1998) External cueing systems in the rehabilitation of executive impairments of action. *Journal of the International Neuropsychological Society 4*: 399–408

Fasotti, L., Kovacs, F., Eling, P. A. T. M., & Brouwer, W. H. (2000) Time pressure management as a compensatory strategy training after closed head injury. *Neuropsychological Rehabilitation 10*: 47–65

Fernandez-Duque, D., & Posner, M. (2001) Brain imaging of attentional networks in normal and pathological states. *Journal of Clinical and Experimental Neuropsychology 23*: 74–93

Ferro, J. M., & Crespo, M. D. (1988) Young adult stroke: Neuropsychological dysfunction and recovery. *Stroke 19*: 982–986

Fleet, W. S., Valenstein, E., Watson, R. T., & Heilman, K. M. (1987) Dopamine agonist therapy for neglect in humans. *Neurology 37*: 1765–1770

Fullerton, K. J., Mackenzie, G., & Stout, R. W. (1988) Prognostic indices in stroke. *Quarterly Journal of Medicine 66*: 147–162

Gabrieli, J. D. E. (1998) Cognitive neuroscience of human memory. *Annual Review of Psychology 49*: 87–115

Gasparrini, B., & Satz, P. (1979) A treatment for memory problems in left hemisphere CVA patients. *Journal of Clinical Neuropsychology 1*: 137–150

Geminiani, G., Bottini, G., & Sterzi, R. (1998) Dopaminergic stimulation in unilateral neglect. *Journal of Neurology, Neurosurgery, and Psychiatry 65*: 344–347

Gianutsos, R., & Gianutsos, J. (1979) Rehabilitating the verbal recall of brain-injured patients by mnemonic training: An experimental demonstration using single-case methodology. *Journal of Clinical Neuropsychology 1*: 117–135

Gillen, R., Tennen, H., & McKee, T. (2005) Unilateral spatial neglect: Relation to rehabilitation outcomes in patients with right hemisphere stroke. *Archives of Physical Medicine and Rehabilitation 86*: 763–767

Gillespie, D. C., Bowen, A., & Foster, J. K. (2006) Memory impairment following right hemisphere stroke: A comparative meta-analytic and narrative review. *The Clinical Neuropsychologist 20*: 59–75

Glisky, E. L., Schacter, D. L., & Tulving, E. (1985) Computer learning by memory impaired patients: Aquistion and retention of complex knowledge. *Neuropsychologia 24*: 313–328

Glisky, E. L., Schacter, D. L., & Tulving, E. (1986) Learning and retention of computer-related vocabulary in memory-impaired patients: Method of vanishing cues. *Journal of Clinical and Experimental Neuropsychology 8*: 292–312

Godfrey, H. P. D., & Knight, R. G. (1985) Cognitive rehabilitation of memory functioning in amnesiac alcoholics. *Journal of Consulting and Clinical Psychology 53*: 555–557

Gordon, W. A., Hibbard, M. R., Egelko, S., Diller, L., Shaver, M. S., et al. (1985) Perceptual remediation in patients with right brain damage: A comprehensive program. *Archives of Physical Medicine and Rehabilitation 66*: 353–359

Gouvier, W. D., Bua, B. G., Blanton, P. D., & Urey, J. R. (1987). Behavioral changes following visual scanning training: Observations of five cases. *The International Journal of Clinical Neuropsychology 9*: 74–80.

Greener, J., Enderby, P., & Whurr, R. (1999) Speech and language therapy for aphasia following stroke. *The Cochrane Database of Systematic Reviews* Issue 4: Art. No.: CD000425. DOI: 10.1002/14651858. CD000425

Grujic, Z., Mapstone, M., Gitelma, D. R., Johnson, N., Weintraub, S., et al. (1998) Dopamine agonists reorient visual exploration away from the neglected hemispace. *Neurology 51*(5): 1395–1398

Halligan, P. W., & Marshall, J. C. (1991) Left neglect for near but not far space in man. *Nature 350*: 498–500

Heilman, K. M. (1979) Neglect and related disorders. In: *Clinical neuropsychology*, (K. M. Heilman and E. Valenstein, eds.1st ed.) NY: Oxford, 268–307

Heilman, K. M. (2004) Intentional neglect. *Frontiers in Bioscience: a Journal and Virtual Library 9*: 694–705

Henley, S., Pettit, S., Todd-Pokropek, A., & Tupper, A. (1985) Who goes home? Predictive factors in stroke recovery. *Journal of Neurology, Neurosurgery, and Psychiatry 48*: 1–6

Hildebrandt, H., Bussmann-Mork, B., & Schwendemann, G. (2006) Group therapy for memory impaired patients: A partial remediation is possible. *Journal of Neurology 253*: 512–529

Hillis, A. E. (2007) Aphasia. Progress in the last quarter of a century. *Neurology 69*: 200–213

Hochstenbach, J., Mulder, T., van Limbeek, J., Donders, R., & Schoonwaldt, H. (1998) Cognitive decline following stroke: A comprehensive study of cognitive decline following stroke. *Journal of Clinical and Experimental Neuropsychology 20*: 503–517

Hochstenbach, J., Prigatano, G., & Mulder, T. (2005) Patients' and relatives' reports of disturbances 9 months after stroke: subjective changes in physical functioning, cognition, emotion, and behavior. *Archives of Physical Medicine and Rehabilitation 86*: 1587–1593

Hochstenbach, J. B., den Otter, R., & Mulder, T. W. (2003) Cognitive recovery after stroke: A 2-year follow-up. *Archives of Physical Medicine and Rehabilitation 84*: 1499–1504

Hoffmann, M. (2001) Higher cortical function deficits after stroke: An analysis of 1,000 patients from a dedicated cognitive stroke registry. *Neurorehabilitation and Neural Repair 15*: 113–127

Honda, T. (1999) Rehabilitation of executive function impairments after stroke. *Topics in Stroke Rehabilitation 6*: 15–22

Hyndman, D, & Ashburn, A. (2003) People with stroke living in the community: Attention deficits, balance, ADL ability and falls. *Disability and Rehabilitation 25*: 817–822

Jutai, J. W., Bhogal, S. K., Foley, N. C., Bayley, M., Teasell, R. W., et al. (2003) Treatment of visual perceptual disorders post stroke. *Topics in Stroke Rehabilitation 10*: 77–106

Kalra, L. (1994) The influence of stroke unit rehabilitation on functional recovery from stroke. *Stroke 25*: 821–825

Kaschel, R., Della Sala, S., Cantagallo, A., Fahlboeck, A., Laaksonen, R., & Kazen, M. (2000) Imagery mnemonics for the rehabilitation of memory: A randomised group controlled trial. *Neuropsychological Rehabilitation 12:* 127–53

Katz, N., Hartman-Maeir, A., Ring, H., & Soroker, N. (1999) Functional disability and rehabilitation outcome in right hemisphere damaged patients with and without unilateral spatial neglect. *Archives of Physical Medicine and Rehabilitation 80*: 379–384

Kelly, M., & Ostreicher, H. (1985) Environmental factors and outcomes in hemineglect syndromes. *Rehabilitation Psychology, 30*, 35–37

Làdavas, E. (1994) The role of visual attention in neglect: a dissociation between perceptual and directional motor neglect. *Neuropsychological Rehabilitation 4*(2): 155–159

Làdavas, E., Berti, A., Ruozzi, E., & Barboni, F. (1997) Neglect as a deficit determined by an imbalance between multiple spatial representations. *Experimental Brain Research 116*: 493–500.

Levine, B., Robertson, I. H., Clare, L., Carter, G., Hong, J., et al. (2000) Rehabilitation of executive functioning: an experimental-clinical validation of goal management training. *Journal of the International Neuropsychological Society 6*: 299–312

Lillie, R., & Mateer, C. A. (2006) Constraint-based therapies as a proposed model for cognitive rehabilitation. *Journal of Head Trauma Rehabilitation 21*: 119–130

Lincoln, N. B., Majid, M.J., & Weyman, N. 2000. Cognitive rehabilitation for attention deficits following stroke. *Cochrane Database of Systematic Reviews* Issue 4: Art. No.: CD002842. DOI: 10.1002/14651858.CD002842

Lincoln, N. B., & Bowen, A. (2006) The need for randomised treatment studies in neglect research. *Restorative Neurology & Neuroscience 24*(4–6): 401–408

Lincoln, N. B., Dent, A., Harding, J., Weyman, N., Nicholl, C., et al. (2002) Evaluation of cognitive assessment and cognitive intervention for people with multiple sclerosis. *Journal of Neurology, Neurosurgery and Psychiatry 72*: 93–98

Luauté, J., Halligan, P., Rode, G., Rossetti, Y., & Boisson, D. (2006) Visuo-spatial neglect: a systematic review of current interventions and their effectiveness. *Neuroscience and Biobehavioral Reviews 30*(7): 961–982

Madureira, S., Guerreiro, M., & Ferro, J. M. (2001) Dementia and cognitive impairment three months

after stroke. *European Journal of Neurology 8*: 621–627

Majid, M. J., Lincoln, N. B., & Weyman, N. (2000) Cognitive rehabilitation for memory deficits following stroke (Cochrane Review). *Cochrane Database of Systematic Reviews*: Art. No.: CD002293. DOI:10.1002/14651858.CD002293

Malouin, F., Belleville, S., Richards, C. L., Desrosiers, J., & Doyon, J. (2004) Working memory and mental practice outcomes after stroke. *Archives of Physical Medicine and Rehabilitation 85*: 177–183

Manly, T., Hawkins, K., Evans, J., Woldt, K., & Robertson, I. H. (2002) Rehabilitation of executive function: Facilitation of effective goal management on complex tasks using periodic auditory alerts. *Neuropsychologia 40*: 271–281

Mark, V. W. (1993) Extrapersonal neglect. *Neurology 43*: 1859–1860

Marshall, J. (2005) Can speech and language therapy with aphasic people affect activity and participation levels. In P. W. Halligan & D. T. Wade (Eds.) *Effectiveness of rehabilitation for cognitive deficits*, (pp. 195–207). Oxford: Oxford University Press

Marshall, J. F. (1979) Somatosensory inattention after dopaminedepleting intracerebral 6-OHDA injections: Spontaneous recovery and pharmacological control. *Brain Research 177*: 311–324

Mazur, B. L., Sofer, S., Korner-Bitensky, N., Gelinas, I., Hanley, J., & Wood-Dauphinee, S. (2003) Effectiveness of a visual attention retraining program on the driving performance of clients with stroke. *Archives of Physical Medicine and Rehabilitation 84*: 541–550

McDowd, J. M., Filion, D. L., Pohl, P. S., Richards, L. G., & Stiers, W. (2003) Attentional abilities and functional outcomes following stroke. *Journal of Gerontology: Psychological Sciences 58B*: 45–53

Meinzer, M., Djundja, D., Barthel, G., Elbert, T., & Rockstroh, B. (2005) Long-term stability of improved language functions in chronic aphasia after constrint-induced aphasia therapy. *Stroke 36*: 1462–1466

Michel, J. A., & Mateer, C. A. (2006) Attention rehabilitation following stroke and traumatic brain injury. *Europa Medicophysica 42*: 59–67

Milton, A. L., Marshall, J. W. B., Cummings, R. M., Baker, H. F., & Ridley, R. M. (2004) Dissociation of hemi-spatial and hemi-motor impairments in a unilateral primate model of Parkinson's disease. *Behavioural Brain Research 150*: 55–63

Mok, V. C. T., Wong, A., Lam, W. W. M., Fan, Y. H., & Tang, W. K., et al. (2004) Cognitive impairment and functional outcome after stroke associated with small vessel disease. *Journal of Neurology, Neurosurgery and Psychiatry 75*: 560–566

Na, D. L., Adair, J. C., Kang, Y., Chung, C. S., Lee, K. H., & Heilman, K. M. (1999) Motor perseverative behavior on a line cancellation task. *Neurology 52*: 1569–576.

Na, D. L., Adair, J. C., Williamson, D. J., Schwartz, R. L., Haws, B., & Heilman, K. M. (1998) Dissociation of sensory-attentional from motor-intentional neglect. *Journal of Neurology, Neurosurgery and Psychiatry 64*: 331–338.

Nico, D. (1996) Detecting directional hypokinesia: the epidiascope technique. *Neuropsychologia 34*: 471–474.

Niemann, H., Ruff, R. M., & Baser, C. A. (1990) Computer-assisted attention retraining in head-injured individuals: A controlled efficacy study of an outpatient program. *Journal of Consulting and Clinical Psychology 58*: 811–817

Nys, G. M. S., Van Zandvoort, M. J. E., De Kort, P. L. M., Jansen, B. P. W., Van Der Worp, H. B, Algra, A.,. et al. (2005a) Domain-specific cognitive recovery after first-ever stroke: A follow-up study of 111 cases. *Journal of the International Neuropsychological Society 11*: 795–806

Nys, G. M. S., Van Zandvoort, M. J. E., de Kort, P. L. M., van der Worp, H. B., Jansen, B. P. W., Algra, A., et al. (2005b) The prognostic value of domain-specific cognitive abilities in acute first-ever stroke. *Neurology 64*: 821–827

Ott, B. R., & Saver, J. L. (1993) Unilateral amnesic stroke: Six new cases and a review of the literature. *Stroke 24*: 1033–1042

Ownsworth, T. L., McFarland, K., & Young, R. M. (2000) Self-awareness and psychosocial functioning following acquired brain injury: An evaluation of a group support program. *Neuropsychological Rehabilitation 10*: 465–484

Paolucci, S., Antonucci, G., Grasso, M. G., & Pizzamiglio, L. (2001) The role of unilateral spatial neglect in rehabilitation of right brain-damaged ischemic stroke patients: A matched comparison. *Archives of Physical Medicine and Rehabilitation 82*: 743–749.

Park, N. W., & Ingles, J. L. (1999) *Effectiveness of attention rehabilitation after an acquired brain injury: A meta-analysis.* Presented at Rotman Research Institute Annual Meeting

Park, N. W., & Ingles, J. L. (2001) Effectiveness of attention rehabilitation after an acquired brain injury: A meta analysis. *Neuropsychology 15*: 199–210

Park, N. W., Proulx, G. B., & Towers, W. M. (1999) Evaluation of the attention process training program. *Neuropsychological Rehabilitation 9*: 135–154

Patel, M., Coshall, C., Rudd, A. G., & Wolfe, C. D. (2003) Natural history of cognitive impairment after stroke and factors associated with its recovery. *Clinical Rehabilitation 17*: 158–166

Payne, B. R., & Rushmore, R. J. (2004) Functional circuitry underlying natural and interventional cancellation of visual neglect. *Experimental Brain Research 154*: 127–153

Plohmann, A. M., Kappos, L., Ammann, W., Thordai, A., Wittwer, A., Huber, S. et al. (1998) Computer assisted retraining of attentional impairments in patients with multiple sclerosis. *Journal of Neurology, Neurosurgery and Psychiatry 64*: 455–462

Posner, M. I., & Petersen, S. E. (1990) The attention system of the human brain. *Annual Review of Neuroscience 13*: 25–42

Pulvermuller, F., Neininger, B., Elbert, T., Mohr, B., Rockstroh, B. Koebbel, P., et al. (2001) Constraint-induced therapy of chronic aphasia after stroke. *Stroke 32:* 1621–1626

Rasquin, S. M. C., Lodder, J., Ponds, R. W. H. M., Winkens, I., Jolles, J., & Verhey, F. R. J. (2004) Cognitive functioning after stroke: A one-year follow-up study. *Dementia and Geriatric Cognitive Disorders 18*: 138–144

Rath, J. F., Simon, D., Langenbahn, D. M., Sherr, R. L., & Diller, L. (2003) Group treatment of problem-solving deficits in outpatients with traumatic brain injury: A randomised outcome study. *Neuropsychological Rehabilitation 13*: 461–488

Riepe, M. W., Riss, S., Bittner, D., & Huber, R. (2004) Screening for cognitive impairment in patients with acute stroke. *Dementia and Geriatric Cognitive Disorders 17*: 49–53

Robertson, I. H., & North, N. (1992) Spatio-motor cueing in unilateral left neglect: The role of hemispace, hand and motor activation. *Neuropsychologia 30*: 553–563

Robertson, I., Halligan, P. W., & Marshall, J. C. (1993) Prospects for the rehabilitation of unilateral neglect. In I. Roberston & J.C. Marshall (Eds.), *Unilateral neglect: Clinical and experimental studies* (pp. 279–292). Hove, UK: LEA.

Robertson, I., & North, N. (1993) Active and passive activation of left limbs: Influence on visual and sensory neglect. *Neuropsychologia 31*: 293–300

Robertson, I. H., North, N. T., & Geggie, C. (1992) Spatio-motor cueing in unilateral left neglect: Three case studies of its therapeutic effects. *Journal of Neurology, Neurosurgery and Psychiatry 55*: 799–805

Robertson, I. H., Ridgeway, V., Greenfield, E., & Parr, A. (1997) Motor recovery after stroke depends on intact sustained attention: A 2-year follow-up study. *Neuropsychology 11*: 290–295

Robertson, I. H., Mattingley, J. B., Rorden, C., & Driver, J. (1998) Phasic alerting of neglect patients overcomes their spatial deficit in visual awareness. *Nature 395*: 169–172

Robey, R. R. (1998) A meta-analysis of clinical outcomes in the treatment of aphasia. *Journal of Speech, Language and Hearing Research 41*: 172–187

Rossetti, Y., Rode, G., Pisella, L., Farne, A., Boisson, D., & Perenin, M-T. (1998) Prism adaptation to a rightward optical deviation rehabilitates left hemispatial neglect. *Nature 395*: 166–169

Rothi, L. J. G., & Barrett, A. M. (2006) The changing view of neurorehabilitation: A new era of optimism. *Journal of the International Neuropsychological Society 12*: 812–815

Schmitter-Edgecombe, M., Fahy, J. F., Whelan, J. P., & Long, C. J. (1995) Memory remediation after severe closed head injury: Notebook training versus supportive therapy. *Journal of Consulting and Clinical Psychology 63:* 484–489

Schneider, J. S., McLaughlin, W. W., & Roeltgen, D. P. (1992) Motor and non-motor behavioral deficits in monkeys made hemi-parkinsonian by intracarotid MPTP infusion. *Neurology 42:* 1565–1572

Schneider, M. B., Murrir, L. C., Pfeiffer, R. F., & Deupree, J. D. (1984) Dopamine receptors: Effects of chronic I-DOPA bromocriptine treatment in an animal model of Parkinson's disease. *Clinical Neuropharmacology 7:* 247–257

Schwarting, R. K., & Huston, J. P. (1996) The unilateral 6-hydroxydopamine lesion model in behavioral brain research. Analysis of functional deficits, recovery and treatments. *Progress in Neurobiology 50*(2–3): 275–331

Schwartz, R. L., Barrett, A. M., Kim, M. H., & Heilman, K. M. (1999) Ipsilesional intentional neglect and the effect of cueing. *Neurology 53*(9): 2017–2022

Singer, J. D., & Willett, J.B. (2003) *Applied Longitudinal Data Analysis.* New York: Oxford University Press

Sohlberg, M., & Mateer, C. (1989a) *Introduction to Cognitive Rehabilitation: Theory and Practice.* New York: Guildford Press

Sohlberg, M. M., & Mateer, C. A. (1987) Effectiveness of an attention-training program. *Journal of Clinical and Experimental Neuropsychology 9:* 117–30

Sohlberg, M. M., & Mateer, C. A. (1989b) Theory and remediation of attention disorders. In *Introduction to Cognitive Rehabilitation: Theory and Practice.* New York: The Guilford Press

Sohlberg, M. M., & Mateer, C. A. (2001a) *Cognitive Rehabilitation: An Integrative Neuropsychological Approach.* New York: The Guildford Press. 492 pp

Sohlberg, M. M., & Mateer, C. A. (2001b) Improving attention and managing attentional problems. Adapting rehabilitation techniques to adults with ADD. *Annals New York Academy of Sciences 931:* 359–375

Sohlberg, M. M., McLaughlin, K. A., Pavese, A., Heidrich, A., & Posner, M. I. (2000) Evaluation of attention process training and brain injury education in persons with acquired brain injury. *Journal of Clinical and Experimental Neuropsychology 22:* 656–676

Squire, L. R. (1986) Mechanisms of memory. *Science 232:* 1612–1619

Squires, E. J., Hunkin, N. M., & Parkin, A. J. (1996) Memory notebook training in a case of severe amnesia: Generalising from paired associate learning to real life. *Neuropsychological Rehabilitation 6:* 55–65

Stablum, F., Umilta, C., Mogentale, C., Carlan, M., & Guerrini, C. (2000) Rehabilitation of executive deficits in closed head injury and anterior communication artery aneurysm patients. *Psychological Research 63:* 265–278

Stapleton, T., Ashburn, A., & Stack, E. (2001) A pilot study of attention deficits, balance control and falls in the subacute stage following stroke. *Clinical Rehabilitation 15:* 437–444

Stephens, S., Kenny, R. A., Rowan, E., Kalaria, R. N, Bradbury, M., et al. (2005) Association between mild vascular cognitive impairment and impaired activities of daily living in older stroke survivors without dementia. *Journal of the American Geriatrics Society 53:* 103–107

Stewart, F. M., Sunderland, A., & Sluman, S. M. (1996) The nature and prevalence of memory disorder late after stroke. *British Journal of Clinical Psychology 35:* 369–379

Stone, S. P., Halligan, P. W., & Greenwood, R. J. (1993) The incidence of neglect phenomena and related disorders in patients with an acute right or left hemisphere stroke. *Age and Ageing 22:* 46–52

Stone, S. P., Halligan, P. W., Marshall, J. C., & Greenwood, R. J. (1998) Unilateral neglect: A common but heterogeneous syndrome. *Neurology 50:* 1902–1905

Sturm, W., Fimm, B., Cantagallo, A., Cremel, N., North, P., et al. (2002) Computerized training of specific attention deficits in stroke and traumatic brain injured patients: A multicentric efficacy study. In M Leclercq, P Zimmermann (Eds.) *Applied Neuropsychology of Attention,* (pp. 365–380) Tübingen: Günther Narr Verlag: Hove: Psychology Press

Sturm, W., Hartje, W., Orgass, B., & Willmes, K. (1993) Computer-assisted rehabilitation of attention impairments. In F. J. Stachowiak & R. de Bleser (Eds.) *Developments in the assessment and rehabilitation of brain-damaged patients. Perspectives from a European Concerted Action,* (pp. 49–54). Tubingen: Gunther Narr Verlag

Sturm, W., & Willmes, K. (1991) Efficacy of a reaction training on various attentional and cognitive functions in stroke patients. *Neuropsychological Rehabilitation 1:* 259–280

Sturm, W., Willmes, K., Orgass, B., & Hartje, W. (1997) Do specific attention deficits need specific training? *Neuropsychological Rehabilitation 7:* 81–103

Stuss, D. T. (2007) New approaches to prefrontal lobe testing. In B. Miller & J. Cumming (Eds.), *The Human Frontal Lobes.* New York: Guildford

Tatemichi, T. K., Desmond, D. W., Stern, Y., Paik, M., Sano, M., & Bagiella, E. (1994) Cognitive impairment after stroke: Frequency, patterns, and relationship to functional abilities. *Journal of Neurology, Neurosurgery, and Psychiatry 57:* 202–207

Taub, E., Uswatte, G., & Pidigiti, R. (1999) Constraint-induced movement therapy: A new family of techniques with broad application to physical rehabilitation - a clinical review. *Journal of Rehabilitation Research and Development 36:* 237–251

Taub, E., Uswatte, G., Mark, V. W., & Morris, D. M. (2006) The learned nonuse phenomenon: Implications for rehabilitation. *Europa Medicophysica 42*: 241–255

Teasell, R., Foley, N., Bhogal, S., Salter, K., Jutai, J., & Speechley, M. (2006) *Evidence-based review of stroke rehabilitation*, University of Western Ontario, London, Ontario

Teasell, R., Foley, N., Salter, K., Bhogal, S., Bayona, N., et al. (2007a) Evidence-Based Review of Stroke Rehabilitation, 8th edition. London, UK: St. Joseph Health Care & London, Ontario, Canada: University of Western Ontario. http://www.ebrsr.com/ Last update September 2007 (a). Accessed November 1, 2007.

Teasell, R., Korner-Bitensky, N., Jutai, J., Desrosiers, J., Swaine, B., et al. (2007b) Ottawa, Ontario, Canada: Canadian Stroke Network & Montreal, Quebec: McGill University.StrokEngine: Systematic stroke rehabilitation and intervention reviews. http://www.medicine.mcgill.ca/Strokengine/ Last update Menon-Nair and Korner-Bitensky, March 2007(b). Accessed February 26, 2007

Tegnér, R., & Levander, M. (1991) Through a looking glass. A new technique to demonstrate directional hypokinesia in unilateral neglect. *Brain 114*: 1943–1951

Tham, W., Auchus, A. P., Thong, M., Goh, M.-L., Chang, H.-M., Wong, M.-C. et al. (2002) Progression of cognitive impairment after stroke: One year results from a longitudinal study of Singaporean stroke patients. *Journal of the Neurological Sciences 203–204*: 49–52

Towle, D., Edmans, J. A., & Lincoln, N. B. (1988) Use of computer-presented games with memory-impaired stroke patients. *Clinical Rehabilitation 2*: 303–307

Tulving, E., & Schacter, D. L. (1990) Priming and human memory systems. *Science 247*: 301–306

Ungerstedt, U. (1976) 6-hydroxydopamine-induced degeneration of the nigrostriatal dopamine pathway: the turning syndrome. *Pharmacology and Therapeutics: Part B – General and Systematic Pharmacology 2*(1): 37–40

von Cramon, D. Y., Mathes-von Cramon, G., & Mai, N. (1991) Problem-solving deficits in brain injured patients: a therapeutic approach. *Neuropsychological Rehabilitation 1*: 45–64

Vuilleumier, P., Valenza, N., Mayer, E., Reverdin, A., & Landis, T. (1998) Near and far visual space in unilateral neglect. *Annals of Neurology 43*: 406–410

Wade, D. T., Parker, V., & Hewer, R. L. (1986) Memory disturbance after stroke: Frequency and associated losses. *International Rehabilitation Medicine 8*: 60–64

Wagenaar, R. C., Van Wieringen, P. C. W., Netelenbos, J. B., Meijer, O. G., & Kuik, D. J. (1992) The transfer of scanning training effects in visual inattention after stroke: Five single-case studies. *Disability and Rehabilitation 14*: 51–60

Walker, R., Young, A. W., & Lincoln, N. B. (1996) Eye patching and the rehabilitation of visual neglect. *Neuropsychological Rehabilitation 6*: 219–231

Webster, J. S., Jones, S., Blanton, P., Gross, R., Beissel, G. F., & Wofford, J. D. (1984) Visual scanning training with stroke patients. *Behavior Therapy 15*: 129–143

Webster, J. S., McFarland, P. T., Rapport, L. J., Morrill, B., Roades, L. A., & Abadee, P. S. (2001) Computer-assisted training for improving wheelchair mobility in unilateral neglect patients. *Archives of Physical Medicine and Rehabilitation 82*: 769–775

Weinberg, J., Diller, L., Gordon, W. A., Gerstman, L. J., Lieberman, A., et al. (1977) Visual scanning training effect on reading-related tasks in acquired right brain damage. *Archives of Physical Medicine and Rehabilitation 58*: 479–486

Weinberg, J., Diller, L., Gordon, W. A., Gerstman, L. J., Lieberman, A., et al. (1979) Training sensory awareness and spatial organization in people with right brain damage. *Archives of Physical Medicine and Rehabilitation 60*: 491–496

Wilson, B. A. (1997) Cognitive rehabilitation: How it is and how it might be. *Journal of the International Neuropsychological Society 3*: 487–496

Wilson, B. A. (2002) Towards a comprehensive model of cognitive rehabilitation. *Neuropsychological Rehabilitation 12*: 97–110

Wilson, B. A., Emslie, H. C., Quirk, K., & Evans, J. J. (2001) Reducing everyday memory and planning problems by means of a paging system: a randomised control crossover study. *Journal of Neurology, Neurosurgery and Psychiatry 70*: 477–482

Zinn, S., Dudley, T. K., Bosworth, H. B., Hoenig, H. M., Duncan, P. W., & Horner, R. D. (2004) The effect of poststroke cognitive impairment on rehabilitation process and functional outcome. *Archives of Physical Medicine and Rehabilitation 85*: 1084–1090

Index

Printed in the United States of America